Orthopaedic Knowledge Update

Trauma

American Academy of Orthopaedic Surgeons

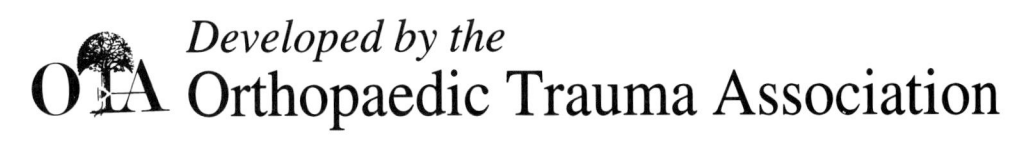

Orthopaedic Knowledge Update
Trauma

Edited by
Alan M. Levine, MD

With 121 illustrations

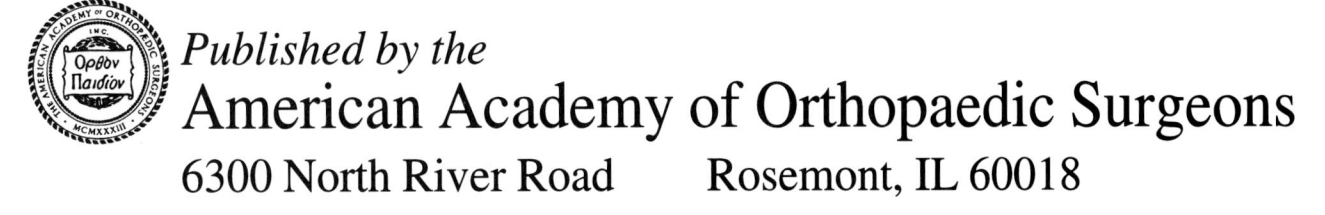

Developed by the
Orthopaedic Trauma Association

Published by the
American Academy of Orthopaedic Surgeons
6300 North River Road   Rosemont, IL 60018

Orthopaedic Knowledge Update: Trauma

American Academy of Orthopaedic Surgeons

The material presented in *Orthopaedic Knowledge Update: Trauma* has been made available by the American Academy of Orthopaedic Surgeons for educational purposes only. This material is not intended to present the only, or necessarily best, methods or procedures for the medical situations discussed, but rather is intended to represent an approach, view, statement, or opinion of the author(s) or producer(s), which may be helpful to others who face similar situations. The information presented in this volume does not reflect the opinions of the Academy, editorial board, or contributors, but is merely intended to be a complete review of the peer literature.

Some drugs and medical devices demonstrated in Academy courses or described in Academy print or electronic publications have FDA clearance for use for specific purposes or for use only in restricted settings. The FDA has stated that it is the responsibility of the physician to determine the FDA status of each drug or device he or she wishes to use in clinical practice, and to use the products with appropriate patient consent and in compliance with applicable law.

Furthermore, any statements about commercial products are solely the opinion(s) of the author(s) and do not represent an Academy endorsement or evaluation of these products. These statements may not be used in advertising or for any commercial purpose.

The material contained in this volume was submitted as previously unpublished material, except in the instances in which credit has been given to the source from which some of the illustrative material was derived.

Materials appearing in this book prepared by individuals as part of their official duties as U.S. Government employees are not covered by the above-mentioned copyright.

All rights reserved. No part of this publication may be reproduced, stored in a retrieval system, or transmitted, in any form, or by any means, electronic, mechanical, photocopying, recording, or otherwise, without prior written permission from the publisher.

First Edition
Copyright© 1996 by the
American Academy of Orthopaedic Surgeons

ISBN 0-89203-126-3

Acknowledgments

Orthopaedic Trauma Association Executive Committee, 1995
Alan M. Levine, MD
Lawrence B. Bone, MD
James B. Carr, MD
M. Bradford Henley, MD
Kenneth D. Johnson, MD
Peter J. O'Brien, MD
Paul J. Duwelius, MD
Thomas F. Varecka, MD
Donald A. Wiss, MD

Editorial Board, OKU: Trauma
Alan M. Levine, MD
Paul A. Anderson, MD
Robert J. Brumback, MD
David L. Helfet, MD
James F. Kellam, MD

American Academy of Orthopaedic Surgeons Board of Directors, 1995
James W. Strickland, MD, *President*
S. Terry Canale, MD
Charles R. Clark, MD
Paul C. Collins, MD
William C. Collins, MD
Robert D. D'Ambrosia, MD
Kenneth E. DeHaven, MD
Robert N. Hensinger, MD
James H. Herndon, MD
Douglas W. Jackson, MD
Richard F. Kyle, MD
George L. Lucas, MD
David R. Mauerhan, MD
Bernard F. Morrey, MD
Bernard A. Rineberg, MD
D. Eugene Thompson, MD
William W. Tipton, Jr, MD (*ex officio*)

Staff
Marilyn L. Fox, PhD, *Director, Department of Publications*
Bruce Davis, *Senior Editor*
Jane Baque, *Associate Senior Editor*
Loraine Edwalds, *Production Manager*
Susan Baim, *Editorial Assistant*
Sophie Tosta, *Editorial Assistant*
Jana Ronayne, *Production Assistant*
Geraldine Dubberke, *Publications Secretary*

Contributors

Paul A. Anderson, MD
Associate Clinical Professor
Department of Orthopaedics
University of Washington
Seattle, Washington

David Asprinio, MD
Clinical Instructor of Orthopaedic Surgery
New York Medical College
Valhalla, New York

Michael J. Bosse, MD
Orthopaedic Trauma Surgeon Director, Clinical Research
Department of Orthopaedic Surgery
Carolinas Medical Center
Charlotte, North Carolina

Michael J. Brennan, MD
Arizona Orthopaedic and Sports Medicine Specialists
Phoenix, Arizona

Robert J. Brumback, MD
Attending Orthopaedic Traumatologist
The R. Adams Cowley Shock Trauma Center
University of Maryland Medical Center
Baltimore, Maryland

John Kenneth Burkus, MD
Hughston Orthopedic Clinic
Columbus, Georgia

Jens R. Chapman, MD
Assistant Professor
Chief, Orthopaedic Spine Service
Department of Orthopaedic Surgery
Harborview Medical Center
University of Washington
Seattle, Washington

Patrick J. Connolly, MD
Assistant Professor of Orthopaedic Surgery
SUNY Health Science Center
Syracuse, New York

Carol E. Copeland, MD
Attending Orthopaedic Traumatologist
The R. Adams Cowley Shock Trauma Center
University of Maryland Medical Center
Baltimore, Maryland

Charles N. Cornell, MD
Associate Professor of Surgery
Cornell University Medical College
New York, New York

Aleksandar Curcin, MD
Assistant Professor of Orthopaedic Surgery
University of Maryland
Baltimore, Maryland

Rick B. Delamarter, MD
Co-Director, UCLA Comprehensive Spine Center
Associate Clinical Professor
UCLA School of Medicine
Los Angeles, California

Paul J. Duwelius, MD
Associate Professor
Division of Orthopaedics and Rehabilitation
Oregon Health Sciences University
Portland, Oregon

W. Andrew Eglseder, Jr, MD
Attending Orthopaedic Traumatologist
The R. Adams Cowley Shock Trauma Center
University of Maryland Medical Center
Baltimore, Maryland

Bruce E. Fredrickson, MD
Professor, Orthopaedic and Neurologic Surgery
SUNY Health Science Center
Syracuse, New York

Michelle Gerwin, MD
Attending Surgeon
The Hospital for Special Surgery
New York, New York

Leonard E. Goldstock, MD
Hand and Upper Extremity Surgery Fellow
Massachusetts General Hospital
Boston, Massachusetts

James A. Goulet, MD
Associate Professor
Section of Orthopaedic Surgery
The University of Michigan
Ann Arbor, Michigan

M. Sean Grady, MD
University of Washington
Harborview Medical Center
Department of Neurological Surgery
Seattle, Washington

Paul R. Gregory, MD
Orthopaedic Trauma Services
Tampa General Hospital
Florida Orthopaedic Institute
Tampa, Florida

David L. Helfet, MD
Director of Orthopaedic Trauma
Associate Professor of Orthopaedic Surgery
The Hospital for Special Surgery
Cornell University Medical College
New York, New York

John G. Heller, MD
Associate Professor of Orthopaedic Surgery
Emory University School of Medicine
Director of Education
The Emory Spine Center
Atlanta, Georgia

Alan L. Jones, MD
Assistant Professor
Department of Orthopaedics
University of Texas
Southwestern Medical Center
Dallas, Texas

Jesse B. Jupiter, MD
Director, Orthopaedic Hand Service
Massachusetts General Hospital
Associate Professor, Orthopaedic Surgery
Harvard Medical School
Boston, Massachusetts

Kenneth L. Kaylor, MD
Lt. Col, USAF, MC
Deputy Department Chairman
Department of Orthopaedics
Wilford Hall Medical Center
Lackland AFB, Texas

James F. Kellam, MD, FRCS(C), FACS
Director of Orthopaedic Trauma
Department of Orthopaedic Surgery
Carolinas Medical Center
Charlotte, North Carolina

Kenneth J. Koval, MD
Chief, Fracture Service
Hospital for Joint Diseases
New York, New York

Jonathan Landsman, MD
Florida Orthopaedic Institute
Tampa, Florida

Richard H. Lange, MD
Associate Professor
Division of Orthopaedic Surgery
University of Wisconsin
Madison, Wisconsin

Alan M. Levine, MD
Professor of Orthopaedic Surgery and Oncology
Consultant, Spinal Injury
The R. Adams Cowley Shock Trauma Center
University of Maryland Medical Center
Baltimore, Maryland

Ronald W. Lindsey, MD
Department of Orthopedic Surgery
Baylor College of Medicine
Houston, Texas

Robert E. Lins, MD
Hand and Upper Extremity Surgery Fellow
Massachusetts General Hospital
Boston, Massachusetts

Robert A. McGuire, Jr, MD
Professor
Department of Orthopaedic Surgery
University of Mississippi Medical Center
Jackson, Mississippi

Theodore Miclau, MD
Assistant Professor of Orthopaedic Surgery
University of California, San Francisco
San Francisco, California

Christopher D. Miller, MD
Kansas Orthopaedic Center
Wichita, Kansas

Michael E. Miller, MD
Chairman, Orthopaedic Surgery
Carraway Methodist Medical Center
Birmingham, Alabama

Berton R. Moed, MD
Chief, Division of Orthopaedic Traumatology
Henry Ford Hospital
Detroit, Michigan

Pasquale X. Montesano, MD
Mercy, Roseville and Sutter Hospitals
Carmichael, California

Elvert F. Nelson, MD
Mercy, Roseville and Sutter Hospitals
Carmichael, California

Glenn R. Rechtine, MD, FACS
Florida Orthopaedic Institute
Tampa, Florida

J. Spence Reid, MD
Assistant Professor
Department of Orthopaedics
Pennsylvania State University
    College of Medicine
Milton S. Hershey Medical Center
Hershey, Pennsylvania

Barry L. Riemer, MD
Director, Orthopaedic Fracture Division
Professor of Surgery (Orthopaedic)
Allegheny Campus
Medical College of Pennsylvania
Pittsburgh, Pennsylvania

M.L. Chip Routt, Jr, MD
Associate Professor of Orthopaedic Surgery
Harborview Medical Center
Seattle, Washington

Thomas A. Russell, MD
Associate Professor, Orthopaedic Surgery
Department of Orthopaedic Surgery
University of Tennessee
Memphis, Tennessee

Roy W. Sanders, MD
Director, Orthopaedic Trauma Services
Chief, Department of Orthopaedics
Tampa General Hospital and the Florida
 Orthopaedic Institute
Tampa, Florida

Stephen H. Sims, MD
Miller Orthopaedic Clinic
Head, Fracture Service
Carolinas Medical Center
Charlotte, North Carolina

Paul Tornetta III, MD
Director, Orthopedic Trauma
Kings County Hospital
Assistant Professor
SUNY-Downstate
Brooklyn, New York

Clifford H. Turen, MD
Attending Orthopaedic Traumatologist
The R. Adams Cowley Shock Trauma Center
University of Maryland Medical Center
Baltimore, Maryland

Mark S. Vrahas, MD
Director, Orthopaedic Trauma
Assistant Professor
Louisiana State University Medical Center
 School of Medicine
New Orleans, Louisiana

Robert L. Waters, MD
Director, Regional Spinal Cord Injury Care
 Systems of South California
Rancho Los Amigos Medical Center
Downey, California

Andrew J. Weiland, MD
Attending Surgeon
Hospital for Special Surgery
Professor of Orthopaedics
Cornell University Medical College
New York, New York

S. Steven Yang, MD, MPH
Attending Orthopaedic Surgeon
Hand Surgery Services
The Lenox Hill Hospital
New York, New York

Gregory M. Yoshida, MD
Co-Chief, Spinal Deformity Program
Rancho Los Amigos Medical Center
Downey, California

Hansen A. Yuan, MD
Professor, Orthopaedic and Neurological Surgery
SUNY Health Science Center
Syracuse, New York

Stephen J. Zabinski, MD
Senior Clinical Associate in Orthopaedic Surgery
Cornell University Medical College
New York, New York

Thomas A. Zdeblick, MD
Associate Professor, Orthopaedic Surgery
University of Wisconsin
Madison, Wisconsin

Preface

The American Academy of Orthopaedic Surgeons developed the *Orthopaedic Knowledge Update* (*OKU*) concept as a response to the need for "learner-centered education programs." The first volume appeared in 1984 and AAOS' task since then has been to provide "a useful, comprehensive, and accessible synthesis of the latest information and knowledge available in the literature related to orthopaedic surgery." This task becomes increasingly difficult each year as the volume of scientific publications increases exponentially. Even with the advent of electronic media and learning techniques, the concept of the *OKU* remains valid and is perhaps even more important than it was at the time of its origin. A recent survey by the American Academy of Orthopaedic Surgeons demonstrated that more than 70% of Academy members felt that their practice was in either general orthopaedic surgery or general orthopaedic surgery with a specialty interest. This indicates that the task of keeping current requires a significant commitment. With the rapid increase in both general and specialty publications, it is virtually impossible for the practicing orthopaedic surgeon to remain current with the literature in all areas that affect his or her practice. Whereas textbooks frequently represent the author's opinion, the *OKU* is a synthesis, by authors knowledgeable in specific areas, of the most current peer-reviewed scientific publications.

With expansion of the knowledge base and the trend in orthopaedic surgery toward specialty fellowship training, the American Academy of Orthopaedic Surgeons has responded with a specialty-oriented *OKU* series. The first two volumes, *Orthopaedic Knowledge Update: Sports Medicine* and *Orthopaedic Knowledge Update: Foot and Ankle*, were published in 1994. The executive boards of the Orthopaedic Trauma Association and the American Academy of Orthopaedic Surgeons felt that the publication of *Orthopaedic Knowledge Update: Trauma* would be a useful and important addition to this series. The face of orthopaedic traumatology and fracture care in North America has changed dramatically over the last 20 years, and along with it the practice of orthopaedic surgery. While care of the small group of critically injured polytraumatized patients rests generally with orthopaedic traumatologists, fracture care remains a critical component of the practices of a large portion of orthopaedic surgeons. Both the treatment techniques and the literature related to these aspects of orthopaedics have changed substantially in the last 10 years.

In *Orthopaedic Knowledge Update: Trauma*, we have attempted to establish a baseline for the discussion of orthopaedic fracture care by reviewing the pertinent literature and changes in care over the last 10 years. The discussion is divided into anatomic sections: upper extremity, lower extremity, pelvis and acetabulum, and spine. These sections are further subdivided to allow groupings of similarly treated injuries. Each chapter then addresses the anatomy and clinical and radiographic evaluation pertinent to the current advances in care. The classification system or systems most widely used to identify the various subtypes of injury are illustrated in each section. Within this framework, each author discusses the types of treatment and results of treatment that have been supported by the peer-reviewed literature over the last 10 years. Each section concludes with a discussion of complications followed by a selected bibliography of the current literature, often with annotations for the most significant or unique contributions. As with all other *OKU*s, the success of this volume rests with the selfless contributions and energy of the section editors, Paul A. Anderson, MD, Robert J. Brumback, MD, David L. Helfet, MD, and James F. Kellam, MD, FRCS(C), FACS. The individual authors not only contributed their expertise in the areas of their chapters, but assisted with overall consistency and content of each section during section editorial meetings. Certainly, the contributions of the Academy staff cannot be forgotten and our thanks go especially to Jane Baque for her adroit project management and expert manuscript editing. In addition, Marilyn Fox, PhD, Bruce Davis, Loraine Edwalds, Susan Baim, Jana Ronayne, Sophie Tosta, and Geraldine Dubberke contributed their efforts and skills.

All of us who have contributed to the completion of this work hope that you, the reader, will find this to be a rich source of information as you seek to update your knowledge in the area of orthopaedic trauma and fracture care.

Alan M. Levine, MD

Table of Contents

Section 1: Upper Extremity
Section Editor — David L. Helfet, MD

1	Injuries to the Shoulder Girdle: Fractures of the Scapula, Clavicle, Acromioclavicular Joint, and Sternoclavicular Joint	Michael E. Miller, MD Christopher Miller, MD	3
2	Fractures of the Proximal Humerus and Dislocation of the Glenohumeral Joint	Charles N. Cornell, MD	15
3	Fractures of the Humeral Shaft	Richard H. Lange, MD	25
4	Fractures of the Distal Humerus	David Asprinio, MD David L. Helfet, MD	35
5	Elbow Trauma	Leonard E. Goldstock, MD Jesse B. Jupiter, MD Robert E. Lins, MD	47
6	Forearm Fractures	Berton R. Moed, MD	57
7	Fractures of the Distal Radius	Stephen J. Zabinski, MD Andrew J. Weiland, MD	67
8	Carpal Fractures and Dislocations	W. Andrew Eglseder, Jr, MD	83
9	Fractures of the Hand	S. Steven Yang, MD, MPH Michelle Gerwin, MD	95

Section 2: Lower Extremity
Section Editor — Robert J. Brumback, MD

10	Intracapsular Hip Fractures	Clifford H. Turen, MD	113
11	Intertrochanteric Femur Fractures	Michael J. Brennan, MD	121
12	Fractures of the Femoral Diaphysis, Including the Subtrochanteric Region	Alan L. Jones, MD	127
13	Supracondylar and Intercondylar Fractures of the Distal Femur	Kenneth J. Koval, MD	137
14	Knee Dislocation	Paul Tornetta III, MD	145
15	Injuries to the Patella and Extensor Mechanism	Kenneth L. Kaylor, MD	153

16	Fractures of the Tibial Plateau	J. Spence Reid, MD	159
17	Fractures of the Tibial Diaphysis	Thomas A. Russell, MD	171
18	Fractures of the Tibial Plafond	Robert J. Brumback, MD	183
19	Ankle and Foot Injuries	Paul R. Gregory, MD Roy W. Sanders, MD	191

Section 3: Pelvis and Acetabulum
Section Editor — **James F. Kellam, MD, FRCS(C), FACS**

20	Fractures of the Pelvis and Acetabulum: An Overview	James F. Kellam, MD, FRCS(C), FACS	213
21	The Acute Management of Pelvic Ring Injuries	Michael J. Bosse, MD	217
22	Acute Care and Evaluation of Acetabular Fractures	Paul J. Duwelius, MD	227
23	Biomechanics of Injuries of the Acetabulum and Pelvic Ring, and Fracture Fixation	Mark S. Vrahas, MD	235
24	Fixation of Pelvic Ring Disruptions	M.L. Chip Routt, Jr, MD	241
25	Functional Outcomes of Pelvic Ring Injuries	Barry L. Riemer, MD	249
26	Posterior Wall, Posterior Column, and Transverse Acetabular Fractures: Surgical Indications and Techniques	James A. Goulet, MD	253
27	Complex Fractures of the Acetabulum	Carol E. Copeland, MD	263
28	Acetabular Fractures: Postoperative Management and Complications	Stephen H. Sims, MD	273
29	Hip Dislocations and Fractures of the Femoral Head	James F. Kellam, MD, FRCS(C), FACS	281

Section 4: Spine
Section Editor — **Paul A. Anderson, MD**

30	Patient Assessment in Spinal Injury	Robert A. McGuire, Jr, MD	289
31	Pathophysiology and Experimental Treatment of Spinal Cord Injury	M. Sean Grady, MD	297
32	Prognosis of Spinal Cord Injuries	Robert L. Waters, MD Gregory M. Yoshida, MD	303
33	Occipital Cranial Injuries	Pasquale X. Montesano, MD Elvert F. Nelson, MD	311
34	The Atlas Vertebra: Fractures and Ligamentous Injuries	John G. Heller, MD	317
35	Fractures of the Axis	Glenn R. Rechtine, MD, FACS Jonathan Landsman, MD	323
36	Lower Cervical Injuries: Classification and Initial Management	Rick B. Delamarter, MD	329

37	Lower Cervical Spine Injuries: Surgical Management	Ronald W. Lindsey, MD Theodore Miclau, MD	335
38	Thoracolumbar Fractures: Injury Evaluation and Classification	Aleksandar Curcin, MD	341
39	Thoracic and Lumbar Fractures: Nonsurgical Management	Bruce E. Fredrickson, MD Hansen A. Yuan, MD Patrick J. Connolly, MD	347
40	Fractures of the Thoracolumbar Junction	John Kenneth Burkus, MD	351
41	Anterior Thoracolumbar Instrumentation for Burst Fracture	Thomas A. Zdeblick, MD	361
42	Sacral Fractures	Jens R. Chapman, MD Paul A. Anderson, MD	365

I
Upper Extremity

David L. Helfet, MD
Section Editor

1

Injuries to the Shoulder Girdle: Fractures of the Scapula, Clavicle, Acromioclavicular Joint, and Sternoclavicular Joint

Introduction

The shoulder joint owes its unique axial and rotational mobility to the unconstrained structure of its articulations. With the exception of the sternoclavicular joint, only the muscular supports of the scapula and clavicle link the shoulder girdle with the rest of the skeleton. The inherent bony instability of the scapula, humerus, and clavicle is supported by a complex web of 18 muscular origins and insertions that serve to suspend the humerus from the scapula and the entire shoulder girdle from the spine and thorax. This particular anatomy allows for a degree of mobility that is unmatched anywhere else in the human body.

Recent advances have focused on the concept of scapulothoracic dislocation, which occurs as a result of a severe traumatic injury to the shoulder girdle. This involves severe injury to the vascular and neurologic supply to the upper extremity as a result of a severe traction injury through the plane of the scapulothoracic joint. In addition, a classification system for scapular fractures has been developed, and there is an increasing role for surgical treatment in the management of these injuries. Many of these indications have emerged with a clearer understanding of fracture anatomy as a result of the use of advanced imaging techniques such as computed tomography (CT). Three-dimensional reconstruction software for computed CT scans allows for a more complete understanding of the fracture patterns of the scapula, as well as the measures that are required for reduction and fixation.

Scapular Fractures and Dislocations

The earliest treatise on scapular fractures is probably that of Desault. Since then, a small number of studies have been published, all of which note the rarity of these fractures and the high incidence of associated injuries.[1-11]

Closed management of the vast majority of these fractures has been the rule. This custom has been based on a belief that the results of nonsurgical treatment were functionally and symptomatically good. The results of more recent studies have raised questions regarding these observations.

Fracture Patterns and Classification

Ada and Miller[12] have developed a classification system based on a series of 148 fractures in 116 scapulae, summarized in Figure 1. The most common fracture type is in the body of the scapula, and seldom requires more than symptomatic treatment. Fractures of the scapular neck were second in frequency, with injuries of the scapular spine, glenoid,

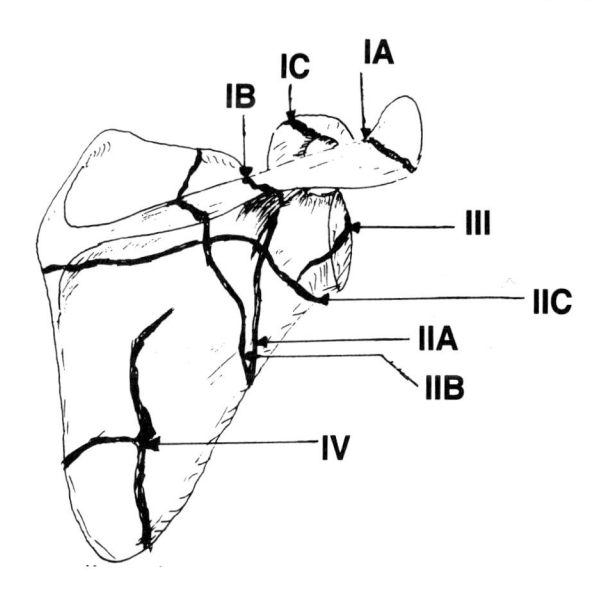

Fig. 1 Classification of scapular fractures. **IA,** Acromion. **IB,** Base of acromion, spine. **IC,** Coracoid. **IIA,** Neck lateral to base of acromion, spine. **IIB,** Neck, extending to base of acromion or spine. **IIC,** Neck, transverse type. **III,** Glenoid, intra-articular. **IV,** Body. (Adapted with permission from Miller ME, Ada JR: Injuries to the shoulder girdle, in Browner BD, Jupiter J, Levine AM, et al (eds): *Skeletal Trauma.* Philadelphia, PA, WB Saunders, 1992, vol 2, pp 1291-1310.)

Table 1. Classification of scapular fracture, based on 148 fractures in 116 scapulae

Site	Fracture Type	No. %
Acromion	I-A	18 (12)
Spine	I-B	17 (11)
Coracoid	I-C	7 (5)
Neck	II-A, II-B, II-C	39 (27)
Glenoid	III	15 (10)
Body	IV	52 (35)

(Adapted with permission from Miller ME, Ada JR: Injuries to the shoulder girdle, in Browner BD, Jupiter J, Levine AM, et al (eds): *Skeletal Trauma*. Philadelphia, PA, WB Saunders, 1992, vol 2, pp 1291-1310.)

and acromion all of about equal occurrence (Table 1). Complete multiple fracture patterns were common. The only indirect injury was an avulsion fracture of the acromion, which occurred in a patient with renal osteodystrophy.

Associated Injury

Ada and Miller[12] reviewed 148 fractures in 116 scapulae. Included in this retrospective study were 24 patients with displaced scapular neck, spine, and intra-articular fractures. Follow-up ranged from 2 to 8 years (average, 36 months). Patient age averaged 25.9 years, consistent with the usual age of multiple blunt trauma patients today. Ninety-six percent of these patients had associated injuries, with upper thoracic rib fractures being most common. This is to be expected, as most scapular fractures occur in high-energy polytrauma accidents as a result of direct impact over the scapular region. Pulmonary injuries were also frequent, with 37% overall, including a 29% incidence of hemopneumothorax and pulmonary contusion in 8%. Thirty-four percent had head injuries, including nine skull fractures. Ipsilateral clavicle fractures occurred in 25%, and 12% of patients had cervical spine injuries, with four permanent cord injuries overall. Of four associated brachial plexus injuries, three recovered spontaneously.

Of the six acromioclavicular sprains that occurred, five were ipsilateral to the scapular fracture, and all were grade I or II. Four of these acromioclavicular injuries were associated with coracoid process fractures, a finding reported in the past with isolated acromioclavicular injuries.

Diagnosis

Scapular fractures and dislocations are often diagnosed incidentally from chest radiographs of the polytrauma patient. Any patient with polytrauma and complaints of shoulder pain, especially in the presence of rib or pulmonary injury, should be examined closely for fractures of the scapula.

Simple anteroposterior (AP) tomography may suffice for most cases, but in complex fractures, CT may be useful for defining displacements in the transverse plane. CT, especially with three-dimensional reconstruction (Fig. 2), is also a valuable planning and educational tool in providing the surgeon with a three-dimensional understanding of the fracture patterns.

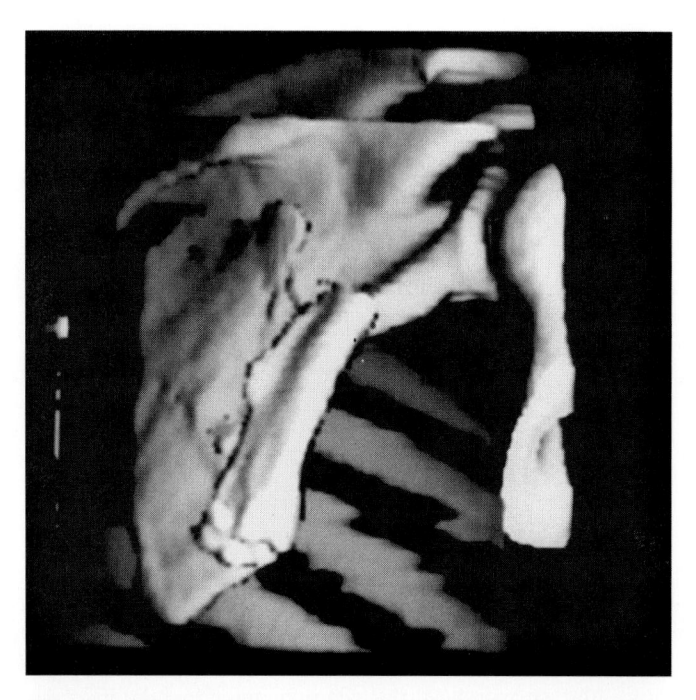

Fig. 2 Three-dimensional reconstruction of complex scapular neck and body fracture.

Management of Scapular Fracture

The problems caused by scapular fractures depend on the location of the fracture, the presence of comminution, and displacement. Union is commonplace, and nonunion is only rarely reported. The vast majority of problems are due to pain and loss of function following closed treatment.

Fragments of the body of the scapula (type IV) do well with closed treatment. Even in the presence of severe displacement, most patients will have neither pain nor loss of motion. A few patients in Ada and Miller's study did note painless popping or grating with motion at the scapulothoracic interface, but had no functional deficits.

Displaced scapular neck fractures frequently cause abduction weakness and also subacromial pain. This may be especially pronounced when these patients lie on the affected side for sleep.

Results

Displaced fractures of the neck and spine of the scapula have been associated with a high rate of associated disability. In Ada and Miller's series, weakness of abduction was associated with displaced scapular neck fractures and comminuted scapular spine fractures. Decreased range of motion was seen in all patients with displaced glenoid fractures. Fifty-seven percent of these patients had night pain, mostly in the subacromial area. Many of these posttraumatic complaints are thought to be related to rotator cuff dysfunction (Table 2).

Table 2. Follow-up study of 24 patients with displaced fractures of the neck and spine of the scapula

Fracture Type	N	Decreased range of motion No. (%)	Pain No. (%)	Weakness with exertion No. (%)	Pain with exertion No. (%)	Popping No. (%)
Displaced neck fractures	16	3 (20)	8 (50) Night: 6 (75)*	6 (40)	7 (46)	4 (25)
Intra-articular fractures	6	6 (100)	4 (66)		4 (66)	4 (66)
Comminuted spine fractures	11	5 (45)	7 (63) Night: 4 (57)	5 (45)	2 (20)	3 (30)

* The night entries are the percentage of those with pain who had pain at night
(Reproduced with permission from Miller ME, Ada JR: Injuries to the shoulder girdle, in Browner BD, Jupiter J, Levine AM, et al (eds): *Skeletal Trauma*. Philadelphia, PA, WB Saunders, 1992, vol 2, pp 1291-1310.)

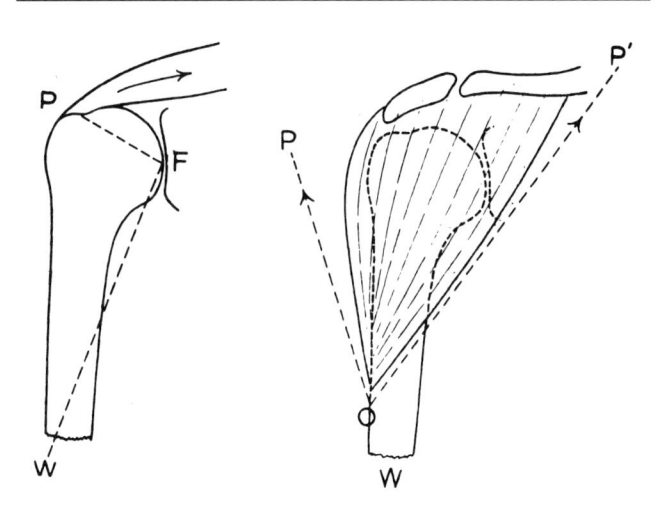

Fig. 3 Muscular forces against the glenoid surface from the rotator cuff and deltoid. (Reproduced with permission from Codman EA (ed): *The Shoulder: Rupture of the Supraspinatus Tendon and Other Lesions in or About the Subacromial Bursa*. Boston, MA, T Todd & Co, 1934, pp 32-64.)

Table 3. Indications for surgical treatment of scapular fractures

Fracture type	Displacement
I-A, I-B	More than 5 to 8 mm
II-A, -B, -C	More than 40° angular displacement in transverse or coronal plane; 1 cm or more displacement of glenoid surface
III	3- to 5-mm step-off of joint surfaces

(Reproduced with permission from Miller ME, Ada JR: Injuries to the shoulder girdle, in Browner BD, Jupiter J, Levine AM, et al (eds): *Skeletal Trauma*. Philadelphia, PA, WB Saunders, 1992, vol 2, pp 1291-1310.)

Rotator Cuff Dysfunction After Scapular Fracture

At less than 90° of abduction, the glenoid reactive force of the deltoid results in a shear vector.[13] The transverse orientation of the rotator cuff muscles in the scapula creates a normalizing or compressive force across the glenoid that neutralizes this destabilizing tendency (Fig. 3). An angular or translational change from the normal position of the glenoid caused by fracture displacement will affect the lever arm of the rotator cuff muscles and the generation of these compressive forces. With increasing tilt of the glenoid, some of the compressive forces of the rotator cuff will be converted to a shear or sliding vector. Because this conversion to shear forces approximates the tangent of the tilt angle, the situation would worsen sharply at about 45° of glenoid tilt.

Fractures of the spine of the scapula can also cause rotator cuff dysfunction, with patients complaining of pain and weakness with abduction, and night pain. When found in combination with scapular neck and body fractures, these scapular spine injuries can produce the so-called Z deformity and collapse of the scapula. In such a situation, one must assume a degree of direct injury to the rotator cuff musculature, proportional to the displacement and comminution evident on radiography. Neviaser[6] described a problem of "pseudorupture" of the rotator cuff in patients with scapular fractures, and thought this due to hemorrhage into the cuff musculature with resulting paralysis.

Treatment Recommendations Management of scapular fractures should be aimed toward restoring and preserving rotator cuff function. Based on our review of available studies, we believe that there is a role for the surgical management of some displaced fractures of the scapula. In addition to cases of intra-articular derangement caused by displaced glenoid (type III) fractures, surgical indications include scapular neck fractures with more than 40° of angulation in either the transverse or coronal plane, and fractures of the scapular neck with 1 cm or more of displacement (Table 3). Scapular spine fractures at the base of the acromion and those with more than 5 mm of displacement may be at risk for the development of nonunion and thus should also be considered for surgical treatment.

The surgical management of scapular fractures has been reported almost exclusively by European surgeons,[14,15] with isolated cases seen in North America.[16] The series of Hardegger and associates[14] is among the largest surgical experiences reported, with 70% of their 37 patients having good to excellent results. In the past few years, an increasing number of reports have appeared documenting the favorable long-term outcome of surgically treated fractures of the glenoid.[17,18]

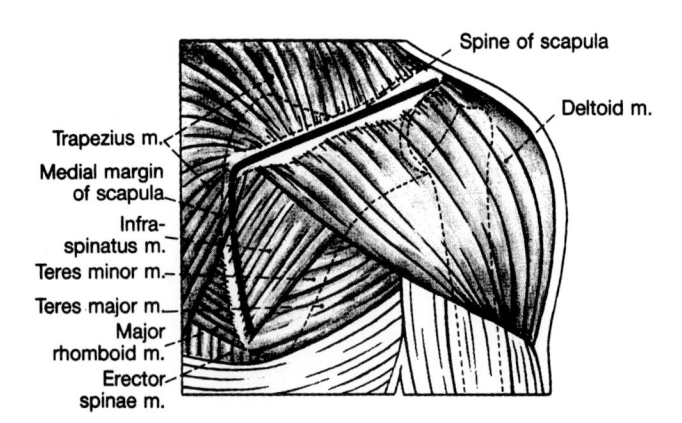

Fig. 4 Judet incision for posterior extensile exposure of the scapula. (Reproduced with permission from von Torklus D, Nicola T (eds): *Atlas of Orthopaedic Exposures*. Baltimore, MD, Urban & Schwarzenberg, 1986.)

Surgical Approaches and Techniques Accurate radiographic assessment and presurgical planning are a minimum requirement in surgical treatment of these fractures. A true AP radiograph and a lateral Y view to assess displacement of the glenoid in the coronal plane are essential minimum studies. In cases with obvious or suspected fractures of the glenoid, CT provides needed information as to the best surgical approach. Glenoid fractures with an anterior fragment, for example, should be treated through an anterior dissection, whereas any fracture involving the body or spine, or a displaced posterior fragment must be approached from the dorsal route.

Anterior glenoid fragments can be seen well through the standard Bankart dissection using a deltopectoral incision. In addition, the articular surface of the glenoid is more clearly seen from the anterior approach because of the anteversion of the scapula and glenoid face on the thorax. In large or muscular patients, the coracoid process or the conjoint tendon of the short head of the biceps-coracobrachialis must be taken down to afford satisfactory visualization of the medial extent of the neck of the glenoid. Fixation may generally be obtained using 3.5-mm AO cortical screws, although in some instances this may also require small plates as well.

The majority of injuries must be viewed and treated from a posterior approach, as they are often complex fracture patterns involving more than one area of the scapula. Most frequently, displaced fractures of the scapular neck and glenoid are associated with fractures of the scapular spine and body. Limited surgical exposures will prove frustrating; thus the extensile exposure of the Judet incision is recommended (Fig. 4) for almost all complex fractures. The robust blood supply to the scapula aids in fracture healing, even in the face of extensive soft tissue dissection. With reasonable care, the two major vascular structures, the suprascapular and circumflex scapular arteries, can be avoided.

Reduction maneuvers and fixation patterns will vary with fracture types, but a few useful points should be considered.

It is very helpful to have two assistants for these demanding cases. Purchase on scapular spine fragments is easily gained with a bone-holding clamp inserted through small keyhole incisions along the superior border of the scapular spine. Because of the complex web of muscle attachments on the scapula, reduction of displaced fragments must be done with patience, and with the aid of complete muscle relaxation by the anesthetist. The small Hohman retractors and dental pick in the AO small fragment instrumentation can be used to good advantage for realigning fracture margins.

Fixation of simple scapular neck fractures, even if widely displaced, can be accomplished with one plate along the lateral scapular margin. The AO 3.5-mm compression plates or reconstruction plates should be used, along with 3.5-mm cortical bone screws.

The lateral scapular margin, although only 10 to 14 mm thick, is very dense cortical bone that provides surprisingly strong purchase for the newer, AO 3.5-mm cortical screws. More complex fractures may require bidirectional fixation with two plates.

Fixation of scapular spine fractures should be done from the inferior surface of the spine so as not to endanger the suprascapular neurovascular bundle or impinge on the relatively tight confines of the supraspinatus muscle itself.

Extremely complex fractures, which include fractures of the glenoid, neck and spine of the scapula, and the clavicle, may require fixation of the clavicle. The intact coracoclavicular ligaments may displace fragments contiguous with the coracoid, making reduction and maintenance of fixation more difficult. Such fractures may require a combined anterior and posterior approach, but the majority of even the most complex fractures of the scapula can be treated through the posterior dissection alone.

Three recent reports discussed complex combined injuries to the scapula and clavicle. Ipsilateral fractures of the scapular neck and clavicle result in disruption of the suspensory mechanism of the shoulder, and the weight of the arm then pulls the glenoid distally and anteromedially. Late deformity and afunctional deficit are prevented by open reduction and internal fixation of the clavicle and occasionally the scapula. Twenty-one of 22 patients in two series achieved good or excellent results at short-term follow-up.[19-21]

With reasonable care, good results should be expected in most cases. Experience in North America is quite limited, with only a few reports. Further long-term follow-up of a greater number of cases is needed to refine surgical indications.

Scapulothoracic Dislocation

The scapula may be dislocated by high-energy trauma, and patients with these injuries have exceedingly complex

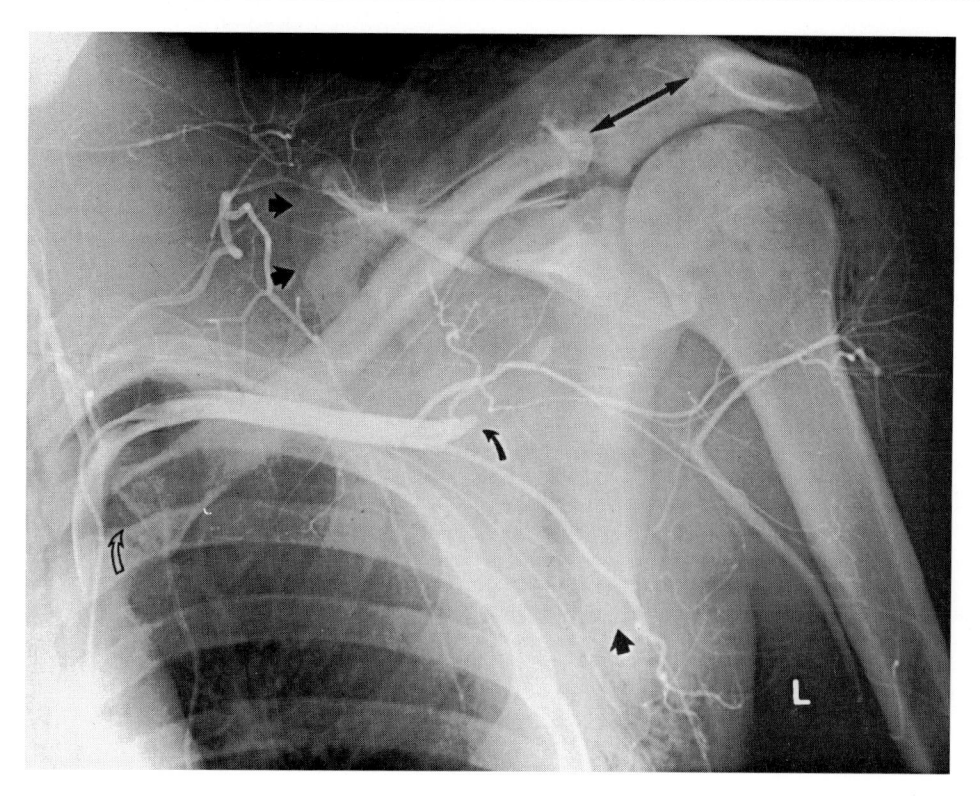

Fig. 5 Arteriogram of capulothoracic dissociation. There is complete disruption of the axillary-brachial artery (small curved arrow). The entire medial scapular border (small arrows) is seen *lateral* to the thoracic wall and the AC joint is widely distracted by the injury (double-ended arrow). (Courtesy of Dr. Ron Clements, Birmingham, AL.)

multisystem problems. Dislocations may be characterized as intrathoracic or lateral. These injuries are rare.

Intrathoracic dislocation with the inferior scapular angle traumatically inserted between two ribs is managed by abduction of the arm and direct manipulation of the scapula, followed by immobilization for 3 to 6 weeks. The vascular and neurologic status of the upper extremity must be carefully assessed.

More ominous is the lateral scapulothoracic dislocation. This injury has been described as the harbinger of a major neurovascular disruption of the forequarter and can be thought of as a partial, closed amputation.[22] The diagnosis is based on lateral displacement of the scapula seen on a well-centered plain radiograph of the chest. Arteriography (Fig. 5) and immediate vascular repair are recommended in both reports. An additional report, however, found no difference in outcome or hemorrhagic complications based on treatment of the arterial injury, and advocated a conservative policy toward revascularization of the affected extremity.[23] Additional treatment options for these devastating injuries include some combination of amputation, shoulder arthrodesis, prosthetic fitting, and reconstructive tendon transfers, but the long-term outcome of these injuries is uniformly disappointing.

Sternoclavicular Dislocations

These uncommon injuries are of two general types, anterior and posterior. In addition, patients less than 25 years old may sustain these injuries as a growth plate fracture-dislocation.

The mechanism of injury is usually a direct force or blow on the point of the shoulder or on the clavicle itself. At least one case of sternoclavicular dislocation has also been reported as a sequel to seizure activity.[24]

Anterior Dislocation of the Sternoclavicular Joint

Most cases of anterior sternoclavicular joint dislocation are easily diagnosed by physical examination, with the prominent medial end of the clavicle visible subcutaneously. The patient will usually complain of pain localized to the joint with abduction-external rotation, and the joint is usually quite tender. The difficulty in some cases is in discerning whether the dislocation is anterior or posterior.[25] The patient must be given a thorough neurovascular examination, but few anterior dislocations have any major associated injuries.

Radiography using apical lordotic views may be helpful, but only CT is accurate enough to fully characterize these lesions.[26,27] In patients aged 25 years or less, these injuries may constitute a Salter type I or II physeal injury, a finding difficult to substantiate with any study other than tomography or CT.

Treatment of Anterior Dislocations

The major considerations in the treatment of acute, chronic, or recurrent anterior sternoclavicular joint dislocations are symptomatic and cosmetic, because such dislocations are generally of little long-term functional impact. The clavicle itself is pinioned by powerful muscular insertions of the pectoralis major, sternocleidomastoid, and trapezius. Loss of stability at its least mobile end is thus damped. Further, the contribution of the clavicle to most daily activities is minimal. Complete claviculectomy may result in little functional limitation of the forequarter.

Closed Reduction

Despite the inherent instability of anterior dislocations, a closed reduction should be tried, particularly in view of the functionally benign nature of these injuries. The reduction maneuver consists of abduction of the affected shoulder, with a sandbag or towel roll placed under the patient's thoracic spine to act as a fulcrum. For reasons of kindness as well as muscle relaxation, general anesthesia is recommended. In the event that the reduction is stable, the limb should be held with a Velpeau-type dressing for a period of 6 weeks, with exercises of the elbow and glenohumeral rotation begun at 3 weeks during daily furloughs from the Velpeau. If a posteriorly directed distraction force on the shoulder girdle is required to maintain reduction, a plaster jacket or figure-of-eight brace may be tried. Commercially available soft figure-of-eight dressings exert insufficient force for the management of clavicle fractures in adults[28] and are just as ineffectual for these injuries.

Anterior dislocation of the sternoclavicular joint is highly unstable when reduced. In the probable event that the anterior dislocation cannot be held reduced by closed means, three alternatives must be considered: acceptance of the deformity, with the small likelihood of a functional deficit; resection of the medial end of the clavicle; and last, and least preferable, surgical stabilization of the medial end of the clavicle.

Treatment of Posterior Dislocations

Posterior dislocations of the sternoclavicular joint are produced by the same mechanisms of injury as the more benign anterior types—a blow on the point of the shoulder or direct trauma to the clavicle. Because of the subjacent mediastinal and cervical structures, these injuries are potentially more serious and require more aggressive diagnosis and management.

Diagnosis based on physical and radiographic findings is similar to the description above of anterior dislocations, with some important differences. Besides pain, the patient may complain of dysphagia or dyspnea due to compression of the esophagus or trachea. Major vascular structures are also at risk for compression. Thus a careful neurovascular assessment is required.

Closed Reduction

Posterior dislocations of the sternoclavicular joint are reduced by a maneuver similar to the one described above. Often, a towel clip or pointed bone-holding forceps must be used percutaneously to gain enough purchase to coax the clavicle back to its desired position. In the majority of cases, these injuries will be stable when reduced, and the patient can then be managed with a sling and swathe for approximately 3 weeks before active exercises are begun. Full activities and contact sports should be restricted for at least 12 to 16 weeks.

Surgical Management

Surgical stabilization of acute or chronically dislocated sternoclavicular joints can only be justified in the presence of posterior dislocations that cannot be managed by a closed technique. Although primary open treatment of anterior dislocations has its advocates,[29] open management is to be reserved for those patients who have intractable pain or in whom the lesion appears to be amenable to soft tissue repair for stabilization. Because of the widely reported complications of Kirschner wire fixations of the sternoclavicular joint, such misadventures are to be condemned. One author, in his report of intrathoracic dislocation of Kirschner wires after fixation of these injuries, suggested that this problem "requires treatment by a surgeon with good experience in thoracic surgery."

Fixation of the medial end of the clavicle with the manubriosternal end of the sternocleidomastoid has been described.[30] The tenodesis transfer of the subclavius described by Burrows,[31] which appears to be physiologically sound, shares the same set of problems with other methods of fixation: surgery done in an area potentially hazardous because of vital structures apposed to the surgical field, and possibly disfiguring scar tissue replacing the medial prominence of the clavicle. While Burrows reported excellent results, there have been too few of these repairs reported by any other surgeons to know whether such soft tissue procedures are efficacious in other hands—thus, in cases undertaken for cosmetic reasons, the pithy warning of Booth and Roper: "the scar looks worse than the lump."

If excision of the medial end of the clavicle is chosen because of persistent pain, care must be taken to avoid removal of too much clavicle, with resultant ablation of the costoclavicular ligament. Not more than 1 to 1.5 cm of the medial end of the clavicle should be resected. The situation is analogous to the removal of the distal end of the clavicle for treatment of a painful acromioclavicular (AC) joint, in which resection of bone sufficient to disturb the intact coracoclavicular ligaments may unnecessarily destabilize the clavicle.

Because the medial clavicular growth plate is among the last to close at the end of growth, any patient less than 25 years old with a sternoclavicular dislocation should be suspected of having a growth plate separation. In younger patients, extensive bone remodeling can be expected.[32]

Fractures of the Clavicle

Clavicle fractures in adults, like those in children, will heal with minimal treatment in the vast majority of cases. Nonunion rates of between 0.1% and 5% have been reported,[25,33] but for reasons discussed below, those reports probably underestimate the occurrence in adults.

Although a fall on an outstretched hand is often cited as the common mechanism of injury, Stanley and associates[34] found that direct trauma was the more likely cause in the majority of cases in adults. In either case, when the sternoclavicular joint remains intact, a posteriorly directed force on the entire shoulder or the scapula itself may bend and break the clavicle over the fulcrum of the first rib.

In an analysis of healing problems in 140 clavicle fractures in adults, White and associates[35] found a much higher incidence of delayed and nonunions (23%) than had previously been appreciated, and analyzed their patients by several criteria. They found significantly higher rates of delayed and nonunion in high-energy injuries, but did not find a significant effect within the high- or low-energy groups of displacement or comminution. They did not recommend initial surgical care even in their high-energy group, because the results of delayed surgery have generally been excellent. A higher rate of delayed healing was found for patients treated with slings compared to a figure-of-eight brace, but this observation was based on only a small group of patients. No difference in results in adults has been found with plain sling treatment compared with figure-of-eight bracing;[28] however, others believe that a sling and swathe is best for adults with clavicle fractures.[12]

Most series of acute fixation of clavicle fractures have been reported from western Europe and have typically reported complication rates in excess of 10%.[36]

Indications for Acute Surgical Treatment

Injuries to the underlying vascular structures associated with clavicle fractures require exploration and stabilization as a logical part of the vascular repair, and protection of the vessels after surgery. In cases of brachial plexus injury, restraint should be exercised, since as many as two thirds of these patients will recover spontaneously.[37]

Open fractures of the clavicle, depending on the degree of surrounding soft tissue trauma, are also candidates for stabilization. In these cases, as well as in some cases of established nonunion, external fixation has been successfully employed by at least one group.[38]

There have been isolated cases of surgical treatment of acute fractures with severe displacement in high-performance athletes with symptomatic nonunion who did not wish to delay returning to play. Surgical treatment can be recommended only in a patient who thoroughly understands the risks, advantages, and disadvantages of treatment options, and then only at the patient's insistence.

In head-injured and seizure patients, tenting of the skin by sharp bone fragments becomes worrisome. In neurologically normal patients, the major skin injury occurs at the time of initial trauma and is not likely to progress. In patients lacking normal proprioception or pain inhibition, fixation of clavicle fractures that are tenting the skin may be indicated. Depending on the nursing needs of the patient, a shoulder spica cast may suffice if a good closed reduction is obtained.

Clavicle Fractures That Fail to Unite

Most ununited clavicle fractures are in the middle third of the bone.[3] Here, the medial and lateral compound S curves unite in a region almost totally devoid of cancellous bone and muscle coverage, and are subject to the most pronounced bending and rotational stresses in the entire bone. Indications for surgical intervention in chronic cases are relatively simple. Most surgical candidates have a painful nonunion that limits function and range of motion. Also, cases of brachial plexus compression and thoracic outlet syndrome have been reported. Most painful nonunions are of the hypertrophic type and atrophic nonunions are frequently asymptomatic.[39] Surgery for cosmetic reasons alone is likely to be disappointing and should be avoided.

Recent reviews of surgery for chronic nonunion or pseudoarthrosis are in general agreement as to indications for surgery and method of treatnent.[3,39-41] Although intramedullary pin fixation has had its proponents, most authors agree that plate fixation is far better, and more likely to produce a satisfactory outcome. Because resection of the nonunion will be necessary in many cases, great care should be taken to avoid shortening the clavicle, as this will result in weakness of abduction. This weakness may be attributed to restriction of the scapula in an adducted position by the shortened clavicle. The technique of sculptured bicortical interposition bone graft described by Jupiter and Leffert[3] should thus be considered in cases with resection gaps of more than 10 mm. The AO 3.5-mm compression or reconstruction plates should be used for most cases. The implants must be carefully shaped because of the complex curves and twists of the clavicular surface. After fixation, motion should be restricted for not more than 3 to 4 weeks, unless bone quality or tenuous fixation indicate a need for more prolonged support.

The fixation of ununited clavicle fractures is to be undertaken with caution, and the patient must have a clear conception of the risks of continued nonunion, loss of fixation, and infection. A hypertrophic scar may result, regardless of the care exercised in wound planning and closure. Despite these admonitions, the series cited above reported an 85% to 95% rate of good to excellent results overall, and a careful surgeon with a reasonably compliant patient should expect to match these favorable outcomes.

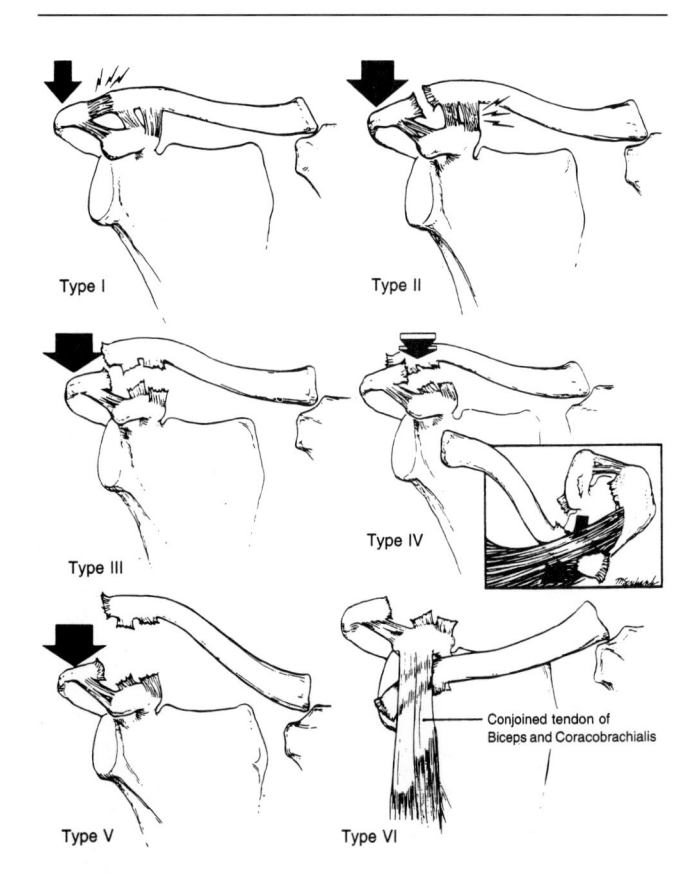

Fig. 6 Six grades of AC joint separation. (Reproduced with permission from Rockwood CA Jr: Subluxation and dislocations about the shoulder, in Rockwood CA Jr, Green DP (eds): *Fractures in Adults*. Philadelphia, PA, JP Lippincott, 1988, pp 722-985.)

Table 4. Classification of AC separations

Fracture Type	Injury Pattern*	Surgery
I	AC joint capsule, partially disrupted	Not indicated
II	AC joint capsule and CC ligaments partially disrupted	Not indicated
III	AC joint capsule and CC ligaments completely disrupted	Optional (see text)
IV	Type III + avulsion of CC ligament from clavicle, penetration of clavicle through periosteal sleeve, or major soft-tissue injury	Indicated
V	Type III + posterior dislocation of clavicle behind acromion	Indicated
VI	Type II + inferolateral dislocation of lateral end of clavicle	Indicated

* AC, acromioclavicular; CC, coracoclavicular
(Reproduced with permission from Miller ME, Ada JR: Injuries to the shoulder girdle, in Browner BD, Jupiter J, Levine AM, et al (eds): *Skeletal Trauma*. Philadelphia, PA, WB Saunders, 1992, vol 2, pp 1291-1310.)

Dislocations of the AC Joint and Fractures of the Lateral End of the Clavicle

For more than 40 years, the treatment of acute AC joint subluxation and dislocation has been a source of controversy among orthopaedic surgeons. At present, orthopaedists still constitute two equally committed and vociferous camps: those who pridefully report their good results after surgical treatment using one of the numerous methods of fixation developed with or without biomechanical research, and those who disdainfully report their excellent results after closed (or non) treatment and point to open management of these injuries as "tantamount to shooting a dove with an elephant hunter's rifle . . . the antithesis of sound practice."

Classification

The classification system proposed by Post[42] and Rockwood[43] is now commonly used and describes six types of injury, which are illustrated in Figure 6. Closed treatment methods are almost universally recommended for types I, II, and III, as recovery from these injuries results in few long-term problems. Any of the rare, severe injuries of types IV–VI may be accompanied by fracture of the coracoid process, and few authors disagree with a need for surgical treatment of these injuries (Table 4).

Treatment of Acute AC Joint Dislocations

Any discussion of the management of acute injuries to the AC joint must confront not only the question of which of the more than 30 methods of surgical treatment described is best, but whether surgery should be considered at all for injury types I–III. Of the few statistically valid, prospective series comparing closed with surgical treatment of acromioclavicular dislocations, none show superior results after surgical management. The majority of surgeons are content to treat type I and II lesions with a sling and swathe and early motion based on symptoms.

When read closely, most studies have the same results, regardless of the authors' conclusions—longer recovery times and high local complication rates for surgically treated patients without any improvement in long-term function[44-48] yet most authors hedged their conclusions, suggesting surgical treatment for patients whose work required frequent abduction to 90° with forward flexion.

Surgical Techniques

Of the many types of surgical treatment described in the literature, there are basically two general approaches: fixation of the AC joint directly with transfixing wires, with or without cerclage or tension band wiring; or indirect purchase on the AC joint with coracoclavicular fixation such as screw, wire loop, woven Dacron loop, or other ligament substitutes. These procedures may be combined with debridement of the AC joint and repair of the coracoclavicular ligaments, ligament transfer, and/or plication of the torn deltotrapezius mechanisms at the distal clavicle.[47,49,50]

An orthopaedic surgeon considering open management of any AC injury of type I–III severity must feel compelled to justify surgical management, because end result studies simply do not support surgical intervention.

Type IV–VI injuries, which probably account for less than 10% to 15% of the total number of AC dislocations, should be managed surgically. For this, we prefer coracoclavicular fixation using a screw, which can be easily removed through a small stab incision after healing.[51]

Treatment of Nonacute Injuries

For the patient with a chronic AC joint dislocation or subluxation that remains painful after 3 to 6 months of closed treatment and rehabilitation, surgery is indicated to improve function and comfort. Only a minority of patients with untreated AC joint injuries will actually choose to have surgical treatment.

Most authors agree that resection of the lateral end of the clavicle will provide excellent relief for a painful AC joint. This has been confirmed by long-term follow-up as well.[52] In neglected type II–III injuries, supplementary reconstruction of the coracoclavicular ligament complex should be based on the surgeon's perception of instability at the time of surgery. Such reconstruction is needed only if instability of the distal clavicle is contributing to the patient's pain or loss of function, and this will rarely be the case.

For sequelae of untreated type IV–VI injuries, a combination of distal clavicle resection and coracoclavicular ligament substitution is called for. The technique of Weaver and Dunn,[53] widely used in North America and simple to perform, is mechanically sound and fulfills its originators' criteria that "The ideal operative procedure should eliminate the possibility of migration of pins or failure of AC reduction. Late degenerative changes should not be seen, and any further or secondary operative procedures should be unnecessary. In addition, the result should be cosmetically acceptable, and should allow the patient to have a fully functional shoulder in a short period of time."

Fractures of the Distal Clavicle

In adults, fractures of the distal clavicle may be classified by the system of Neer and Rockwood[44] to be of three types. Surgical treatment is occasionally indicated for only one of these types.

The distal clavicle is pinioned in place by the static stabilization of the coracoclavicular ligament complex and the AC joint capsule. Acting against these are the relatively weak dynamic downward forces of the pectoralis major and the stronger upward forces of the trapezius and sternocleidomastoid. Depending on the location of a fracture of the lateral end of the clavicle relative to these static and dynamic stabilizers, certain displacements and functional problems can be expected. Fracture types are based on these considerations.

Type I injuries, which occur lateral to the coracoclavicular ligament complex and are therefore quite stable, will heal with sling and swathe support. These fractures may be complicated by an undisplaced intra-articular component at the AC joint, leading to some postfracture arthrosis and pain. This can be treated by distal clavicle resection if it remains symptomatic, using open or arthroscopic methods.

Type III injuries are intra-articular fractures of the distal clavicle at the AC joint and are sometimes an occult source of posttraumatic arthritis and pain in cases that might otherwise have been diagnosed as grade 1 AC joint subluxations. The diagnosis may be made from AP tomography in patients with an unusual level of pain after an apparently trivial AC joint injury, but acute treatment is supportive only.

Type II injuries are complex fracture-dislocations that leave the distal clavicle and the AC joint intact but separate the clavicle from the underlying coracoclavicular ligament complex through an oblique fracture. Sometimes a small fragment of bone is left attached to the coracoclavicular ligaments, avulsed from the clavicle. The deformity is marked, and Neer[54] favors open treatment with Kirschner wires transfixing the AC joint into the displaced clavicle or suture-loop fixation of the clavicle to the coracoid with #5 nonabsorbable material. Experience with these rare injuries is necessarily limited, but surgical treatment for these lesions is probably unwarranted in most cases.

These injuries can be treated with a sling or a Kenny Howard splint, with excellent functional results. The deformity can be reduced somewhat, but a sizable lump will still be present, which in young women may be cosmetically distressing. The fact remains that these injuries, like other more routine clavicle fractures, heal readily, and splintage may be discontinued at 3 to 4 weeks. The result is generally a strong, painless shoulder with a cosmetic deformity.

References

1. Froimson AI: Fracture of the coracoid process of the scapula. *J Bone Joint Surg* 1978;60A:710-711.

2. Ishizuki M, Yamaura I, Isobe Y, et al: Avulsion fracture of the superior border of the scapula: Report of five cases. *J Bone Joint Surg* 1981;63A:820-822.

3. Jupiter JB, Leffert RD: Non-union of the clavicle: Associated complications and surgical management. *J Bone Joint Surg* 1987;69A:753-760.

4. Mathews RE, Cocke TB, D'Ambrosia RD: Scapular fractures secondary to seizures in patients with osteodystrophy: Report of two cases and review of the literature. *J Bone Joint Surg* 1983;65A:850-853.

5. Heyse-Moore GH, Stoker DJ: Avulsion fractures of the scapula. *Skeletal Radiol* 1982;9:27-32.

6. Neviaser JS: Injuries in and about the shoulder joint, in Raney RB (ed): American Academy of Orthopaedic Surgeons *Instructional Course Lectures XIII*. Ann Arbor, MI, JW Edwards, 1956, pp 187-216.

7. Protass JJ, Stampfli FV, Osmer JC: Coracoid process fracture diagnosis in acromioclavicular separation. *Radiology* 1975;116:61-64.

8. Tarquinio T, Weinstein ME, Virgilio RW: Bilateral scapular fractures from accidental electric shock. *J Trauma* 1979;19:132-133.

9. Wolf AW, Shoji H, Chuinard RG: Unusual fracture of the coracoid process: A case report and review of the literature. *J Bone Joint Surg* 1976;58A:423-424.

10. Zettas JP, Muchnic PD: Fractures of the coracoid process base in acute acromioclavicular separation. *Orthop Rev* 1976;5:77-79.

11. Zilberman Z, Rejovitzky R: Fracture of the coracoid process of the scapula. *Injury* 1981;13:203-206.

12. Ada JR, Miller ME: Scapular fractures: Analysis of 113 cases. *Clin Orthop* 1991;269:174-180.

13. Codman EA (ed): *The Shoulder: Rupture of the Supraspinatus Tendon and Other Lesions in or About the Subacromial Bursa*. Boston, MA, T Todd & Co, 1934.

14. Hardegger FH, Simpson LA, Weber BG: The operative treatment of scapular fractures. *J Bone Joint Surg* 1984;66B:725-731.

15. Izadpanah M: Osteosynthesis in scapula fractures. *Arch Orthop Unfall Chir* 1975;83:153-164.

16. Aulicino PL, Reinert C, Kornberg M, et al: Displaced intra-articular glenoid fractures treated by open reduction and internal fixation. *J Trauma* 1986;26:1137-1141.

17. Leung KS, Lam TP, Poon KM: Operative treatment of displaced intra-articular glenoid fractures. *Injury* 1993;24:324-328.

18. Kavanagh BF, Bradway JK, Cofield RH: Open reduction and internal fixation of displaced intra-articular fractures of the glenoid fossa. *J Bone Joint Surg* 1993;75A:479-484.

19. Leung KS, Lam TP: Open reduction and internal fixation of ipsilateral fractures of the scapular neck and clavicle. *J Bone Joint Surg* 1993;75A:1015-1018.

20. Goss TP: Double disruptions of the superior shoulder suspensory complex. *J Orthop Trauma* 1993;7:99-106.

21. Herscovici D Jr, Fiennes AG, Allgower M, et al: The floating shoulder: Ipsilateral clavicle and scapular neck fractures. *J Bone Joint Surg* 1992;74B:362-364.

22. Oreck SL, Burgess A, Levine AM: Traumatic lateral displacement of the scapula: A radiographic sign of neurovascular disruption. *J Bone Joint Surg* 1984;66A:758-763.

23. Sampson LN, Britton JC, Eldrup-Jorgensen J, et al: The neurovascular outcome of scapulothoracic dissociation. *J Vascular Surg* 1993;17:1083-1089.

24. Dastgeer GM, Mikolich DJ: Fracture-dislocation of the manubriosternal joint: An unusual complication of seizures. *J Trauma* 1987;27:91-93.

25. Neer CS II: Non-union of the clavicle. *JAMA* 1960;172:1006-1011.

26. Deutsch AL, Resnick D, Mink JH: Computed tomography of the glenohumeral and sternoclavicular joints. *Orthop Clin North Am* 1985;16:497-511.

27. Levinsohn EM, Bunnell WP, Yuan HA: Computed tomography in the diagnosis of dislocations of the sternoclavicular joint. *Clin Orthop* 1979;140:12-16.

28. Andersen K, Jensen PO, Lauritzen J: Treatment of clavicular fractures: Figure-of-eight bandage versus a simple sling. *Acta Orthop Scand* 1987;58:71-74.

29. Eskola A: Sternoclavicular dislocation: A plea for open treatment. *Acta Orthop Scand* 1986;57:227-228.

30. Booth CM, Roper BA: Chronic dislocation of the sternoclavicular joint: An operative repair. *Clin Orthop* 1979;140:17-20.

31. Burrows HJ: Tenodesis of subclavius in the treatment of recurrent dislocation of the sterno-clavicular joint. *J Bone Joint Surg* 1951;33B:240-243.

32. Lemire L, Rosman M: Sternoclavicular epiphyseal separation with adjacent clavicular fracture. *J Pediatr Orthop* 1984;4:118-120.

33. Zenni EJ Jr, Krieg JK, Rosen MJ: Open reduction and internal fixation of clavicular fractures. *J Bone Joint Surg* 1981;63A:147-151.

34. Stanley D, Trowbridge EA, Norris SH: The mechanism of clavicular fracture: A clinical and biomechanical analysis. *J Bone Joint Surg* 1988;70B:461-464.

35. White RR, Anson PS, Kristiansen T, et al: Adult clavicle fractures: The relationship between mechanism of injury and healing. *Orthop Trans* 1989;13:514-515.

36. Poigenfurst J, Reiler T, Fischer W: Plating of fresh clavicular fractures: Experience with 60 operations. *Unfallchirurg* 1988;14:26-37.

37. Sturm JT, Perry JF Jr: Brachial plexus injuries from blunt trauma: A harbinger of vascular and thoracic injury. *Ann Emerg Med* 1987;16:404-406.

38. Schuind F, Pay-Pay E, Andrianne Y, et al: External fixation of the clavicle for fracture or non-union in adults. *J Bone Joint Surg* 1988;70A:692-695.

39. Wilkins RM, Johnston RM: Ununited fractures of the clavicle. *J Bone Joint Surg* 1983;65A:773-778.

40. Eskola A, Vainionpaa S, Myllynen P, et al: Surgery for ununited clavicular fracture. *Acta Orthop Scand* 1986;57:366-367.

41. Manske DJ, Szabo RM: The operative treatment of mid-shaft clavicular non-unions. *J Bone Joint Surg* 1985;67A;1367-1371.

42. Post M: Curent concepts in the diagnosis and management of acromioclavicular dislocations. *Clin Orthop* 1985;200:234-247.

43. Rockwood CA Jr: Injuries to the acromioclavicular joint, in *Fractures in Adults*, ed 2. Philadelphia, PA, JB Lippincott, 1984, vol 1, pp 860-910.

44. Neer CS II, Rockwood CA Jr: Fractures and dislocations of the shoulder, in Rockwood CA Jr, Green DP (eds): *Fractures in Adults*, ed 2. Philadelphia, PA, JP Lippincott, 1984, vol 1, pp 675-985.

45. Bjerneld H, Hovelius L, Thorling J: Acromio-clavicular separations treated conservatively: A 5-year follow-up study. *Acta Orthop Scand* 1983;54:743-745.

46. Larsen E, Bjerg-Nielsen A, Christensen P: Conservative or surgical treatment of acromioclavicular dislocation: A prospective, controlled, randomized study. *J Bone Joint Surg* 1986;68A:552-555.

47. Galpin RD, Hawkins RJ, Grainger RW: A comparative analysis of operative versus nonoperative treatment of grade III acromioclavicular separations. *Clin Orthop* 1985;193:150-155.

48. Taft TN, Wilson FC, Oglesby JW: Dislocation of the acromioclavicular joint: An end-result study. *J Bone Joint Surg* 1987;69A:1045-1051.

49. Heitemeyer AU, Hierholzer G, Schneppendahl G, et al: The operative treatment of fresh ruptures of the acromioclavicular joint (Tossy III). *Arch Orthop Trauma Surg* 1986;104:371-373.

50. Lancaster S, Horowitz M, Alonso J: Complete acromioclavicular separations: A comparison of operative methods. *Clin Orthop* 1987;216:80-88.

51. Neviaser RJ: Injuries to the clavicle and acromioclavicular joint. *Orthop Clin North Am* 1987;18:433-438.

52. Petersson CJ: Resection of the lateral end of the clavicle: A 3- to 30-year follow-up. *Acta Orthop Scand* 1983;54:904-907.

53. Weaver JK, Dunn HK: Treatment of acromioclavicular injuries, especially complete acromioclavicular separation. *J Bone Joint Surg* 1972;54A:1187-1194.

54. Neer CS: Injuries to the AC Joint, in Rockwood CA Jr, Green DP (eds): *Fractures in Adults*. Philadelphia, PA, JB Lippincott, 1984, p 895.

2

Fractures of the Proximal Humerus and Dislocation of the Glenohumeral Joint

Introduction

The frequency of fractures of the proximal humerus has increased since the 1950s, keeping pace with the increased growth of the elderly population.[1-3] Over the past decade, improved techniques for open reduction and internal fixation (ORIF) of osteoporotic fractures have been developed and applied to the shoulder with gratifying results. Simultaneously, methods of closed reduction and percutaneous fixation of the proximal humerus have been reported, offering a less-invasive and perhaps more biologically friendly approach.

Recently, the validity of the Neer classification system, which is based on plain radiographic studies, has been questioned because of interobserver inconsistency. More-detailed subclassification of fractures has been advocated and the use of computerized scanning has been suggested to improve the reliability of classification systems.[4,5] In fact, subclassification of four-part fractures, combined with an improved understanding of the vascular anatomy to the humeral head, has renewed interest in ORIF, preserving the humeral head in certain four-part fractures.

Finally, the importance of early mobilization following severe injury has focused additional interest on fixation of proximal humeral fractures in polytrauma patients. Although significant risk of multisystem organ failure cannot be blamed on proximal humeral fractures alone, the importance of early functional use of the upper extremities is evident. There is, therefore, a new interest in stabilization of the proximal humerus in polytrauma patients by methods that allow early motion and weightbearing on the injured limb.

Dislocations of the glenohumeral joint continue to be exceedingly common, affecting all age groups. The goal of treatment is stable reduction with recovery of full function. Young patients with violent injury mechanisms are those most likely to develop recurrent instability. In these patients, arthroscopic evaluation may play a role in defining lesions associated with late instability and may allow for early repair, decreasing the number of patients who develop late, chronic instability. In elderly patients, a high index of suspicion for associated injury to the rotator cuff is recommended and, if present, surgical repair should be considered. Early mobilization of the shoulder following dislocation may not in and of itself be a risk factor for late instability and therefore prolonged immobilization of the shoulder should be discouraged.

Anatomy

The skeletal, muscular, and neurovascular aspects and relationships of the proximal humerus must be clearly understood[6] as well as the changes in this anatomy associated with aging. With advancing age the medullary cavity expands and advances proximally, replacing the metaphyseal cancellous bone. The humeral cortex thins and trabecular density in the head diminishes, increasing the vulnerability to fracture.

The ascending branch of the anterior humeral circumflex artery and its intraosseous continuation, the arcuate artery, provide the main arterial supply to the humeral head. The humeral head can be completely perfused following ligation of the ascending branch by an abundant intraosseous anastomosis of posteromedial metaphyseal vessels.[7] In four-part fractures, these vessels can maintain perfusion of the humeral head if the soft-tissue attachments to the posteromedial aspect of the head are maintained. The data have obvious implications for the management of certain four-part fractures.

Recent interest in surgical management of posterior fracture-dislocations, internal fixation of the scapula, biopsy and removal of foreign bodies, and drainage of septic arthritis has led to a need for improved posterior surgical exposure of the glenohumeral joint. The evaluation of the posterior approach has evolved from the early extensile dissections described by Kocker in 1911, McWherter in 1932, and Benneh in 1941. These exposures usually resulted in considerable deltoid weakness. A limited deltoid splitting posterior approach is currently advocated. The posterior deltoid splitting incision[8] provides utility access to the posterior aspect of the joint. The incision runs vertically from the posterior acromion to the posterior axillary crease. The underlying oblique fibers of the deltoid are split without bony detachment. The infraspinatus and capsule are

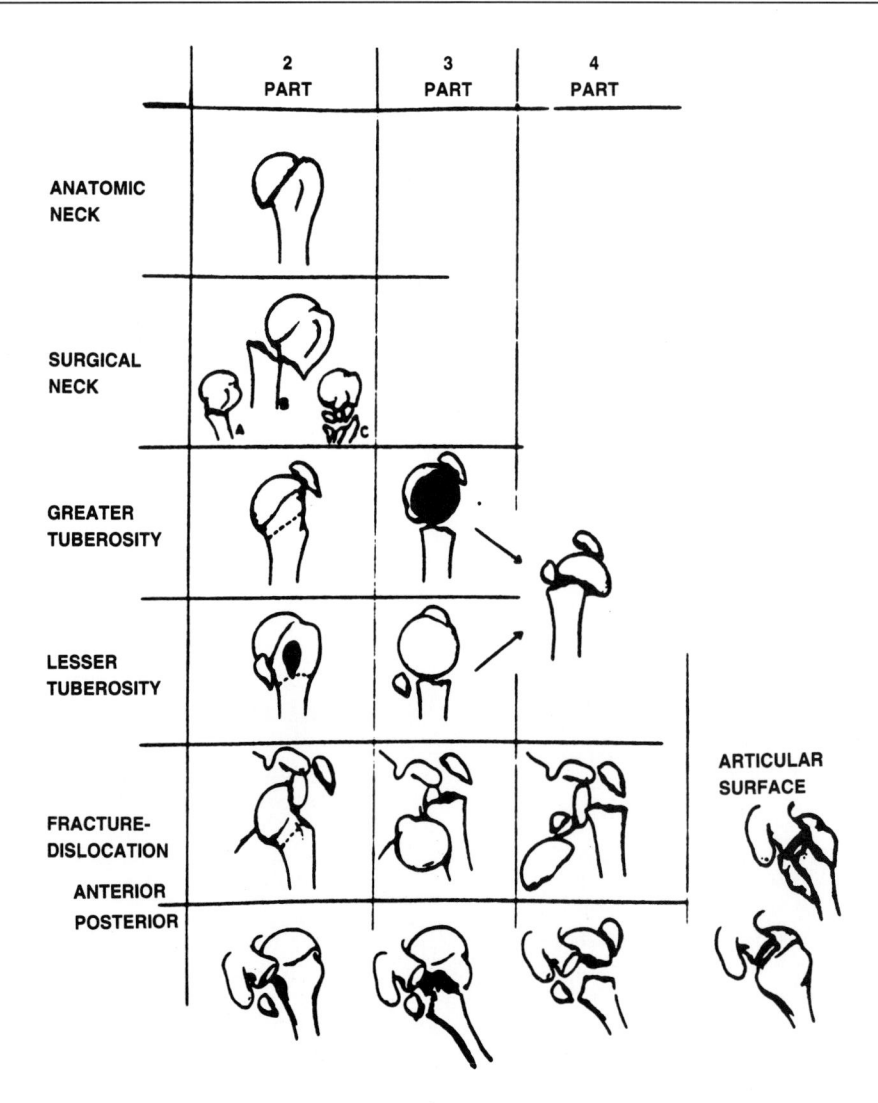

Fig. 1 The Neer classification of proximal humeral fractures. (Reproduced with permission from Neer CS II: Displaced proximal humeral fractures: Part I. Classification and evaluation. *J Bone Joint Surg* 1970;52A:1077–1089.)

incised for exposure of the posterior glenoid. Care must be taken to avoid injury to the axillary nerve as it exits the quadrilateral space just below the teres minor as well as the suprascapular nerve, which runs as near as 15 mm medial to the posterior glenoid rim. When exposure is needed for repair of posterior fracture dislocations, a superior subacromial approach[9] provides superior access to both the posterior and anterior aspects of the joint. This approach has advantages over the pure anterior or posterior approaches. This approach splits the deltoid between its anterior one third and posterior two thirds and detaches the anterior deltoid subperiosteally. More deeply, the supraspinous muscle is split medial to its tendonous portion for limited, but useful, exposure of the glenoid and humeral articular surface.

Clinical and Radiographic Evaluation

The patient with fractures or dislocations of the proximal humerus typically presents following either a direct blow to the shoulder (an axial loading mechanism) or by indirect trauma (as might occur from a fall or an outstretched, abducted arm or following a grand mal seizure). Deformity and swelling are noted during physical examination. Careful palpation will suggest the dislocated position of the humeral head. A careful neurologic assessment should be performed to rule out associated injury to the axillary nerve or brachial plexus. Fractures with gross displacement can result in injury to the axillary artery, as suggested by an expanding axillary hematoma and loss of pulses at the wrist.

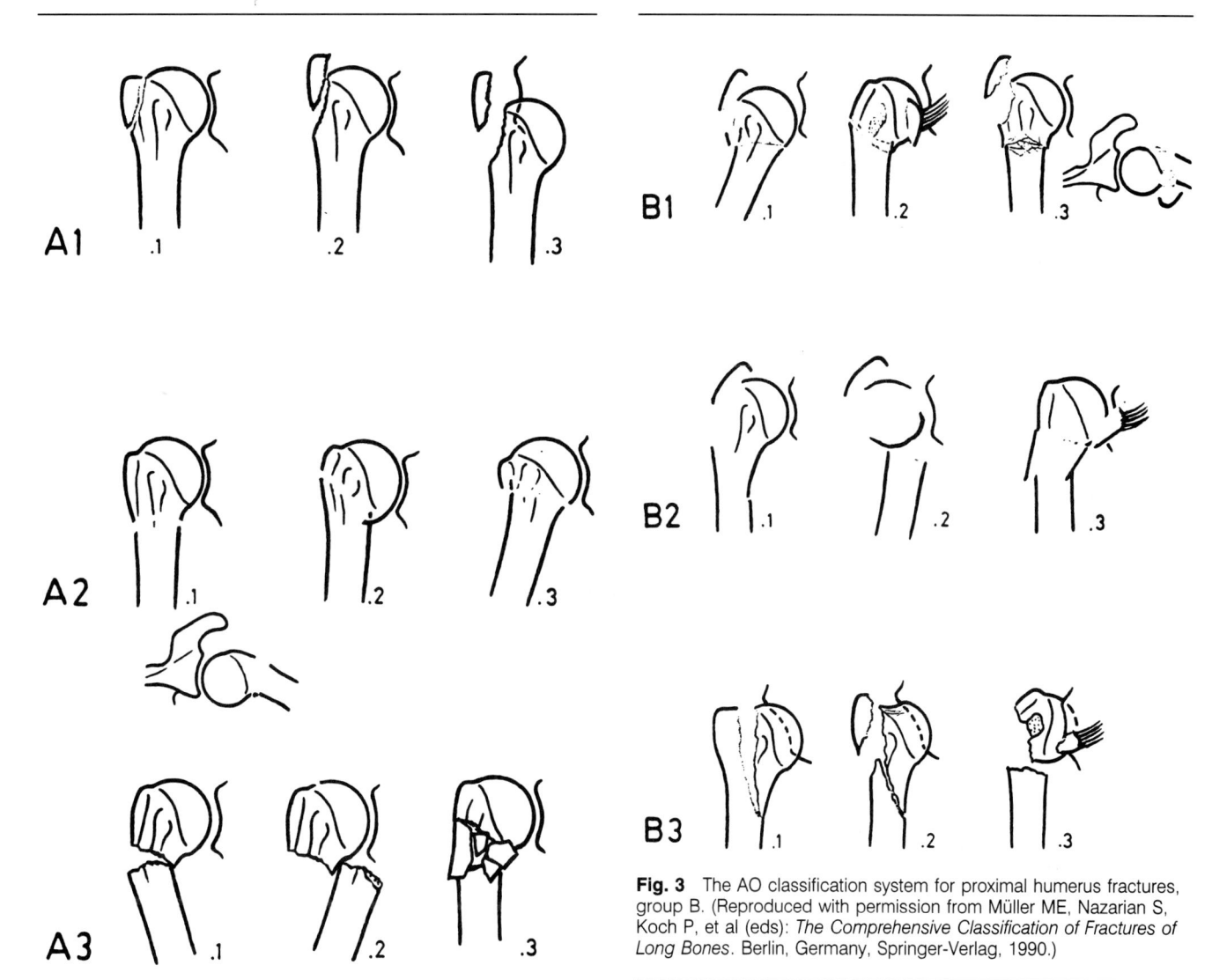

Fig. 2 The AO classification system for proximal humerus fractures, group A. (Reproduced with permission from Müller ME, Nazarian S, Koch P, et al (eds): *The Comprehensive Classification of Fractures of Long Bones*. Berlin, Germany, Springer-Verlag, 1990.)

Fig. 3 The AO classification system for proximal humerus fractures, group B. (Reproduced with permission from Müller ME, Nazarian S, Koch P, et al (eds): *The Comprehensive Classification of Fractures of Long Bones*. Berlin, Germany, Springer-Verlag, 1990.)

Accurate assessment of the fracture configuration requires three radiographic views. An anteroposterior view of the glenohumeral joint and a lateral view taken in the place of the scapula can be obtained in all patients and does not require arm movement. Even though fracture fragments might be moved, an axillary view taken with the arm in 20° to 40° of abduction is essential[6] for three reasons. First, it contributes valuable information regarding fracture angulation and comminution. Second, it reliably demonstrates posterior dislocation. Third, it allows assessment of the glenoid margins. Additional views, such as the West Point view, Stryker notch view, or Didiee views are usually obtained when assessing chronic instability.[10] Computed tomography (CT) is helpful in determining exact fragment displacement and helps evaluate the presence of comminution of the humeral head.[11]

Dislocations of the Glenohumeral Joint

The design of the glenohumeral joint sacrifices inherent stability to gain a large arc of motion. Functional stability is provided by muscles and their attachments. The most common dislocation occurs in the anterior direction and is caused by excessive external rotation and hyperextension of the arm in the overhead direction. As the humeral head is levered out of the glenoid, the anterior capsule and labrum may be torn, the rotator cuff can be torn or avulsed, and the glenoid rim may be fractured.[12] The cuff may separate along the rotator interval, causing pain, rotator cuff dysfunction, and chronic instability.[13] The Hill-Sachs defect of the posterolateral humeral head is produced by recoil of the humeral head against the anterior glenoid rim.

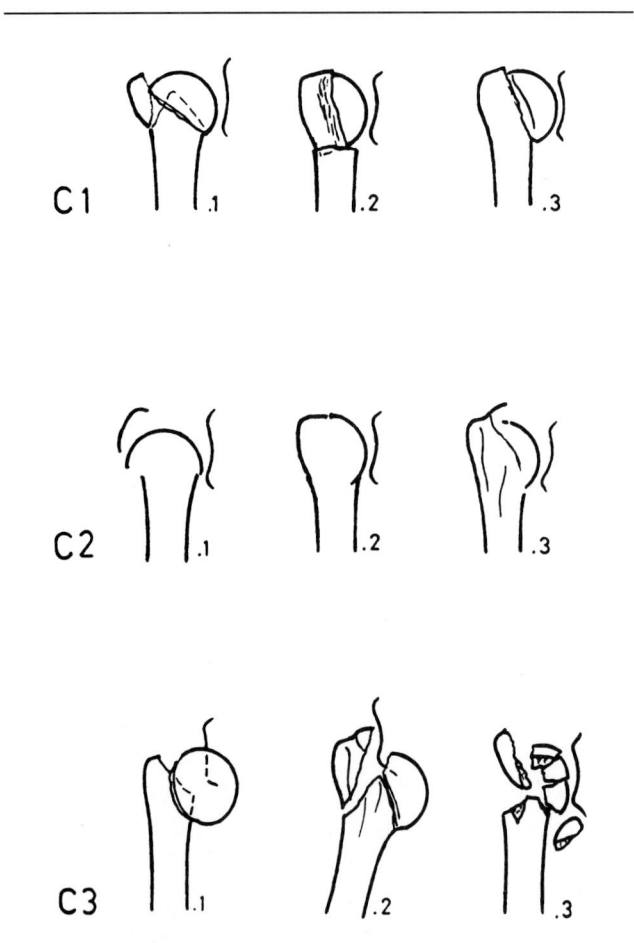

Fig. 4 The AO classification system for proximal humerus fractures, group C. (Reproduced with permission from Müller ME, Nazarian S, Koch P, et al (eds): *The Comprehensive Classification of Fractures of Long Bones*. Berlin, Germany, Springer-Verlag, 1990.)

This lesion is best seen on the internal rotation view of the glenohumeral joint. The axillary and Stryker notch views are also helpful in defining this lesion.[10]

It is important to consider the mechanism of injury when evaluating the patient with an anterior dislocation. Dislocations caused by little or no trauma probably result from chronic instability. In younger patients, dislocations caused by high-energy violence are more likely to result in recurrent instability. Older patients and those with luxatio ercetae are likely to sustain rotator cuff avulsions.[12,14,15] The incidence of axillary nerve palsy following anterior dislocation is 9% to 10%.[15] In the setting of luxatio erectae, however, the incidence of neurovascular injury is 60%.[14] Because the length of immobilization following dislocation is not related to chronic instability, early range of motion is encouraged in the postreduction period.[12]

Patients unable to abduct the arm following anterior shoulder dislocation should be evaluated for avulsion of the rotator cuff.[15] There should be a high degree of suspicion for this injury complex in older patients with anterior shoulder dislocation. Because surgical repair leads to good results, early diagnosis and timely treatment are important.

Recently, the role of arthroscopy in evaluating acute anterior dislocations has been debated.[10] The factors associated with risk of recurrent dislocation are age of the patient, the degree of violence producing the injury, and the nature of the damage to the anterior labrum and capsular attachments. Although arthroscopic examination soon after acute dislocation may help identify those patients with high-risk lesions, allowing early repair, the role of early arthroscopy and repair remain unknown.[16]

Current management of the acute anterior dislocation calls for rapid relocation of the shoulder by gentle closed reduction. There are a variety of helpful techniques, such as installation of intra-articular lidocaine and other gentle reduction maneuvers.[17] Immobilization of the shoulder in a sling in internal rotation should not exceed 3 weeks and rehabilitation exercises focusing on regaining range of motion and rotator cuff strength should be prescribed.

Posterior dislocations of the glenohumeral joint[18] are rare, representing less than 5% of dislocations in most series. The diagnosis of an uncomplicated posterior dislocation is often delayed, but early closed reduction is rarely difficult and recurrent instability is uncommon. In 50% of posterior dislocations there can be an impaction fracture of the humeral head, leading to the locked dislocation or giving rise to late instability. The impaction fracture most commonly occurs between the articular margin and the lesser tuberosity. Locked posterior dislocations often require open reduction.[9] Stableforth has presented a superior subacromial approach nicely suited to this surgical problem.

Fractures of the Proximal Humerus

Classification

Fractures of the proximal humerus are classified according to the presence of displacement or angulation of each of the four major segments: the humeral head, greater tuberosity, lesser tuberosity, and shaft. A segment is considered displaced if displacement is greater than 1 cm or 45° of angulation.

Since it was first described in 1970, the Neer classification system has gained wide acceptance.[19] The Neer classification describes a two-, three-, or four-part fracture pattern based on the number of displaced segments. The presence of a dislocation is described by the direction of displacement of the humeral head. Comminution and the number of fracture fragments are irrelevant unless they fit into the previously described classification (Fig. 1). Hawkins and associates[20] further clarified the classification by focusing on the key segment that is displaced. For example, a two-part anatomic neck fracture, where the key segment is the articular head, would be correctly classified as a two-part articular segment fracture rather than as a surgical neck fracture, where the humeral shaft is the key fragment. The surgical neck fracture is correctly referred to as the two-part shaft displacement pattern. In three-part

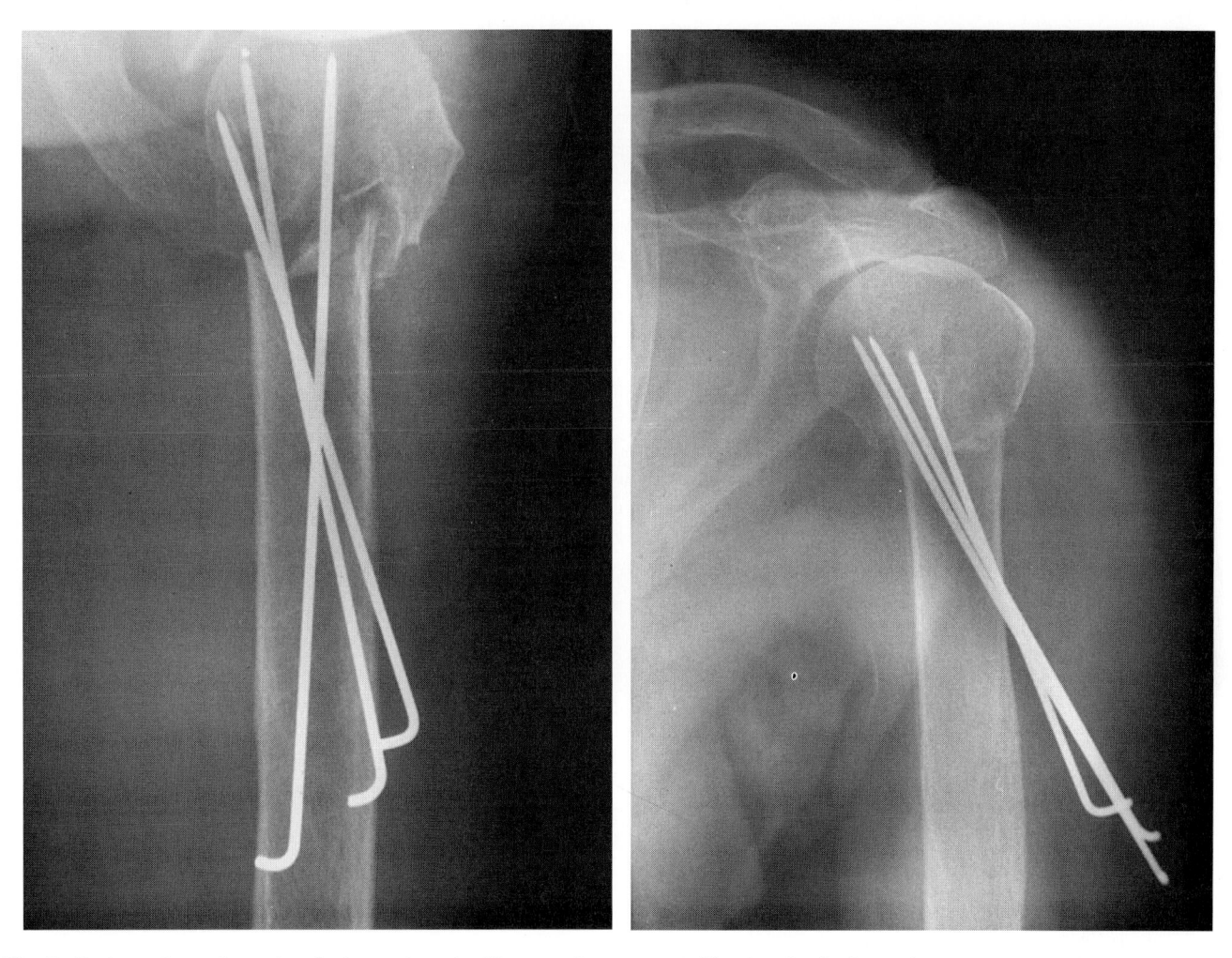

Fig. 5 Postoperative radiographs of a two-part proximal humerus fracture treated by closed reduction and percutaneous pinning. (Reproduced with permission from Müller ME, Nazarian S, Koch P, et al (eds): *The Comprehensive Classification of Fractures of Long Bones*. Berlin, Germany, Springer-Verlag, 1990.)

fractures, the greater tuberosity is always the key segment. The Neer classification system is based on plain radiographic views obtained with the trauma series. The difficulty experienced when applying the Neer system is that interobserver variability can be significant, suggesting a low level of reproducibility and reliability.[4,5] Exercising greater care when obtaining the trauma series of radiographs and perhaps the addition of CT might be helpful in improving the reproducibility of the Neer system.

The AO classification system places a greater emphasis on the blood supply to the humeral head and has group subdivisions that allow more specific classification of fractures.[21] The AO classification is an alpha numeric system. Group A fractures are extracapsular fractures involving only two main fragments (Fig. 2). In group B fractures, there is partial intracapsular extension involving two or three fragments (Fig. 3). Group C fractures have intracapsular extension involving two, three, or four fragments and the risk of avascularity to the humeral head is high (Fig. 4).

Both the Neer and AO classification systems are useful in suggesting the approach to treatment, but they fail to stratify treatment schemes according to age or the presence of metabolic bone disease. Many recent reviews report poor results after ORIF in elderly osteoporotic patients compared to younger patients with good bone quality.[20–25]

Treatment

In general, treatment of proximal humeral fractures requires an assessment of the fracture classification, bone quality, age, and functional demands of the patient, dominance, preexisting cognitive or physical deficits, patient expectations, and the ability of the patient to comply with a rehabilitation program. Elderly patients require and benefit

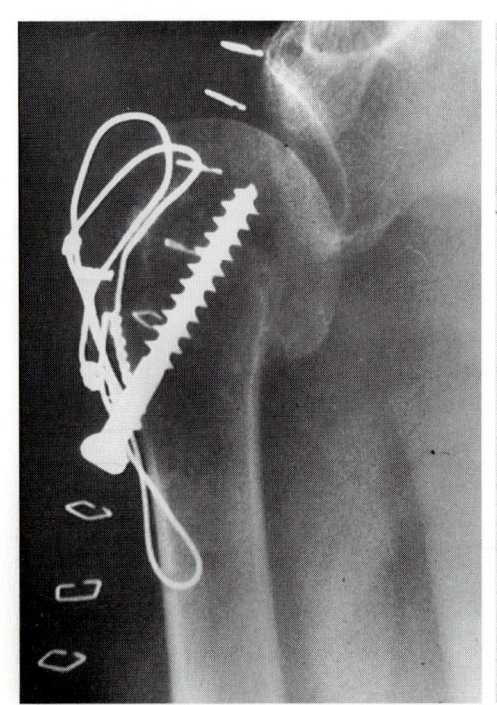

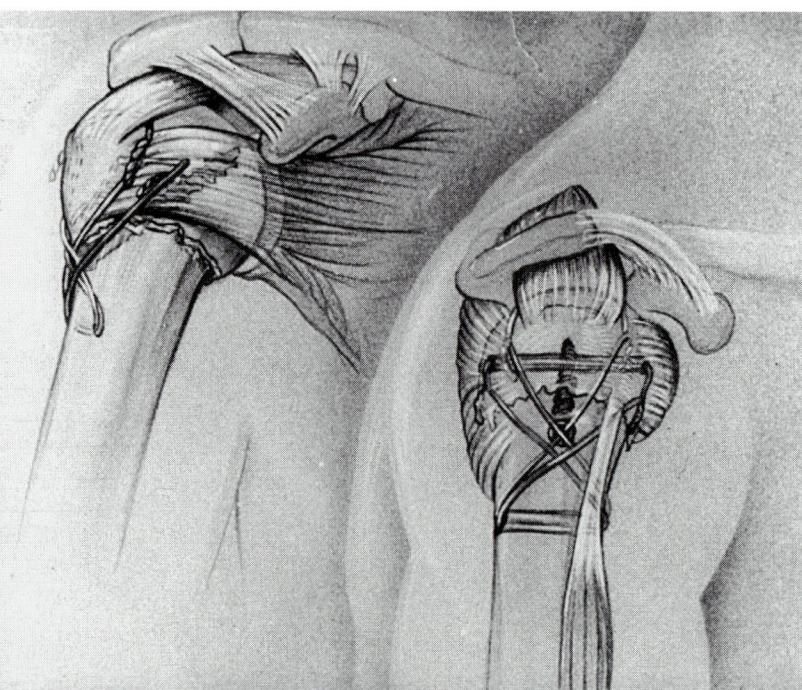

Fig. 6 A two-part proximal humeral fracture treated with a tension band technique with an accompanying diagram of the method. (Reproduced with permission from Müller ME, Nazarian S, Koch P, et al (eds): *The Comprehensive Classification of Fractures of Long Bones*. Berlin, Germany, Springer-Verlag, 1990.)

from restoration of functional shoulder range of motion and strength following these injuries. Loss of significant shoulder motion can strongly reduce one's ability to dress and maintain personal hygiene. A poor outcome following fractures of the proximal humerus in the elderly can lead to significant loss of independence with subsequent need for expensive social services. Advanced age alone, therefore, should not be considered an indication for conservative, nonsurgical treatment.[26]

Eighty percent of proximal humeral fractures are impacted and relatively nondisplaced. These fractures can be managed nonsurgically, immobilizing the arm in a sling and instituting range of motion exercises when pain permits. Early institution of therapy speeds recovery but residual deformity determines the ultimate range of motion. More than 45° of angulation or 1.5 cm of displacement contribute to poor functional outcome if the Neer rating system of shoulder function is applied as the outcome standard.[27] Based on the results of two studies on a series of elderly patients with displaced proximal humeral fractures treated nonsurgically despite significant displacement, the authors advocate a nonsurgical approach.[28,29] The authors relied primarily on the patient's degree of satisfaction and the argument that only 60° of forward flexion is needed for activities of daily living in elderly patients. On the other hand, in other studies, surgical intervention to reduce and stabilize these injuries provided superior range of motion and function with little surgical risk or morbidity.[23,30,31] It is therefore advisable to manage the significantly displaced or unstable fracture surgically.

Two-part lesser tuberosity fractures are usually associated with posterior dislocations. Large fragments of the lesser tuberosity may require open reduction and fixation if they are displaced. Two-part greater tuberosity fractures (AO classification: A1) usually displace posteriorly and superiorly and are associated with a rotator cuff tear. Open reduction and internal fixation of these fractures with repair of the rotator cuff should be performed for displacements of 1 cm or greater.[32]

Displaced or unstable two- and three-part fractures are those with greater than 45° of angulation or 1 cm of displacement of the humeral head and greater tuberosity from the shaft: types A3, B1, B2, B3 of the AO classification. Although closed management can be attempted for these fractures, some form of closed or open reduction and internal fixation speeds rehabilitation with better overall results.

Closed reduction and percutaneous pin fixation[33] under fluoroscopic guidance is a technique that is rapidly gaining popularity. Because it is a closed technique, it encourages rapid healing and avoids surgical devascularization of the fracture site. It is very helpful in the multiple trauma setting because it avoids the need for an incision and its associated blood loss. Furthermore, because the technique is performed with the patient in the supine position, it allows multiple teams to work simultaneously, which is not possible with the beach chair position. Use of threaded 2.5-mm Schanz pins, which are cut off subcutaneously, have been recommended (Fig. 5).

The technique is technically very demanding. It is useful in young patients with good bone quality, especially in the multiple trauma situation. It should not be used routinely in four-part fractures or in elderly patients.

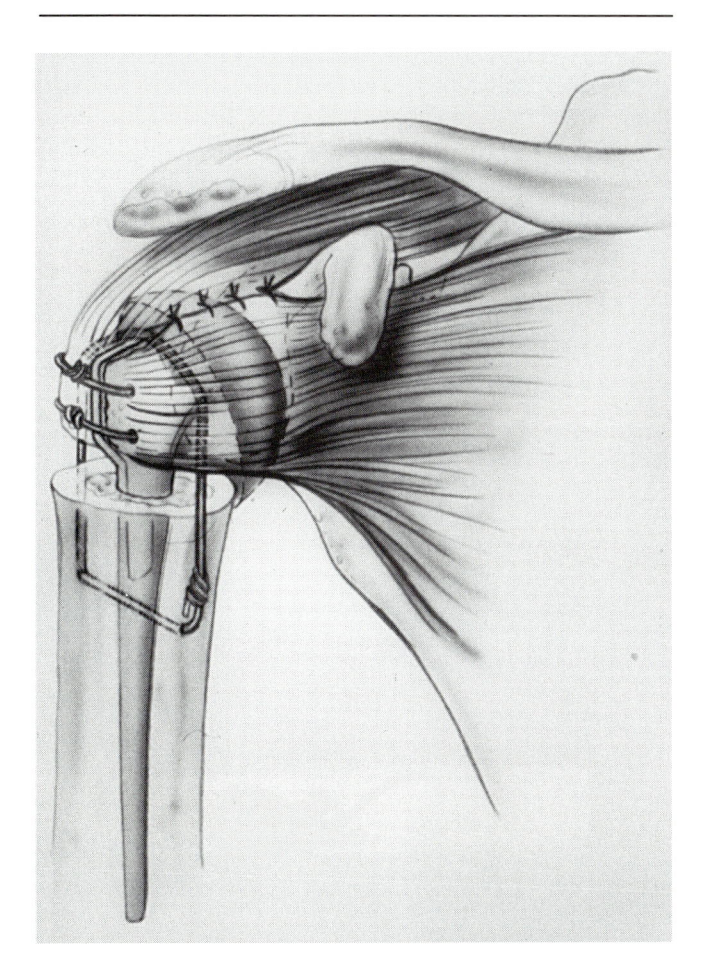

Fig. 7 A diagram of the technique recommended to achieve secure fixation of the tuberosities to the humeral head prosthesis and shaft. (Reproduced with permission from Müller ME, Nazarian S, Koch P, et al (eds): *The Comprehensive Classification of Fractures of Long Bones*. Berlin, Germany, Springer-Verlag, 1990.)

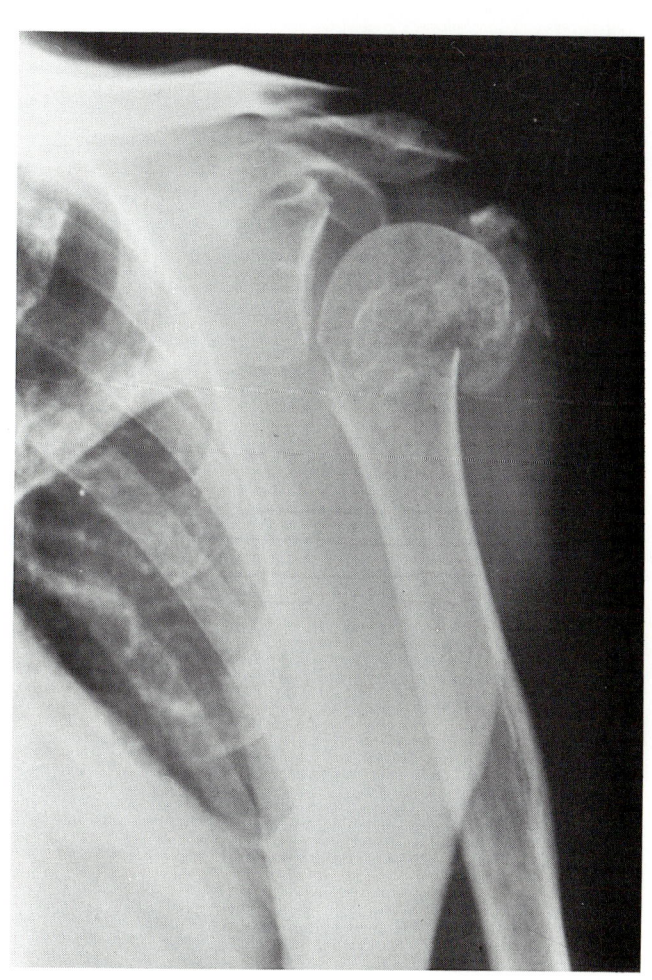

Fig. 8 The valgus impact four part fracture of the proximal humerus. This fracture configuration appears to have a lower incidence of osteonecrosis when treated by open reduction and internal fixation. (Reproduced with permission from Müller ME, Nazarian S, Koch P, et al (eds): *The Comprehensive Classification of Fractures of Long Bones*. Berlin, Germany, Springer-Verlag, 1990.)

Open reduction and internal fixation is the procedure of choice for two- and three-part fractures that cannot be reduced, those in which there is significant comminution of the metaphysis and in the elderly patient. Over the past decade there has been a trend toward using smaller implants, which cause less circulatory compromise and avoid intrusion into the subacromial space. Although plates and screws achieved good purchase in young patients, better results are now obtained with tension band wiring techniques, especially in elderly patients with osteoporosis. Hawkins pioneered the use of tension band fixation for these fractures, pointing out that the soft tissues of the rotator cuff often have better holding power and strength than the bone of the humeral head and tuberosities[30] (Fig. 6). In addition, tension bands do not cause subacromial impingement and can be applied with minimal surgical disruption of soft-tissue attachments to the humeral head and tuberosities.[30,31]

Four-part fractures of the proximal humerus (AO type C) are associated with significant risk of vascularity of the humeral head. Neer[34] noted the very unsatisfactory results of nonsurgical management of these injuries, which has recently been corroborated by other authors.[35,36] In addition, because of high risk of osteonecrosis of the head, and the difficulty of performing open reduction and internal fixation of these injuries, Neer proposed that prosthetic replacement should be performed in this setting. Since the early 1970s, many series of patients treated by prosthetic replacement of the four-part fracture have been reported.[37,38] The results consistently suggest that the technique is successful in that it provides a relatively painfree shoulder with satisfaction in most patients; however, functional results are generally poor. Active forward flexion in most series averages 70° with poor external rotation. The majority of patients lose the ability to use the arm for overhead activities. The technique is extremely demanding and requires proper positioning of the prosthesis and secure healing of the tuberosities to the humeral shaft. Techniques that are believed to encourage the best results include use of cement to prevent subsidence of the stem and to secure the proper retroversion of the head as well as achieving secure healing of the tuberosities to the shaft with tension band sutures and bone grafting (Fig. 7). Finally, a prolonged and intensive rehabilitation program must be followed by the patient.

In several studies it has been suggested that the risk of avascular necrosis following open reduction and internal fixation of four-part fractures is lower than previously predicted. In two studies no evidence of osteonecrosis was found in long-term follow-up of 45 patients treated with preservation of the head.[23,36] Other authors argue that certain four-part fractures maintain soft-tissue attachments to the posteromedial neck, preserving some circulation to the head (Fig. 8). For this reason, some authors advocate open reduction and internal fixation in young patients or in those with valgus-impacted fracture patterns (AO type C2).[22,23]

Summary

Better understanding of the subtypes of four-part fractures has suggested that the valgus impacted fracture (type C2) may be amenable to internal fixation with little risk of osteonecrosis. In an effort to provide better functional results, especially in younger patients, many authors are selecting open reduction and internal fixation over prosthetic replacement for these injuries. However, head splitting fractures, fracture-dislocations of the head, and fractures in the setting of severe osteoporosis probably still require prosthetic reconstruction.

Annotated References

1. Horak J, Nilsson BE: Epidemiology of fracture of the upper end of the humerus. *Clin Orthop* 1975;112:250–253.

2. Bengner U, Johnell O, Redlund-Johnell I: Changes in the incidence of fracture of the upper end of the humerus during a 30-year period: A study of 2125 fractures. *Clin Orthop* 1988;231:179–182.

3. Rose SH, Melton LJ III, Morrey BF, et al: Epidemiologic features of humeral fractures. *Clin Orthop* 1982;168:24–30.

4. Sidor ML, Zuckerman JD, Lyon T, et al: The Neer classification system for proximal humeral fractures: An assessment of interobserver reliability and intraobserver reproducibility. *J Bone Joint Surg* 1993;75A:1745–1750.

    The authors test the reliability and reproducibility of the Neer classification of proximal humerus fractures. The mean interobserver reproducibility was 66%.

5. Siebenrock KA, Gerber C: The reproducibility of classification of fractures of the proximal end of the humerus. *J Bone Joint Surg* 1993;75A:1751–1755.

    Ninety-five fractures of the proximal humerus were classified using the Neer and AO/ASIF systems. Interobserver reproducibility was extremely poor for both classification systems and became worse as the number of subgroups was increased.

6. Hawkins RJ, Angelo RL: Displaced proximal humeral fractures: Selecting treatment, avoiding pitfalls. *Orthop Clin North Am* 1987;18:421–431.

7. Brooks CH, Revell WJ, Heatley FW: Vascularity of the humeral head after proximal humeral fractures: An anatomical cadaver study. *J Bone Joint Surg* 1993;75B:132–136.

8. Wirth MA, Butters KP, Rockwood CA Jr: The posterior deltoid-splitting approach to the shoulder. *Clin Orthop* 1993;296:92–98.

9. Stableforth PG, Sarangi PP: Posterior fracture-dislocation of the shoulder: A superior subacromial approach for open reduction. *J Bone Joint Surg* 1992;74B:579–584.

10. Pavlov H, Warren RF, Weiss CB Jr, et al: The roentgenographic evaluation of anterior shoulder instability. *Clin Orthop* 1985;194:153–158.

11. Kilcoyne RF, Shuman WP, Matsen FA III, et al: The Neer classification of displaced proximal humeral fractures:

Spectrum of findings on plain radiographs and CT scans. *Am J Radiol* 1990;154:1029–1033.

Computed tomographic scans can be an important adjunct to plain radiographs in evaluation of proximal humerus fractures. Determination of the degree of displacement or rotation of fragments and assessment of impression or head splitting fractures can be easily evaluated.

12. Zarins B, McMahon MS, Rowe CR: Diagnosis and treatment of traumatic anterior instability of the shoulder. *Clin Orthop* 1993;291:75–84.
13. Harryman DT II, Sidles JA, Harris SL, et al: The role of the rotator interval capsule in passive motion and stability of the shoulder. *J Bone Joint Surg* 1992;74A:53–66.
14. Mallon WJ, Bassett FH III, Goldner RD: Luxatio erecta: The inferior glenohumeral dislocation. *J Orthop Trauma* 1990;4:19–24.
15. Neviaser RJ, Neviaser TJ, Neviaser JS: Concurrent rupture of the rotator cuff and anterior dislocation of the shoulder in the older patient. *J Bone Joint Surg* 1988;70A:1308–1311.

The authors recently reviewed 31 patients with this combination of injuries. The patients were older than 35 years of age. The diagnosis was initially missed in 29 patients because the weakness was incorrectly attributed to axillary nerve palsy. Only 8% of the patients in this series suffered axillary nerve palsy. In 20 patients, the rotator cuff tear involved avulsion of the supraspinatus and infraspinatus from the greater tuberosity. In 8 patients, the subscapulary was avulsed from the lesser tuberosity. All of these patients had recurrent instability, whereas those with isolated supraspinatus injury tended to remain stable. Successful repair of the rotator cuff eliminated pain, prevented further instability, and restored excellent function to the arm in most patients. The authors strongly advise a high degree of suspicion for this injury complex in older patients with anterior shoulder dislocation.

16. Baker CL, Uribe JW, Whitman C: Arthroscopic evaluation of acute, initial anterior shoulder dislocations. *Am J Sports Med* 1990;18:25–28.

The authors have reported on the findings of a preliminary study of 45 patients who underwent early arthroscopic examination following acute dislocation. Half of the patients in this series had complete labral tears; however, no follow-up of these patients was reported. Therefore, the role of early repair of these lesions cannot be evaluated and the role of early arthroscopy following acute dislocation remains unknown.

17. Noordeen MH, Bacarese-Hamilton IH, Belham GJ, et al: Anterior dislocation of the shoulder: A simple method of reduction. *Injury* 1992;23:479–480.
18. Pollock RG, Bigliani LU: Recurrent posterior shoulder instability: Diagnosis and treatment. *Clin Orthop* 1993;291:85–96.
19. Neer CS II: Displaced proximal humerus: Part I. Classification and evaluation. *J Bone Joint Surg* 1970;52A:1077–1089.
20. Hawkins RJ, Kiefer GN: Internal fixation techniques for proximal humeral fractures. *Clin Orthop* 1987;223:77–85.
21. Szyszkowitz R, Seggl W, Schleifer P, et al: Proximal humeral fractures: Management techniques and expected results. *Clin Orthop* 1993;292:13–25.

The type C2 fractures achieved excellent results when treated by open reduction and internal fixation. These accounted for 22% of the four-part fractures in the series. Head splitting fractures or those with dislocation of the humeral head did poorly. The authors review 10 years of experience of their treatment of proximal humerus fractures. Of 1,386 patients, 143 required surgical treatments. Fifty percent of patients treated surgically had good results. The remainder had poor or fair outcome. A move toward minimal fixation away from traditional plate fixation is recommended.

22. Hawkins RJ: Displaced proximal humeral fractures. *Orthopedics* 1993;16:49–53.
23. Esser RD: Open reduction and internal fixation of three- and four-part fractures of the proximal humerus. *Clin Orthop* 1994;299:244–251.

The author achieved excellent results in 8 patients using a modified clover-leaf plate. All patients in this series achieved 140° or better forward flexion. None had osteonecrosis. Two patients had four-part fractures with dislocation of the head. These did poorly in this series.

24. Fleischmann W, Kinzl L: Philosophy of osteosynthesis in shoulder fractures. *Orthopedics* 1993;16:59–63.
25. Kristiansen B, Christensen SW: Plate fixation of proximal humeral fractures. *Acta Orthop Scand* 1986;57:320–323.
26. Mills HJ, Horne G: Fractures of the proximal humerus in adults. *J Trauma* 1985;25:801–805.
27. Keene JS, Huizenga RE, Engber WO, et al: Proximal humerus fractures: A correlation of residual deformity with long term function. *Orthopedics* 1993;6:173–178.
28. Young TB, Wallace WA: Conservative treatment of fractures and fracture-dislocations of the upper end of the humerus. *J Bone Joint Surg* 1985;67B:373–377.
29. Rasmussen S, Hvass I, Dalsgaard J, et al: Displaced proximal humeral fractures: Results of conservative treatment. *Injury* 1992;23:41–43.
30. Hawkins RJ, Bell RH, Gurr K: The three-part fracture of the proximal humerus: Operative treatment. *J Bone Joint Surg* 1986;68A:1410–1414.

In this and the following reference, two series of elderly patients with two- and three-part fractures stabilized with tension band techniques are reported. Sufficient stability was achieved at the time of surgery to allow immediate postoperative physical therapy. Good to excellent results were achieved in the majority of patients. The authors argue that the technique can be widely applied, except in cases where significant comminution of the shaft requires use of a plate to maintain length. In this series of patients with a three-part fracture all were treated with tension band fixation. In 14 patients, there was no loss of fixation and no patients suffered acromial impingement. The merits of tension band fixation are discussed by the authors.

31. Cornell CN, Levine D, Pagnani MJ: Internal fixation of proximal humerus fractures using the screw-tension band technique. *J Orthop Trauma* 1994;8:23–27.

Thirteen elderly patients with two- and three-part proximal humerus fractures were treated with open reduction and internal fixation using a screw tension band technique. The fixation was sufficiently stable to allow immediate postoperative rehabilitation. Average forward flexion 1 year after surgery was 160°. All fractures healed. Ten of 13 patients had good function according to the Hawkins functional score.

32. Flatow EL, Cuomo F, Maday MG, et al: Open reduction and internal fixation of two-part displaced fractures of the greater tuberosity of the proximal part of the humerus. *J Bone Joint Surg* 1991;73A:1213–1218.

The authors report on a series of 12 patients with two-part greater tuberosity fractures with dislocation treated by exposure of the injury through a deltopectoral incision with fixation of the tuberosity using heavy nonabsorbable suture along with suture of the rotator cuff. This treatment allows early range of motion exercises. All patients treated in this manner had at least a good result. The average forward flexion achieved was 170°. Intraosseous suture was found to be superior to screws or pins in fixing these injuries.

33. Jaberg H, Warner JJ, Jakob RP: Percutaneous stabilization of unstable fractures of the humerus. *J Bone Joint Surg* 1992;74A:508–515.

   The authors report on a series of 48 patients treated by closed reduction and percutaneous pinning. Good to excellent results were obtained in 34 patients and fair to poor, in 14. Ten patients developed osteonecrosis. The authors recommend using terminally threaded 2.5-mm Schanz pins, which are cut off subcutaneously. Pin removal was required and range of motion exercises were delayed until 3 weeks after surgery. Poor results occurred in comminuted fractures and in elderly patients with osteoporotic bone. The procedure was noted to be technically demanding but comparable results to other techniques of fixation of the proximal humerus could be realized.

34. Neer CS II: Displaced proximal humerus fractures: Part II. Treatment of three-part and four-part displacement. *J Bone Joint Surg* 1970;52A:1090–1103.

35. Stableforth PG: Four-part fractures of the neck of the humerus. *J Bone Joint Surg* 1984;66B:104–108.

36. Lee CK, Hansen HR: Post-traumatic avascular necrosis of the humeral head in displaced proximal humeral fractures. *J Trauma* 1981;21:788–791.

37. Hawkins RJ, Switlyk P: Acute prosthetic replacement for severe fractures of the proximal humerus. *Clin Orthop* 1993;289:156–160.

   In a series of 19 patients, the results of prosthetic replacement of the humeral head were reviewed. Average age of the patients was 64 years. Active forward flexion averaged only 74°. Poor function appeared to be directly related to lack of rotator cuff integrity. Surgical techniques designed for secure tuberosity union are essential.

38. Compito CA, Self EB, Bigliani LU: Arthroplasty and acute shoulder trauma: Reasons for success and failure. *Clin Orthop* 1994;307:27–36.

3
Fractures of the Humeral Shaft

Introduction

Fractures of the humeral diaphysis historically have been characterized as relatively simple to treat, usually nonsurgically, with predictably satisfactory outcomes. There was a strong bias against surgical intervention because of an unacceptable rate of complications and failures. However, there has been a significant evolution of thought relative to these injuries. Nonsurgical treatment has been refined, further evaluated, and the limits of its applicability better defined. Simultaneously, the science and techniques of internal fixation have been the subject of considerable laboratory and clinical investigation. Intramedullary fixation has undergone the most dramatic proliferation of devices and techniques, all with the hope of improving on the comparatively dismal results previously reported with this technique. A more critical assessment of fracture and patient variables has led to a better understanding of the general indications, both absolute and relative, for surgical intervention. An appreciation of this recent literature is critical to the development of an appropriate treatment plan for these injuries.

Relevant Anatomy

The humeral diaphysis extends from the upper border of the insertion of the pectoralis major proximally to the supracondylar ridge distally. The fracture alignment can be determined and the resultant deformity can be predicted by the location of the fracture relative to major muscle attachments, most notably the pectoralis major and deltoid insertions (Fig. 1).[1] The imbalance in muscle pull will determine angulation and displacement of the fracture relative to the intact proximal humerus. These deforming forces must be considered when developing a treatment plan for a given injury. Appreciation of the unique anatomy of the medullary canal is also important when intramedullary fixation is being considered for fracture fixation.

Classification

Fractures of the humeral shaft have most commonly been classified based on fracture descriptors, including the nature and location of the primary fracture lines, an estimation of the kinetics of the injury (low-energy versus high-energy mechanisms), and associated soft-tissue trauma (open fracture grading and associated neurovascular injury). Together, these factors are thought to present a unique fracture personality for each injury. These variables are largely descriptive in nature, however, and have limited usefulness in critical research and outcome assessments.

The AO classification is gaining acceptance as a precise anatomic classification scheme for all long bone fractures, including those of the humerus.[2,3] The alpha-numeric coding system used for the AO classification presents the humeral diaphysis as bone 1, segment 2. After classification by anatomic location, the fracture is further defined by its morphologic characteristics (Fig. 2). Fracture types are simple (type A), wedge (type B), and complex (type C). Each type is further classified into three groups (1, 2, 3), which represent a further refinement of fracture geometry. For type A and type B fractures, these groups can then be further classified into three subgroups, representing fractures of proximal (.1), middle (.2), and distal (.3) zones. For type C fractures, subgroups define the number and characteristics of the intermediate fragments. For example, a coding of 12-C1.2 defines a humeral (1) diaphyseal (2) fracture, complex spiral configuration (C1) with three intermediate fragments (.2). Thus, the fracture is defined by two numbers to express anatomic location, followed by a letter and two numbers to express the fracture morphology. Additional fracture qualifiers may be added as parentheticals to convey even more information about the location, extent, and morphology of the fracture.

In general, types A, B, and C fractures represent a spectrum of increasing fracture severity and worsening prognosis. This does not always correspond to the complexity of managing these fractures, however. For example, a simple transverse midshaft fracture (12-A3.2) is often one of the most problematic humeral shaft fractures to manage. A clinically useful, comprehensive classification of fractures of the humeral diaphysis ideally should be more than anatomically precise. The decision-making factors of soft-tissue injury, neurovascular status, associated injuries, and individual patient variables are also important in defining an appropriate treatment plan. These determinants will be

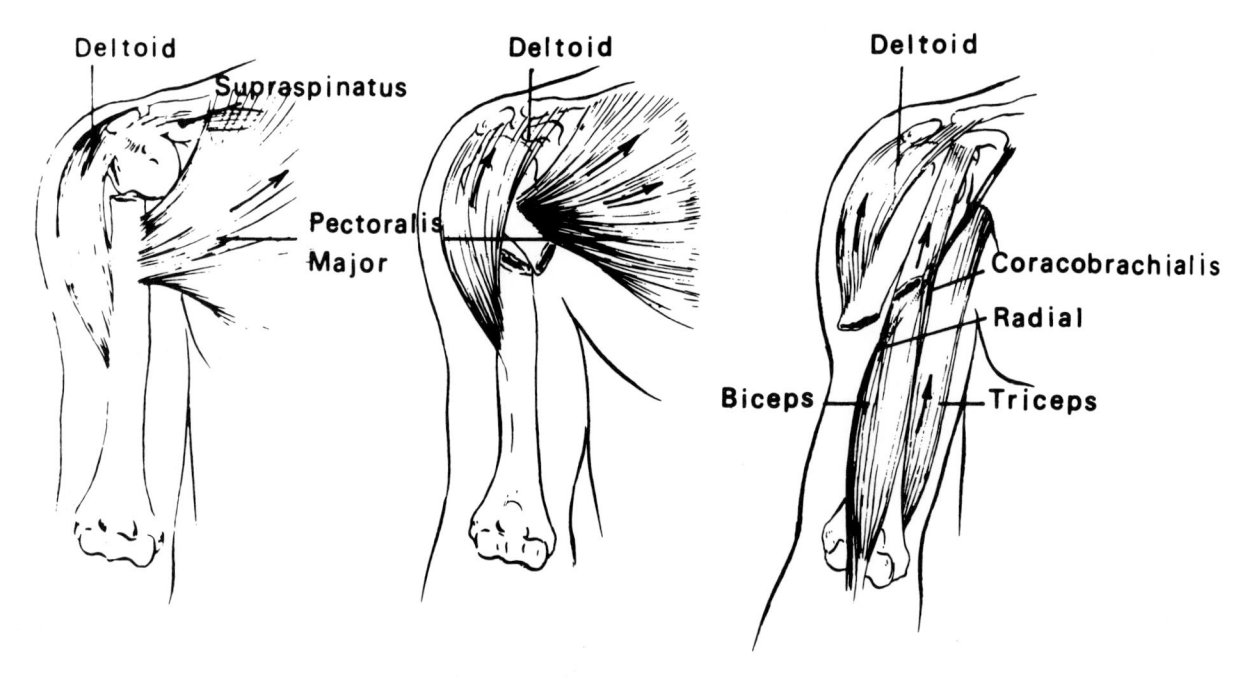

Fig. 1 Anatomic factors that influence deformities in typical fractures of the humeral shaft. **Left,** Fracture between rotator cuff and pectoralis major, causing abduction and rotation of proximal fragment. **Center,** Fracture between the pectoralis major insertion and deltoid, producing adduction of proximal fragment. **Right,** Fracture below the deltoid insertion, causing abduction of proximal fragment. (Reproduced with permission from Epps H Jr, Grant RE: Fractures of the shaft of the humerus, in Rockwood CA Jr, Green DP, Bucholz RW (eds): *Rockwood and Green's Fractures in Adults*, ed 3. Philadelphia, PA, JB Lippincott, 1991, vol 1, pp 843–869.)

further defined in the course of outlining treatment options and anticipating potential associated complications.

Clinical and Radiographic Evaluation

Fractures of the humeral shaft may result from either direct or indirect forces caused by motor vehicle accidents, falls, industrial trauma, direct blows, or penetrating injuries. Fractures secondary to violent muscle contraction have been reported occasionally, most frequently caused by torsional forces associated with the throwing motion.[4] These fractures characteristically have spiral fracture patterns in the middle to distal thirds of the humerus.

The patient with a humeral shaft fracture will typically have all of the cardinal signs of a long bone fracture: pain, swelling, deformity, shortening, and abnormal motion. This rarely presents a challenge to diagnosis except for polytrauma patients, especially those who are unresponsive. In these patients, the fracture can be overlooked unless a comprehensive examination of the extremity is routinely performed.

Also critical to determining the appropriate treatment is a careful assessment of the entire extremity for the extent of associated soft-tissue injury. The kinetics of injury should be determined and closed and open fractures should be graded. A complete neurovascular assessment is necessary, not only to document associated injuries to these structures, but also to serve as a baseline should the neurologic or vascular status of the limb deteriorate during the course of evaluation and treatment. The anatomic relationships of the radial nerve to the humeral shaft places the nerve at highest risk of injury with fractures of the middle or distal thirds of the shaft. The implications of this association to fracture management will be reviewed later. Compartment syndrome of the arm, although uncommon, must always be considered.

Radiographic evaluation must include two full-length views of the entire humerus, at 90° to each other, with clear delineation of the shoulder and elbow joints. Additional studies are rarely necessary, except where associated intra-articular extension requires tomographic evaluation or, in the case of pathologic lesions, where staging evaluation by bone scans, magnetic resonance imaging (MRI), or computed tomography (CT) might be indicated.

Treatment

A basic premise in the care of humeral shaft fractures is that the majority of these injuries are amenable to nonsurgical treatment. Surgical treatment has been characterized in the literature as being associated with a higher rate of delayed union, nonunion, infection, radial nerve palsy, and pro-

12- Humerus Diaphysis

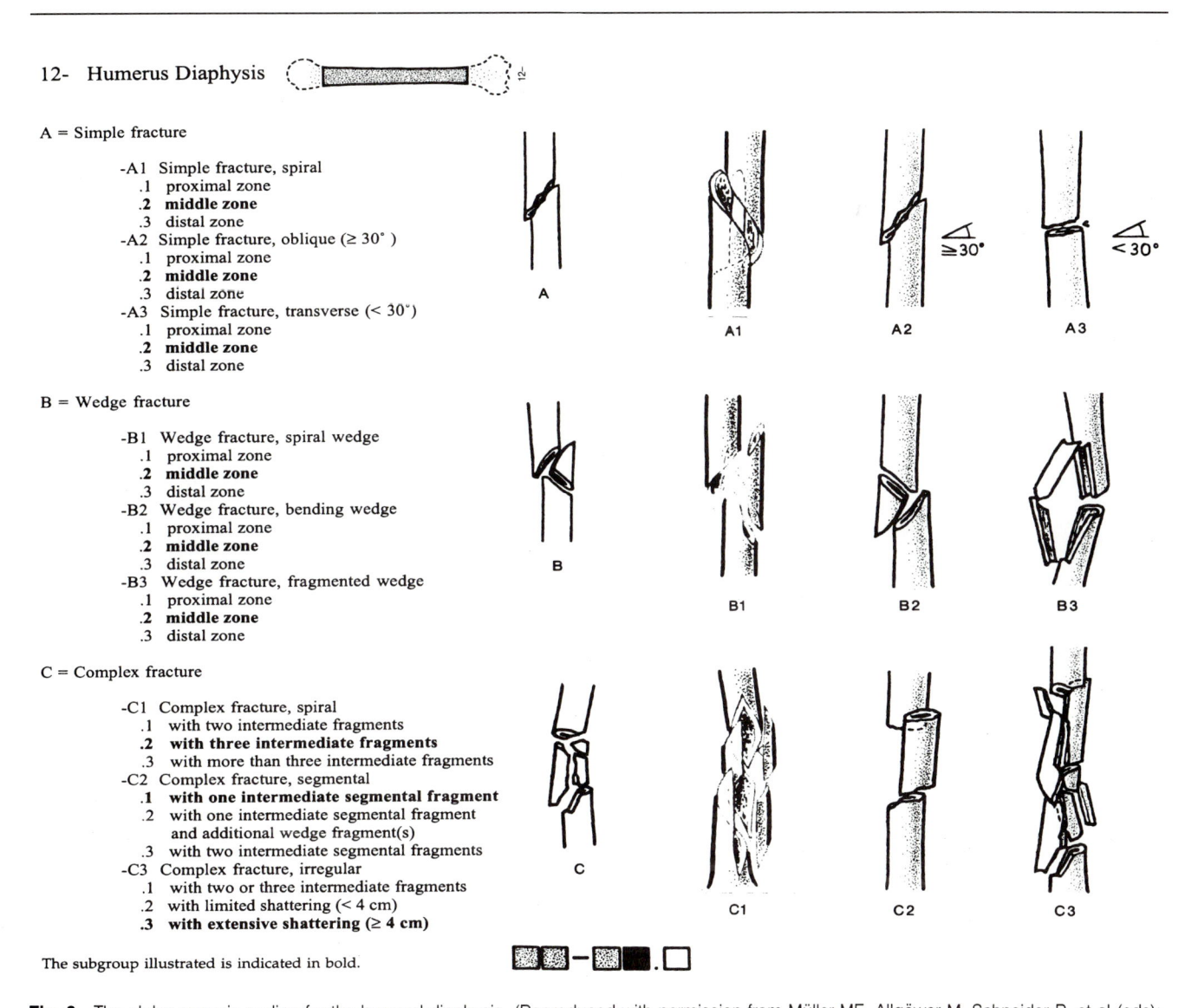

A = Simple fracture
- A1 Simple fracture, spiral
  - .1 proximal zone
  - **.2 middle zone**
  - .3 distal zone
- A2 Simple fracture, oblique (≥ 30°)
  - .1 proximal zone
  - **.2 middle zone**
  - .3 distal zone
- A3 Simple fracture, transverse (< 30°)
  - .1 proximal zone
  - **.2 middle zone**
  - .3 distal zone

B = Wedge fracture
- B1 Wedge fracture, spiral wedge
  - .1 proximal zone
  - **.2 middle zone**
  - .3 distal zone
- B2 Wedge fracture, bending wedge
  - .1 proximal zone
  - **.2 middle zone**
  - .3 distal zone
- B3 Wedge fracture, fragmented wedge
  - .1 proximal zone
  - **.2 middle zone**
  - .3 distal zone

C = Complex fracture
- C1 Complex fracture, spiral
  - .1 with two intermediate fragments
  - **.2 with three intermediate fragments**
  - .3 with more than three intermediate fragments
- C2 Complex fracture, segmental
  - **.1 with one intermediate segmental fragment**
  - .2 with one intermediate segmental fragment and additional wedge fragment(s)
  - .3 with two intermediate segmental fragments
- C3 Complex fracture, irregular
  - .1 with two or three intermediate fragments
  - .2 with limited shattering (< 4 cm)
  - **.3 with extensive shattering (≥ 4 cm)**

The subgroup illustrated is indicated in bold.

Fig. 2 The alpha-numeric coding for the humeral diaphysis. (Reproduced with permission from Müller ME, Allgöwer M, Schneider R, et al (eds): *Manual of Internal Fixation*, ed 3. Berlin, Germany, Springer-Verlag, 1991, pp 118–150.)

longed disability times compared to nonsurgical treatment. Overall, better results with fewer complications have been demonstrated with nonsurgical management. Nonsurgical treatment is generally successful for most fractures of the humeral shaft because rigid immobilization is not necessary for healing and perfect alignment is not essential for an acceptable result. The bias in the early literature against surgical treatment is not particularly helpful in current decision-making, however, because the most difficult fractures were generally treated surgically and early reported fixation techniques were often unsound.

The requirements for nonsurgical treatment include an understanding by the treating physician of the postural and muscular forces that must be controlled, a dedication to close patient supervision and follow-up, and a cooperative and preferably upright or mobile patient. The arm is thought to be able to accommodate up to 20° of anterior angulation, 30° of varus, and 1 inch of shortening without a significant compromise of function or appearance.[5] For this reason, many forms of nonrigid immobilization have been successfully used to treat these fractures.

Hanging arm casts, coaptation splints, and prefabricated functional braces all have been associated with high rates of union and acceptable functional outcomes.[6-9] Velpeau dressings, shoulder spica casts, and skeletal traction are advocated less frequently. The most common nonsurgical treatment scheme is initial immobilization with either a hanging arm cast or a coaptation splint with conversion to

Outline 1. Indications for surgical intervention

Extremity Indications
    Failed closed treatment
        Loss of reduction
        Poor patient tolerance/compliance
    Open fractures
    Vascular injury/neurologic injury*
    Segmental fractures
    Floating elbow (associated fractures of the forearm)
    Associated intra-articular fractures
    Associated injuries to the brachial plexus
        Chronic problems
        Delayed union
        Nonunion/malunion
        Infection

Patient Indications
    Bilateral fractures of the humerus
    Pathologic fractures
    Parkinson's disease
    Polytrauma
        Head injuries
        Burns
        Chest trauma
        Multiple fractures

*Controversial indication (see text)

a functional brace in the subacute phase when swelling and pain have improved (generally 7 to 10 days after injury). The principles of functional bracing for the humerus were introduced in 1977.[8] A subsequent review of 170 patients treated with a prefabricated fracture brace (43 open and 127 closed fractures) demonstrated a 98% rate of union with good functional restoration and minimal angular deformity.[9] Nearly full range of motion of the extremity was restored and complications were minimal.

Despite concluding that functional bracing is the treatment of choice for diaphyseal fractures of the humerus, three contraindications to fracture bracing were identified: (1) massive injury to soft tissue or bone loss, (2) lack of patient reliability or cooperation, and (3) inability to obtain or maintain acceptable alignment. The number of patients with humeral shaft fractures who were excluded from this treatment protocol for these contraindications was not given. Comminuted fractures of the distal third of the humerus are thought to be the most problematic to reduce or hold in a brace. An analysis of functional bracing for these fractures in 65 patients, however, demonstrated a 96% rate of union, with an average varus deformity of 9° in 81% of the patients.[7] Functional outcomes were characterized as good for the majority of patients.

Although most humeral shaft fractures are appropriately, and successfully, managed nonsurgically, there are several clinical scenarios in which surgical intervention is preferable. Surgical indications may be best understood by differentiating those determined by the nature of the extremity injury itself and those defined overall by patient variables, as listed in Outline 1. Of this list, only open fractures and those with vascular injury present absolute indications for surgical intervention, however, there are compelling data to support a surgical approach for the other relative indications to be reviewed.

Failure of closed treatment, either to obtain or maintain an acceptable reduction, or poor patient tolerance or compliance is a clear indication to proceed with surgical stabilization as long as no medical contraindication is identified and the patient is likely to cooperate with the postoperative care. A suboptimal outcome from nonsurgical treatment, even nonunion, may occasionally be preferable to surgical treatment for a very elderly and medically frail individual or for a patient who clearly will not participate appropriately during the postoperative period.

Open fractures and those associated with vascular injury are absolute indications for surgical intervention. Most vascular trauma is associated with open fractures.[10] As with all open fractures, emergent irrigation and meticulous debridement, adjunctive antibiotic therapy, and appropriate soft-tissue coverage decision-making is critical to the outcome. The preferred technique of fracture stabilization is controversial, with supporters of both internal and external fixation. Vascular repair may precede or follow fracture stabilization, depending on the nature of the fracture, surgical approach required, pattern of vascular injury, and warm ischemia time for the extremity. Temporary intraluminal vascular shunts occasionally may be useful to perfuse the arm during wound debridement and fracture stabilization. Fasciotomies are frequently necessary after reperfusion of the ischemic limb.

Ipsilateral humeral shaft and forearm fractures (floating elbow) have been associated with a high rate of malunion or nonunion when the humeral shaft is managed nonsurgically.[11] The argument for surgical intervention is similar for shaft fractures associated with intra-articular fractures because closed management does not permit full, early, active mobilization of all joints in these severely injured extremities.

Fractures of the humeral shaft associated with ipsilateral injury to the brachial plexus, although uncommon, is a problematic combination.[12] Conventional nonsurgical treatment with a hanging cast or functional brace is contraindicated with a flail extremity. Internal fixation is associated with the highest rate of fracture union in these patients.

Chronic problems associated with fractures of the humeral shaft, such as nonunions, malunions, and infections, also generally require surgical intervention. These will be reviewed below in *Complications*.

In addition to the extremity-specific indications for surgical intervention, there are patient-specific factors that should be considered as well. The management of bilateral humeral fractures without fixation of at least one of the fractures is very problematic if the patient is to have any level of independent function. Similarly, in most patients, even simple fracture patterns that are pathologic are best managed with stable internal fixation, often augmented by methylmethacrylate, to manage pain and optimize the quality of the remaining lifetime for the patient. Patients with Parkinson's disease also tend to have difficulty dealing with nonsurgical treatment and generally do better with internal fixation.

Polytrauma patients present with a variety of relative contraindications to nonsurgical treatment. Numerous constellations of injuries may make nonsurgical management of the humeral shaft fracture extremely difficult, or perhaps impossible. Enforced recumbency or the inability of the patient to actively participate in the care of the fracture are problematic for splint, cast, or brace management. Patients with chest wall trauma or burns may not be amenable to external immobilization of the arm. A comparative study of surgical stabilization, traction, and bracing evaluated outcomes of these different treatment modalities relative to the severity of associated injuries.[13] In isolated humeral fractures, bracing gave the best results. Conversely, in polytrauma patients (injury severity score [ISS] 18), the results of surgical stabilization were clearly superior and this treatment approach was strongly advocated for this patient group. Overall patient care is facilitated and mobilization is easier when stable fixation is provided in this clinical setting.

Humeral Shaft Fractures With Associated Radial Nerve Palsy

Radial nerve palsies associated with humeral shaft fractures, primary or secondary to closed or open management, have been the subject of numerous reviews and conflicting opinions.[6,7,13-21] The reported incidence of radial nerve palsies varies from 1.8% to 24% of shaft fractures. Nerve contusion with neurapraxia is the most common injury pattern, however, the nature of individual nerve damage is dependent on the associated fracture characteristics. Transverse fractures of the middle third are most commonly associated with neurapraxia, whereas spiral fractures of the distal third present a higher risk of laceration or entrapment of the radial nerve.

Spontaneous recovery of nerve function is found in more than 70% of reported cases, and a recovery time of over 3 months is not uncommon. Even secondary palsies, those associated with fracture manipulation, have a high rate of spontaneous recovery.

Considerable controversy and disparate opinion have been expressed over the preferred management of fractures with associated radial nerve palsy. The three most frequently stated indications for immediate surgical intervention for fractures associated with radial nerve palsies include open fractures, Holstein-Lewis distal-third spiral fractures, and secondary palsies developing after closed reduction. Exploration for palsies associated with open fractures is the only indication that is not associated with conflicting data.[18] Although there are frequent references to the need for surgical exploration of the radial nerve for the other two indications, they often represent opinion without solid supporting data. It may seem most compelling to proceed with surgical intervention for secondary palsies that develop during the course of closed reduction, however, even in these cases, it is not clearly established that surgical intervention will improve the ultimate overall recovery rate compared to nonsurgical management.

In a review of 59 cases of immediate (primary) and 16 delayed (secondary) radial nerve palsies, watchful expectance was recommended as the initial management for both types of palsy.[15,16] No difference was noted in recovery rates for those lesions that required neurorrhaphy between early or delayed exploration. Further, it was noted that early exploration may risk additional injury to the nerve and potentially impair recovery if the nerve is only contused.

Considering the potential of iatrogenic nerve injury with exploration and the impression that the results of delayed nerve repair are comparable to primary repair, caution should be exercised before early exploration for these injuries is considered. In general, nerve exploration generally requires the addition of a second appropriate indication for surgical intervention for the fracture.

Surgical Treatment

If surgical treatment is elected, plate osteosynthesis, intramedullary fixation, and external fixation all play a role. There is no support, however, for stabilization of the humeral shaft by screw fixation alone. This form of stabilization cannot resist the torsional and bending forces imposed on the humerus during mobilization of the extremity and patient.

Three recent investigations have attempted to define the biomechanical characteristics of currently available fixation systems.[22-24] All three studies were similar in design and utilized a midshaft transverse humeral osteotomy as the experimental model. The individual studies evaluated the mechanical properties of various combinations of compression plating, intramedullary fixation with flexible pins, and interlocking nailing systems incorporating locking screws, distal endosteal fins, or fluted design for interference stabilization. Interpretation of the results is difficult, however, because of variability based on whether the testing was performed nondestructively or to failure. A comparison of the mechanical properties of plating and nailing techniques requires an appreciation of the differences in the characteristics of bone healing associated with plate versus nail fixation in general. The various nailing systems that were tested performed in a fashion that may be intuitively apparent: statically locked nails with screws afford more torsional stability than other design alternatives that utilize various forms of intramedullary interference with fins or flutes. Flexible nails perform with a fair degree of mechanical "give" in terms of bending and torsion at the osteotomy or fracture site. Unfortunately, none of these data can be readily extrapolated to the clinical setting or sheds light on the actual clinical performance or indication for a given device.

Surgical stabilization with plating techniques has been the subject of several recent reviews (Table 1).[17,25-28] Union rates averaged 96% with significant complications ranging from 3% to 13%. Functional restoration was generally good, with motion restrictions at the elbow or shoulder

Table 1. AO plating results

Source	Fractures	Union	Complications
Bell et al[25]	34	33	4
Foster et al[26]	45	43	3
Vander Griend et al[28]	34	33	4
Dabezies et al[17]	44	43	3
Heim et al[27]	127	120	13
Totals	284	272 (96%)	27 (9.5%)

usually seen in patients who had other severe bony or soft-tissue injuries to the same extremity.

Both the anterolateral and posterior approaches for plate stabilization are supported by the literature, the individual determination often a matter of training and preference. Advocates of the posterior approach note that it affords a more direct exploration of the radial nerve. This approach, however, may increase the risk of intraoperative radial nerve palsy, for the nerve must be mobilized to allow for plate application beneath it. The posterior approach also generally requires lateral or prone positioning of the patient, which may be problematic for the patient with multiple injuries. Finally, although not routinely recommended, plate removal is more hazardous to the radial nerve if the posterior approach has been utilized.

Radial nerve palsy is identified as a surgical complication in almost every review of plate fixation; however, most cases are characterized as transient, with good recovery as the rule. Infection and loss of fixation comprise most of the remaining complications of plate fixation. Loss of fixation is most often the result of technical errors culminating in inadequate fixation. The broad 4.5-mm dynamic compression plate has been recommended for the humeral diaphysis. This implant was thought to be necessary to control the torsional forces on these fractures and to offset the screws to prevent intraoperative development and propagation of a cortical crack. In practice this plate often may be too bulky for the humerus and recent literature suggests that the narrow 4.5-mm dynamic compression plate, limited contact plates, and even 3.5-mm plates may be acceptable implants with proper attention to the details of reduction and stabilization.

An early report of multiple techniques of intramedullary fixation for humeral shaft fractures demonstrated a complication rate of 67% and a reoperation rate of 64%.[29] Although most of the patients in this series presented problem fractures or multiple trauma, the authors thought that their results reconfirmed the previous literature perspective of significant morbidity associated with the surgical treatment of fractures of the humeral shaft. Despite identifying an unacceptable rate of infection, failed fixation, adhesive capsulitis of the shoulder, and delayed or nonunion, intramedullary fixation was thought to be a viable treatment alternative if the technique could be improved. Subsequent evaluations of unlocked nailing techniques have identified more favorable results.[26,30,31]

Two basic techniques of intramedullary fixation have evolved; flexible nailing and locked nailing. Flexible nailing takes several forms, Rush rods, Ender rods, or the Hackethal technique of filling the canal with multiple small flexible pins.[32–35] A review of the results of these techniques indicates that union is rapid and predictable (averaging 97%), especially if the closed technique is used. Despite this high rate of union there is a variable but relatively high incidence of implant-related problems, often requiring secondary procedures to correct.

Attention to the nuances of the surgical technique for each device is critical to avoiding problems. Both antegrade (proximal starting point) and retrograde (distal starting point) techniques have proponents. If an antegrade approach is elected, most techniques attempt to avoid the rotator cuff to minimize potential postoperative shoulder problems. For the retrograde technique, a starting point proximal to the olecranon fossa is recommended and close attention to detail is necessary to avoid the catastrophic complication of generating an intercondylar fracture of the distal humerus. Epicondylar starting points are technically easier but not recommended because of an unacceptable complication rate.[9]

Locked nailing is the most recent technique in the evolution of surgical stabilization for the humeral shaft. In large part, this represents an attempt to develop a closed technique of fracture stabilization that overcomes the historical perspective against intramedullary techniques and addresses the implant problems inherent in unlocked rigid nailing or flexible nailing techniques.

Static-locked nailing with screws, locking with endosteal fins, and fluted-geometry interference fit nails are all in clinical use. As previously noted, these systems behave very differently when evaluated mechanically with fracture models. In clinical practice, the preliminary results have been favorable, but implant-related problems persist.[36–41] Impaired shoulder function, instrumentation problems, iatrogenic comminution, and implant or locking failure have all been reported. A cadaveric investigation has identified potential risk to the axillary vein, artery, or nerve associated with proximal locking screw placement.[42] Screws that protrude beyond the medial cortex were noted to potentially impinge on the axillary nerve with internal rotation. Anterior-to-posterior screw placement was not recommended because of the potential for injury to the main trunk of the axillary nerve. Further investigation is necessary to better define the exact role and design preference for locked nailing of humeral shaft fractures.

External fixation is infrequently utilized, problematic, and generally reserved for fractures that present contraindications to other forms of management. Severe open fractures with extensive soft-tissue injury or bone loss, associated burns, or infected nonunions are the principal indications for external fixation. The fixator can be used provisionally with conversion to internal fixation or functional bracing after any associated soft-tissue problems are resolved.

Pin-tract problems,[43] muscle or tendon impalement, and delayed or nonunion all plague external fixation of the humerus. To minimize pin-related problems, attention to the safe zones for pin placement and open insertion techniques are recommended. Meticulous pin care, stable frame constructs, and liberal use of bone grafting to speed healing will further reduce the problems associated with external fixation.

Complications

Although most isolated humeral shaft fractures heal uneventfully, the results for high-energy fractures and other problem injury combinations are not as uniformly favorable. Complications of nonsurgical treatments include nonunion, malunion, radial nerve palsy, and joint stiffness. Surgical management is associated with all of these potential complications plus the risk of infection, iatrogenic neurovascular injury, and implant-related problems as previously described.

Delayed union or nonunion are caused by biologic and mechanical factors, including significant bone gaps secondary to fracture distraction, soft-tissue interposition or bone loss, uncontrolled fracture motion, or impaired blood supply. Infection also contributes significantly to the potential for nonunion.

A nonunion may be an acceptable outcome for a fracture in an elderly osteopenic patient with low functional demands, if pain is not problematic. A lightweight orthosis may provide acceptable function in this clinical situation.[44] More often, however, the nonunion presents a significant disability to the patient and more active intervention is required. Electric stimulation for humeral nonunions has met with limited success.[44-46] Union rates of 0% to 60% have been noted and because of this, there is little enthusiasm or current support for this technique for these nonunions.

Stable internal fixation is the treatment of choice for most nonunions, with proponents of plate fixation and intramedullary fixation (Table 2).[26,44,46-49] Compression plate fixation provides favorable results overall while intramedullary fixation with flexible or standard Küntscher nails has been less successful. The efficacy of locked nailing for nonunion management requires further investigation. Biologic stimulation with drilling, shingling, and autogenous bone grafting is an important adjunct to the internal fixation construct, especially for atrophic nonunion patterns.

Infected nonunions require additional attention to complete debridement of all pathologic tissue, often with antibiotic bead placement and provisional external fixation. When the infection has been defined and controlled, definitive management can then include additional bone grafting and internal fixation.

Complex nonunions associated with significant bone loss, osteopenia, synovial cavities, or failed prior surgical procedures may require even more elaborate reconstruction efforts.[50,51] Vascularized fibular transfers, used in conjunction with plate fixation, have been reported with favorable results.[50] Ilizarov techniques also may be applicable, but require further investigation.

Table 2. Treatment of nonunions

Source	Treatment	Cases	Union*
Foster et al[26]	Plate (13 cases), nail (13 cases), with or without bone graft	26	17 (65%)
Trotter and Dobozi[49]	Plate, cement, bone graft	5	5 (100%)
Esterhai et al[45]	Electric stimulation	39	17 (44%)
Healy et al[46]	Plate (23 cases), nail (3 cases), bone graft	26	23 (88%)
Barquet et al[47]	Plate, bone graft	25	24 (96%)
Jupiter[50]	Plate, vascularized fibular graft, bone graft	4	3 (75%)
Rosen[44]	Plate, bone graft, with or without cement	32	31 (97%)
Wright et al[51]	Plate, fibular graft, bone graft	9	8 (89%)

*Union after index operation

Controversial Issues

The management of humeral shaft fractures continues its refinement of both nonsurgical and surgical techniques. Nonsurgical treatment, with relatively simple immobilization techniques, remains the treatment of choice for the majority of these fractures. Further controlled investigation is necessary to clarify the role of surgical exploration for fractures associated with radial nerve palsy. It would be helpful for the clinician to have better guidelines as to which injury combinations would benefit most predictably from exploration, and if not early then the appropriate timing needs to be better defined for delayed interventions.

The indications for surgical stabilization have evolved over the past decade to reasonably well-established guidelines. Clinical judgment remains important, because many of the indications are relative, not absolute, and must be applied after careful consideration of individual patient and extremity injury characteristics. Numerous techniques of internal fixation have merit, although with technique-specific associated problems. Interlocking intramedullary nailing, in particular, continues to evolve relative to implant design and technique. Definition of the optimal design for these devices requires further investigation.

As with all diaphyseal fractures and nonunions, the future promises exciting alternatives to our present treatment options. Noninvasive stimulation of fracture healing, refinement of bone graft substitutes, and new implant alternatives are certain to enhance and refine the management of these injuries.

Annotated References

1. Epps CH Jr, Grant RE: Fractures of the shaft of the humerus, in Rockwood CA Jr, Green DP, Bucholz RW (eds): *Rockwood and Green's Fractures in Adults*. Philadelphia, PA, JB Lippincott, 1991, vol 1, pp 843–869.

2. Müller ME, Allogöwer M, Schneider R, et al: *Manual of Internal Fixation: Techniques Recommended by the AO-ASIF Group*. Berlin, Germany, Springer-Verlag, 1991, pp 118–150.

3. Müller ME, Nazarian S, Koch P, et al: *Comprehensive Classification of Fractures of Long Bones*. Berlin, Germany, Springer-Verlag, 1990.

4. DiCicco JD, Mehlman CT, Urse JS: Fracture of the shaft of the humerus secondary to muscular violence. *J Orthop Trauma* 1993;7:90–93.

5. Klenerman L: Fractures of the shaft of the humerus. *J Bone Joint Surg* 1966;48B:105-111.

6. Mast JW, Spiegel PG, Harvey JP Jr, et al: Fractures of the humeral shaft: A retrospective study of 240 adult fractures. *Clin Orthop* 1975;112:254–262.

7. Sarmiento A, Horowitch A, Aboulafia A, et al: Functional bracing for comminuted extra-articular fractures of the distal-third of the humerus. *J Bone Joint Surg* 1990;72B:283-287.

   This series described the utilization of functional braces for extra-articular fractures of the distal-third. The authors demonstrated a 96% union rate and minimal residual deformities. Twelve associated radial nerve palsies were managed nonsurgically. At last reported follow-up, nine had complete recovery and three reported improved function.

8. Sarmiento A, Kinman PB, Galvin EG, et al: Functional bracing of fractures of the shaft of the humerus. *J Bone Joint Surg* 1977;59A:596–601.

9. Zagorski JB, Latta LL, Zych GA, et al: Diaphyseal fractures of the humerus: Treatment with prefabricated braces. *J Bone Joint Surg* 1988;70A:607–610.

   The authors evaluated 170 patients treated with prefabricated braces for humeral shaft fractures. Results overall were favorable, with minimal complications and only three nonunions. Contraindications to this form of management were defined. The authors concluded that this was the treatment of choice for most diaphyseal fractures of the humerus. All seven associated radial nerve palsies resolved without surgical intervention.

10. Gainor BJ, Metzler M: Humeral shaft fracture with brachial artery injury. *Clin Orthop* 1986;204:154–161.

11. Lange RH, Foster RJ: Skeletal management of humeral shaft fractures associated with forearm fractures. *Clin Orthop* 1985;195:173–177.

12. Brien WW, Gellman H, Becker V, et al: Management of fractures of the humerus in patients who have an injury of the ipsilateral brachial plexus. *J Bone Joint Surg* 1990:72A:1208–1210.

13. Bleeker WA, Nijsten MW, ten Duis H-J: Treatment of humeral shaft fractures related to associated injuries: A retrospective study of 237 patients. *Acta Orthop Scand* 1991;62:148–153.

    The authors demonstrated that humeral shaft fracture treatment should be defined in relation to the severity of associated injuries. Isolated humeral fractures were best managed by bracing, whereas polytrauma patients fared better with surgical stabilization. Surgical exploration did not appear to be a significant influence over the outcome for either 21 primary or 19 secondary radial nerve palsies.

14. Amillo S, Barrios RH, Martinez-Peric R, et al: Surgical treatment of the radial nerve lesions associated with fractures of the humerus. *J Orthop Trauma* 1993;7:211–215.

    Delayed surgical repair for radial nerve injuries averaging 6 months in 12 patients resulted in excellent or good results in 91% of cases. The nerve pathology at exploration included perineural fibrosis (four patients), entrapment in callus (three), partial laceration (two), and complete laceration (three). Surgical exploration is recommended if there are no clinical or electromyographic signs of recovery after 3 months.

15. Böstman O, Bakalim G, Vainionpää S, et al: Immediate radial nerve palsy complicating fracture of the shaft of the humerus: When is early exploration justified? *Injury* 1985;16:499–502.

16. Böstman O, Bakalim G, Vainionpää S, et al: Radial palsy in shaft fracture of the humerus. *Acta Orthop Scand* 1986;57:316–319.

    This 20-year review of radial nerve injuries identified 59 primary and 16 secondary palsies. Early surgical exploration did not appear to have any predictable or necessarily favorable influence over the potential for nerve recovery for either group. The authors further suggested that exploration of what proves to be an intact contused nerve can compromise the ultimate recovery. Their literature review highlights the problems in comparing results of early exploration versus "watchful expectance."

17. Dabezies EJ, Banta CJ II, Murphy CP, et al: Plate fixation of the humeral shaft for acute fractures, with and without radial nerve injuries. *J Orthop Trauma* 1992;6:10–13.

    The authors of this study identified a 97% union rate for closed fractures and 100% for open fractures with plate fixation. With experience, the authors preferred the posterior approach except for fractures of the proximal third. Two cases of radial nerve neurapraxia were associated with using the posterior approach. Implants of variable sizes were utilized, depending on fracture geometry and bone size.

18. Foster RJ, Swiontkowski MF, Bach AW, et al: Radial nerve palsy caused by open humeral shaft fractures. *J Hand Surg* 1993;18A:121–124.

    The authors present a strong argument for surgical exploration for radial nerve palsy associated with an open fracture of the humeral shaft. Unlike closed fractures, the majority of nerve injuries in open fractures involve either laceration or nerve entrapment between the fracture fragments. Epineural nerve repair was associated with good return of motion function for the lacerated nerves.

19. Holstein A, Lewis GB: Fractures of the humerus with radial-nerve paralysis. *J Bone Joint Surg* 1963;45A:1382–1388.

    This is the classic article that is repeatedly referenced as identifying the spiral fracture of the distal third of the humerus as notorious for its association with radial nerve palsy. The authors personally treated only four cases, identified three others in consultation, and reviewed the records of a private hospital to identify a radial nerve palsy in five of 85 fractures of the distal third.

20. Samardzic M, Grujicic D, Milinkovic ZB: Radial nerve lesions associated with fractures of the humeral shaft. *Injury* 1990;21:220–222.

21. Sonneveld GJ, Patka P, van Mourik JC, et al: Treatment of fractures of the shaft of the humerus accompanied by paralysis of the radial nerve. *Injury* 1987;18:404–406.

22. Dalton JE, Salkeld SL, Satterwhite YE, et al: A biomechanical comparison of intramedullary nailing systems for the humerus. *J Orthop Trauma* 1993;7:367–374.

23. Henley MB, Monroe M, Tencer AF: Biomechanical comparison of methods of fixation of a midshaft osteotomy of the humerus. *J Orthop Trauma* 1991;5:14–20.

24. Zimmerman MC, Waite AM, Deehan M, et al: A biomechanical analysis of four humeral fracture fixation systems. *J Orthop Trauma* 1994;8:233–239.

25. Bell MJ, Beauchamp CG, Kellam JK, et al: The results of plating humeral shaft fractures in patients with multiple injuries: The Sunnybrook experience. *J Bone Joint Surg* 1985;67B:293–296.

    The authors reported that 33 of 34 fractures treated with plate fixation healed with excellent functional restoration and minimal complications. They specifically recommended this technique for the polytrauma patient to obtain an upright patient and to facilitate better nursing care.

26. Foster RJ, Dixon GL Jr, Bach AW, et al: Internal fixation of fractures and non-unions of the humeral shaft: Indications and results in a multi-center study. *J Bone Joint Surg* 1985;67A:857–864.

    Many techniques of internal fixation for humeral fractures and nonunions were reviewed. AO compression plating resulted in 100% union for acute fractures in 27 polytrauma patients and union in eight (80%) of 10 treated for nonunions. Rush rods and Küntscher nails were associated with more implant-related problems, yet were recommended for select surgical indications.

27. Heim D, Herkert F, Hess P, et al: Surgical treatment of humeral shaft fractures: The Basel experience. *J Trauma* 1993;35:226–232.

    The largest series of plate fixation reviewed in the literature demonstrated union in 120 of 127 patients with 13 significant complications. The anterolateral approach was preferred. Fixation failures were attributed to "insufficient technique" and the "short-plate syndrome." Indications for surgical intervention were reviewed.

28. Vander Griend R, Tomasin J, Ward EF: Open reduction and internal fixation of humeral shaft fractures: Results using AO plating techniques. *J Bone Joint Surg* 1986;68A:430–433.

    This series demonstrated union in 33 of 34 fractures managed with AO plating techniques with minimal associated complications. The anterolateral approach was preferred.

29. Stern PJ, Mattingly DA, Pomeroy DL, et al: Intramedullary fixation of humeral shaft fractures. *J Bone Joint Surg* 1984;66A:639–646.

    Intramedullary fixation utilizing a variety of implants and techniques was associated with a 67% complication rate, with 64% of the patients requiring at least one additional operation. Fracture healing problems were more common with open fractures, open reduction nailing techniques, and with fracture fixation more than 6 weeks after injury. Antegrade nailing was associated with a 56% incidence of painful adhesive capsulitis of the shoulder.

30. Vander Griend RA, Ward EF, Tomasin J: Closed Küntscher nailing of humeral shaft fractures. *J Trauma* 1985;25:1167–1169.

31. Watanabe RS: Intramedullary fixation of complicated fractures of the humeral shaft. *Clin Orthop* 1993;292:255–263.

32. Brumback RJ, Bosse MJ, Poka A, et al: Intramedullary stabilization of humeral shaft fractures in patients with multiple trauma. *J Bone Joint Surg* 1986;68A:960–970.

    The benefits of surgical fixation of humeral shaft fractures in polytrauma patients are reviewed. Flexible nailing utilizing Rush or Ender rods resulted in a 94% rate of union with excellent clinical results in 62%. The surgical technique is well described. Implant-related problems were most commonly associated with antegrade insertion through the rotator cuff or retrograde insertion with epicondylar starting points.

33. Durbin RA, Gottesman MJ, Saunders KC: Hackethal stacked nailing of humeral shaft fractures: Experience with 30 patients. *Clin Orthop* 1983;179:168–174.

    The Hackethal technique of stacked flexible pins is reviewed, outlining the nuances of the surgical technique. Although the union rate was 92%, the reoperation rate for nonunion or pin-related pain was 14%. Good results were noted with a small number of patients (five) with pathologic fractures stabilized with this technique.

34. Hall RF Jr, Pankovich AM: Ender nailing of acute fractures of the humerus: A study of closed fixation by intramedullary nails without reaming. *J Bone Joint Surg* 1987;69A:558–567.

    Closed intramedullary fixation utilizing multiple Ender nails was prospectively evaluated with 85 of 86 fractures uniting. Nail backout was the most frequent problem but was thought to have been eliminated by wiring the eyelets of the nails together. Both antegrade and retrograde techniques were evaluated.

35. Henley MB, Chapman JR, Claudi BF: Closed retrograde Hackethal nail stabilization of humeral shaft fractures. *J Orthop Trauma* 1992;6:18–24.

    A retrospective review of closed retrograde Hackethal nailing demonstrated excellent healing (32 of 33) with a low incidence of reoperation for nail migration (two of 33). Heterotopic ossification at the entry portal was noted in three patients but limited elbow motion was found in only one. The nuances of the technique are also reviewed.

36. Barnes CE, Shuler TE: Complications associated with the Seidel nail. *Orthop Rev* 1993;22:699–706.

37. Habernek H, Orthner E: A locking nail for fractures of the humerus. *J Bone Joint Surg* 1991;73B:651–653.

38. Ingman AM, Waters DA: Locked intramedullary nailing of humeral shaft fractures: Implant design, surgical technique, and clinical results. *J Bone Joint Surg* 1994;76B:23–29.

    A modified Gross-Kemph 9-mm tibial nail was utilized for locked nailing of the humeral shaft. With experience, the retrograde technique was preferred for almost all fractures. The authors felt that this technique of internal fixation was the treatment of choice for osteoporotic and pathologic fractures.

39. Riemer BL, Foglesong ME, Burke CJ III, et al: Complications of Seidel intramedullary nailing of narrow diameter humeral diaphyseal fractures. *Orthopedics* 1994;17:19–29.

40. Robinson CM, Bell KM, Court-Brown CM, et al: Locked nailing of humeral shaft fractures: Experience in Edinburgh over a two-year period. *J Bone Joint Surg* 1992;74B:558–562.

    This series of 30 fractures treated with locked Seidel nailing identified frequent technical problems, most commonly with the locking mechanism. Compromise of shoulder function was common, even when the nail was not prominent, suggesting that the entry point through the rotator cuff was a problem. Modification of nail design was recommended.

41. Seidel H: Humeral locking nail: A preliminary report. *Orthopedics* 1989;12:219–226.

42. Riemer BL, D'Ambrosia R: The risk of injury to the axillary nerve, artery, and vein from proximal locking screws of humeral intramedullary nails. *Orthopedics* 1992;15:697–699.

43. Neumann HS, Brug E, Winckler S, et al: The surgical treatment of diaphyseal fractures of the humerus: Stabilization with plate osteosynthesis, Hackethal nailing, locking nail and external fixation. *Int J Orthop Trauma* 1993;3(suppl):25–28.

    As part of a larger study of humeral fixation, a dynamic axial fixator was used in 27 patients with severe closed or open fractures or polytrauma. A union rate of 93% (average time to union, 13.1 weeks) associated with a pin-tract infection rate of 7.5% was reported.

44. Rosen H: The treatment of nonunions and pseudarthroses of the humeral shaft. *Orthop Clin North Am* 1990;21:725–742.

    The etiology of humeral nonunions is thought to be related to any combination of "unbridled motion, gap between fragments, and loss of blood supply." This comprehensive review of humeral nonunions outlines the objectives of therapy, emphasizes preoperative planning, and describes a surgical protocol that is associated with a success rate of more than 95%.

45. Esterhai JL, Brighton CT, Heppenstall RB, et al: Nonunion of the humerus: Roentgenographic, scintigraphic, and response characteristics to treatment with constant direct current stimulation of osteogenesis. *Clin Orthop* 1986;211:228–234.

46. Healy WL, White GM, Mick CA, et al: Nonunion of the humeral shaft. *Clin Orthop* 1987;219:206–213.

    Factors predisposing to humeral shaft nonunion were transverse and short oblique fracture patterns and initial treatment of the fracture with either a hanging arm cast or open reduction. Successful healing of the nonunions in 23 (88%) of 26 cases was identified with their protocol of preparation of the nonunion site (combination of resection, shortening, and drilling), stable plate fixation, and cancellous bone grafting.

47. Barquet A, Fernandez A, Luvizio J, et al: A combined therapeutic protocol for aseptic nonunion of the humeral shaft: A report of 25 cases. *J Trauma* 1989;29:95–98.

    Stable internal fixation with broad AO plates combined with decortication and autologous cancellous bone grafting was used for 25 cases of aseptic nonunion of the humeral shaft. Healing was achieved in 24 patients with 21 good functional outcomes.

48. Pietu G, Raynaud G, Letenneur J: Treatment of delayed and nonunions of the humeral shaft using the Seidel locking nail: A preliminary report of five cases. *J Orthop Trauma* 1994;8:240–244.

49. Trotter DH, Dobozi W: Nonunion of the humerus: Rigid fixation, bone grafting, and adjunctive bone cement. *Clin Orthop* 1986;204:162–168.

50. Jupiter JB: Complex non-union of the humeral diaphysis: Treatment with a medial approach, an anterior plate, and a vascularized fibular graft. *J Bone Joint Surg* 1990;72A:701–707.

51. Wright TW, Miller GJ, Vander Griend RA, et al: Reconstruction of the humerus with an intramedullary fibular graft: A clinical and biomechanical study. *J Bone Joint Surg* 1993;75B:804–807.

4

Fractures of the Distal Humerus

Introduction

Distal humeral fractures account for only 2% of all adult fractures. However, a disproportionate percentage of both surgically and nonsurgically treated individuals have been reported to have poor outcomes when compared to patients with other injuries. Pain, deformity, instability, stiffness, nonunion, malunion, and ulnar neuropathy are commonly reported treatment sequelae. Fractures involving the articular surface, comminuted fractures occurring in elderly osteopenic patients, and fractures occurring as a result of high-energy trauma have consistently yielded the worst results. The two factors that appear to be most predictable of an acceptable treatment outcome are the ability to achieve and maintain a stable, anatomic reduction and the ability to resume early active motion.[1] There have been no recent advances in methodology that have improved nonsurgical results. Nonsurgical treatment is seldom capable of restoring anatomy following a displaced distal humeral fracture. Joint reaction forces across the elbow may exceed two to three times body weight and may lead to displacement of initially nondisplaced fractures. These same forces may subsequently lead to displacement following initially successful reduction attempts, particularly if early motion is allowed. When displacement occurs, eventual nonunion or malunion are common. Acceptable results are obtained with nonsurgical treatment only when the fracture is nondisplaced or minimally displaced and adequate intrinsic stability allows for early motion.

In contradistinction to the poor results generally reported following nonsurgical treatments, acceptable results are now reported in a majority of patients treated with modern methods of open reduction and internal fixation.[2] No controlled prospective trials have compared patients treated with modern surgical techniques and modern methods of internal fixation to patients treated nonsurgically or those treated with older surgical techniques and implants. Comparison with historic controls strongly suggests current results are superior to those previously reported. One recent series compared 29 patients treated with open reduction and internal fixation to 13 patients treated conservatively. Seventy-six percent of surgically treated patients were reported to have good and excellent results and 8% of nonsurgically treated patients were reported to have similar results.[3] Treatment selection was not randomized.

The primary goal of most early surgical treatments for distal humeral fractures was restoration of anatomy. Surgical technique, which would be considered poor by modern standards, often resulted in wound complications and fibrosis. Implant limitations frequently prevented anatomic reduction and stable fixation. The importance of reestablishing range of motion was often unrecognized or was precluded by unstable fixation. Early resumption of motion following unsuccessful attempts to obtain stable fixation typically resulted in fixation failure and nonunion. Prolonged immobilization resulted in stiffness or ankylosis.

Restoration of anatomy can no longer be considered an acceptable treatment result for most patients. Acceptable outcome now requires both restoration of anatomy and functional recovery. These treatment goals can now be attained in an increasing percentage of patients. Improved surgical technique has decreased the incidence of soft-tissue complications, and small fragment fixation devices now allow fixation of fractures that were previously difficult to treat. Biomechanical studies have defined optimal implant characteristics, placement, and configuration. Improved fixation methods allow earlier resumption of motion.

The increased emphasis on surgical treatment of distal humeral fractures has been accompanied by a revised understanding of distal humeral anatomy. The distal humerus has historically been described in terms of medial and lateral condyles. Increasingly, its osseous anatomy is considered in terms of medial and lateral osseous columns that support an articular surface. Treatment principles and fixation techniques are more easily understood within the framework of a columnar distal humerus.

Anatomic reduction of the articular surface and stable fixation that allows for early active range of motion has become the treatment of choice for most distal humeral fractures. This chapter summarizes those developments that have resulted in an improved treatment outcome for these difficult fractures. Relevant anatomy is reviewed as it pertains to evaluation, fracture classification, and treatment. Treatment is discussed within the framework of single comprehensive classification schema. Treatment results are considered for individual fracture types.

The greater emphasis placed on the surgical treatment of distal humeral fractures has resulted in an increased number of surgical complications.[4] Commonly reported postoperative complications include symptomatic hardware, ulnar neuropathy, malunion, nonunion, loss of motion, and heterotopic ossification. Modalities for the prevention and treatment of complications will be addressed within this chapter.

Anatomy

The elbow joint includes two functionally independent articulations contained within a single synovial capsule. At the ulnotrochlear articulation, the trochlear portion of the distal humerus articulates with the semilunar notch of the proximal ulna. This highly constrained articulation functions as a hinge that allows flexion and extension to occur in a single oblique sagittal plane. The radiocapitellar and radioulnar joints function together, independent of the ulnotrochlear joint, to allow pronation and supination.

The distal humerus is generally regarded as that portion of the humerus distal to and including the origin of the brachialis musculature. The cylindrical humeral diaphysis becomes broad in the medial-lateral dimension and narrow in the anteroposterior dimension at its distal aspect. Traditionally the most distal aspect of the humerus has been considered to be composed of radial and ulna condyles. Unlike the distal femur or metacarpal bones, which are composed of two similar "condyles," the medial and lateral aspects of the distal humerus are anatomically dissimilar. The arbitrary sagittal division into condyles occurs at the capitellotrochlear groove and results in a medial condyle, which is significantly larger than the lateral. The medial and lateral triangular ridges, which flare distally, have been termed supracondylar ridges. These end distally at the so-called medial and lateral epicondyles. The medial flare is greater than lateral, which also contributes to the discrepancy in condylar size. Each "condyle" is composed of an articular and an extraarticular portion.

In the columnar conceptualization of the distal humerus, the supporting columns are of primary structural significance. Within this framework medial and lateral osseous columns diverge to support an intervening "spool-shaped" trochlea articular surface. Together the medial and lateral column and the articular surface form a triangular construct. The generalized goal of treatment is to restore and stabilize the normal triangular anatomic relationship. Restoration of all three limbs of this osseous triangle is thought to be important in restoring and maintaining distal humeral stability. The osseous columns provide reliable sites for screw placement. The columnar concept of the distal humerus is achieving increased acceptance; however, retained terminology often results in confusion. Much literature continues to refer to the distal humeral "condyles." In clinical practice older terminology also remains in common use. Though the remainder of this chapter will consider the evaluation and treatment of distal humeral fractures within the framework of the columnar anatomic description, older terminology will in many cases be necessarily retained (Fig. 1).

The lateral column of the distal humerus diverges 20° from the sagittal axis and projects anteriorly to terminate as the capitellar articular surface. The presence of an articular component to this column has important implications when planning surgical reconstruction and placement of hardware. The medial column diverges at an angle of approximately 45° and ends proximal to the trochlea articular surface. In contradistinction to the lateral column, the terminal portion of the medial column has no articular surface. The posterior olecranon fossa is located proximal to the trochlea between the medial and lateral osseous columns and accommodates the olecranon during terminal elbow extension. Anteriorly, the coronoid fossa is located proximal to the trochlea and a small radial fossa is located proximal to the capitellum. The coronoid and radial fossae accept the coronoid and radial head, respectively, during full elbow flexion. Unlike the olecranon and coronoid fossae, which are located between the two aforementioned bony columns, the radial fossa is a portion of the lateral column. This fossa must be avoided during the placement of screws within the lateral column. In a small percentage of patients the olecranon and coronoid fossae communicate.

The ulnotrochlear articulation is oriented obliquely in relation to the anatomic sagittal and coronal planes. The trochlear axis is internally rotated approximately 3° to 8° relative to the medial and lateral humeral condyles and has a valgus inclination of approximately 94° in males and 98° in females. The so-called "carrying angle" observed with the arm held in the anatomic position has often been attributed to the valgus inclination of the humeral articular surface; however, this is an oversimplification of its true etiology (Fig. 2).

Static elbow stability is primarily a consequence of the constrained nature of the hemicircumferential ulnotrochlear articulation. Stability is augmented by the dynamic opposing forces of the extensor and flexor muscle mechanisms. The radiocapitellar articulation is partially responsible for resisting valgus instability however primary resistance to varus and valgus forces is provided by soft tissues.

The medial collateral ligament provides the primary resistance to valgus forces. Two distinct components of this ligament arise from the medial epicondyle and insert on the proximal ulna. The anterior portion inserts on the sublime tubercle of the coronoid and the posterior component on the medial surface of the olecranon. The anterior portion of the ligament is of greater importance. The flexor-pronator muscle group arising from the medial epicondyle also assists in the resistance of valgus forces.

The lateral collateral ligament provides the primary resistance to varus forces. This fan-shaped ligament arises from the lateral epicondyle and inserts on the orbicular ligament and radial aspect of the proximal ulna. The labral humeral-ulnar component is of primary importance. The extensor and supinator muscle groups arising from the lateral condyle provide additional resistance to varus

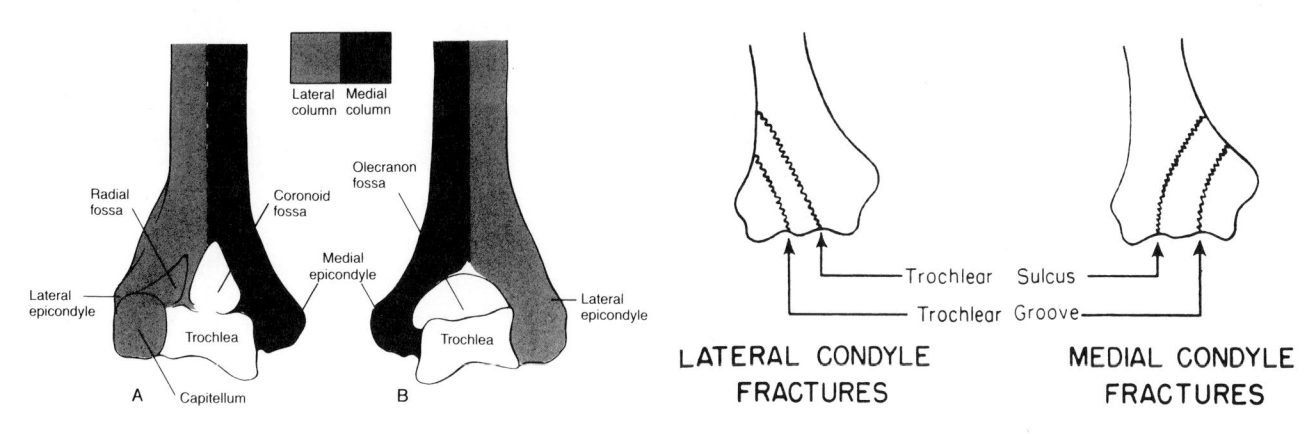

Fig. 1 Left, Anterior and posterior views of distal humerus including columns fossae and articular components. (Reproduced with permission from Mehne DK, Jupiter JB: Fractures of the distal humerus, in Browner BD, Jupiter JB, Levine AM, et al (eds): *Skeletal Trauma*. Philadelphia, PA, WB Saunders, 1992, pp 1146-1176.) **Right,** Typical schematic representation of medial and lateral "condyle" fractures lacking clear anatomic designation of individual condyles. (Reproduced with permission from Milch H: Fractures and fracture dislocations of the humeral condyles. *J Trauma* 1963;3:592-607.)

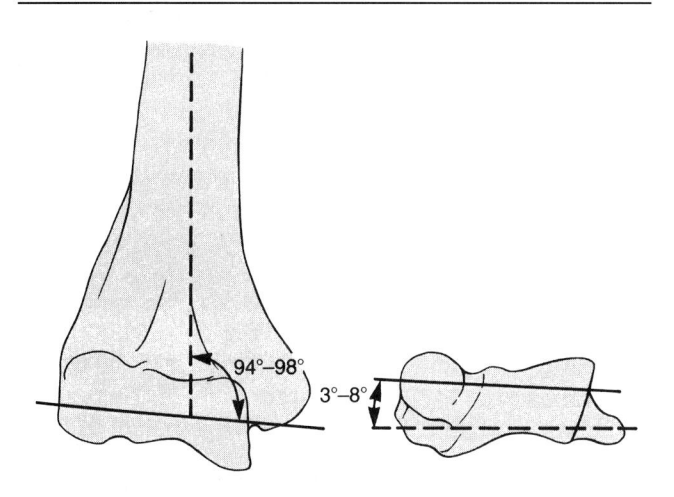

Fig. 2 Left, Anteroposterior view demonstrating longitudinal axis and valgus inclination of trochlea articular surface. **Right,** Coronal view demonstrating internal rotation of trochlea articular surface with respect to transverse axis. (Reproduced with permission from Mehne DK, Jupiter JB: Fractures of the distal humerus, in Browner BD, Jupiter JB, Levine AM, et al (eds): *Skeletal Trauma*. Philadelphia, PA, WB Saunders, 1992, pp 1146-1176.)

forces. Attempts to repair or preserve both collateral ligaments should be made at the time of surgery.

The neurovascular structures that supply the hand and forearm are found in close proximity to the osseous structures about the elbow. All are at risk at the time of injury and at the time of surgery. Although the majority of surgical procedures on the distal humerus are performed via a posterior approach, a thorough knowledge of the cross-sectional anatomy of the elbow and familiarity with alternate surgical approaches is important for all surgeons treating these fractures. Distal humeral fractures often require placement of medial hardware to provide optimal stability and the ulna nerve is at particular risk in its location within the cubital tunnel. The nerve should be clearly identified and, when necessary, anteriorly transposed to prevent neuropathy.[5,6]

Classification

Classification schema for distal humeral fractures have historically been devised based on the condylar concept of the distal humerus. Until recently, no single classification system categorized all possible variations of intra-articular and extra-articular distal humeral fractures. Extra-articular fractures were subclassified as supracondylar and transcondylar or alternatively as high and low based on proximity to joint surface. A majority of adult distal humeral fractures involve the articular surface. Those intra-articular fractures involving both so-called condyles were termed intercondylar or bicondylar and "T," "Y," and "H" variants described. Fractures involving only one condyle have been termed unicondylar. Classification systems based on the condylar concept of the distal humerus failed to consider medial and lateral osseous column involvement. Restoration of these columns along with restoration of the articular segment is now believed to be of primary importance in the treatment of these injuries. The AO/ASIF classification has been considered by many to be an improvement over many of the previously utilized classification systems. Within this system all periarticular distal humeral fractures may be classified; however, detractors believe this system remains deficient in its ability to adequately incorporate columnar involvement.

Extra-articular Fractures

Extra-articular fractures of the distal humerus occur more commonly in children than adults. They have been subdivided into supracondylar and transcondylar types; however, the inability to clearly define the condyle has made the division somewhat arbitrary. These fractures have also been arbitrarily termed high and low based on proximity to the distal humeral articular surface. Kocher initially classified supracondylar fractures as flexion and extension types based on probable mechanism of injury and direction of displacement. Flexion and extension categories were then subdivided based on amount of displacement. Flexion injuries were believed to occur as a result of a force directed against the posterior aspect of the flexed elbow. The more common extension injury is believed to occur as a result of a fall on the outstretched extremity or as a consequence of direct trauma. Additional categories for abduction and adduction type injuries have been suggested; however, many authors disagree with the theory such injuries exist.

Intra-articular Fractures

In retaining the arbitrary division of the distal humerus into medial and lateral condylar components, intra-articular fractures may be designated as either unicondylar or bicondylar.

Unicondylar Fractures The distal humerus is arbitrarily divided into medial and lateral condyles at the capitellotrochlea groove. Milch classified unicondylar fractures into medial and lateral types based on the primarily involved condyle. Milch subdivided medial and lateral condylar fractures based on the location of the primary fracture line relative to the lateral wall of the trochlea. Type 1 fractures were those in which the primary fracture line exited the articular surface of the involved condyle while leaving the lateral trochlea ridge intact. Type 2 injuries were those in which the primary fracture line exited the articular surface on the contralateral side of the lateral trochlea ridge. Except for rare medial condylar fractures, which cross the lateral trochlea ridge and exit the joint distally through the capitellotrochlea groove, all Milch type 2 fractures involve portions of both condyles. The loss of the lateral trochlea ridge was believed to greatly increase the instability imparted by these injuries.

Capitellum and trochlear fractures are by definition partial condylar fractures. The capitellum comprises the articular portion of the lateral condyle and the trochlea the articular portion of the medial condyle. Capitellar and trochlea injuries occur in isolation or as a component of more extensive injuries. Fractures of the capitellum are more common than fractures of the trochlea. These injuries typically result in a devascularized articular segment. Three common types of capitellum fractures have been described. Bryan and Morrey incorporated previously described variants within a single classification system. Bryan and Morrey type 1 fractures are those in which a primary fracture line in the coronal plane separates the entire capitellum from the distal humerus. These have also been termed Hahn-Steinthal fractures. Type 2 fractures, also known as Kocher-Lorenz fractures, are subchondral and result in a fragment consisting of cartilage and subchondral bone. Grantham had previously included a subdivision of comminuted fractures within the type 2 category of injuries. In the classification advocated by Bryan and Morrey comminuted fractures are designated type 3. There is no classification system commonly used for trochlea fractures.

Bicondylar Fractures Bicondylar fractures result in dissociation of the entire articular surface or a majority of the articular surface from the more proximal humerus. These fractures were originally classified as "T" or "Y" types by Reich in 1936 based on fracture configuration. Risenborough and Radin classified bicondylar fractures into four types based on displacement, rotation of fragments, and articular comminution.

Other Classifications Recently, an additional classification system has been described for fractures that involve the entire articular surface. This classification includes six different fracture configurations and has been advocated as more consistent with the columnar concept of the distal humerus and thus of greater utility in guiding treatment. This system has received only limited acceptance in the literature.

The AO/ASIF classification was devised in an attempt to create a single comprehensive system that would be applicable to all long bone fractures. Through application of this system its creators hope to develop and refine treatment guidelines. Through accurate identification of subgroups of injuries prognostic capabilities are also felt possible. The generalized system can be applied to all long bone fractures, including humeral fractures. Separate categories exist for proximal, middle, and distal segments of individual long bones. The primary classification of periarticular fractures is determined by the degree of articular involvement. Type A fractures are entirely extra-articular, type B fractures involve only a portion of the articular surface, and type C fractures the entire articular surface. Further subdivision is related to fracture comminution and orientation. As applied to the distal humerus the system has been criticized for its inability to reliably incorporate columnar involvement. The treatment of distal humeral fractures will, however, be approached within the framework of the comprehensive AO classification as this system appears to be achieving general acceptance.

Periarticular type A extra-articular distal humeral fractures are subdivided into three categories. Type A1 injuries are avulsion fractures with no resulting loss of columnar support to the articular surface. Type A2 injuries are metaphyseal fractures with limited comminution and type A3 injuries with significant metaphyseal comminution. Type B injuries involve a portion of the articular surface with or without columnar involvement. In addition to the injury to the articular surface, type B1 injuries involve the lateral column and type B2 injuries, the medial column. B3 injuries are injuries to the articular surface with no loss of columnar support. Type C injuries involve the entire articular surface and include disruption of both osseous columns. Type C1 injuries have no significant comminution of the articular surface or metaphyseal region. Metaphyseal comminution and an absence of articular comminution distinguish type C2 injuries. Type C3 injuries are characterized by articular comminution irrespective of the metaphysis comminution (Fig. 3).

Evaluation

The clinical and radiographic evaluation of adult distal humeral fractures is generally uncomplicated. There is a wide spectrum of injuries and physical findings vary accordingly. A majority of patients will present with complaints of pain following a traumatic event. Deformity and soft-tissue swelling are common in association with serious injuries. Following less serious injuries, a palpable effusion may be present. Attempted range of motion is generally painful and may be associated with crepitus. Deliberate attempts to elicit crepitus are not advisable because they may cause additional soft-tissue injury. Skin should be inspected carefully for lacerations indicative of an open injury. Distal humeral fractures are often high-energy injuries and associated soft-tissue injury is common. Soft-tissue injury is particularly important to assess as it relates to surgical timing and approach. A thorough neurologic and vascular examination should be performed as a component of all evaluations. Fractures in limbs with vascular compromise should undergo immediate closed reduction and immobilization. Failure to observe prompt improvement necessitates further evaluation and possible surgical intervention. If unfamiliar with techniques of vascular surgery, the treating orthopaedist should obtain appropriate consultation. Subtle injuries, such as isolated anterior interosseous nerve palsy, may be present and must be excluded.

Adequate radiographic assessment generally requires only standard anteroposterior and lateral views of the elbow. Most distal humeral fractures will be readily apparent and classification is possible with these two views. When clinical suspicion of fracture is high and no fracture is obvious, radiographs should be evaluated for subtle findings, such as the presence or absence of a "fat pad sign." Standard radiographic views may be supplemented with the so-called "radial head-capitellar view" if a capitellum or radial head fracture is suspected. In some instances, overlapping structures, rotation of fragments, and displacement make accurate preoperative planning difficult. In these cases, radiographs may be supplemented with a traction anteroposterior view obtained in the operating room prior to surgery.

In rare partial articular fractures and fractures with significant articular comminution, CT scan may be useful. The scan may provide a helpful guide in the choice of a surgical approach and/or in fixation technique. The presence of multiplanar fractures or severe comminution as depicted on CT scan may also lead to the choice of nonsurgical treatment, allograft replacement, or total elbow arthroplasty. Additional studies generally are unnecessary.

Treatment

The two factors that have proven to be most reliably predictive of an acceptable outcome when treating distal humeral fractures are a stable anatomic reduction and a relatively brief period of postoperative immobilization.[3] Nonsurgical treatment is rarely capable of meeting these goals. Displaced fractures are difficult to reduce. Maintaining an anatomic reduction with nonsurgical treatment generally requires a long period of immobilization. Modern methods of open reduction and internal fixation are capable of restoring anatomy and allowing early motion when treating the majority of distal humeral fractures. Current recommendations for surgical treatment are based on an improved understanding of the anatomic characteristics and biomechanical requirements of the distal humerus. Principles of treatment, surgical techniques, and implants that were formerly associated with poor surgical outcome are now considered outdated. Though no controlled trials have compared patients treated with current surgical techniques and stable fixation to those treated nonsurgically or with less rigid fixation techniques, comparison with historic controls suggests that current modalities result in decreased pain, increased stability, and an improved range of motion for many patients. Severe osteoporosis, articular comminution, and multiplanar fracture configurations continue to be associated with the majority of poor results and complications.

A limited number of fractures remain amenable to nonsurgical forms of treatment. Avulsion fractures with no resulting instability may be treated nonsurgically with protected range of motion. Stable nondisplaced fractures with the potential for rapid healing may be treated with a brief period of immobilization followed by protected range of motion. Frequent clinical and radiographic follow-up is necessary when nonsurgical treatment is chosen. Nonsurgical treatment options include splints, functional braces, casts, and traction. Patients with comminuted fractures and/or osteopenia precluding stable fixation may also be more appropriately treated nonsurgically or with alternative surgical modalities, such as prosthetic replacement or allograft replacement.

Absolute indications for surgical treatment include vascular injury requiring repair and open fracture requiring irrigation and debridement. A majority of open fractures are amenable to definitive fixation at the time of initial irrigation and debridement. When large amounts of devitalized tissue or significant contamination are present, limited fixation of the articular surface and a bridging external fixator may be indicated. Definitive fixation may be performed following soft-tissue stabilization.

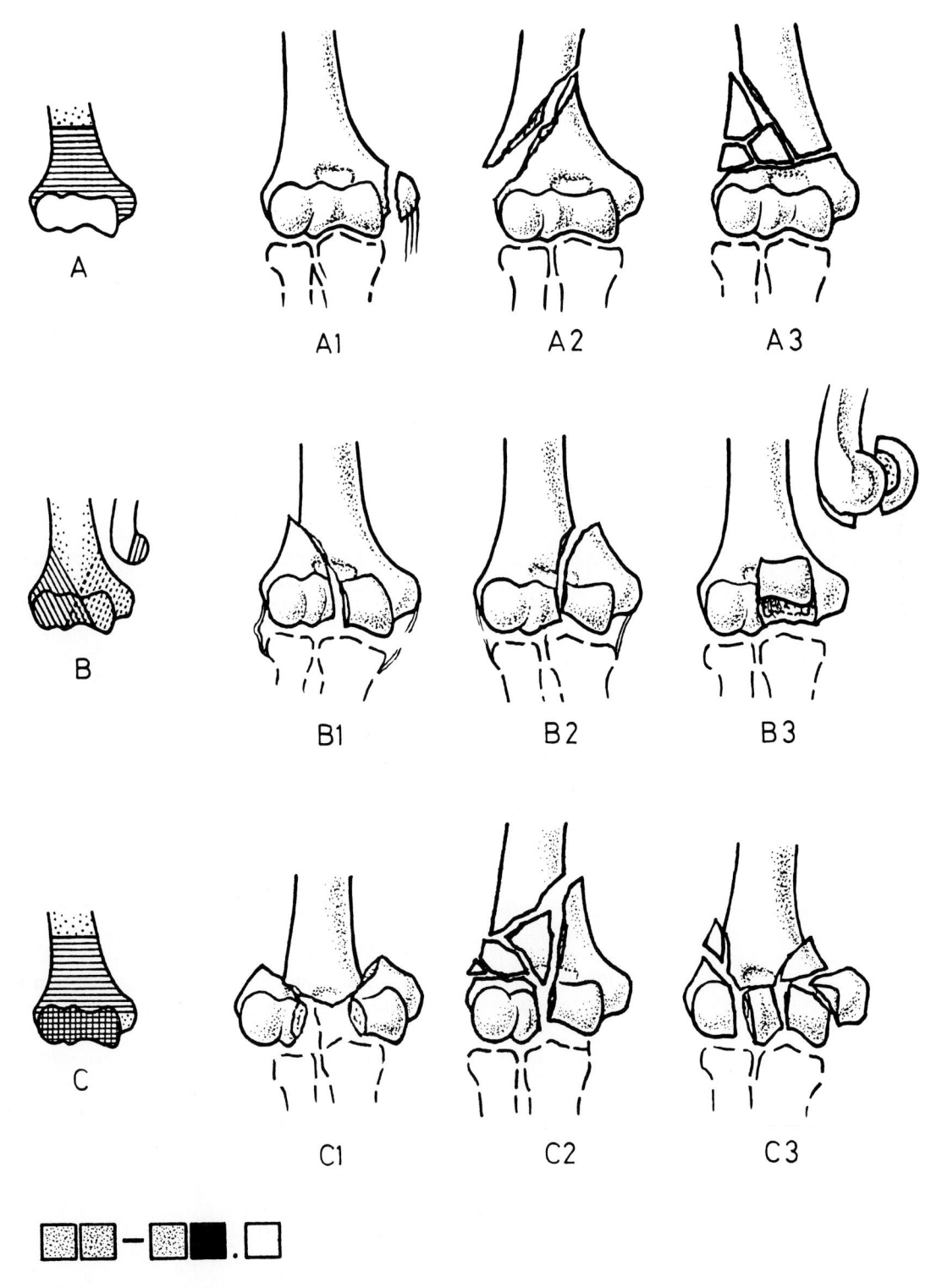

Fig. 3 Comprehensive AO classification of fractures of the distal humerus. A, Periarticular fractures; B, partial articular fractures; C, Complete articular fractures. A1, apophyseal avulsion; A2, metaphyseal simple; metaphyseal fragmentary. B1, lateral sagittal; medial sagittal; frontal. C1, articular simple, metaphyseal simple; C2, articular simple, metaphyseal multifragmentary; C3, multifragmentary. (Reproduced with permission from Müller ME, Nazarian S, Koch P, et al (eds): *The Comprehensive Classification of Fractures of Long Bones*. Berlin, Germany, Springer-Verlag, 1990.)

Surgical Technique for Open Reduction and Internal Fixation

A variation of the posterior surgical approach is commonly used in the treatment of distal humeral fractures. Medial and lateral approaches are used less frequently. Anterior approaches are rarely indicated. Patient positioning is determined by planned surgical approach. For most posterior approaches, the patient is positioned prone or decubitus with the involved extremity draped across the chest. Regional anesthetic may be used; however, general anesthetic is usually preferable due to the potential for long procedures. Use of a tourniquet minimizes blood loss and improves visualization while rarely limiting exposure. Iliac crest bone graft donor site should be available if significant comminution is present. All fractures with significant comminution or bone loss require bone grafting. Fractures with articular involvement are generally treated via a posterior approach with an intra-articular olecranon osteotomy. Extra-articular osteotomies provide a limited exposure of the articular surface. Chevron osteotomy results in greater immediate stability and greater surface contact for healing than transverse osteotomies. Osteotomy may be stabilized using any of the commonly described techniques of tension banding. Posterior triceps splitting and sparing approaches may sometimes be utilized in the treatment of extra-articular fractures and fractures with limited articular involvement. Medial and lateral approaches may also be used in select situations, such as when treating partial articular fractures. The extended medial approach with subperiosteal elevation of the extensor mechanism from the olecranon is advocated by some authors, particularly when primary or subsequent total elbow arthroplasty may be anticipated. Neurovascular structures, particularly the ulna nerve, should be identified and protected during all surgical approaches. Ulna nerve transposition significantly decreases the risk of postoperative neuropathy when medial exposure and placement of hardware are necessary.[6]

The goals of open reduction and internal fixation are to restore anatomy and to provide stable fixation of the articular surface and both osseous columns. Accurate reduction and stable fixation will allow early range of motion. Early resumption of motion is an important component of successful surgical treatment and continuous passive motion appears to be a valuable adjunct in some patients.[7] Recent studies have confirmed inadequate fixation to be the primary cause for nonunion.[8,9] Biomechanical testing has been performed following stabilization of simulated type A and type C fracture configurations in cadavers.[10,11] Plates and screws have been shown to provide optimal stability. Dual plate configurations provide greater resistance to flexion and extension forces than "Y" plates or screw fixation alone. Optimal fixation employs plates placed on the medial and lateral osseous columns. Plates are generally placed in a 90° offset configuration with one placed posterolaterally and another directly medial. Bicolumnar stabilization appears to be of greater importance than 90° plate offset.[11] Rigidity and fatigue testing reveal no difference between the use of one-third tubular and 3.5-mm reconstruction plates when placed in 90° offset configuration.[10] Reconstruction plates provide for ease of contouring. In rare cases with severe comminution or osteopenia, a third plate may be placed direct lateral though no published studies have proven this provides increased stability.[12] The stability of fixation techniques used to treat distal humeral fractures that do not disrupt both osseous columns has not been studied. Fixation techniques for partial articular fractures are advised based on the general principles of fracture management, information extrapolated from the above studies, and the columnar concept of the distal humerus. Stabilization employs screw fixation and plates when possible. Stable fixation of small articular fragments may require multiple Kirschner wires, mini fragment screws, or differentially threaded screws, such as those designed by Fisher and Herbert.

The treatment of specific distal humeral fracture types is considered here within the schema provided by the comprehensive AO/ASIF classification. All patients with articular displacement or potentially unstable fractures are considered to be candidates for open reduction and internal fixation. Alternative surgical and nonsurgical treatments are discussed where appropriate. An attempt is made to summarize the reported results for individual fracture types; however, this is often difficult. These are rare fractures and many series have grouped dissimilar fractures. Until recently no comprehensive system of classification was available. In the literature, fracture configuration is often difficult to determine and treatments are seldom standardized. Outcome has been assessed using a variety of criteria. A limited number of current studies are available for meaningful interpretation.

Type A: Extra-articular Fractures

Extra-articular avulsion fractures (type A1 injuries) do not disrupt the osseous columns supporting the distal humeral articular surface and rarely require surgical intervention. The flexor pronator muscle group arises from the so-called medial epicondyle and the extensor supinator group from the so-called lateral epicondyle. Most avulsion fractures occur medially and many occur in association with additional injuries. Avulsed fragments may be displaced distally by the attached muscle groups. Surgery is necessary only when instability results from loss of muscular and/or ligamentous soft-tissue support or in rare cases when muscle function is compromised due to significant displacement and functional shortening. Though displacement of greater than 1 cm has been suggested to require surgical treatment, brief periods of immobilization followed by protected range of motion have yielded good functional results in patients with greater degrees of displacement. When fixation is required screws alone are usually adequate.

Extra-articular fractures that disrupt the medial and lateral osseous columns (AO/ASIF types A2 and A3) typically present with instability and displacement. Nondisplaced or minimally displaced fractures, typically type A2, may be amenable to closed treatment with splint, cast, or functional brace. Ideally, the period of complete immobilization is limited to less than 3 weeks to minimize long-term stiffness and contracture. Acceptable results have been reported when using functional braces in the treatment of patients with distal one third humeral fractures.[13] One reported series of 85 extra-articular humeral fractures with brace applied an average of 12 days following injury and used for 10 weeks, yielded 96% union and no loss of flexion or extension greater than 25°. The exact location of these distal one third humeral fractures is not detailed and these results may not be applicable to more distal injuries. When nonsurgical treatment is chosen, frequent radiographic follow-up is necessary because displacement is not uncommon. Surgical treatment of extra-articular distal humeral fractures generally requires the use of plates and screws. Crossed Kirschner wires and Steinmann pins provide inadequate fixation and have been associated with a high incidence of fixation failure and nonunion. Screws alone are occasionally adequate for long oblique fractures occurring in nonosteoporotic bone. Screws may also be used in a crossed configuration for treatment of transverse distal fractures. In each instance, screw fixation alone is predominantly uniplanar and provides limited resistance to flexion-extension and torsional forces. Plates and screws together provide optimal fixation and resistance to bending and torsional forces. Dual plate constructs are generally superior. Plate configuration and type are determined based on factors similar to those considered in the treatment of fractures involving the entire articular surface (type C). Plate selection and placement are discussed further in considering the treatment of type C fractures. Distal diaphyseal and proximal metaphyseal extra-articular fractures are subject to stronger bending moments and are ideally treated with the heavier 4.5 narrow and 4.5 broad DC plates, assuming distal fixation can be obtained. Types A2 and A3 fractures are usually approached posteriorly. Triceps splitting or sparing variants are often possible because visualization of the articular surface is not necessary.

Type B: Partial Articular Fractures

Fractures involving a portion of the distal humeral articular surface (type B) generally require surgical intervention. Included within this grouping of fractures are those that disrupt the columnar support to the articular surface (types B1 and B2) and those that disrupt only the capitellar or trochlear surface (type B3). For the purpose of this discussion, the terms condyle and column are used interchangeably. Unicolumnar fractures are more common in children than adults. Most unicolumnar fractures in both children and adults involve the lateral column and are designated (type B1). The less common type B2 fractures disrupt the medial column. Nondisplaced fractures may be treated nonsurgically; however, close clinical and radiographic follow-up is necessary. The period of immobilization should be brief and should be followed by a therapy program designed to restore motion. Injuries in which the articular surface remains attached to a large fragment of the lateral (type B1) or medial (type B2) column may be reduced and stabilized with plates and screws or screws alone. Lateral column plates are typically placed posteriorly and medial column plates medially. Choice of plate and technique for placement are considered further in the discussion of fractures that involve the entire articular surface (type C). The results of treatment for partial articular unicolumnar fractures are generally thought to be superior to those obtained in the treatment of fractures that involve the entire articular surface; however, there are few series detailing the results of treatment for subgroups of patients. The largest single series including only unicolumnar fractures reports 18 of 22 patients to have good or excellent results; however, four patients developed significant degenerative changes.[14]

Fractures of the capitellar and trochlear articular surfaces (type B3) present additional difficulties. Fracture fragments are often devascularized and their small size may make fixation difficult. A majority of these fractures involve the capitellar surface. Truly nondisplaced or minimally displaced fractures involving a large portion of the articular surface can be treated with a cast or splint for a period of 2 to 3 weeks. Tomography or CT may help to verify the nondisplaced nature of these fractures. Displaced fragments generally require open reduction and fixation or excision, particularly when interfering with motion. Closed reduction of larger fragments has been reported; however, this commonly requires prolonged immobilization and recurrent displacement is common. Options for implants include multiple Kirschner wires, recessed interfragmentary screws, and differentially threaded screws, such as those designed by Herbert and Fisher. Differentially threaded screw fixation for fractures of the capitellar and trochlea articular surface has been shown to lead to reliable fracture healing with a limited incidence of osteonecrosis in a number of small series.[15-18] The use of fibrin sealant or glue has also been reported.[19] The treatment of comminuted fractures remains difficult. Comminuted fractures often require excision, particularly when fragments interfere with motion. The results of primary excision appear to be superior to those that follow delayed excision. Surgical approach for the treatment of partial articular injuries is chosen based on location of pathology.

Type C: The Entire Articular Surface

The most difficult distal humeral fractures to treat are believed to be those involving the entire articular surface (type C).[20] Though technically demanding, open reduction with internal fixation is possible in a majority of these injuries. A systematic treatment protocol has yielded the best results.[2] A posterior approach with an intra-articular olecranon osteotomy generally provides optimal exposure of the articular surface, although some authors have advocated an extensile medial exposure. Iliac crest bone graft donor site should be available. In approaching fractures with articular involvement, the initial step is generally reduction and stable fixation of the articular surface. Lag screw fixation is used to stabilize the articular components when treating type C1 and type C2 fractures. In the treatment of fractures with articular comminution (type C3), preservation of trochlea width is necessary to maintain elbow stability. Overzealous lag screw fixation may narrow the trochlea, resulting in instability. Preservation of trochlea width may require placement of a contoured tricortical bone graft. The reconstructed articular component including the trochlea and capitellum is secondarily attached to the humeral shaft with plates and screws. In aligning this component with the more proximal humerus, it is important to maintain a normal valgus inclination. When unilateral comminution of the articular surface precludes articular fixation, it may be necessary to first restore continuity of the contralateral osseous column and then reduce remaining columnar fragments. The osseous columns provide optimal purchase for screws. As noted earlier, biomechanical testing has shown dual plate configurations to provide greater resistance to flexion and extension forces than "Y" plates or screw fixation alone.[10] Fixation generally employs plates placed posterolaterally and directly medial. Rigidity and fatigue testing has revealed no difference between the use of one-third tubular and 3.5-mm reconstruction plates, however. Reconstruction plates provide for ease of contouring.

The results and complications from a number of series have recently been summarized.[2] Good and excellent results are reported in approximately 75% of patients with type C fractures when the above treatment protocol is followed. The criteria generally required for a good or excellent result include a stable elbow, absent or minimal pain, no deformity, range of motion from 15° to 130° or 30° to 120°, and a return to activities similar to those performed prior to injury.

Severe comminution or bone loss may necessitate nonsurgical treatment, allograft replacement, or primary total elbow replacement. Allograft replacement is capable of restoring bone stock in the short term; however, the incidence of infection is high and rigid fixation is required to prevent nonunion. Degenerative changes have been noted at 2-year follow-up and the long-term results are unknown.[21,22] Arthrodesis and resection arthroplasty are generally indicated only as salvage procedures for refractory infections. There is no functional position for arthrodesis and resection arthroplasty results in an unstable elbow. The results of primary total elbow arthroplasty for traumatic conditions have generally been poor.

Complications

Complications of surgical intervention include failure of fixation, nonunion, malunion, infection, restricted range of motion, osteoarthrosis, heterotopic ossification, osteonecrosis, ulnar neuropathy, neurovascular injury, and symptomatic hardware. Surgical technique and experience can minimize the incidence of many of these complications. Supervised postoperative range of motion exercises or continuous passive motion are important in reestablishing motion; however, stable fixation is a prerequisite to early motion. The incidence of radiographic osteonecrosis appears to greatly exceed the incidence of that which is clinically significant.

Nonunion/Malunion/Failure of Fixation

The incidence of nonunion following internal fixation of the distal humerus has ranged from 1% to 11%.[2] Inadequate or unstable fixation has been implicated by most authors.[23-25] A significant percentage of those patients who have early failure of fixation subsequently progress to nonunion. Olecranon osteotomy nonunion has also been reported, particularly following transverse intra-articular osteotomy.[26,27] Nonunion is usually amenable to internal fixation and bone grafting. Rare hypertrophic nonunions may be treated with compression fixation alone. When distal humeral nonunion is present, elbow motion may occur predominantly at the nonunion site. Extensive soft-tissue release is often required at the time of nonunion repair. Through the use of these methods, union can usually be obtained with resolution of pain and improved range of motion.[8,9,28] In difficult or recalcitrant cases, allograft replacement[21,22] or total elbow arthroplasty[29,30] may be necessary. The results of total elbow arthroplasty for traumatic and posttraumatic conditions have historically been poor; however, one recent series of patients treated with semiconstrained total elbow arthroplasty for distal humeral nonunion reported 86% of patients to have satisfactory results at greater than 2-year follow-up.[30] Corrective osteotomies have been described for malunion; however, these are technically demanding and are best performed by individuals with extensive experience in complex elbow reconstructive procedures.[31]

Symptomatic Hardware

Implants used in the repair of olecranon osteotomies account for most reports of symptomatic hardware. The incidence of surgery for removal of symptomatic hardware has been as high as 70% in one series.[32] When possible, low profile hardware should be used and fixation should be as stable as possible to prevent proximal migration. Routine anterior transposition of the ulnar nerve minimizes the incidence of complications due to medial column hardware.[6]

Infection

The incidence of infection following the open treatment of closed distal humeral fractures is surprisingly small. Timing of surgery, meticulous surgical technique, and perioperative antibiotic coverage can minimize the occurrence of infection following closed injuries. When infection does occur, serial irrigation and debridement and treatment with culture-specific antibiotics are necessary. Loose hardware should be removed; however, stable fixation should be retained. Infection following open injuries is significantly more common. This incidence can be minimized by performing an adequate initial debridement. Primary internal fixation can usually be performed following debridement; however, gross contamination may require temporary external fixation. A significant percentage of patients with infection will ultimately have a poor result. Persistent infection may require arthrodesis or resection arthroplasty.

Ulnar Neuropathy

Ulna neuropathy is among the most common complications reported following the treatment of distal humeral fractures.[2,32] This complication is found in a high percentage of patients with nonunion, particularly those who develop valgus deformity. The incidence of neuropathy may be minimized by routine ulnar nerve transposition.[6] In many cases, symptoms are relieved when impinging hardware is removed or nonunion is repaired along with neurolysis and transposition.

Heterotopic Ossification

The incidence of heterotopic ossification following surgical treatment of distal humeral fractures has been estimated at approximately 4%.[2] Head injury, serious soft-tissue injury, anterior surgical approach, and delayed surgery appear to increase the incidence of heterotopic ossification. Passive range of motion exercises have also been implicated, but not continuous passive motion. Although no studies have prospectively evaluated prophylaxis for heterotopic ossification, most authors recommend nonsteroidal anti-inflammatory drugs, particularly indomethacin, based on experience following total hip arthroplasty and acetabular fracture surgery. Radiation treatment has been advocated by a limited number of authors. Surgical excision of heterotopic ossification has been reported but may be technically demanding and the ideal time to perform excision is unclear. Cognitive disability following head injury, elevated alkaline phosphatase, osseous immaturity on plain radiographs and increased activity on bone scan are all believed to adversely influence results.

Conclusion

Intra-articular fractures of the distal humerus are uncommon and complex injuries. Current methods of internal fixation, when followed by appropriate physical therapy, are believed to yield the optimal outcome for most periarticular fractures, including those that involve the distal humerus. No controlled trials have yet been performed; however, comparison with historic controls suggests this conclusion is valid. The ideal treatment for comminuted distal humeral fractures and those that occur in osteopenic patients is unclear. Fixation failure, nonunion, and stiffness remain common in this patient population. Treatment must be selected based on the personality of the fracture, patient expectations and requirements, and a realistic appraisal of the surgeon's experience and expertise. A limited number of authors have reported the use of distal humeral allografts and total elbow prostheses as primary treatment for serious injuries; however, no long-term results are available and the indications for these procedures are not yet clear. Prospective evaluation of patients with well defined fracture types is necessary in order to more accurately assess and improve the results of treatment.

Annotated References

1. Aitken GK, Rorabeck CH: Distal humeral fractures in the adult. *Clin Orthop* 1986;207:191-197.

2. Helfet DL, Schmeling GJ: Bicondylar intraarticular fractures of the distal humerus in adults. *Clin Orthop* 1993;292:26-36.

    The authors describe in detail a protocol for evaluation and treatment of bicondylar (type C) distal humeral fractures. Literature review reveals 75% excellent-to-good results in patients similarly treated. Incidence of complications is summarized.

3. Zagorski JB, Jennings JJ, Burkhalter WE, et al: Comminuted intraarticular fractures of the distal humeral condyles: Surgical vs nonsurgical treatment. *Clin Orthop* 1986;202:197-204.

4. McKee MD, Jupiter JB: A contemporary approach to the management of complex fractures of the distal humerus and their sequelae. *Hand Clinics* 1994;10:479-494.

5. Perry CR, Gibson CT, Kowalski MF: Transcondylar fractures of the distal humerus. *J Orthop Trauma* 1989;3:98-106.

6. Wang KC, Shih HN, Hsu KY, et al: Intercondylar fractures of the distal humerus: Routine anterior subcutaneous transposition of the ulnar nerve in a posterior operative approach. *J Trauma* 1994;36:770-773.

7. Soffer SR, Yahiro MA: Continuous passive motion after internal fixation of distal humeral fractures. *Orthop Rev* 1990;19:88-93.

8. Ackerman G, Jupiter JB: Non-union of fractures of the distal end of the humerus. *J Bone Joint Surg* 1988;70A:75-83.

    In a series of 20 patients, 17 of 18 nonunions ultimately united with repeat ORIF and bone grafting, but continued to have significantly impaired motion.

9. Sanders RA, Sackett JR: Open reduction and internal fixation of delayed union and nonunion of the distal humerus. *J Orthop Trauma* 1990;4:254-259.

10. Helfet DL, Hotchkiss RN: Internal fixation of the distal humerus: A biomechanical comparison of methods. *J Orthop Trauma* 1990;4:260-264.

Double plating techniques with plates placed posterolaterally and medially were found to provide more rigid fixation than crossed screws or single "Y" plates. The particular plate chosen appeared to have little effect on stability.

11. Schemitsch EH, Tencer AF, Henley MB: Biomechanical evaluation of methods of internal fixation of the distal humerus. *J Orthop Trauma* 1994;8:468-475.

12. Jupiter JB: Complex fractures of the distal part of the humerus and associated complications. *J Bone Joint Surg* 1994;76A:1252-1264.

    This is a comprehensive review of fracture classification, operative approach, operative technique, and management of complications.

13. Sarmiento A, Horowitch A, Aboulafia A, et al: Functional bracing for comminuted extra-articular fractures of the distal third of the humerus. *J Bone Joint Surg* 1990;72B:283-287.

14. Jupiter JB, Neff U, Regazzoni P, et al: Unicondylar fractures of the distal humerus: An operative approach. *J Orthop Trauma* 1988;2:102-109.

15. Richards RR, Khoury GW, Burke FD, et al: Internal fixation of capitellar fractures using Herbert screws: A report of four cases. *Canadian J Surg* 1987;30:188-191.

16. Liberman N, Katz T, Howard CB, et al: Fixation of capitellar fractures with the Herbert screw. *Arch Orthop Trauma Surg* 1991;110:155-157.

17. Jupiter JB, Barnes KA, Goodman LJ, et al: Multiplane fracture of the distal humerus. *J Orthop Trauma* 1993;7:216-220.

18. Simpson LA, Richards RR: Internal fixation of a capitellar fracture using Herbert screws: A case report. *Clin Orthop* 1986;209:166-168.

19. Scapinelli R: Treatment of fractures of the humeral capitulum using fibrin sealant. *Arch Orthop Trauma Surg* 1990;109:235-237.

20. Letsch R, Schmit-Neuerburg KP, Sturmer KM, et al: Intraarticular fractures of the distal humerus: Surgical treatment and results. *Clin Orthop* 1989;241:238-244.

21. Urbaniak JR, Black KE Jr: Cadaveric elbow allografts: A six-year experience. *Clin Orthop* 1985;197:131-140.

22. Urbaniak JR, Aitken M: Clinical use of bone allografts in the elbow. *Orthop Clin North Am* 1987;18:311-321.

23. Sodergard J, Sandelin J, Bostman O: Postoperative complications of distal humeral fractures: 27/96 adults followed up for 6 (2-10) years. *Acta Orthop Scand* 1992;63:85-89.

24. Sodergard J, Sandelin J, Bostman O: Mechanical failures of internal fixation in T and Y fractures of the distal humerus. *J Trauma* 1992;33:687-690.

25. Behrman MJ, Bigliani LU: Distal humeral replacement after failed continuous passive motion in a T-condylar fracture. *J Orthop Trauma* 1993;7:87-89.

26. Henley MB: Intra-articular distal humeral fractures in adults. *Orthop Clin North Am* 1987;18:11-23.

27. Henley MB, Bone LB, Parker B: Operative management of intra-articular fractures of the distal humerus. *J Orthop Trauma* 1987;1:24-35.

28. McKee M, Jupiter J, Toh CL, et al: Reconstruction after malunion and nonunion of intra-articular fractures of the distal humerus: Methods and results in 13 adults. *J Bone Joint Surg* 1994;76B:614-621.

29. Figgie MP, Inglis AE, Mow CS, et al: Salvage of non-union of supracondylar fracture of the humerus by total elbow arthroplasty. *J Bone Joint Surg* 1989;71A:1058-1065.

30. Morrey BF, Adams RA: Semiconstrained elbow replacement for distal humeral nonunion. *J Bone Joint Surg* 1995;77B:67-72.

31. Cobb TK, Linscheid RL: Late correction of malunited intercondylar humeral fractures: Intra-articular osteotomy and tricortical bone grafting. *J Bone Joint Surg* 1994;76B:622-626.

32. Jupiter JB, Neff U, Holzach P, et al: Intercondylar fractures of the humerus: An operative approach. *J Bone Joint Surg* 1985;67A:226-239.

5
Elbow Trauma

Anatomy

The management of trauma to the adult elbow must be approached with a comprehensive knowledge of the soft-tissue and bony anatomy. The elbow consists of three articulations within a single synovial-lined cavity. The ulnohumeral hinge joint provides the flexion-extension arc and the radiocapitellar and proximal radioulnar joints allow for forearm rotation.

The most familiar surface of the distal humerus is its posterior one; it is composed of both the medial and lateral columns, which tend to cradle the distal articular surface. The olecranon fossa is bordered by the columns. This fossa is designed to accept the proximal ulna during elbow extension. A layer of fatty tissue, the posterior fat pad, is normally contained within the fossa and is sandwiched between the two layers of the posterior joint capsule. After trauma to the elbow, this structure can become adherent to the proximal ulna, resulting in loss of elbow extension. Anteriorly, the radial and coronoid fossa can be seen articulating with the radial head and coronoid process.

The medial column is the origin of the forearm flexor mass and the important medial collateral ligament (MCL) complex. The ulnar nerve passing through the cubital tunnel at the distal aspect of the medial column is at risk for injury either from the trauma or, should surgical exploration be done, from injury during the surgical procedure. Therefore, prior to any surgical reconstruction of distal humeral fractures, the ulnar nerve must be found distal to the medial epicondyle in the cubital tunnel and transposed anteriorly to avoid injury. The triangular shape of this medial column permits access for purchase of bone screws.

The lateral column of the distal humerus has a broad and flat posterior aspect that facilitates plate and screw application. The lateral column gently slopes anteriorly in its distal extent, serving as the origin for the forearm extensor mass. The capitellum represents the terminal articular surface of the lateral column. Screw penetration of this surface must be avoided.

The trochlea somewhat resembles a spool held in place by the medial and lateral columns. The trochlea features medial and lateral lips as well as a central sulcus for articulation with the semilunar notch of the ulna. This construction offers a considerable degree of intrinsic stability to the elbow.

The articular surface of the distal humerus is angulated 30° anteriorly to the humeral shaft in the sagittal plane with 3° to 8° of internal rotation in the coronal plane as well as 6° of valgus tilt of the condyles with respect to the long axis of the humerus.[1-3]

The valgus angle of the humeral articulation, the long axis of the humerus, and the valgus angle of the proximal ulna account for the creation of the carrying angle; for males, the mean value is between 11° and 14°, and for the female, it is between 13° and 16°.[1-3]

The radial head is covered by hyaline cartilage in its central depression as well as approximately 240° of its outside circumference that articulates with the ulna. The lesser sigmoid fossa of the proximal ulna forms an arc of approximately 60° to 80°, thereby providing an opportunity for roughly 180° of combined pronation and supination of the radius on the fixed ulna.[1-3]

The sigmoid notch of the proximal ulna is not covered by a continuous surface of hyaline cartilage but is commonly divided into anterior and posterior articular segments by a transverse portion of fibrous fatty tissue.

Elbow stability is also dependent on the medial and lateral ligament complex. The medial collateral ligament (MCL) is an important stabilizer of the elbow joint and is composed of the anterior, posterior, and transverse bundles. The anterior bundle is the one that is most important to elbow stability; it has regularly defined margins and can be distinguished from the joint capsule.[3]

The lateral ligamentous complex is less well defined and is a confluence of structures, including the annular ligament, the radial collateral ligament (RCL), the lateral ulnohumeral ligament (LUL), and the accessory collateral ligaments. The stability of the elbow is based on an integration of articular congruity as well as these capsular ligamentous complexes.

Dislocation

Dislocation of the elbow is a relatively common type of dislocation, second in frequency only to shoulder dislocation. Simple dislocations are those without elbow fracture; those involving skeletal, neural, or soft-tissue trauma are defined as complex. Elbow dislocations occur most often in younger individuals, with the peak ages being between

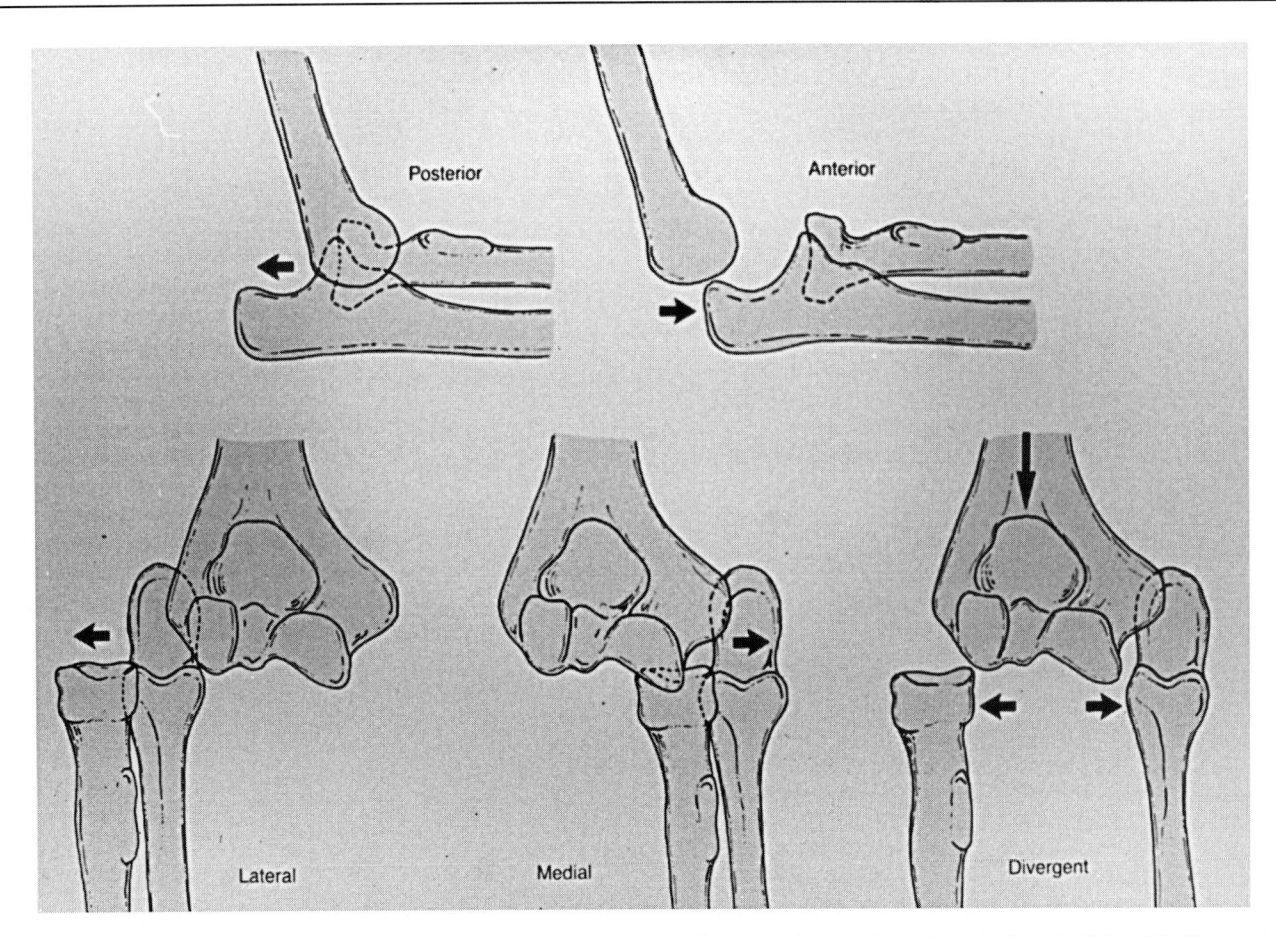

Fig. 1 An elbow dislocation is defined by the direction of the forearm bones. (Adapted with permission from Jupiter JB, Mehne DK: Trauma to the adult elbow and fractures of the distal humerus, in Browner B, Jupiter J, Levine A, et al (eds): *Skeletal Trauma*. Philadelphia, PA, WB Saunders, 1992, vol 2, pp 1125–1175.)

5 and 25 years. Two theories have been suggested to explain the mechanism of injury. The hyperextension theory suggests that a hyperextension force of the elbow levers the olecranon tip into its fossa, thus dislocating the ulnohumeral joint. Simultaneous valgus forces can lead to fractures of the radial head. A second theory suggests that the dislocation occurs as the axial load is directed onto the forearm with the elbow in a slightly flexed position.

The dislocation of the elbow is classified by the position of the forearm segment. The posterior dislocation is the most common; the anterior variant is extremely rare. A divergent dislocation refers to the dislocation in conjunction with separation of the proximal radius from the ulna (Fig. 1). Associated injuries within the elbow are common along with dislocations. Radial head and neck fractures occur in 50% to 60% of cases of dislocation; avulsion fracture of the medial or lateral epicondyle, in 10%; and fracture of the coronoid process, in 10% of dislocations.[4] Intra-articular osteochondral fractures of the distal humerus, which are not always visible on plain radiographs, can also occur during elbow dislocation.

The goal of treating elbow dislocations is to restore articular congruity expeditiously but atraumatically. Adequate anesthesia is essential to minimize the force necessary for reduction. To minimize additional trauma to any medial ligamentous structures that may not be disrupted, it has been recommended that posterior elbow dislocations be reduced in supination to clear the coronoid under the trochlea.[5] Open reduction may be necessary for neglected dislocations and for those that cannot be reduced by closed means. Immediately after reduction the elbow is placed in a well-padded splint at 90° of elbow flexion. The hand should be accessible for neurovascular monitoring. If the elbow is stable to stress following reduction, most would agree to limiting the post-reduction immobilization to a maximum of 7 to 10 days, followed by a supervised program of mobilization. For those elbows that are defined as unstable, immobilization for 2 to 3 weeks may be necessary. Immobilization beyond 3 weeks has been shown to result in residual loss of elbow motion.[6]

Elbow subluxation and dislocation is a spectrum of instability, which can be described by the circle concept, with capsuloligamentous disruption occurring in three stages from lateral to medial.[7] Stage I instability, posterolateral rotatory subluxation, is caused by disruption of the lateral ulnar collateral ligament with the possible addition of the posterolateral capsule and radial collateral ligament (RCL). Stage II instability represents a perched or incomplete dislocation with the coronoid perched on the trochlea and implies additional disruption of the anterior capsule. Either partial or complete disruption of the medial ulnar collateral ligament represents stage III instability. Although the anterior medial collateral ligament (AMCL) is usually torn with elbow dislocation, it is possible for the elbow to dislocate without disrupting this ligament, which is the primary constraint to valgus stress in the elbow.

Pronating the forearm is important when testing for valgus stability after elbow dislocation.[5] This prevents acute posterolateral rotatory instability, which may be mistaken for valgus instability in the presence of an intact AMCL. The AMCL is disrupted when valgus laxity is noted with the forearm pronated. Valgus laxity with the elbow in supination implies disruption of either the lateral ulnar collateral ligament or the AMCL. Posterolateral rotatory instability in young patients most commonly results from radial collateral ligament disruption after elbow dislocation. Thus, it has been recommended that in patients younger than 16 years of age, the elbow be immobilized for 3 weeks.[8] Others have recommended that if the elbow is stable to valgus stress with the forearm pronated, it is acceptable to begin immediate mobilization in a hinged cast-brace with the forearm pronated.[7]

In a study of the long-term sequelae of simple dislocation of the elbow, although no patient had radiographic evidence of loss of the joint space, many of the affected elbows did show radiographic irregularities, and these changes were associated with an above-average decrease in extension.[9] In another review of the long-term results of simple elbow dislocations treated nonsurgically, the authors concluded that a highly significant correlation exists between length of immobilization and the resultant flexion contracture.[6] They recommended active gentle flexion as soon as pain would allow, and that unprotected flexion and extension be initiated before 2 weeks. The results of a study that evaluated the results of surgical versus nonsurgical treatment of elbow dislocations did not support surgical treatment for a simple dislocation of the elbow that could be reduced by closed means.[10]

Fracture-Dislocation

Favorable results are not as common with complex elbow dislocations, particularly those associated with fractures of the radial head, olecranon, or coronoid process. Because these are more likely to be caused by violent trauma and are generally more unstable following reduction, it is more likely that surgical intervention will be necessary.

Elbow dislocation with associated fracture of the radial head results from a fall with the elbow extended and the arm abducted, creating a valgus stress on the elbow. An associated radial head fracture has been reported in 5% to 10% of patients sustaining an elbow dislocation.[4] These injuries can result in recurrent instability because the medial and lateral stabilizing structures may be compromised.

In a study of patients with ulnohumeral dislocation and associated radial head fracture, the authors recommend that these injuries be treated with early reduction of the ulnohumeral joint and treatment of the radial head fracture according to its type.[11]

With elbow dislocation and associated radial head fracture, all attempts should be made to salvage the radial head to preserve its role as a secondary stabilizer of the elbow while the surrounding capsular ligaments heal. If the degree of fracture comminution precludes surgical repair, removal must be considered. The timing of the excision, with or without prosthetic head replacement, remains controversial. If valgus laxity is present after a radial head excision, repair of the medial ligament complex must be considered.

Elbow dislocation with concomitant fracture of the olecranon can be an extremely complex injury, often associated with high-energy trauma and extensive soft-tissue injury. As with any intra-articular fracture, the goal of treatment should be anatomic restoration of the articulations between the olecranon and trochlea followed by early active range of motion.

Fractures of the Coronoid Process

Fractures of the coronoid process of the ulna have been identified in up to 10% of elbow dislocations. In some instances, these fractures have been associated with recurrent instability following elbow reduction. In a review of patients who had a fracture of the coronoid process of the ulna, three types of fractures were identified: type I, avulsion of the tip of the process; type II, a fragment involving 50% of the process or less; and type III, a fragment involving more than 50% of the process (Fig. 2).[12] The authors recommended closed treatment with early mobilization for type I and II coronoid fractures. Open reduction and internal fixation should be considered for type III fractures because the coronoid process provides an attachment for the anterior bundle of the MCL, the middle half of the anterior capsule, and functions as the anterior buttress of the greater sigmoid fossa preventing anterior instability of the ulnohumeral joint.

Fractures of the Olecranon

The olecranon is the subcutaneous portion of the ulna, which, together with the coronoid process, articulates with the trochlea of the distal humerus to allow flexion and extension as well as to provide inherent bony stability to the elbow. The varied fracture patterns are a consequence of its superficial position and multitude of injury mechanisms, including a fall on an outstretched hand with the elbow in

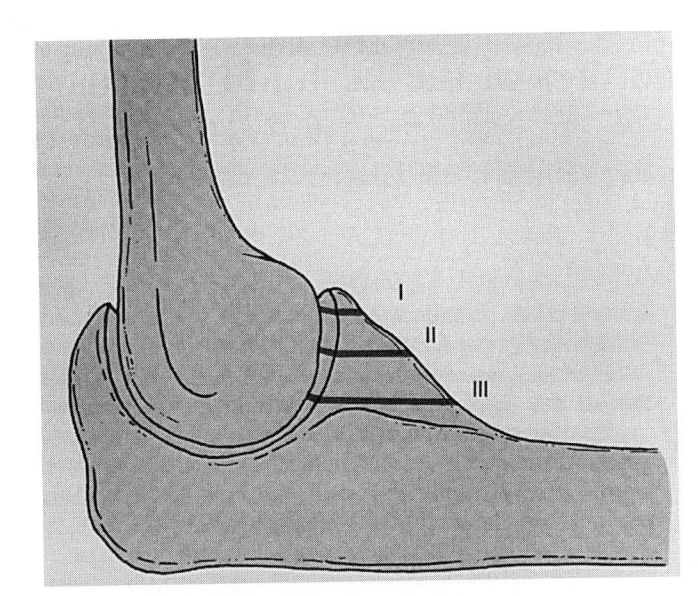

Fig. 2 The coronoid fracture has been classified into three types by Regan and Morrey. (Adapted with permission from Jupiter JB, Mehne DK: Trauma to the adult elbow and fractures of the distal humerus, in Browner B, Jupiter J, Levine A, et al (eds): *Skeletal Trauma.* Philadelphia, PA, WB Saunders, 1992, vol 2, pp 1125–1175.)

flexion, a direct blow to the olecranon, or higher energy trauma with other associated fractures or dislocations.

Several classification schemes have been developed to reflect the unique patterns of injury to the olecranon. Colton proposed a classification scheme dividing fractures into four main groups: (1) avulsion; (2) oblique; (3) fracture-dislocations; and (4) unclassified.[13] The oblique group was further subclassified into four stages, A through D, determined by the position and degree of comminution. Schatzker attempted to address the mechanical considerations of olecranon fractures with specific reference to the requirements placed on the internal fixation.[14] The fractures were designated as transverse (either simple or impacted), oblique, comminuted, or as a fracture-dislocation (Fig. 3).

Nondisplaced fractures, although uncommon, can be effectively managed nonsurgically with casting or splinting with the elbow in a position of midflexion. Radiographic evaluation should be performed 7 to 10 days after injury to ensure that the fracture has not displaced. Avulsion fractures, although extra-articular, should arouse the suspicion of an avulsion of the triceps insertion. If the patient lacks active extension, the triceps should be repaired with nonabsorbable suture into drill holes in the proximal ulna. A tension band wire loop should also be added to reinforce the repair. Oblique fractures should, whenever possible, have an interfragmentary screw placed across the fracture. Angular rotational forces on the screw can be neutralized by a tension band or plate. Comminuted fractures of the olecranon, which extend distally to involve the coronoid process, are not easily managed by the tension band technique. These fractures are best treated by plating, preferably one applied on the dorsal or tension side.

A transverse fracture, whether simple or involving comminution or depression of the articular surface, is amenable to treatment with a tension band technique.[15] This technique is based on the mechanical principle that placement of a wire loop dorsal to the mid axis of the ulna can convert distraction forces into compressive forces at the fracture site. The tension band is supplemented by either K-wires or a screw placed longitudinally into the proximal ulna to neutralize rotational and angular forces while the fracture unites. Concern that this method might open up the fracture at the articular surface of the ulna by causing the compressive forces to be greater posteriorly than anteriorly led Rowland and Burkhart[16] to modify the original AO technique. They placed the transverse hole in the ulna anterior to the center of the longitudinal axis and used a free body diagram to show that the compressive force is then guided anteriorly, causing bone compression without opening the fracture at the articular level.

In a study in which the original tension band wiring technique was used, gaps noted in the intra-articular surface of the semilunar notch of the ulna produced no ill effects and was compatible with excellent results.[15] Good or excellent results were noted in 97% of isolated olecranon fractures treated with this method. In a study using a screw plus wire technique as opposed to traditional tension band wire method in treating transverse or oblique fractures, slightly better results were noted.[17]

Biomechanical analysis of fixation methods in a transverse fracture pattern showed that the screw plus wire combination provided the greatest strength in fixation, although the difference between this technique and AO tension-band fixation was not statistically significant.[18] For transverse fractures, tension band wiring with two tightening knots was reported to be much stronger than intramedullary screw fixation.[19] Comminuted patterns were best held by plate fixation, while in oblique fractures there was no statistical difference between one-third plate fixation and double knot wiring.

An alternative to surgical fixation of olecranon fractures is that of excision of the fracture fragment and triceps reattachment. Advocates of early excision of transverse and oblique fractures claim that this operation eliminates the possibility of incongruent articular surfaces and resultant osteoarthritis, allows for early range of motion exercises, and does not impair the power or stability of the elbow.[20,21]

Complications such as nonunion may result after treatment of olecranon fractures.[22,23]

Fractures of the Radial Head

Fractures of the head of the radius are common injuries associated with almost 20% of cases of elbow trauma and account for about 33% of elbow fractures. Despite the relatively high volume of fractures that are treated, no

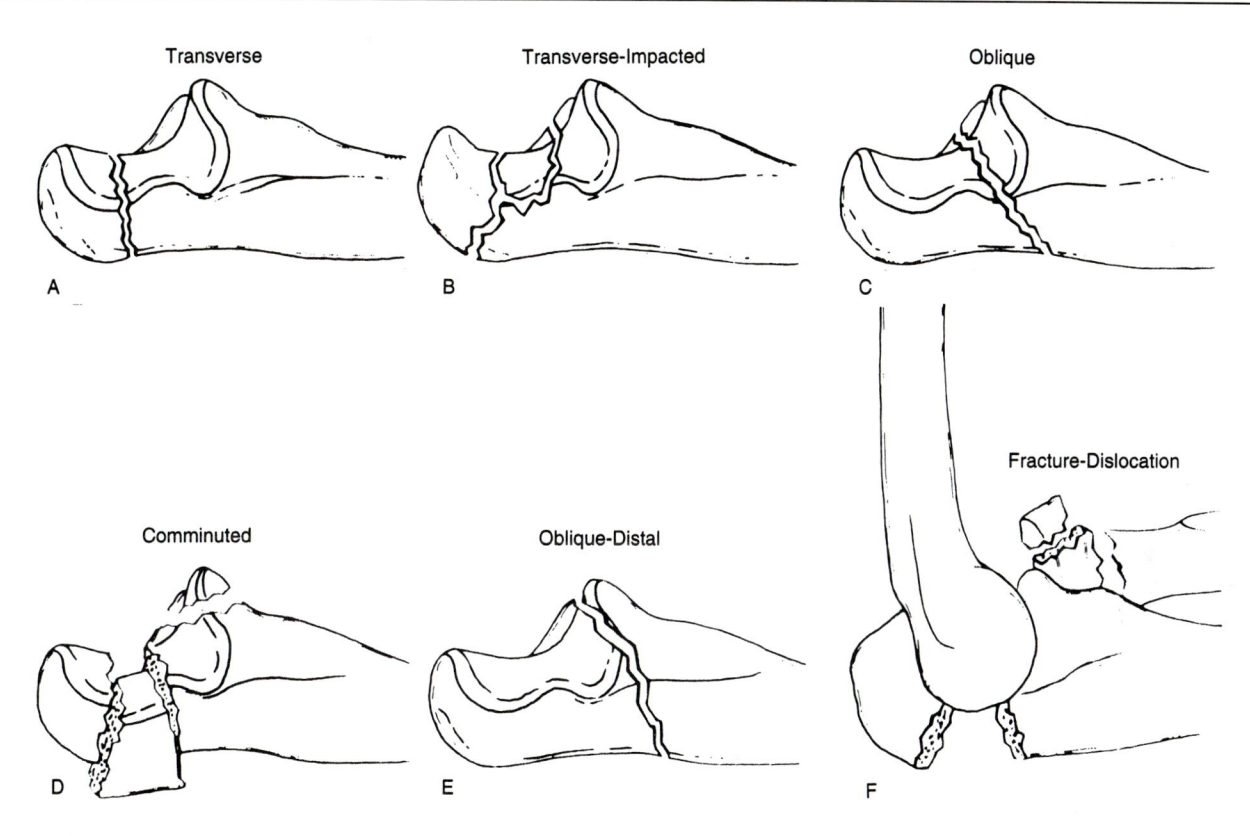

Fig. 3 Schatzker's classification system of olecranon fractures. **A,** Transverse; **B,** Transverse impacted; **C,** Oblique; **D,** Comminuted; **E,** Oblique distal; **F,** Fracture-dislocation. (Adapted with permission from Jupiter JB, Mehne DK: Trauma to the adult elbow and fractures of the distal humerus, in Browner B, Jupiter J, Levine A, et al (eds): *Skeletal Trauma.* Philadelphia, PA, WB Saunders, 1992, vol 2, pp 1125-1175.)

consensus has been reported as to the most advantageous method of treatment. Support can be found for virtually every form of treatment from prolonged immobilization to prosthetic head reconstruction.[24-29]

The mechanism of injury has been described as an axial load on a pronated forearm. The anterolateral quadrant of the articular margin is devoid of articular cartilage and strong subchondral bone, making this area the most common location for fracture. The axial load can be of varying force and direction and can result in a variety of associated soft tissue and skeletal injuries. It is extremely important to evaluate the ipsilateral wrist and distal radioulnar joint both clinically and radiographically when treating fractures of the radial head.[30]

The most commonly used classification for radial head fracture is that proposed by Mason: type I, undisplaced; type II, displaced (often a single fragment); type III, comminuted (Fig. 4).[26] Johnston added a fourth category to Mason's classification, identifying those fractures with elbow dislocation.[24]

There is little controversy regarding treatment of type I radial head fractures. Without concurrent soft-tissue or other osseous injury, these fractures should be managed nonsurgically. Early mobilization has been shown to reduce disability time and enhance elbow motion. Elbow mobilization, however, should be considered cautiously when the fracture involves a large segment of the articular surface. In one review of 30 patients with nondisplaced radial head fractures treated with early motion, the authors found that although most of the patients did well, some of those fractures involving more than one third of the radial head displaced with early motion, leading to less optimal results.[27] The fractures that resulted in loss of elbow motion all became displaced during treatment. In another study of 387 cases of radial head fractures of all types treated by nonsurgical means, the authors found that for fractures in which forearm or elbow motion was not limited, short-term immobilization followed by active range of motion resulted in predominantly good and excellent results.[29]

If a mechanical block to forearm or elbow motion is present due to displacement of the radial head fracture, surgical intervention is often needed. Yet, varied opinions exist with this subgroup as well. Surgical treatment of type II fractures has included fracture fragment excision, open reduction and internal fixation, radial head excision, and radial head excision with radial head replacement. The results of a study on the surgical versus nonsurgical treatment of Mason type II fractures suggested a beneficial

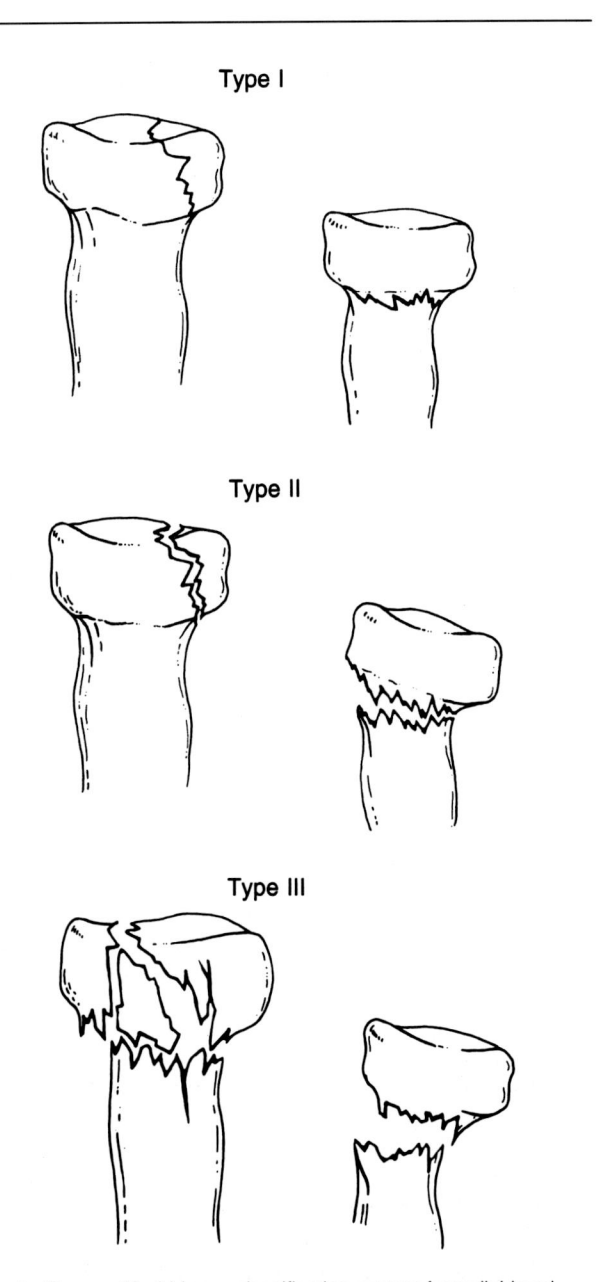

Fig. 4 The modified Mason classification system for radial head fractures. (Adapted with permission from Jupiter JB, Mehne DK: Trauma to the adult elbow and fractures of the distal humerus, in Browner B, Jupiter J, Levine A, et al (eds): *Skeletal Trauma*. Philadelphia, PA, WB Saunders, 1992, vol 2, pp 1125–1175.)

outcome in those treated surgically.[25] The patients so treated were found to have less pain, more motion, improved grip strength, and higher levels of function in activities of daily living.

When faced with the more complex Mason type III (comminuted) or type IV (associated with dislocation fractures), surgical intervention is needed. The surgical timing, method of treatment, and management of associated injuries represent contemporary questions. In most instances, internal fixation is the preferred management if the radial head fracture is amenable. However, because this is not always the case, alternative treatments must be identified. If resection of a fragmented radial head is necessary, the elbow is tested in a valgus stress at 30° of flexion to determine the status of the MCLs. If unstable, primary repair of these ligaments should be considered. In most cases, the ligaments will be found to have been avulsed from their origin on the distal humerus. In addition, a radial head spacer can be used in conjunction with repair of the lateral capsular and ligamentous structures, which function as secondary stabilizers of the elbow joint. If the complex fracture is associated with interosseous membrane and distal radioulnar joint disruption (the "Essex-Lopresti" lesion), realignment and stabilization of the distal radioulnar joint, temporary fixation of the distal ulna to radius with a K-wire for 4 to 6 weeks and either primary fixation of the radial head or temporary use of a radial head implant will be necessary to allow the soft tissues to heal.[30]

Fractures of the Capitellum

Capitellar fractures are extremely rare injuries, accounting for approximately 1% of all elbow fractures and about 6% of all fractures of the distal humerus. When displaced, failure to realign this articular fracture can lead to loss of elbow or forearm mobility and, in some instances, instability. The fractures commonly result from a fall on the outstretched hand with a resultant shear force across the distal humeral articular surface as the radial head is driven against the capitellum. As a result, the fracture tends to be displaced in an anteroposterior (AP) direction.

These fractures have classically been divided into three types: type I, complex capitellar fracture with variable extension into the lateral aspect of the trochlea; type II, which involves a shearing of the articular surface of the capitellum with little underlying subchondral bone; and type III, the comminuted fracture (Fig. 5).[31]

Treatment options advocated have ranged from closed treatment to surgical excision to open reduction and internal fixation. Although some have advocated excision of the fracture fragment, unsatisfactory results at 5-year follow-up using this technique have also been reported.[32-34] Open reduction and internal fixation has become increasingly popular with the development of small fragment fixation techniques.[34,35]

With type I fractures, consideration should be given to closed reduction. If successful, the elbow should be immobilized for 3 to 4 weeks, followed by active mobilization. If the closed reduction fails, one should proceed with open reduction and internal fixation. A lateral approach is recommended utilizing the interval between the anconeus and extensor carpi ulnaris. The radiocapitellar joint is identified and the fracture is reduced and temporarily held with K-wire fixation. The surgeon may then use standard small fragment screws inserted from a posterior to anterior direc-

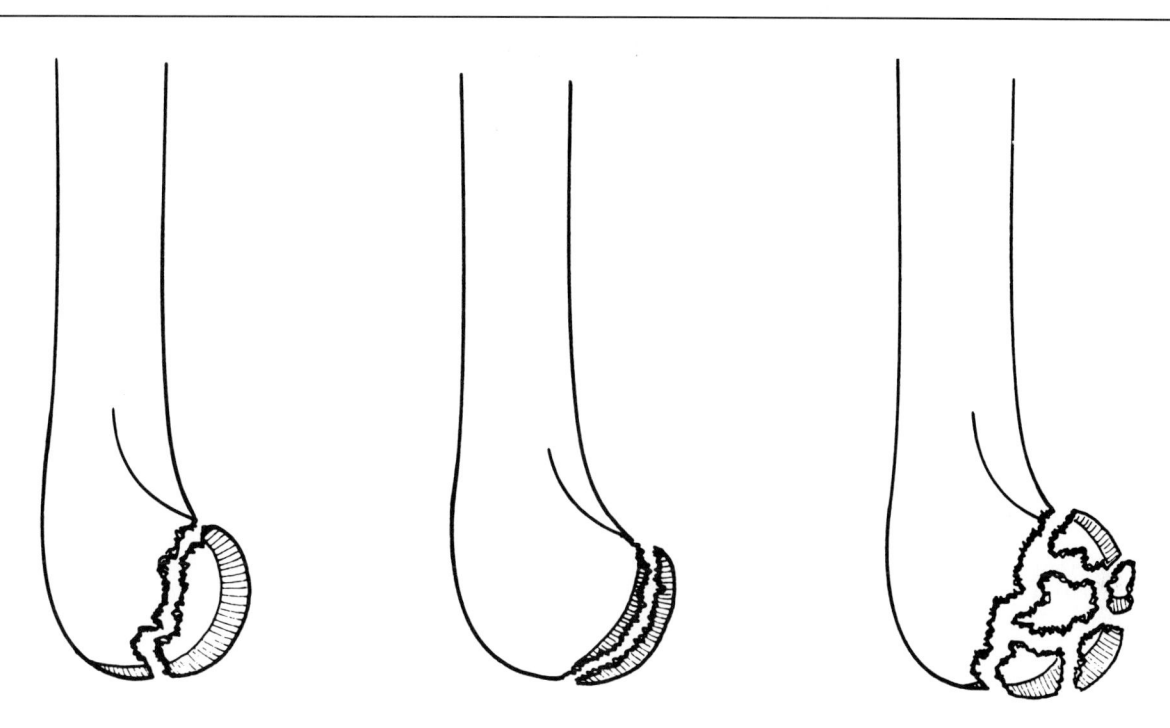

Fig. 5 Fractures of the capitellum. Type I, Complete fracture of the capitellum. Type II, The more superficial lesion of Kocher-Lorenz. Type III, Comminuted fracture of the capitellum. (Adapted with permission from Jupiter JB, Mehne DK: Trauma to the adult elbow and fractures of the distal humerus, in Browner B, Jupiter J, Levine A, et al (eds): *Skeletal Trauma*. Philadelphia, PA, WB Saunders, 1992, vol 2, pp 1125–1175.)

tion or the Herbert screw, which can be introduced from within the articular fragment with the head of the screw buried beneath the cartilage. Type II and III fractures may be less amenable to internal fixation. However, the Herbert screw or a small threaded K-wire may provide sufficient stability. Alternatively, excision of the fragment may be the only other option.

In one study of 29 patients with fractures of the capitellum, with 17 available for follow-up assessment, the authors found that a large number of the patients treated by resection of the capitellum had poor or fair results.[36] Instability and loss of motion were the most common problems that adversely affected the result. They recommend that if capitellar excision is to be performed, it should be done as soon as possible and that enough bone be removed to avoid postoperative impingement of the radial head. The authors' most favorable results were in those patients treated with open reduction and internal fixation followed by elbow mobilization.

A recent study reported on five patients with shear fractures of the distal humerus in whom the majority of the anterior aspect of the articular surface in the coronal plane had separated.[37] This injury was described as a "coronal shear" fracture. In these cases, the capitellum and trochlea were displaced *en masse* anteriorly and proximally, resulting in severe disruption of joint biomechanics. Four fractures were treated by open reduction and internal fixation and one by closed reduction and casting. Four patients required additional surgical procedures. However, all patients eventually obtained good or excellent results. The authors concluded that although surgical intervention is technically demanding and the complication rate is high, acceptable results can be obtained with prompt and rigid fixation and early active postoperative motion.

The most common complication after capitellar fracture is loss of elbow motion.[36,38] This is less frequent with open reduction and internal fixation and more common after fragment excision. A less frequently noted occurrence is osteonecrosis of the capitellar fragment.[30,33] Delayed excision is indicated if this becomes symptomatic.[36] A third potential complication is nonunion of the fracture fragment. This can be removed and an elbow soft-tissue release performed if it results in a significant loss of motion or becomes painful.

Unicondylar Fractures of the Distal Humerus

Isolated fractures of the distal humeral condyles in the adult are uncommon injuries that are often difficult to diagnose and treat effectively. Jupiter and associates,[39] in a retrospective review, report on 22 consecutive unicondylar fractures of the distal humerus treated by open reduction and internal fixation.

Overall, the authors found that 12 patients (55%) had an overall rating of excellent; 6, good; and 4, fair. They conclude that because these fractures often involve fragile articular fragments with limited subchondral bone and soft-tissue attachments, they are best managed by stable internal fixation. This treatment approach may facilitate rapid mobilization of the injured elbow, thereby decreasing the potential for residual contracture and loss of function.

Annotated References

1. Linscheid RL, O'Driscoll SW: Elbow dislocations, in Morrey BF (ed): *The Elbow and its Disorders,* ed 2. Philadelphia, PA, WB Saunders, 1993, pp 441–452.

2. Morrey BF: Anatomy of the elbow joint, in Morrey BF (ed): *The Elbow and its Disorders,* ed 2. Philadelphia, PA, WB Saunders, 1993, pp 16–52.

3. Morrey BF, An KN: Functional anatomy of the ligaments of the elbow. *Clin Orthop* 1985;201:84–90.

4. Jupiter JB, Mehne DK: Trauma to the adult elbow and fractures of the distal humerus, in Browner BD, Jupiter JB, Levine AM, et al (eds): *Skeletal Trauma: Fractures, Dislocations, Ligamentous Injuries.* Philadelphia, PA, WB Saunders, 1992, vol 2, pp 1125–1175.

5. O'Driscoll SW, Bell DF, Morrey BF: Posterolateral rotatory instability of the elbow. *J Bone Joint Surg* 1991;73A:440–446.

6. Melhoff TL, Noble PC, Bennett JB, et al: Simple dislocation of the elbow in the adult: Results after closed treatment. *J Bone Joint Surg* 1988;70A:244–249.

   The patients were evaluated at an average follow-up of 34 months. The authors found that, on examination, the average loss of extension was 12.3°. Although there was no radiographic evidence of substantial degenerative joint disease, they did note that 27 of 52 patients developed periarticular ossification. No elbow was unstable to stress examination. The authors concluded that a correlation exists between length of immobilization and the resultant flexion contracture and suggested a treatment protocol.

7. O'Driscoll SW, Morrey BF, Korinek S, et al: Elbow subluxation and dislocation: A spectrum of instability. *Clin Orthop* 1992;280:186–197.

8. Nestor BJ, O'Driscoll SW, Morrey BF: Ligamentous reconstruction for posterolateral rotatory instability of the elbow. *J Bone Joint Surg* 1992;74A:1235–1241.

9. Josefsson PO, Johnell O, Gentz CF: Long-term sequelae of simple dislocation of the elbow. *J Bone Joint Surg* 1984;66A:927–930

   The authors performed a retrospective review of 52 cases treated nonsurgically with a 24-year follow-up. The elbows were evaluated for their range of motion as well as for radiographic changes. Of 52 patients studied, 19 had decreased elbow motion, although some of the patients were unaware of their loss. Instability was uncommon and when present was asymptomatic. Periarticular calcification was associated with a loss of extension. They noted that only one patient had to change his line of work and that no other patient was forced to change his/her habits with regard to any activity.

10. Josefsson PO, Gentz CF, Johnell O, et al: Surgical versus non-surgical treatment of ligamentous injuries following dislocation of the elbow joint: A prospective randomized study. *J Bone Joint Surg* 1987;69A:605–608.

    The authors conducted a randomized prospective study of 30 consecutive patients who were randomly assigned to either the surgical or nonsurgical protocol. Data did not support surgical treatment for simple dislocation of the elbow that could be reduced by closed means, whatever the underlying degree of ligamentous and muscular damage to the elbow.

11. Broberg MA, Morrey BF: Results of treatment of fracture-dislocations of the elbow. *Clin Orthop* 1987;216:109–119.

    The authors evaluated 24 patients with ulnohumeral dislocation and associated radial head fracture. On the basis of an objective functional grading score that included elements of pain, motion, strength, and stability, results were excellent in 3 (12%), good in 15 (62%), and fair in 6 (25%). The best results were obtained in patients with Mason type 2 injuries treated by closed reduction without fracture excision and with early complete radial head excision for a type 3 fracture. No cases of late instability and only one case of ectopic ossification were found. The poorest results were associated with prolonged immobilization.

12. Regan W, Morrey B: Fractures of the coronoid process of the ulna. *J Bone Joint Surg* 1989;71A:1348–1354.

    The authors retrospectively reviewed 35 patients who had a fracture of the coronoid process of the ulna. They identified three types of fractures and recommended treatment protocols for each type.

13. Colton CL: Fractures of the olecranon in adults: Classification and management. *Injury* 1973;5:121–129.

14. Schatzker J: Fractures of the olecranon, in Schatzker J, Tile M (eds): *The Rationale of Operative Fracture Care.* Berlin, Germany, Springer-Verlag, 1987, pp 89–95.

15. Wolfgang G, Burke F, Bush D, et al: Surgical treatment of displaced olecranon fractures by tension band wiring technique. *Clin Orthop* 1987;224:192–204.

16. Rowland SA, Burkhart SS: Tension band wiring of olecranon fractures: A modification of the AO technique. *Clin Orthop* 1992;277:238–242.

17. Murphy DF, Greene WB, Dameron TB: Displaced olecranon fractures in adults: Clinical evaluation. *Clin Orthop* 1987;224:215–223.

18. Murphy DF, Greene WB, Gilbert JA, et al: Displaced olecranon fractures in adults: Biomechanical analysis of fixation methods. *Clin Orthop* 1987;224:210–214.

19. Fyfe IS, Mossad MM, Holdsworth BJ: Methods of fixation of olecranon fractures: An experimental mechanical study. *J Bone Joint Surg* 1985;67B:367–372.

20. Gartsman GM, Sculco TP, Otis JC: Operative treatment of olecranon fractures: Excision or open reduction with internal fixation. *J Bone Joint Surg* 1981;63A:718–721.

21. McKeever FM, Buck RM: Fracture of the olecranon process of the ulna: Treatment by excision of fragment and repair of triceps tendon. *JAMA* 1947;135:1–5.

    The authors evaluated the results of ten fractures treated by excision. They concluded that instability of the elbow does not result from this procedure as long as the coronoid process and the vertical distal face of the trochlear (semilunar) notch of the ulna remains. They note that up to 80% of the trochlear notch can be excised and result in absolutely no loss in the stability of the elbow joint. This was also supported in a study by Gartsmann and associates.

22. Papagelopoulos PJ, Morrey BF: Treatment of nonunion of olecranon fractures. *J Bone Joint Surg* 1994;76B:627–635.

    The authors report on the treatment of 24 patients using either excision of the olecranon fragment, osteosynthesis, or joint replacement. Three additional patients were treated with activity as tolerated and one with immobilization. Sixteen patients had a good or excellent result.

23. Macko D, Szabo RM: Complications of tension-band wiring of olecranon fractures. *J Bone Joint Surg* 1985;67A:1396–1401.

    In their retrospective review of complications with tension band wiring of olecranon fractures, Macko and Szabo found that pin migration was the most common complication. They noted that 16 of 20 patients developed pain over prominent Kirschner wires at the elbow. The authors conclude that prominence of the wires was usually due to improper seating at the time of surgery and that it could be avoided by careful attention to surgical technique.

24. Johnston GW: A follow-up of one hundred cases of fracture of the head of the radius with a review of the literature. *Ulster Med J* 1962;31:51–56.

25. Khalfayan EE, Culp RW, Alexander AH: Mason type II radial head fractures: Operative versus nonoperative treatment. *J Orthop Trauma* 1992;6:283–289.

    The authors reviewed the treatment of cases of Mason type II radial head fractures. Sixteen cases were treated nonsurgically and 10 cases underwent open reduction and internal fixation. The indication for surgical intervention was a mechanical block to full elbow motion after arthrocentesis and instillation of local anesthetic. Patients treated surgically were found to have less pain, more motion, improved grip strength, and higher levels of function in activities of daily living.

26. Mason ML: Some observations on fractures of the head of the radius with a review of one hundred cases. *Br J Surg* 1954;42:123–132.

27. Radin EL, Riseborough EJ: Fractures of the radial head: A review of eighty-eight cases and analysis of the indications for excision of the radial head and non-operative treatment. *J Bone Joint Surg* 1966;48A:1055–1064.

28. Swanson AB, Jaeger SH, La Rochelle D: Comminuted fractures of the radial head: The role of silicone-implant replacement arthroplasty. *J Bone Joint Surg* 1981;63A:1039–1049.

29. Weseley MS, Barenfeld PA, Eisenstein AL: Closed treatment of isolated radial head fractures. *J Trauma* 1983;23:36–39.

30. Bryan RS: Fractures about the elbow in adults, in Murray DG (ed): American Academy of Orthopaedic Surgeons *Instructional Course Lectures XXX*. St. Louis, MO, CV Mosby, 1981, pp 200–223.

31. Bryan RS, Morrey BF: Fractures of the distal humerus, in Morrey BF (ed): *The Elbow and Its Disorders*. Philadelphia, PA, WB Saunders, 1985, pp 302–339.

32. Deshuttle R, Coyle M, Zawalsky J, et al: Fracture of the capitellum. *J Trauma* 1985;25:317–321.

33. Alvarez E, Patel MR, Nimberg G, et al: Fractures of the capitulum humeri. *J Bone Joint Surg* 1975;57A:1093–1096.

34. Lansinger O, Mare K: Fracture of the capitulum humeri. *Acta Orthop Scand* 1981;52:39–44.

35. Heim V, Pfeiffer KM: *Small Fragment Set Manual*. Berlin, Germany, Springer-Verlag, 1982.

36. Grantham SA, Norris TR, Bush DC: Isolated fracture of the humeral capitellum. *Clin Orthop* 1981;161:262–269.

37. Jupiter J, McKee M, Toh CL: Coronal shear fracture of the distal humerus. *J Shoulder Elbow Surg* 1994;3(suppl):70.

38. Collert S: Surgical management of fracture of the captulum humerus. *Acta Orthop Scand* 1977;48:603–606.

39. Jupiter JB, Neff U, Regazzoni P, et al: Unicondylar fractures of the distal humerus: An operative approach. *J Orthop Trauma* 1988;2:102–109.

6

Forearm Fractures

Introduction

In the management of displaced diaphyseal fractures of the forearm, treatment objectives are clear-cut. Anatomic fracture reduction, to restore the normal relationship between the radius and ulna, and stable fracture fixation, to facilitate the early return of forearm motion, are essential in obtaining a satisfactory functional outcome. The methods used to accomplish these objectives have remained essentially unchanged over the past decade. However, open fracture treatment recommendations have been substantially altered. Additionally, concerns regarding the advisability and timing of the removal of forearm plates and the treatment of radioulnar synostosis have recently been addressed.

Classification

Forearm fractures are most often characterized using general descriptive terms and eponymic labels. Overall, this type of "fracture classification" has been instrumental in formulating an appropriate treatment plan. Important factors include fracture location, fracture configuration, the presence of any radioulnar or radiohumeral articular involvement, and the status of the surrounding soft-tissue envelope.

Ideally, a specific classification scheme should provide better documentation of forearm injuries, thereby allowing a more critical analysis of treatment methods and further delineation of the expected clinical outcome. Two such systems have been developed. A classification system proposed by the Orthopaedic Trauma Association[1] has been revised and currently awaits formal publication. The AO/ASIF group, as part of their Comprehensive Classification of Fractures of Long Bones,[2] have presented a well-organized method that is currently in use (Fig. 1). Unfortunately, preliminary reports suggest that, in general, this system is overly complex and has the potential for a high degree of interobserver variability.[3,4] Specific deficiencies noted in the forearm portion of this classification include an inability to document the degree of fracture displacement and angular deformity or to describe the injury to the soft tissues.[4]

Separate classification systems exist for the grading of the soft-tissue injury in both open and closed fractures. For open fractures, the method of Gustilo and Anderson, later modified by Gustilo and associates,[5] is commonly used (Outline 1). However, its reliability as a basis for decision-making has recently been questioned.[6] Grading of the soft-tissue injury in closed fractures has had limited applicability for diaphyseal fractures of the forearm. The AO/ASIF group has recently proposed an extensive soft-tissue grading system[7] that incorporates specific skin, muscle-tendon, and neurovascular injury groups (Table 1) for use in conjunction with their fracture classification. This system may prove useful in eliminating the deficiencies of other methods.

Patient Evaluation

Diaphyseal fractures of the forearm are commonly caused by high-energy trauma, caused either by a direct blow (which is often the result of a motor vehicle accident) or by a fall from a height. Associated systemic and musculoskeletal injuries are frequent. Therefore, examination of the injured extremity, even in those with an apparently isolated injury, should be just one part of a well-organized overall patient evaluation.

Examination of the extremity must include a detailed neurologic and vascular evaluation, as well as a careful assessment of the soft tissues. Although the Monteggia (fracture of the ulna associated with dislocation of the radial head) and Galeazzi (fracture of the radius associated with dislocation of the distal radioulnar joint) lesions are well known, a myriad of other bone and soft-tissue combination injuries have been described that involve a fracture of one or both forearm bones.[8,9] Therefore, the initial radiographic evaluation requires anteroposterior and lateral views of the entire forearm, wrist, and elbow.

Patients with Multiple Injuries

Forearm fractures often occur in conjunction with additional injuries to the musculoskeletal or other systems.[1,10,11] The treatment objectives are no different in these patients than in those with an isolated injury. Early surgical treatment is desirable.[1,11] Delayed surgery is more difficult and appears to increase the risk of radioulnar synostosis.[10-12] However, in the severely injured polytrauma patient, surgi-

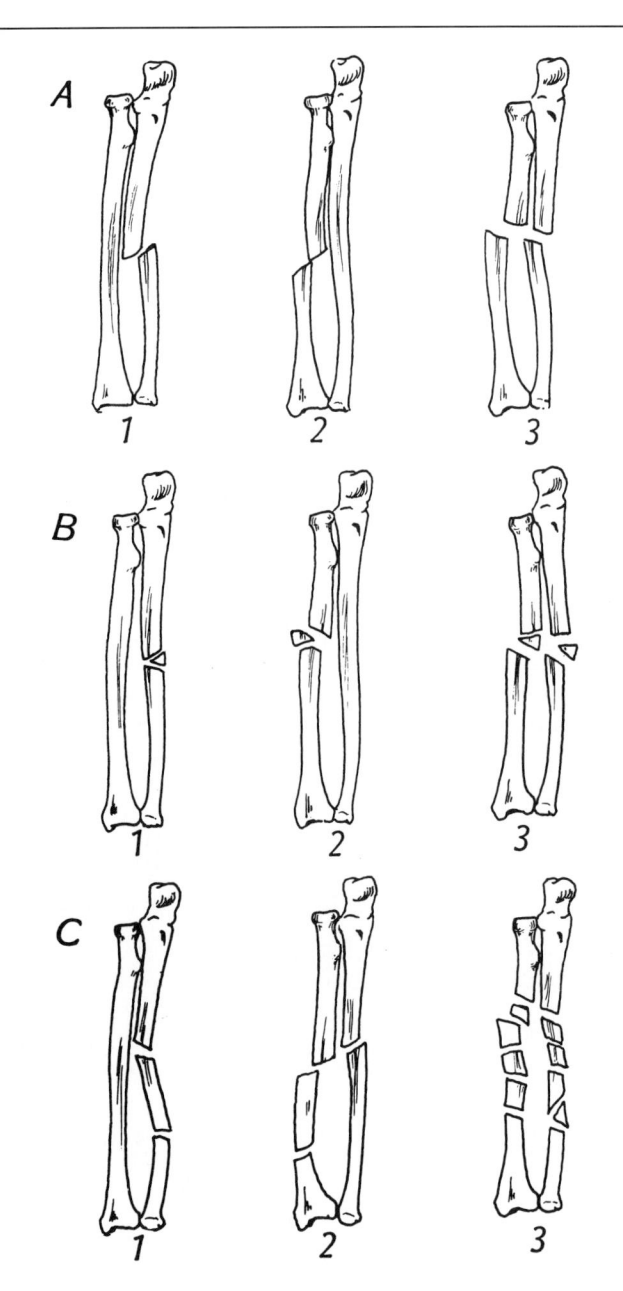

Fig. 1 AO/ASIF classification of diaphyseal forearm fractures. **A**, Simple fracture: 1, ulna (radius intact); 2, radius (ulna intact); 3, both bones. **B**, wedge fracture: 1, ulna (radius intact); 2, radius (ulna intact); 3, both bones (wedge of one, simple or wedge of the other). **C**, complex fracture (segmental or comminuted): 1, ulna (radius intact, simple or wedge); 2, radius (ulna intact, simple or wedge); 3, both bones. (Adapted with permission from Müller ME, Nazarian S, Koch P, et al (eds): *The Comprehensive Classification of Fractures of Long Bones*. Berlin, Germany, Springer-Verlag, 1990, pp 96–105.)

Outline 1 Gustilo classification of open fractures[5]

Type

I A wound less than 1 cm long with little soft-tissue damage; the fracture pattern is simple with little comminution

II A wound more than 1 cm long without extensive soft-tissue damage, flaps, or avulsion; contamination and fracture comminution are moderate

III Extensive soft-tissue damage, contamination, and fracture comminution
   IIIA Soft-tissue coverage is adequate; comminuted and segmental high-energy fractures are included regardless of wound size
   IIIB Extensive soft-tissue injury with massive contamination and severe fracture comminution requiring a local or free flap for coverage
   IIIC Arterial injury requiring repair

cal intervention for the forearm fracture is best delayed until systemic conditions have improved.

Associated Musculoskeletal Injury As previously mentioned, a great number of ipsilateral ligamentous and bony injuries can occur along with the diaphyseal fracture of one or both bones of the forearm.[8] Over time, the "classic" Galeazzi and Monteggia fracture-dislocation patterns have been expanded and redefined. The Galeazzi eponym, originally defined as fracture of the distal third of the radial shaft with an associated dislocation of the distal radioulnar joint (DRUJ), has been applied when referring to a fracture anywhere along the radial shaft as well as to fractures to both radius and ulna that occur in conjunction with a DRUJ injury.

Likewise, in addition to the four main "variations" of the Monteggia fracture-dislocation described by Bado, there are also "equivalent" lesions to consider[13] (Outline 2). Other described combinations of bony and ligamentous injury are basically variations on the same theme—a previously unreported association of fracture of one or both forearm bones in conjunction with a proximal and/or distal injury of the elbow, forearm, or wrist. The importance of these reports lies not so much in the description of the particular injury, but in the recognition that additional injury can occur with any diaphyseal forearm fracture and can easily be missed.[8,14] In general, these are all unstable injuries that require surgical intervention for reduction and stabilization of both the forearm fracture and the associated injury. A delay in diagnosis often has an adverse effect on functional outcome. In some cases, the site of the associated injury is not initially evident radiographically.[8] Therefore, a high index of suspicion is required, along with quality radiographs of the entire forearm, elbow, and wrist. In one small series of patients who had apparently isolated fractures of one forearm bone, radionuclide bone scanning was used successfully to screen for a second site of injury.[8]

Radiographic signs of injury to the DRUJ include fracture at the base of the ulnar styloid, widening of the joint space on the anteroposterior radiograph, dislocation of the radius relative to the ulna on the lateral radiograph, and radial shortening greater than 5 mm.[15] If the radial head is properly located, a line drawn through the radial head and shaft in any radiographic projection should align with the capitellum. A lateral radiograph of the elbow with the arm in supination can also be used to evaluate the position of

Table 1 AO/ASIF classification of soft-tissue injury[7]

Skin Injury		Musculotendinous Injury	
Integument Closed (IC)	Integument Open (IO)	(MT)	Neurovascular Injury (NV)
IC1 No injury	IO1 Inside out puncture	MT1 No injury	NV1 No injury
IC2 Contusion	IO2 Outside in < 5 cm wound	MT2 Localized injury, one compartment	NV2 Isolated nerve injury
IC3 Local degloving	IO3 > 5 cm wound with contused devitalized edges, local degloving	MT3 Two compartment involvement	NV3 Localized vascular injury
IC4 Extensive degloving	IO4 Full-thickness contusion, abrasion, or skin loss	MT4 Extensive muscle defect, tendon laceration	NV4 Combined neurovascular injury
IC5 Skin necrosis from contusion	IO5 Extensive degloving	MT5 Extensive crush or compartment syndrome	NV5 Subtotal or complete amputation

Outline 2 Monteggia lesions[13]

Type

1 Anterior dislocation of the radial head with an anteriorly angulated fracture of the ulnar diaphysis
  Equivalent: Fracture of the ulnar diaphysis and fracture of the radial head or neck

2 Posterior or posterolateral dislocation of the radial head with a posteriorly angulated fracture of the ulnar diaphysis
  Equivalent: Posterior dislocation of the elbow with a posteriorly angulated fracture of the ulnar diaphysis and fracture of the radial head or neck

3 Lateral or anterolateral dislocation of the radial head and fracture of the proximal ulnar metaphysis

4 Anterior dislocation of the radial head with a proximal third diaphyseal fracture of both bones of the forearm

the radial head.[13] Two lines are drawn: one tangential to the bicipital tuberosity and the anterior border of the radial head extending beyond the distal humerus, the other tangential to the posterior border of the radial head parallel to the first line (Fig. 2). These two lines should enclose the entire capitellum.

A less subtle combination injury is the so-called "floating elbow." Ipsilateral fractures of the humeral shaft and forearm are severe high-energy injuries. These often occur in conjunction with multiple other injuries, and open fractures are common.[16,17] The best results are obtained by open reduction and internal fixation of both the humerus and the forearm fractures.[16,17]

Open Fractures Irrigation and debridement of an open fracture with the institution of appropriate intravenous antibiotics should be performed on an emergent basis. Initially, the traumatic wounds are left open. Subsequent treatment depends on the time delay between injury and surgical intervention, the magnitude of the soft-tissue injury, and, as noted earlier, the presence of any additional injuries.

Despite recent concerns regarding the reliability of the Gustilo classification of open fractures,[6] reported series do indicate that wound severity graded according to this method is the most important prognostic factor in the treatment of open forearm fractures.[11,18-21] Assuming a treatment delay of less than 24 hours, open reduction and plate fixation is currently preferred for the acute stabilization of types I, II, and IIIA open fractures.[11,18,19] Autogenous cancellous bone grafting should be performed at the time of definitive wound closure in comminuted fractures when interfragmentary compression cannot be obtained.[1,11]

For type IIIB and IIIC injuries, treatment must be individualized. External fixation[20,21] and plating[1,11,19] both have a place in the treatment armamentarium. For patients who have extensive soft-tissue loss and severe wound contamination, or for those in whom multiple injuries preclude early definitive surgical treatment, primary external fixation should be considered.[21] Conversion to plate fixation, if indicated, should be performed after wound healing.[21] Overall, results are much poorer for these severe injuries than for types I, II, and IIIA injuries.

Open fractures caused by gunshots present a special situation. Low-velocity gunshot fractures do not require formal debridement, but should otherwise be handled as type I injuries.[22] Although these are low-energy injuries, associated problems such as neurovascular injury, compartment syndrome, and fracture comminution are common.[22,23] Furthermore, while the mechanism remains unclear, isolated gunshot fractures of one forearm bone can be associated with ipsilateral ligamentous injury. One report included four Galeazzi lesions.[22] Two were missed, which resulted in a poor clinical outcome.[22] High-energy injuries, such as close-range shotgun blasts and high-velocity gunshots, should be managed as type IIIB injuries.

Compartment Syndrome Compartment syndrome of the forearm is usually thought of as being associated with high-energy trauma.[24] However, it is not uncommon following low-velocity gunshot wounds.[22,23] Other open fractures are also at risk.[24] Predisposing factors include vascular injury, coagulopathy, and a history of external limb compression. Early diagnosis and subsequent fasciotomy are mandatory in order to provide the best chance for recovery.[24,25] The most reliable physical findings are marked pain on passive digital extension and reduced hand sensibility or paresthesias.[25] A high index of suspicion and judicious use of compartment pressure monitoring are essential.

Neurovascular Injury Neurovascular injury is uncommon following a closed forearm fracture. One well-described injury pattern is the loss of posterior interosseous nerve function in association with a Monteggia lesion. Prognosis

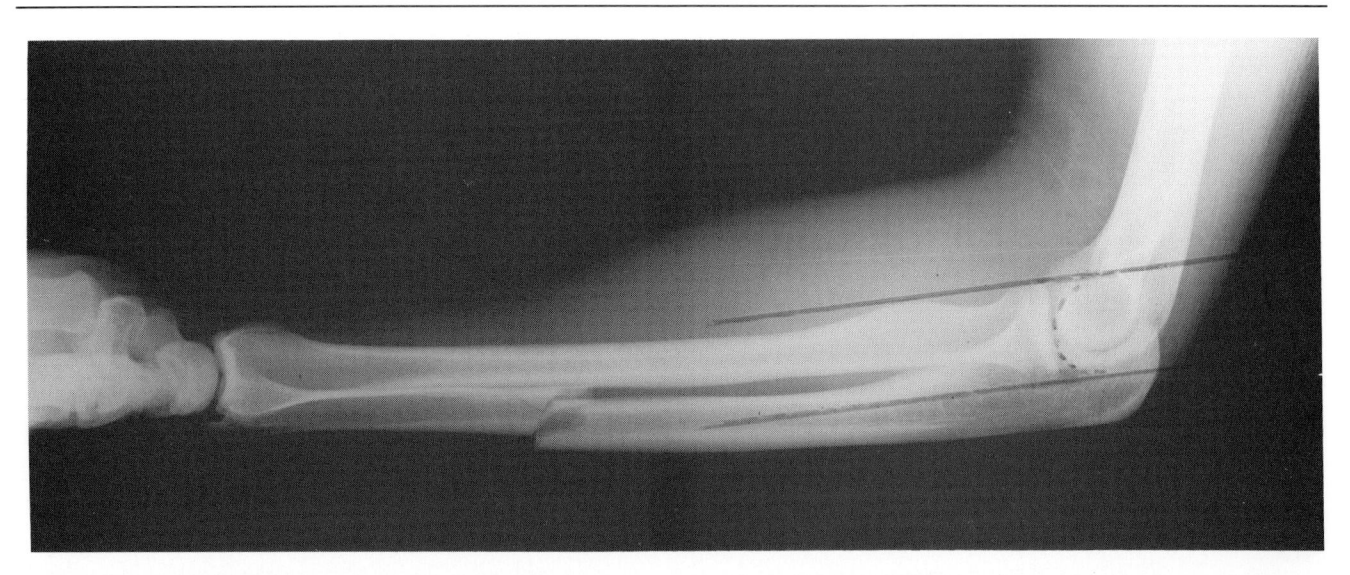

Fig. 2 Lateral radiograph with the forearm in full supination. The two parallel lines are drawn and the outline of the capitellum is highlighted, demonstrating a normal relationship between the radial head and capitellum. This injury, a stable, nonangulated fracture of the ulna, was caused by a direct blow. Closed treatment was followed by uneventful fracture healing and return of full function.

for recovery is good. Open fractures present an entirely different situation. Nerve injury is frequent, especially in type III open fractures.[19,20] In one report, 6 of 18 patients with type III open wounds sustained a major peripheral nerve injury that required repair.[19] The nerve injury often has an adverse effect on functional outcome.[19,20]

Arterial injury is a frequent sequela of penetrating forearm trauma.[26] Injury to both forearm arteries with distal ischemia requires immediate vessel repair. Injuries to one artery with adequate distal blood flow to the hand do not present clear-cut indications for vessel repair. Recent reports citing improved patency rates support preserving a dual arterial supply to the hand.[26,27] Single vessel ligation should be considered when the repair cannot be accomplished readily or when a more pressing associated injury demands priority.[26] After successful arterial repair, functional results are usually dictated by the severity of associated nerve or musculoskeletal injury.[26,28]

Treatment

The treatment of diaphyseal fractures of the forearm is predicated on the belief that anatomic fracture reduction is required to restore normal forearm motion. This supposition is supported by a number of cadaver studies, indicating that forearm motion is limited by angular deformity of one or both bones of greater than 10.[29–31] Clinical data appear to corroborate this laboratory finding.[31,32] However, angular deformity alone, as determined by routine biplanar radiography, cannot provide a completely accurate correlation with limited forearm motion, especially for fractures that involve the radius.[31] Other factors such as the plane, level, and displacement of the fracture play a role.[29,31] It is no surprise, then, that the restoration of the normal radial bow, which encompasses all of these anatomic factors, is an extremely important prognostic indicator of functional outcome.[33]

Early active forearm motion is also thought to be important in the treatment of forearm fractures. Injuries involving both bones appear to derive the most benefit from this early motion therapy.[34]

Nonsurgical Care

Despite some reports recommending a wider range of applicability, closed treatment of diaphyseal fractures of the forearm is best applied to stable isolated fractures of the distal two thirds of the ulna with 10 or less of angular deformity.[32,35] Stable fractures have been defined as those displaced less than 50% of the shaft diameter.[36,37] Their treatment does not involve any attempt at fracture reduction. In these selected cases, results are generally excellent, with the return of normal motion and fracture union reported in over 96% of patients (Fig. 2).[35,37] Functional bracing, as opposed to cast immobilization, appears to offer the advantage of greater patient satisfaction.[35] As noted previously, however, the potential for occult instability must always be considered. Fractures of the distal two thirds of the ulna with greater angulation or displacement and those involving the proximal one third of the ulnar shaft are best treated by other means.[32,35,37]

Closed treatment has an extremely limited role in the care of fractures of the radial shaft. Nondisplaced isolated fractures maintaining a normal radial bow, such as those caused by a low-energy gunshot wound, may be considered for this method of treatment.[22] Once again, care must be taken to ensure that there is no associated radioulnar instability.[22] Fractures of both bones of the forearm are unstable (prone to shortening and angulation) and require surgical management.

External Fixation

External fixation is not indicated for the routine treatment of diaphyseal fractures of the forearm. Its main indication is in the management of open fractures with severe soft-tissue injury (types IIIB and C).[20,21] The objective is to stabilize the limb while minimizing the risk of infection. Although it has been shown that the Hoffman C-series external fixator can maintain near anatomic fracture alignment (84% with less than 5 of angulation in one series), re-reduction is often required (approximately 10%).[38] Other secondary procedures are routinely needed (as high as 50% in one report[21]) in order to obtain fracture union. Pin site colonization is also a frequent problem. However, its progression to clinical soft-tissue infection and osteomyelitis is uncommon.[20,21,38] Despite a low infection rate (less than 5%), good or excellent functional results can be expected in less than two thirds of these severely injured patients.[20,35,38] Currently, these results are attributed more to the magnitude of the initial injury than to any intrinsic deficiencies of external fixation.

Intramedullary Nailing

Since the 1950s, intramedullary (IM) devices of varying shapes and sizes have been advocated for use in the forearm. Although investigators using these implants have more recently reported improved results, current concerns, as in the past, include rotational instability, loss of the normal radial bow, shortening of axially unstable oblique and comminuted fractures, and fracture nonunion.[39-41] The development of locked IM devices applicable to fractures of the forearm may address these concerns adequately.[42] At present, the indications for IM nailing of forearm fractures are not clearly defined.

Plate Fixation

Open reduction and internal plate fixation as advocated by the AO/ASIF group remains the surgical method of choice for the management of closed and types I, II, and IIIA open diaphyseal fractures of the forearm.[1,11,13,15,16-19,22,32,43] The high rates of fracture union (greater than 96%) and overall satisfactory limb function (greater than 85%) reported by Anderson and associates[43] in 1975 have been duplicated subsequently by many investigators.[1,11] Infection rates are also low (less than 3%). This surgical technique, as supported by these results, appears to satisfy the treatment objectives of anatomic and stable fracture fixation and is the standard to which all other treatment methods must be compared.

The reported numbers are small and the situation is not as clear-cut for types IIIB and IIIC open fractures. It appears that better fracture alignment and union rates are obtained in exchange for an increased risk of infection.[18,38] In one series, despite a relatively low infection rate (9%), functional results were good or excellent in only six (55%) of the 11 types IIIB and C injured patients.[19] Many of the unsatisfactory outcomes could be attributed to residual nerve deficits, pointing again to the magnitude of the initial injury as the limiting factor.

Monteggia and Galeazzi lesions constitute a special subset of forearm injury. These fracture-dislocations and their equivalents require anatomic reduction of the diaphyseal fracture component in order to restore the normal axial interrelationship of the forearm bones and allow reduction of the dislocation.[13,44] Fracture fixation is accomplished best by plating. In most cases, the anatomic reduction and fixation of the diaphyseal fracture result in an indirect anatomic and stable reduction of the joint dislocation, allowing early motion of the extremity.[44] Instability or failure to achieve a reduction of the dislocation may be caused by malreduction of the diaphyseal fracture. An irreducible joint dislocation after anatomic fracture fixation indicates the need for open reduction of the joint.[13,44] Residual instability of a reduced DRUJ after anatomic plating of the radius can usually be addressed by immobilizing the limb in supination for 6 weeks postoperatively.[13] Temporary pin fixation of the DRUJ is rarely required. Cast immobilization after surgical treatment of closed, unstable single bone forearm injuries has not been shown to have any detrimental effect on functional outcome.[34]

Autogenous iliac crest cancellous bone grafting is generally recommended for comminuted fractures or those with bone loss.[1,11,43] For open fractures treated by immediate plate fixation, the bone graft is usually applied at the time of wound closure.[1,11] Depending on the investigator, the recommended criteria for bone grafting vary. Anderson and associates[43] advise the use of bone graft if comminution involves more than one third of the cortical circumference, while Moed and associates[11] recommend bone grafting whenever fracture comminution precludes interfragmentary compression. Chapman and associates[1] grafted all open fractures and all comminuted fractures, as well as those with bone loss—68 (53%) of 129 fractures in the series. Their fracture union rate was 98%. In series reporting poor results, some published essentially for the purpose of demonstrating errors in judgment and plating technique, injudicious failure to bone graft is a common theme.[45,46] Despite the fact that more recent investigators have stated otherwise,[33] the aggressive use of autogenous cancellous bone graft seems warranted.

Complications of Plate Fixation

Infection Deep infection is uncommon after plating of closed and low-grade open forearm fractures. Acute infection requires irrigation and debridement of all nonviable tissue. The plate should be maintained if it has not loosened and continues to provide stabilization of the fracture fragments. Late infections, presenting after fracture union, can be addressed by debridement and plate removal.[11] In either an acute or late infection presenting with failed hardware and/or requiring extensive bony debridement, the hardware should be removed and the forearm stabilized by casting or external fixation. When the infection has cleared and the tissues are supple, reconstruction by replating and bone grafting can be undertaken.[46,47]

Iatrogenic Nerve Injury When nerve injury occurs as a result of surgical treatment, it commonly involves a branch of the radial nerve.[33,43] Injury to the posterior interosseous nerve is associated with the use of the dorsal Thompson surgical approach. This injury is mainly caused by excessive retraction during the reduction and fixation of a fracture of the proximal radius. The nerve deficit is usually transient. Injury to the sensory branch of the radial nerve is associated with the volar Henry approach.[33,43] Failure to identify and protect the nerve during the surgical approach increases the risk of injury. Transected nerves have a poor prognosis. The return of sensation in stretched or contused nerves is variable.

Iatrogenic injury to the anterior interosseous nerve is thought to be caused by traction or by entrapment by bone forceps during radial fracture fixation.[48] Rarely reported, its true frequency may be underestimated. When a deficit is discovered in the postoperative period, documentation is often lacking regarding the nerve function at the time of the initial fracture trauma. Often the patient is the first to notice the nerve deficit as a weakness in pinch strength. This deficit is usually transient. Care should be taken to document the status of anterior interosseous nerve function in both the immediate pre- and postoperative periods.

Fixation Failure and Nonunion The postoperative complications of fixation failure and nonunion are interrelated, as one usually follows the other. In the forearm, the AO/ASIF group recommends a 3.5 mm dynamic compression plate (DCP) with a screw through at least seven cortices of each main fracture fragment, including an interfragmentary lag screw.[49] A six- or seven-hole plate is used depending upon whether the interfragmentary screw is placed through or independent of the plate. Although a short fracture fragment may limit the extent of fixation, an eight-hole plate (eight cortices in each main fragment) is recommended in comminuted fractures and whenever an interfragmentary screw cannot be used.[1,49] Biomechanical documentation is lacking, and, in actual clinical practice, use of six cortices of screw fixation in each main fracture fragment is often accepted. However, early fixation failure can usually be attributed to the failure to follow the recommendations of the AO/ASIF group.[1,45,46] Poor fixation technique is one cause of nonunion.[11,45,46] Infection and failure to recognize the need for bone grafting are other contributory factors.[1,11,45,46] Although the specific management sequence for these problems must be individualized, ultimately, revision fracture fixation and/or bone grafting are required.

Synostosis While the incidence of radioulnar synostosis following forearm plating has ranged from 0% to 11% in reported series, the most commonly reported figure is approximately 3%.[1,11,33,43,45,46,50] Risk factors for its development include: fracture of both bones at the same level, high-energy trauma, head injury, infection, operation on both bones through a single Boyd-type surgical approach, delayed operation (approximately 2 weeks or more), bone graft placed in proximity to the interosseous membrane, and the use of screws that are too long and protrude into the interosseous membrane.[12,50] A classification system has been devised based on the anatomic location of the synostosis within the forearm: type 1, distal intra-articular; type 2, diaphyseal; and type 3, proximal third.[12] Resection of the cross-union with or without the insertion of an interpositional barrier, such as silicone sheeting, can restore useful rotation of the forearm in approximately 50% of patients.[12,51] Type 1 lesions appear to have the worst prognosis, type 2 the best.[12,51] Timing of the surgical resection is thought to be important, best performed after one year, but no later than three years following the injury.[51] Adjunctive postoperative low-dose radiation as an alternative to the use of interpositional materials has been successful in a small number of cases.[52] Single-fraction, low-dose (800 cGy) limited-field postoperative radiation may improve results and eliminate the necessity for a 1- to 3-year treatment window.[52]

Plate Removal

Despite the concerns of stress protection under the plate and stress concentration at the end of the plate, the available data indicate that the complications of plate removal outweigh the potential consequences of retaining the plate.[53–55] One widely recognized complication is refracture after plate removal, with an incidence ranging from 4% to 20%.[1,33,53,55,56] The main causes of refracture are the use of too large a plate (4.5 mm DCP) and premature plate removal.[1,33,56,57] Most refractures after plate removal occur through the original fracture site or through a screw hole,[33,56,57] indicating more a problem with incomplete fracture healing and weakness at the screw holes than generalized cortical atrophy.[58] Bone density does not return to its prefracture level until approximately 21 months after fixation.[59] Furthermore, retained plates do not appear to have an adverse effect on bone mass or bone mineral density.[54,59] Therefore, if a forearm plate is to be removed, it seems prudent to allow this time interval to pass. Other reported complications of plate removal include infection and nerve injury. Their incidence ranges between 10% and 20% and increases when the surgical procedure is not performed by an experienced surgeon.[53,55] Plate removal is often performed in "symptomatic" patients—those complaining of barometric pain, exercise pain, proximity of the plate to the skin, etc. In one series, however, 67% of the patients noted residual symptoms after plate removal, and 9% believed their condition had deteriorated.[55] The routine removal of forearm plates is not recommended.[1,53,54]

Annotated References

1. Chapman MW, Gordon JE, Zissimos AG: Compression-plate fixation of acute fractures of the diaphyses of the radius and ulna. *J Bone Joint Surg* 1989;71A:159–169.

   This retrospective review of 129 diaphyseal forearm fractures in 87 patients plated using AO/ASIF techniques demonstrated union in 98% and an excellent or satisfactory functional result in 92%. Refracture occurred in only 2 patients, both fixed with 4.5 mm DCPs. Forty-nine fractures were open. The overall infection rate was less than 3%. Immediate fixation of open fractures had a low complication rate. Routine autogenous bone grafting was performed in all comminuted and open fractures.

2. Müller ME, Nazarian S, Koch P, et al: *The Comprehensive Classification of Fractures of Long Bones.* Berlin, Germany, Springer-Verlag, 1990, pp 96–105.

3. Johnstone DJ, Radford WJ, Parnell EJ: Interobserver variation using the AO/ASIF classification of long bone fractures. *Injury* 1993;24:163–165.

4. Newey ML, Ricketts D, Roberts L: The AO classification of long bone fractures: An early study of its use in clinical practice. *Injury* 1993;24:309–312.

5. Gustilo RB, Merkow RL, Templeman D: Current concepts: Review of the management of open fractures. *J Bone Joint Surg* 1990;72A:299–304.

6. Brumback RJ, Jones AL: Interobserver agreement in the classification of open fractures of the tibia: The results of a survey of two hundred and forty-five orthopaedic surgeons. *J Bone Joint Surg* 1994;76A:1162–1166.

   The reliability of the Gustilo and Anderson classification of open fractures was tested on the basis of responses to a survey by 245 orthopaedic surgeons. The accepted supposition is that the subdivisions of this classification correlate with the level of wound contamination and/or impaired vascularity, allowing them to serve as a basis for decision-making and prognosis. Participant demographics were obtained and were correlated with their responses in classifying 12 open tibia fractures, which were displayed on videotape. The average agreement was 60% (range, 42% to 94%). In the participant subgroup of those with the most experience (trauma trained academicians), average agreement was only 66%. It was concluded that interobserver agreement is poor and that this classification system may not be adequate.

7. Rüedi TH, Border JR, Allgöwer M: Classification of soft tissue injuries, in Müller ME, Allgöwer M, Schneider R, et al (eds): *Manual of Internal Fixation: Techniques Recommended by the AO-ASIF Groups,* ed 3. Berlin, Germany, Springer-Verlag, 1991, pp 151–158.

8. Goldberg HD, Young JW, Reiner BI, et al: Double injuries of the forearm: A common occurrence. *Radiology* 1992;185:223–227.

   The various patterns of combined ipsilateral ligamentous and bony injury to the forearm as well as the potential for occult instability are emphasized. Of 119 patients studied, 80 had sustained a combination injury. Thirty-seven injuries were classic Galeazzi lesions. Thirteen patients had fractures of both forearm bones in association with either a dislocation of the radial head or disruption of the DRUJ. Eight patients had a fracture and dislocation involving the same bone. Six patients had Monteggia lesions and 4 had sustained a bipolar fracture-dislocation. In 12 of the 17 patients with radiographic evidence of only an isolated fracture of one bone, a second site of injury was subsequently demonstrated. In 8 of these, the occult second site was identified by using radionuclide bone scanning.

9. Jupiter JB, Kour AK, Richards RR, et al: The floating radius in bipolar fracture-dislocation of the forearm. *J Orthop Trauma* 1994;8:99–106.

10. Garland DE, Dowling V: Forearm fractures in the head-injured adult. *Clin Orthop* 1983;176:190–196.

11. Moed BR, Kellam JF, Foster RJ, et al: Immediate internal fixation of open fractures of the diaphysis of the forearm. *J Bone Joint Surg* 1986;68A:1008–1017.

    Fifty patients with 79 open fractures were retrospectively evaluated. Results were excellent or good in 85% with infection in 4% and nonunion in 7%. Immediate open reduction and internal fixation was recommended for open fractures. Of note, type III injuries were not further subclassified, as type III A, B, and C divisions were not described until 1987.

12. Vince KG, Miller JE: Cross-union complicating fracture of the forearm: Part I. Adults. *J Bone Joint Surg* 1987;69A:640–653.

13. Reckling FW: Unstable fracture-dislocations of the forearm (Monteggia and Galeazzi lesions). *J Bone Joint Surg* 1982;64A:857–863.

14. Trousdale RT, Amadio PC, Cooney WP, et al: Radio-ulnar dissociation: A review of twenty cases. *J Bone Joint Surg* 1992;74A:1486–1497.

15. Moore TM, Klein JP, Patzakis MJ, et al: Results of compression-plating of closed Galeazzi fractures. *J Bone Joint Surg* 1985;67A:1015–1021.

    Thirty-six closed Galeazzi fractures were treated with compression plating. Anatomic reduction was accomplished in 35 (97%) and 35 returned to regular activities. Based on the results, the technique was recommended despite a 39% complication rate.

16. Rogers JF, Bennett JB, Tullos HS: Management of concomitant ipsilateral fractures of the humerus and forearm. *J Bone Joint Surg* 1984;66A:552–556.

17. Lange RH, Foster RJ: Skeletal management of humeral shaft fractures associated with forearm fractures. *Clin Orthop* 1985;195:173–177.

18. Duncan R, Geissler W, Freeland AE, et al: Immediate internal fixation of open fractures of the diaphysis of the forearm. *J Orthop Trauma* 1992;6:25–31.

19. Jones JA: Immediate internal fixation of high-energy open forearm fractures. *J Orthop Trauma* 1991;5:272–279.

    Eighteen open fractures (7 type IIIA, 8 type IIIB, and 3 type IIIC) were treated with immediate open reduction and internal fixation. Bone grafting was performed after wound healing in fractures with bone loss or comminution. The deep infection rate was 5%. Functional results (good or excellent in 66%, overall) were best in patients with type IIIA injuries.

20. Levin LS, Goldner RD, Urbaniak JR, et al: Management of severe musculoskeletal injuries of the upper extremity. *J Orthop Trauma* 1990;4:432–440.

21. Smith DK, Cooney WP: External fixation of high-energy upper extremity injuries. *J Orthop Trauma* 1990;4:7–18.

22. Lenihan MR, Brien WW, Gellman H, et al: Fractures of the forearm resulting from low-velocity gunshot wounds. *J Orthop Trauma* 1992;6:32–35.

23. Moed BR, Fakhouri AJ: Compartment syndrome after low-velocity gunshot wounds to the forearm. *J Orthop Trauma* 1991;5:134–137.

24. Broström L-A, Stark A, Svartengren G: Acute compartment syndrome in forearm fractures. *Acta Orthop Scand* 1990;61:50–53.

    Sixteen patients with acute compartment syndrome complicating forearm fractures were evaluated. High-energy trauma was the cause in eleven. Emergent treatment included fasciotomy and fracture fixation. Fracture healing was not impaired, however, weakness and stiffness of the arm were common complaints. Mean decrease in grip strength was 54% and only 8 patients returned to their previous occupation.

25. Gelberman RH, Garfin SR, Hergenroeder PT, et al: Compartment syndromes of the forearm: Diagnosis and treatment. *Clin Orthop* 1981;161:252–260.

26. Lee RE, Obeid FN, Horst HM, et al: Acute penetrating arterial injuries of the forearm: Ligation or repair? *Am Surg* 1985;51:318–324.

27. Rothkopf DM, Chu B, Gonzalez F, et al: Radial and ulnar artery repairs: Assessing patency rates with color Doppler ultrasonographic imaging. *J Hand Surg* 1993;18A:626–628.

28. Cikrit DF, Dalsing MC, Bryant BJ, et al: An experience with upper-extremity vascular trauma. *Am J Surg* 1990;160:229–233.

29. Matthews LS, Kaufer H, Garver DF, et al: The effect on supination-pronation of angular malalignment of fractures of both bones of the forearm: An experimental study. *J Bone Joint Surg* 1982;64A:14–17.

30. Tarr RR, Garfinkel AI, Sarmiento A: The effects of angular and rotational deformities of both bones of the forearm: An in vitro study. *J Bone Joint Surg* 1984;66A:65-70.

31. Sarmiento A, Ebramzadeh E, Brys D, et al: Angular deformities and forearm function. *J Orthop Res* 1992;10:121–133.

32. Zych GA, Latta LL, Zagorski JB: Treatment of isolated ulnar shaft fractures with prefabricated functional fracture braces. *Clin Orthop* 1987;219:194–200.

33. Schemitsch EH, Richards RR: The effect of malunion on functional outcome after plate fixation of fractures of both bones of the forearm in adults. *J Bone Joint Surg* 1992;74A:1068–1078.

    Fifty-five patients with both-bone fractures of the forearm treated by plating were evaluated at an average of 6 years after injury. Ninety-eight percent of the fractures healed. Recovery of grip strength and forearm motion correlated with the restoration of the normal radial bow.

34. Grace TG, Eversmann WW Jr: Forearm fractures: Treatment by rigid fixation with early motion. *J Bone Joint Surg* 1980;62A:433–438.

35. Gebuhr P, Hülmich P, Ørsnes T, et al: Isolated ulnar shaft fractures: Comparison of treatment by a functional brace and long-arm cast. *J Bone Joint Surg* 1992;74B:757–759.

36. Dymond IWD: The treatment of isolated fractures of the distal ulna. *J Bone Joint Surg* 1984;66B:408–410.

37. Ostermann PAW, Ekkernkamp A, Henry SL, et al: Bracing of stable shaft fractures of the ulna. *J Orthop Trauma* 1994;8:245–248.

38. Schuind F, Andrianne Y, Burny F: Treatment of forearm fractures by Hoffmann external fixation: A study of 93 patients. *Clin Orthop* 1991;266:197–204.

39. Aho AJ, Nieminen SJ, Salo U, et al: Antebrachium fractures: Rush pin fixation today in the light of late results. *J Trauma* 1984;24:604–610.

40. Street DM: Intramedullary forearm nailing. *Clin Orthop* 1986;212:219–230.

41. Ono M, Bechtold JE, Merkow RL, et al: Rotational stability of diaphyseal fractures of the radius and ulna fixed with Rush pins and/or fracture bracing. *Clin Orthop* 1989;240:236–243.

42. Schemitsch EH, Jones D, Henley MB, et al: A comparison of malreduction after plate and intramedullary nail fixation of forearm fractures. *J Orthop Trauma* 1995;9:8–16.

43. Anderson LD, Sisk T, Tooms RE, et al: Compression-plate fixation in acute diaphyseal fractures of the radius and ulna. *J Bone Joint Surg* 1975;57A:287–297.

44. Strehle J, Gerber C: Distal radioulnar joint function after Galeazzi fracture-dislocations treated by open reduction and internal plate fixation. *Clin Orthop* 1993;293:240–245.

45. Stern PJ, Drury WJ: Complications of plate fixation of forearm fractures. *Clin Orthop* 1983;175:25–29.

46. Langkamer VG, Ackroyd CE: Internal fixation of forearm fractures in the 1980s: Lessons to be learnt. *Injury* 1991;22:97–102.

47. Grace TG, Eversman WW: The management of segmental bone loss associated with forearm fractures. *J Bone Joint Surg* 1980;62A:1150–1155.

48. Hope PG: Anterior interosseous nerve palsy following internal fixation of the proximal radius. *J Bone Joint Surg* 1988;70B:280–282.

49. Heim U: Forearm and hand/mini-implants, in Müeller ME, Allgöwer M, Schneider R, et al (eds): *Manual of Internal Fixation*, ed 3. Berlin, Germany, Springer-Verlag, 1991, pp 453–484.

50. Bauer G, Arand M, Mutschler W: Post-traumatic radioulnar synostosis after forearm fracture osteosynthesis. *Arch Orthop Trauma Surg* 1991;110:142–145.

51. Failla JM, Amadio PC, Morrey BF: Post-traumatic proximal radio-ulnar synostosis: Results of surgical treatment. *J Bone Joint Surg* 1989;71A:1208–1213.

52. Cullen JP, Pellegrini VD Jr, Miller RJ, et al: Treatment of traumatic radioulnar synostosis by excision and postoperative low-dose irradiation. *J Hand Surg* 1994;19A:394–401.

    Four cases of posttraumatic radio-ulnar synostosis (three type II and one type III) were treated by excision followed by low-dose limited-field radiation. The surgery was performed outside the "treatment window" in all four cases—at less than 12 months in 3 and at 6 years in one. At follow-up, 1 to 4 years after excision, the average range of forearm rotation was 118° (range, 115° to 120°). There were no recurrences.

53. Langkamer VG, Ackroyd CE: Removal of forearm plates: A review of the complications. *J Bone Joint Surg* 1990;72B:601–604.

54. Lindsey RW, Fenison AT, Doherty BJ, et al: Effects of retained diaphyseal plates on forearm bone density and grip

strength. *J Orthop Trauma* 1994;8:462–467.

Fourteen patients with retained forearm plates were evaluated for residual grip strength and bone mineral density (BMD) between 2 and 12 years after injury. No significant differences were detected between the plated and the contralateral uninjured forearm bones. BMD was well preserved both adjacent to and removed from the plate.

55. Mih AD, Cooney WP, Idler RS, et al: Long-term follow-up of forearm bone diaphyseal plating. *Clin Orthop* 1994;299:256–258.

    In this retrospective review, 113 of 175 patients studied retained their forearm plates and 62 had plate removal at an average of 19 months after injury. Ten (16%) patients sustained major complications after plate removal, including refracture (11%), compartment syndrome, and infection. Sixty-seven percent reported continued symptoms despite plate removal, and 9% felt they were worse.

56. Deluca PA, Lindsey RW, Ruwe PA: Refracture of bones of the forearm after the removal of compression plates. *J Bone Joint Surg* 1988;70A:1372–1376.

57. Rosson JW, Shearer JR: Refracture after the removal of plates from the forearm: An avoidable complication. *J Bone Joint Surg* 1991;73B:415–417.

58. Rosson JW, Egan J, Shearer J, et al: Bone weakness after the removal of plates and screws: Cortical atrophy or screw holes? *J Bone Joint Surg* 1991;73B:283–286.

59. Rosson JW, Petley GW, Shearer JR: Bone structure after removal of internal fixation plates. *J Bone Joint Surg* 1991;73B:65–67.

7
Fractures of the Distal Radius

Introduction

Fractures of the distal radius are among the most common of all orthopaedic injuries. The reported incidence is approximately one in 500 persons and they account for nearly one sixth of all fractures seen in the emergency room. A bimodal age distribution exists, with one peak in early adolescence and a second in the older age population. Reviews of these injuries have documented that 50% or more of these fractures involve either the radiocarpal or distal radioulnar joints, in addition to the radial metaphyseal fracture.[1]

Unique among periarticular and intra-articular fractures, however, the standard of treatment for most fractures of the distal radius has been, and unfortunately remains, closed reduction and immobilization. Colles' oft-quoted statement that deformity does not correlate with functional limitation[2] remains a widely held belief among orthopaedists. Additionally, the predominance of injury to the elderly population, often with concomitant medical problems, perceived low functional demands, and significant osteoporosis, has helped to further establish closed management as the treatment of choice for the majority of these injuries.

During the past 10 years, however, there has been a dramatic improvement in our knowledge of fracture patterns as well as the long-term effects of intra-articular and extra-articular malunion of the distal radius. Additionally, the surgical equipment and techniques necessary to successfully manage these injuries has been further studied and refined. As a result of motor vehicle accidents and recreational activities such as in-line skating, there has been an increase in the number of high-energy fractures of the distal radius seen in young adults. In combination, these events bring into question the management of many of the distal radius fractures that are seen in the emergency room and have led to many recent reports that document the surgical management of these injuries.

This chapter will review recent attempts to more accurately classify these injuries as well as principles of clinical and radiographic evaluation. Treatment rationale, especially reviewing recent evidence supporting anatomic reduction of these injuries, treatment alternatives, and results will be similarly discussed. Finally, complications of injury management as well as populations deserving special treatment considerations will be explored.

Classification of Injuries

The use of eponyms to describe various fracture patterns of the distal radius is an imprecise and confusing method of classifying these injuries. These limitations have led to the recent development of more specific classification schemes. The goal of these systems is to provide a means of categorizing fractures of the distal radius that will provide the orthopaedist with a guide to treatment options and expected outcome. Unfortunately, there are as many modern classification systems as there are eponyms for these injuries, and, ultimately, the individual surgeon must choose the one or two systems that he or she finds most useful. At present, none of the systems can be regarded as completely accurate or descriptive of all injuries of the distal radius and for this reason, no classification is universally accepted among orthopaedic traumatologists.

Current classification schemes may broadly be divided into those based on the mechanism of injury and those based on the anatomy of the fracture. Fernandez[3] has advocated a scheme based on mechanism of injury, believing that the mechanics of fracture reduction and fixation (whether open or closed) depend strictly on those forces at the time of injury. Type I fractures result from bending forces and represent extra-articular metaphyseal tensile failure (Colles' and Smith fractures). These fractures are further subdivided into stable and unstable patterns based on the degree of metaphyseal comminution and fracture displacement. Type II fractures result from shearing forces across the joint surface and include Barton's and radial styloid fractures. Compression forces result in type III fractures, and are categorized by impaction of subchondral and metaphyseal bone; several intra-articular fracture fragment patterns are possible (ie, die-punch injuries). Type IV fractures result from avulsion forces with fracture at the site of ligament attachment. These injuries include a wide spectrum of radiocarpal sprains, subluxations, and dislocations. Type V fractures result from high-energy injuries and combinations of the above forces and are categorized by marked displacement, comminution, and instability.

Since Gartland and Werley first divided these injuries into extra-articular and intra-articular fractures, the majority of fracture classification schemes have been based on fracture anatomy. As methods of evaluating and treating these injuries have become more sophisticated, so too have the classification schemes become more complex. The Frykman classification, which divides injuries based on involvement of the radiocarpal and/or the distal radioulnar joint as well as by the presence or absence of an ulnar styloid fracture, unfortunately does not include variables, such as direction and degree of displacement or comminution. These variables are vital in guiding fracture treatment as well as in determining expected outcome.

Recent anatomic classifications have been expansions of the original Gartland scheme. McMurtry and Jupiter[4] have retained the division of extra-articular and intra-articular injuries. Extra-articular injuries are further subdivided into stable and unstable fractures based on the amount of comminution and angulation. Unstable injuries are characterized by extensive dorsal comminution, comminution extending volar to the mid-axial plane of the radius, dorsal angulation of greater than 20°, or significant volar angulation. Intra-articular injuries are divided on the basis of the number of articular fracture fragments (Fig. 1). A two-part fracture is one in which the opposite portion of the radiocarpal joint remains in continuity with the remainder of the radius (ie, dorsal and volar Barton's, radial styloid, and isolated lunate fossa die-punch fractures). A three-part fracture is one in which the intact lunate and scaphoid facets separate both from each other and from the radius. A four-part fracture is one in which the lunate fossa fragment of the three-part fracture splits into dorsal and volar fragments. Comminuted injuries (having five or more parts), in which high-energy trauma completely disrupts the distal radius and its articulations, may occur.

Trumble and associates[5] instead divide intra-articular injuries into four groups, based on patterns of involvement: simple intra-articular and extra-articular; simple articular with metaphyseal comminution; simple metaphyseal with articular comminution; and comminution of both articular and metaphyseal surfaces. An initial injury severity score is also determined for each injury based on the number of fracture fragments and associated carpal injuries. From this classification, a treatment algorithm and prognosis can be assigned to each injury.

Melone has further classified four part intra-articular fractures based on the pattern of displacement (Fig. 2).[6] Type I fractures are minimally displaced. In type II fractures, dorsal or volar displacement of the lunate fossa fragments occurs as a unit and the individual fragments are neither rotated nor widely separated. Melone divides type II injuries into type IIa and type IIb, recognizing fractures in which both the scaphoid and lunate impact the lunate fossa. In type II injuries, if excessive dorsal or volar comminution or significant radiocarpal step-off, shortening, or angulation exists, closed reduction will often fail. In type III fractures, displacement of the lunate fossa fragments is similar to that seen in type II injuries; however, there is an associated metaphyseal spike (typically volar in dorsally displaced fractures), which further increases fracture instability and may create soft-tissue complications. Finally, in type IV injuries, there is wide separation of the lunate fossa fragment, often with rotation of the palmar medial fragment as much as 180°. The type V, or explosion, fracture represents high-energy, highly comminuted injuries similar to the five-part or more class of fractures in the Jupiter classification.

The most comprehensive, and perhaps cumbersome, anatomic classification scheme is the AO system (Fig. 3).[7] This system divides injuries into type A (extra-articular), type B (simple articular), and type C (complex articular). Fractures are further subclassified within each type based on the presence and direction of displacement, the status of the ulna, and the presence and location of comminution. Even the most complex of distal radius injuries may be classified using this system.

Clinical and Radiographic Evaluation

As with most fractures, a systematic and thorough clinical evaluation of the patient's injury is vital prior to initiating treatment. The mechanism of injury is important in predicting the extent of injury and associated soft-tissue damage. Falls from height and motor vehicle accidents are likely to result in more severe injury patterns. The position of the extremity and hand at the time of impact can also aid in understanding the mechanism of injury and displacement patterns. Additionally, it is important to assess whether the patient has any systemic (ie, rheumatoid arthritis) or local (ie, previous fracture) disease or injury that may adversely affect outcome. Finally, it is important to appreciate the socioeconomic importance of the injury to the individual patient. Is the injured limb the dominant extremity? Does the patient engage in vocational or recreational activities that rely extensively on the wrist-hand unit that has been injured? Is the patient willing and able to comply with treatment restrictions and rehabilitation?

After a physical examination for evidence of other bony injury, attention should be directed to the injured extremity. Careful palpation and passive range of motion of the ipsilateral shoulder, arm, elbow, forearm, and hand is vital to rule out associated skeletal injury. Particular attention should be directed to the elbow and carpus, where most associated fractures will occur. In a review of 565 distal radius fractures, four scaphoid, two radial head, and one Bennett's fracture were unrecognized at the time of injury.[8]

Associated soft-tissue injury is also common and must be considered during the examination. Although fractures of the distal radius are usually closed injuries, open fractures (especially in the setting of widely displaced or high-energy injuries) do occur and therefore skin integrity must be inspected and documented. Radial and ulnar pulses should be evaluated and if absent despite reduction, Doppler ultrasound evaluation is warranted. Although complete division of these structures is exceedingly rare, laceration or entrapment by fracture fragments can occur and is best managed by early repair or release.

A complete median, radial, and ulnar motor and sensory examination is in order as well during the initial evaluation.

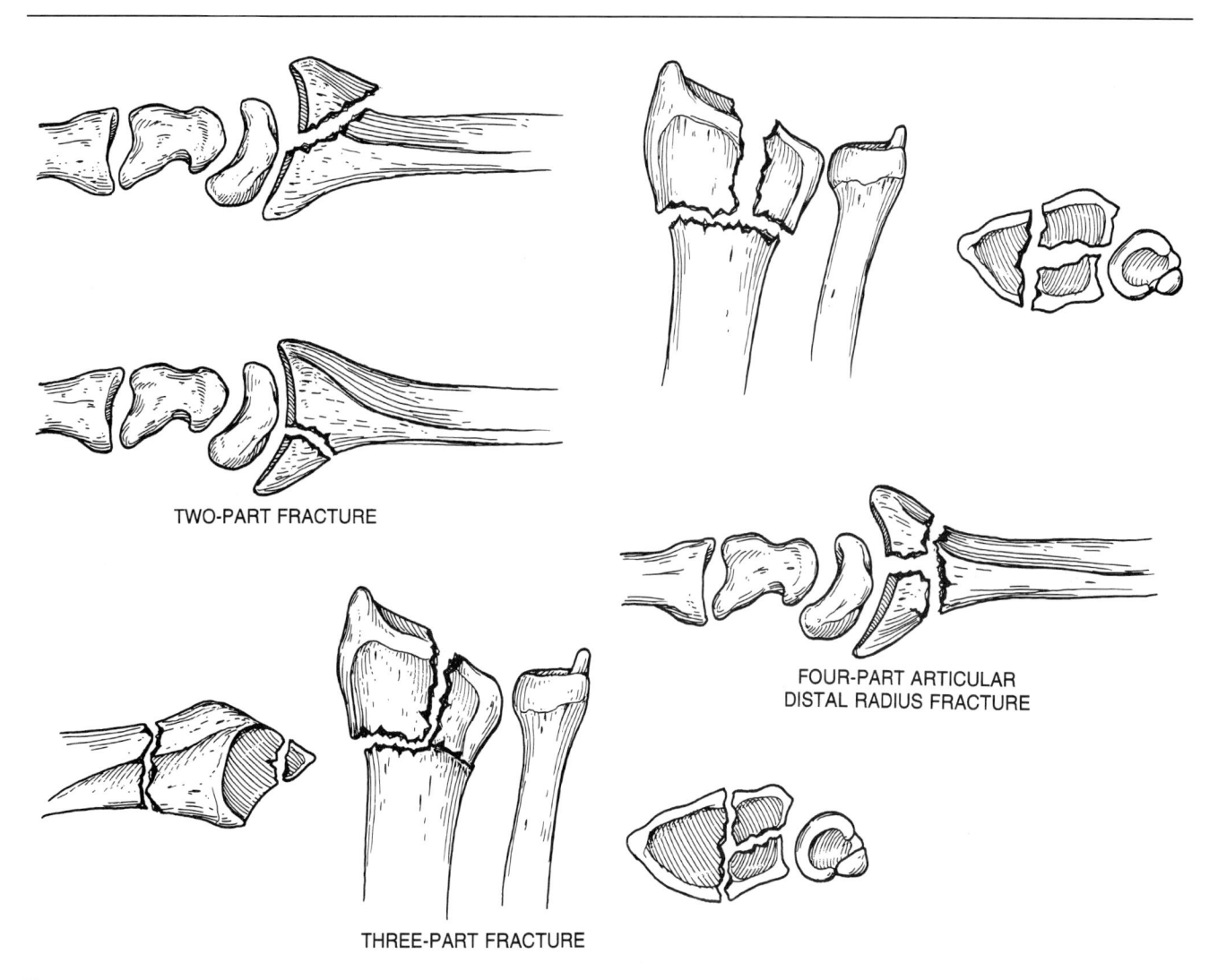

Fig. 1 Intra-articular fracture classification of McMurtry and Jupiter based on number of articular fragments. (Reproduced with permission from McMurtry RY, Jupiter JB: Fractures of the distal radius, in Browner B, Jupiter JB, Levine A, et al (eds): *Skeletal Trauma*. Philadelphia, PA, WB Saunders, 1992, pp 1063-1094.)

The median nerve is the most commonly injured nerve following distal radius fractures. Neuropraxia secondary to contusion at the time of maximum fracture displacement and after injury swelling remains the most common cause of nerve dysfunction after injury, however, complete disruption of the median and ulnar nerves has been reported. Initial documentation of neurologic status is vital should neurologic sequelae develop later in treatment. In high-energy injuries or injuries in patients at risk (ie, altered mental status secondary to head trauma), careful follow-up of swelling and neurologic function is vital to rule out a compartment syndrome.

Despite pain and swelling, tendon evaluation is also important and, with some gentle encouragement, a rapid evaluation of tendon function is easily performed. Although late attritional tendon rupture (usually the extensor pollicis longus) is most commonly seen, acute tendon laceration can occur at the time of injury. Additionally, in injuries involving disruption of the distal radioulnar joint, the extensor carpi ulnaris tendon may become entrapped.

Good quality posteroanterior (PA), lateral, and oblique radiographs are sufficient for evaluating most distal radius fractures. The PA view is facilitated by abducting the patient's humerus so that the elbow is at the same level as the shoulder. The lateral view is taken with the humerus adducted and the elbow flexed at 90°. The oblique view is obtained with the forearm supinated approximately 45°.

Four radiographic measurements are routinely recorded in regard to displacement of distal radius injuries. In the lateral view, the volar tilt of the distal radial articular surface should be measured. The normal value is approximately 11°. In the PA view, the radial length (or height),

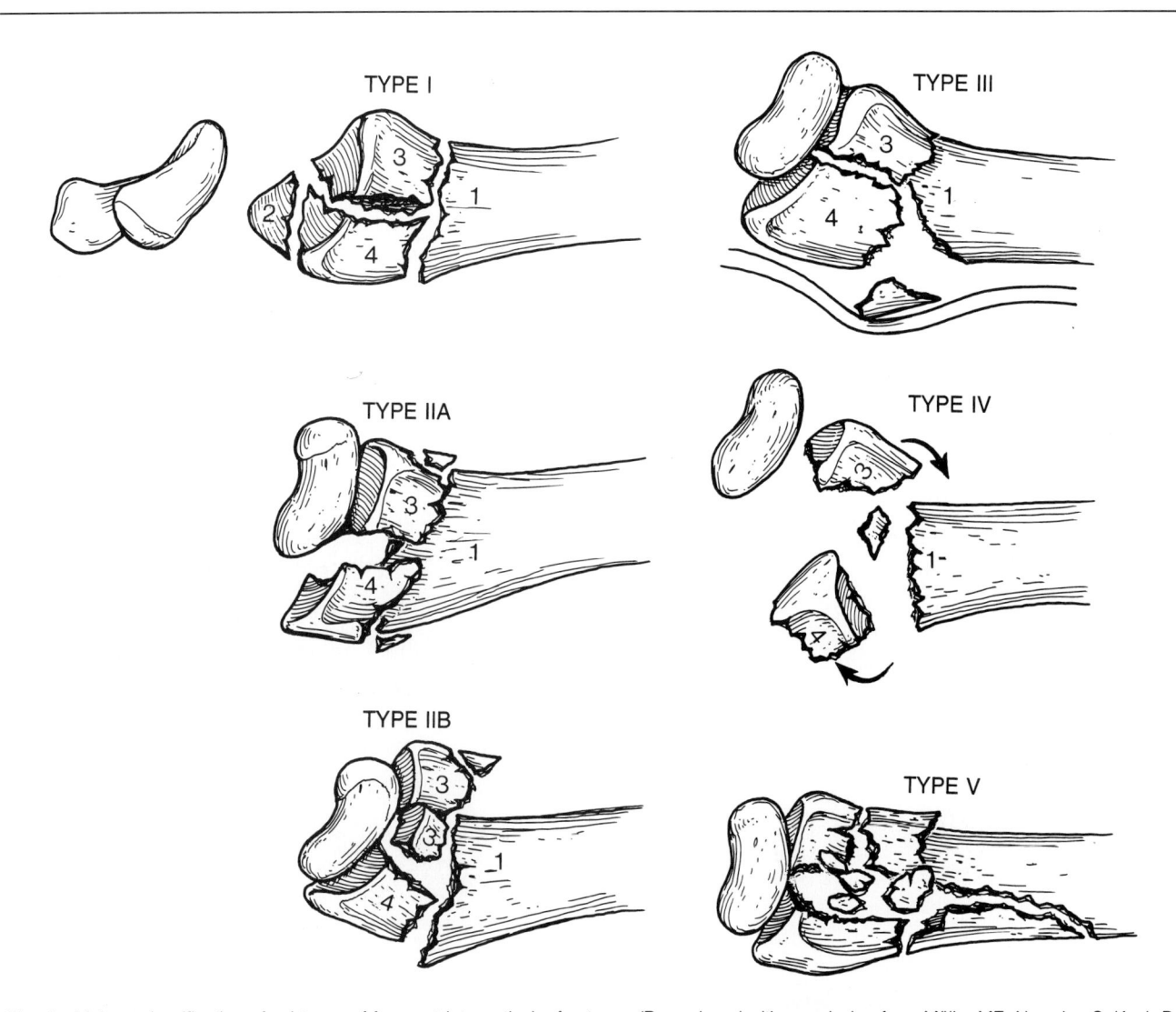

Fig. 2 Melone classification of subtypes of four-part intra-articular fractures. (Reproduced with permission from Müller ME, Nazarian S, Koch P, et al (eds): *The Comprehensive Classification of Fractures of Long Bones.* Berlin, Germany, Springer-Verlag, 1990.)

inclination, and width are routinely recorded. The radial length is measured as the distance between two lines perpendicular to the long axis of the radius, one drawn at the tip of the radial styloid and another drawn at the distal ulnar articular surface. The normal value is approximately 11 to 12 mm. Alternatively, the radial length may be measured as the relative ulnar variance (vertical distance between the ulnar articular surface and the medial corner of the lunate facet) and compared to the opposite wrist. It has been suggested that this is a more accurate reflection of shortening because this value is independent of alterations in the radial inclination. As ulnar variance changes with differing positions of pronation and supination however, the views must be highly controlled for positional changes. Radial inclination is measured as the angle formed between a line drawn through the tip of the radial styloid and the medial corner of the lunate facet and a line perpendicular to the long axis of the radius. The normal value is 22° to 23°. Finally, the radial width is measured as the distance between the central long axis of the radius and a line parallel to it drawn at the radial edge of the styloid process. This distance is then compared to the opposite wrist.

Additional factors should be considered when evaluating distal radius fractures. The degree and location of comminution is vital to predicting the outcome of management. Severe dorsal comminution is associated with shortening and redisplacement, while a volar butterfly fragment may be associated with median neurapraxia. Articular involvement and displacement must also be assessed, both in classifying these injuries as well as in therapeutic decision-making. Ulnar styloid fractures should be noted because they suggest higher degrees of fracture displacement. In

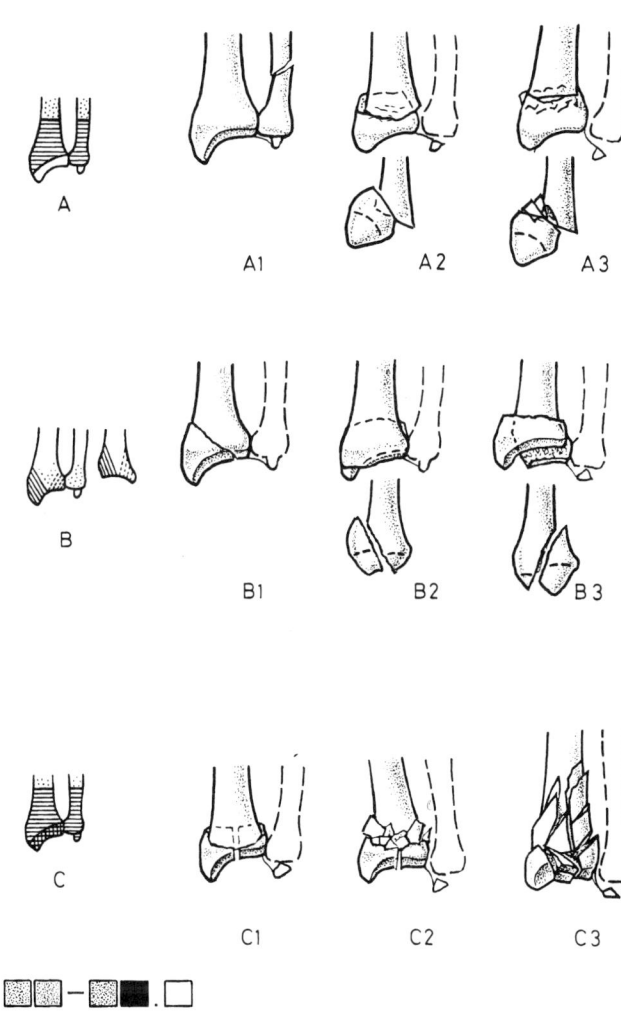

A1 Extra-articular fracture, of the ulna, radius intact
A2 Extra-articular fracture, of the radius, simple and impacted
A3 Extra-articular fracture, of the radius, multifragmentary

B1 Partial articular fracture, of the radius, sagittal
B2 Partial articular fracture, of the radius, dorsal rim (Barton)
B3 Partial articular fracture, of the radius, volar rim (reverse Barton, Goyrand-Smith II)

C1 Complete articular fracture, of the radius, articular simple, metaphyseal simple
C2 Complete articular fracture, of the radius, articular simple, metaphyseal multifragmentary
C3 Complete articular fracture, of the radius, multifragmentary

Fig. 3 AO classification system for distal radius fractures. (Reproduced with permission from Müller ME, Nazarian S, Koch P, et al (eds): *The Comprehensive Classification of Fractures of Long Bones*. Berlin, Germany, Springer-Verlag, 1990, p109.)

one study, dorsal angulation of greater than 15° or radial shortening of greater than 4 mm could not be produced without fracturing the ulnar styloid.[9] Carpal anatomy should be evaluated for evidence of fracture as well as for intercarpal ligament disruption.

Tomography and computed tomography (CT) are indicated to assess the location and degree of articular fracture displacement. Splint materials and osteoporosis often make tomography difficult, however, and, given its availability at most centers, CT is now more commonly used in the evaluation of distal radius fractures. CT is also indicated to evaluate the distal radioulnar joint and can assist in preoperative planning in complex, comminuted injuries. One- to 2-mm thick sections in the axial, sagittal, and coronal planes are usually sufficient to define the relationships and integrity of the lunate and scaphoid facets, the congruity of the distal radioulnar joint, the degree of dorsal and/or palmar comminution, and the position and size of depressed articular fragments. Three-dimensional reconstructions can be obtained for the most complex injuries and provide additional information about fracture anatomy.

The ability of magnetic resonance imaging (MRI) to define bony anatomy is not as good as CT; however, MRI does have a role in the management of some distal radius fractures. For patients with associated median neuropathy, rupture of flexor or extensor tendons, or carpal ligament disruption, MRI offers distinct advantages in further defining soft-tissue injury. MRI has also been used extensively to evaluate the triangular fibrocartilage that may be disrupted in a significant number of distal radial fractures.

Rationale for Treatment

Despite Colles' words of consolation, there has been dramatic evidence since the mid 1980s that function is intimately related to form in regard to distal radial fractures. Both extra-articular and intra-articular malunion have been shown in the laboratory, as well as in clinical studies, to alter patient function as well as their satisfaction with treatment outcome.

Extra-articular malunion relates primarily to three considerations: (1) the degree of dorsal or palmar angulation of the distal radial articular surface present in the sagittal plane; (2) the degree of radial inclination as well as radial shift present in the coronal plane; and (3) the degree of shortening of the distal radius as compared to the relative ulnar variance of the uninjured extremity. Cadaveric experiments utilizing pressure-sensitive film have demonstrated that alterations in any of these anatomic values will alter loading patterns and concentration in the radiocarpal joint. Excessive dorsal or palmar angulation of the distal radius (greater than 30°) was found to result in increased forces at a position dorsal to their normal location in the radiocarpal joint.[9] Loss of radial inclination beyond 10° increases loads at the lunate fossa as does radial shortening of as little as 2 mm. Triquetroulnar impingement occurred beyond 6 mm of shortening. Loss of radial inclination and radial shortening have also been shown to alter the kinematics of the distal radioulnar joint and to produce deformity within the triangular fibrocartilage.[10] This may relate to the prevalence of distal radioulnar arthrosis after distal radial fracture. Similarly, with a 45° dorsal articular angulation, 65% of carpal loads are borne by the ulna (versus 20% in the normal wrist) and the remainder of the loads are transmitted in high concentration dorsally in the scaphoid fossa.[11]

A variety of clinical studies have confirmed laboratory data correlating malunion with poor function. Pain, decreased range of motion, decreased grip strength, and poor patient function/satisfaction have been consistently associated with poor anatomic results after fracture.[12-14] Importantly, the position of the fracture at union rather than the position at time of presentation has the greatest correlation with long-term functional results. In attempting to define specific effects of malunion, it appears that intra-articular fractures and dorsal articular angulation coincide with decreased range of motion, while radial shortening and shift are associated with decreased grip strength and pain. In regard to the magnitude of deformity seen in these patients, patients with as little as 10° of dorsal angulation or 2 mm of radial shift are much more likely to experience pain, stiffness, weakness, and poor function 4 years after fracture than are those patients with an anatomic reduction.[14] In a study of 29 extra-articular fractures reviewed after a period of more than 30 years, shortening of as little as 1 mm was found to increase the risk of radiocarpal arthrosis by 20%.[15] Shortening of 2 mm increased this risk to 50%. Pain and stiffness were frequently present among the patients with arthrosis.

Dorsal articular angulation after fracture in young adults has also been associated with dynamic midcarpal instability and pain, leading Taleisnik and Watson[16] to perform corrective osteotomy in nine patients. Correction of the extra-articular malunion relieved symptoms and restored carpal alignment in these patients. Bickerstaff and Bell[17] also found that malunion with excessive dorsal angulation of the distal radius caused painful midcarpal instability and lower functional scores in patients who had sustained a distal radius fracture.

Intra-articular malunion has also been recognized as a factor in poor outcome in patients with distal radius fractures. In reviewing 47 patients at 30 or more years after intra-articular fracture, as little as 1 mm of joint incongruity was found to significantly increase the risk of long-term degenerative changes both in the radiocarpal and distal radioulnar joint. The presence of radiocarpal degenerative changes was strongly correlated with persistent symptoms of pain and motion loss. Despite adequate extra-articular restoration, failure to restore intra-articular anatomy has been reported to be the most critical factor in patients who do poorly.[18] Additionally, soft-tissue, intercarpal ligament, and distal radioulnar joint disruption in these patients further worsens outcome. Although residual articular malalignment may be better tolerated in older patients who sustain lower energy injuries, the longer life span and increased activity of our growing elderly population heightens the importance of anatomic articular restoration in this population as well.

Treatment Goals and Considerations

There are four principles in the treatment of distal radius fractures: (1) restoration of articular congruity and axial alignment; (2) maintenance of reduction; (3) achievement of bony union; and (4) restoration of hand and wrist function. These principles may be violated to an extent, however, depending on patient variables. Other factors, such as low functional demand, significant medical illness, inability to comply with postoperative instructions, or previous fracture and deformity, may justify acceptance of less than anatomic results. It must be emphasized, however, that chronologic age does not correlate with functional age and many of these fractures, even in older patients, will benefit from aggressive treatment.

Given recent evidence to support the role of anatomic reduction in improving functional results in these injuries, the following criteria for an acceptable reduction may be defined: (1) change in volar (palmar) tilt of no more than 10° (ie, neutral or 20° palmar slope); (2) radial shortening no more than 2 mm; and (3) change in radial angle of no more than 5°. Additionally, when intra-articular fracture is present, no more than 1 to 2 mm of articular step-off should be accepted. Reduction may be attempted under local (hematoma block) anesthesia or with the assistance of intravenous narcotics and sedation. Because of its inherent risk for local anesthetic systemic toxicity, the Bier block should be avoided, if possible. Reduction should be achieved primarily by axial traction augmented by reduction of the specific deformity present through manual pressure over the fracture fragments. Excessive traction and gross exaggeration of the deformity have been associated with further soft-tissue injury and their use should be avoided.

If the fracture is not reduced, surgical management with limited or formal open reduction and percutaneous, external and/or internal fixation is indicated. If fracture reduction is achieved, however, a reliable method of maintaining this reduction must be chosen. Initially, nondisplaced injuries are almost always amenable to closed treatment. Fractures that require reduction, however, must be further classified as stable or unstable injuries. Stable fractures can be successfully held by closed means; unstable fractures will require external and/or internal fixation to maintain reduction.

Fracture stability may be self-evident during the course of treatment. Irreducible fractures and reducible fractures that redisplace during closed treatment are obviously unstable. Early gross redisplacement of these injuries is less common than slow loss of reduction over the first 2 to 3 weeks of treatment.[19] Because the results of surgical treatment of fractures that have displaced late in treatment have been less rewarding than immediate surgical intervention, attempts have been made to predict fracture stability based on the pattern and degree of displacement on initial radiographs. Criteria for instability cited by a variety of authors have included widely displaced intra-articular fractures, excessive dorsal or volar comminution, dorsal angulation of greater than 20°, and osteoporosis in elderly patients. Recent studies have shown that instability, as defined by failure to maintain reduction by closed methods, most closely correlates with initial fracture displacement, specifically with shortening greater than 5 mm and dorsal comminution.[20,21] Additionally, it has been evident that articular margin injuries (Barton and Chauffeur fractures), palmarly displaced and comminuted extra-articular injuries (Smith fractures), and high-energy, highly comminuted intra-articular injuries are often unstable and will fail nonsurgical management.

Treatment Options and Results

Cast Immobilization

Following acceptable closed reduction, cast immobilization remains the treatment of choice for most stable fractures of the distal radius. Although commonly practiced at many centers in the United States, above-elbow immobilization has not been demonstrated to benefit fracture maintenance or functional outcome in any controlled study. The position of immobilization has also been widely debated. The Cotton-Loder position of extreme flexion and ulnar deviation has been abandoned because of median nerve complications; however, some degree of palmarflexion and ulnar deviation is still utilized by most orthopaedists. Better anatomic and functional results are obtained through immobilization with the wrist in extension.[22] Three-point molding at the fracture site is compatible with carpal dorsiflexion; this not only utilizes the dorsal periosteal hinge but also places the hand and carpus in a functional position that will maintain reduction. In regard to forearm rotation, supination has been proposed to be superior to pronation because it negates the radial displacing force of the brachioradialis and allows for greater functional recovery after a displaced fracture,[23] although other authors have failed to document a benefit for either pronation or supination.[24] The theoretical benefits of supination also extend to the maintenance of distal radioulnar joint reduction following dorsal subluxation; indeed, in fractures involving disruption of this joint, supination may be the position of choice. For most fractures of the distal radius, however, forearm rotation does not appear to be important in regard to final outcome.

A painless, functional wrist and hand can be expected in the vast majority of patients treated in a cast, as long as the principles of maintaining acceptable alignment are followed. Redisplacement of fractures either in an acute or slowly progressive loss of reduction should be managed by relocation and maintenance of reduction through percutaneous pinning, external fixation, or internal fixation. Repeated attempts at nonsurgical maintenance of reduction will meet with 50% or less satisfactory outcome.[19] Precise casting technique leaving the metacarpophalangeal joints free, with early attention to edema control and surrounding joint range of motion, is also important to achieving full functional recovery in these patients.

Functional Bracing

Functional bracing of distal radius fractures maintains some advocates, although its use at present is not widespread. The same criteria of adequate fracture reduction and stability necessary for successful results with casting must be met to achieve similar results with functional bracing.

Advocates of functional bracing have cited advantages of this technique over casting. Better anatomic and early functional results have been documented in patients treated with a cast brace;[25] unfortunately, the casted group in this study was inadequately immobilized with a simple dorsal plaster. The benefit of functional bracing over casting has not been confirmed in other prospective trials.[26] Superficial radial nerve irritation by the brace has been reported as a complication of this technique. As with casting, fracture reduction must be achieved and maintained in order to consistently return function in fractures treated by this method.

Pins and Plaster

Although pins and plaster have been used with success in the past, significant problems have been reported with this technique. Carrozzella and Stern[27] documented a 52% complication rate after treating 95 distal radius fractures with pins and plaster. Complications included loss of reduction, pin site loosening, pin tract infection, and neurapraxia. With the advent of new external fixation devices and given the number of unacceptable anatomic results and complications, the use of pins and plaster for the treatment of these injuries has largely been abandoned.

Percutaneous Pinning

Percutaneous pinning of unstable fractures of the distal radius remains an excellent treatment choice for many of these injuries. It represents a relatively simple, minimally invasive, and widely applicable form of treatment. Percutaneous pinning is ideally suited to maintain fracture sagittal alignment in unstable extra-articular injuries in which the volar cortex remains intact. It may also be used for simple intra-articular injuries in which the articular surface is undisplaced or is in two large fragments. Percutaneous pinning will not reliably maintain fracture length when volar or bicortical comminution is present. Significant intra-articular displacement or comminution or inability to obtain closed reduction also represent contraindications to the procedure.

A variety of techniques of pin insertion have been described. The most common of these is radial styloid pinning, either alone or in combination with dorsal radial pinning. Additionally, techniques in which pins are passed through both the distal radius and ulna, and in which pins are placed directly through the dorsal fracture line into the proximal fragment have been described. Regardless of technique used, the standard of care includes a variable period of supplemental immobilization with a cast or splint. In cases where significant swelling or open wound care contraindicate a cast, external fixation may be used instead.

Complications commonly reported with percutaneous pinning include fracture redisplacement, tendon or nerve injury, pin site infection, pin migration, pin breakage, and reflex sympathetic dystrophy.

Recent reports have clearly documented the superiority of percutaneous pinning over traditional casting techniques for unstable fractures of the distal radius in regard to both anatomic and functional results.[28] Unfortunately, there are no studies as yet to compare the results of the variety of pinning techniques to each other or to external or internal fixation. Excellent anatomic results were reported in 82%[29] and 90%[30] and excellent or good functional results with minimal complications using two radial styloid pins were reported in 100%.[29] In a study on radial styloid pinning combined with dorsal radial pinning, excellent anatomic results were reported in 90%. There were two cases of pin migration and one of tendon entrapment.[30] Rayhack's technique of passing multiple small K-wires across the ulna into the distal radius was reported to produce superior fixation, allowing lightweight splinting at 3 weeks while avoiding risk to the radial sensory nerve.[31] Although no long-term loss of pronation or supination, pin breakage, or pin migration were reported, loss of reduction did occur in some patients. Finally, in the intrafocal pinning technique of Kapandji, which is widely used in Europe and South America, pins are introduced into the proximal fracture fragment dorsally through the fracture site, thus acting as a buttress against displacement. Acceptable radiographic results were reported in only 60% of patients older than 65, while better anatomic but poorer functional results were seen in younger patients.[32]

Percutaneous pins have also been used by a variety of authors in conjunction with external or internal fixation of more highly comminuted injuries. After application of an external fixator, limited or formal open reduction of articular fragments may be performed, followed by fixation of these fragments by K-wires. These may be placed transulnarly, through the dorsal radial surface, or through the radial styloid. Small fragments or marked osteoporosis may necessitate combining pin fixation with plating techniques. The use of polyglycolic acid rods in an attempt to avoid pin removal has been associated with soft-tissue inflammation and osteolysis, and further study of this technique is required before widespread clinical use.

External Fixation

External fixation has been used increasingly to treat unstable fractures of the distal radius. Indeed, fracture care *in part* involving the use of external fixation is probably the treatment of choice for unstable extra-articular injuries with extensive comminution (in which percutaneous pinning techniques have a significant incidence of failure) and for the majority of unstable, comminuted intra-articular injuries. Several retrospective and prospective studies have documented that both the anatomic and functional results with external fixation are superior to cast treatment of these fractures.[33-35] However, enthusiasm over the use of external fixation in these fractures must be tempered by a thorough understanding of the indications, theoretical basis, limitations, and complications of these devices.

Commonly cited indications for external fixation of distal radius fractures include unstable extra-articular fractures with significant comminution, comminuted intra-articular fractures, fractures that have failed to maintain reduction with other treatment modalities, open fractures, and fractures in a polytrauma patient. Volarly displaced and comminuted injuries usually require formal volar exposure and open reduction and internal fixation (ORIF); however, external fixation is often used to augment stability when less than rigid fixation is achieved because of small bony fragments or osteoporosis.

External fixation devices provide fracture reduction and maintenance of that reduction through constant ligamentotaxis. Various fixator designs are available and these vary greatly in their biomechanical properties as well as in their specific techniques. Advantages offered by more recent fixator designs include the ability to apply the fixator prior to fracture reduction, a system for controlled adjustment of traction force during the course of treatment, ability to apply traction force in multiple planes, ability to place pins in a converging pattern, and ability to position the wrist in extension while maintaining fracture reduction. The comparison of reported results with these various fixators is not yet possible because a controlled study comparing these devices has not been conducted.

Despite excellent reduction of radial length and inclination, it had become evident from early reports that restoration of palmar tilt of the distal radius as well as anatomic reduction of the radiocarpal joint surface often were not achieved with external fixation. The strong palmar ligaments have been shown to become taut and limit radiocarpal distraction, while the weaker, Z-shaped dorsal ligament complex has yet to reach maximum length.[36] This prevents purely longitudinal traction from restoring palmar tilt. Similarly, the dorsomedial radiocarpal fragment is not reduced.

Complications with the use of these devices have been many, ranging from 15% to as high as 60% in early reports. Complications related to achieving and maintaining reduction include failure to restore palmar tilt or radiocarpal alignment, overdistraction, late fracture displacement, and nonunion. Complications related to the pins include pin tract infection, pin breakage, pin loosening, fracture through pin sites, and injury to the iatrogenic nerve and to tendons. Complications related to distal radius fractures in general include median neuropathy, reflex sympathetic dystrophy, and decreased motion and grip strength.

Recent reports of the results of external fixation for distal radial fractures have shown a dramatic decrease in the complication rate because potential complications are better appreciated. The failure of longitudinal traction to restore palmar slope and radiocarpal alignment in some injuries must be recognized at the time the fixator is placed. Agee has introduced the concept of triplanar ligamentotaxis with palmar translation of the carpus utilized to achieve restoration of palmar slope in response to this problem.[37] Supplementing longitudinal traction with limited open reduction techniques and internal fixation in order to correct both palmar slope and radiocarpal alignment has been described.[38,39] These techniques involve reduction through a small dorsal incision and radiographically controlled elevation of articular fragments with an awl or elevator followed by pin fixation of these fragments. As greater duration and magnitude of distraction force have been shown to be associated with posttreatment stiffness and decreased strength regardless of anatomic result (especially when associated with resultant radiocarpal lengthening or positioning of the wrist in flexion during fixator treatment), care has been taken to limit radiocarpal distraction to 5 mm or less and to maintain the wrist in neutral or extension during the course of external fixation.[40,41] The theoretical value of segmentally decreasing traction force after 3 weeks has not yet been specifically documented, and this practice has been associated with loss of reduction by some authors. Cancellous bone grafting of the metaphyseal region has been advocated in order to improve reduction and decrease the duration of external fixation to 3 weeks without this complication.[42] Pin complications may be minimized by meticulous detail to identification of nerves and tendons, predrilling, appropriate pin sizing, and release of skin tension.[43] The importance of early aggressive treatment of pain, limited motion, and median neuropathy cannot be overstated and includes organized and frequent occupational therapy, edema control, adequate pain control, and carpal tunnel release when indicated. In 1987, the concept of dynamic external fixation of these injuries as a means of allowing radiocarpal flexion and extension during treatment was introduced. Potential advantages cited included better restoration of function as well as improved cartilage healing. Studies of cadaveric specimens, however, have documented fracture site movement during wrist motion with these devices. A prospective study comparing dynamic fixation to static fixation with the AO frame documented a higher incidence of loss of reduction and technical complications, as well as poorer functional results in the dynamic fixator group.[44] At present, no study favors these devices over conventional fixators.

Utilization of these new concepts has led to improved results and a dramatic decrease in complications with external fixation. Successful anatomic and functional outcomes have been documented in 80% to 90% of patients studied with few major complications despite high-energy comminuted injuries.[37,45,46] The choice of fixator at this time remains up to the individual surgeon. The principles of anatomic extra-articular and intra-articular reduction, strict attention to fixator application, and augmentation with internal fixation and/or bone grafting, when needed, should be followed closely.

Open Reduction and Internal Fixation (ORIF)

Despite the difficulty involved in formal ORIF of fractures of the distal radius, there are injuries for which it is advised. Concerns about ORIF include difficult surgical exposure; risks to local nerves, tendons, and vessels; multiple articular fragments that are difficult to reduce; and poor fixation in osteoporotic bone. These issues are valid and it is advisable that only surgeons familiar with both the regional anatomy and a variety of internal fixation options attempt such management.

There are two primary indications for ORIF. First among these are articular marginal injuries, such as dorsal and volar lip fractures (Barton's fractures). These shearing fractures are often associated with carpal dislocation, intercarpal ligament injury, and carpal fractures. Although closed reduction may be possible, the articular surface is usually difficult to reduce anatomically, and, because of muscle tension across the oblique fracture line, redisplacement is common. Radial styloid avulsion fractures may be managed by percutaneous pinning and cast treatment. However, when associated with perilunate dislocation (and scapholunate ligament disruption or scaphoid fracture) or when severe displacement or soft-tissue interposition make closed reduction impossible, ORIF may be required.

The second major indication for ORIF is in complex, comminuted intra-articular fractures. These represent a unique subset of distal radius injuries that often are the result of high-energy trauma, are associated with significant soft-tissue and concomitant skeletal injuries, and have significant rotation and impaction of articular fragments. These fractures include Melone type 4 fractures, AO type C3 fractures, and Fernandez combined injuries. Because of the underlying complexity of these injuries, ORIF has been increasingly combined with external fixation and bone grafting in order to achieve the goal of anatomic intra-articular and extra-articular reduction, which is vital to functional recovery.

Additional indications for primary or supplemental ORIF in distal radius fractures include associated distal ulnar shaft fractures, fractures with displaced volar cortical comminution, and fractures with metaphyseal–diaphyseal extension.

Surgical exposure may be achieved through dorsal or palmar approaches or by a combined approach. Choice of exposure is generally dictated by fracture anatomy as well as by the need for exploration and release of neurovascular structures. Choice of internal fixation includes buttress plate application, lag screw fixation, and/or K-wires. The 2.7-mm minifragment plates and screws may be used as alternatives to the 3.5-mm small fragment set. Because of extensor tendon irritation and risk of attritional rupture, many authors recommend removing dorsal plates. The lower profile of isolated lag screw(s) fixation is therefore attractive for fixation of radial styloid and dorsal lip fractures; however, small fragment size and regional osteoporosis limit their usefulness.

Results of ORIF of articular marginal fractures have been generally excellent. In one report on the management of 12 palmar marginal fractures managed with a buttress plate, complications were few and functional recovery was high.[47] However, when associated with carpal ligament injury or carpal fracture, results of treatment will not be as rewarding.[48] Careful evaluation for and appropriate treatment of associated carpal injuries is vital in the management of these fractures.

Results of treatment of comminuted intra-articular fractures have been surprisingly good.[49,50] Despite the severity of these injuries, preoperative planning, combined dorsal and palmar exposure if needed, supplemental external fixation to neutralize compressive forces, and bone grafting yield excellent anatomic results in more than 85% of patients. Trumble as well reviewed his experience treating AO C2 and C3 injuries with similar combination of surgical procedures and reported excellent anatomic and functional recovery in most of his 43 patients.[51] Patients with residual articular step-off, radial shortening, and a higher number of initial fracture fragments fared the worst. After a 3-year follow-up period, only one patient had developed symptomatic radiocarpal arthritis and remarkably few had experienced difficulties during or after treatment. A variety of complications may occur during treatment, however, including forearm compartment syndrome, median and ulnar neurovascular compromise, and wound infection. Early aggressive treatment of these problems, when coupled with anatomic joint reduction, has been shown to have a greater than 80% successful outcome in most series. High functional recovery and a low incidence of late radiocarpal arthritis can be expected, although results in older patients may not be as good after these injuries.[52]

Arthroscopy

Arthroscopy has been advocated as a minimally invasive means of assessing and facilitating intra-articular fracture reduction thereby avoiding extensile exposure and palmar capsular incision.[53] Arthroscopy also serves as a means of identifying and potentially treating associated intercarpal ligament and triangular fibrocartilage lesions. Concerns with arthroscopy include the extravasation of fluid into the forearm after acute fracture, limited ability of the arthroscope to guide reduction accurately, and risk to displaced neurovascular structures. The true role of arthroscopy in the management of these injuries has yet to be defined, and no prospective studies demonstrating its efficacy or safety exist at present.

Complications

Soft Tissue

Neuropathy remains among the most common complications following distal radius fracture. Its reported incidence ranges from 1% to 12% in most large series and as high as 30% in recent series specifically reviewing comminuted high-energy injuries.[7,39,49,51,54,55] Median nerve involvement is most common, followed by ulnar neuropathy. Radial sensory neuropathy is most often iatrogenic secondary to external fixator pin placement or cast-brace pressure (as previously discussed). Diffuse, poorly localized pain, and swelling may make the diagnosis of neuropathy difficult and late diagnosis has been frequently reported in the literature. Specific motor and sensory testing with electromyelographic confirmation, if needed, should be performed in patients in whom neuropathy is suspected.

Neuropathy may be seen acutely at the time of injury, subacutely within the initial 6 weeks of treatment, or late. Although complete disruption of both the median and ulnar nerve have been reported, acute neuropathy is usually secondary to nerve contusion at the time of injury. Median subacute neuropathy has been attributed to hematoma and swelling within the distal forearm and carpal canal as well as immobilization in excessive wrist flexion. Displaced volar fracture fragments also may cause median neuropathy by compression of the nerve against the forearm flexor retinaculum. Volar subluxation of the ulna in the event of distal radioulnar joint disruption has been associated with ulnar neuropathy.[7,39,49,51,54,55] Fracture callus in this same position may contribute to late median neuropathy. Both late median and ulnar nerve dysfunction increase in the event of fracture malunion. Although temporary median or ulnar neuropathy may follow hematoma block, this probably represents a local anesthetic effect and there is no evidence to support permanent neuropathy on this basis.

Observation was once the rule for treatment; however, recent reviews have documented the need for a more aggressive approach to this difficult problem. The initial treatment of acute neuropathy is gentle fracture reduction. Paresthesias and hypesthesias that fail to respond to closed reduction should undergo exploration and decompression within 24 to 48 hours of injury. Ulnar nerve decompression is performed at Guyon's canal, while median decompression involves release of both the carpal canal and the volar forearm flexor retinaculum. Partial lesions that fail to resolve within 1 week also should be considered for decompression. If neuropathy develops in the immobilization period following fracture reduction elevation, cast splitting and repositioning of the wrist in neutral position are in order. Neutral wrist positioning has been associated with the lowest pressure within the carpal canal. If neuropathy persists or worsens despite these interventions, decompression is indicated. The association of neuropathy with displaced volar fragments and volar ulnar head subluxation should guide the surgeon to earlier decompression with reduction of the fragment or relocation of the distal radioulnar joint in patients in whom this exists. Finally, in high-energy, comminuted intra-articular distal radius fractures that will require open reduction, median and/or ulnar nerve decompression should be routinely performed when a volar approach is utilized. Routine decompression regardless of the surgical approach or the presence or absence of symptoms has been advocated in these injuries.[49] Although the relationship between postfracture reflex sympathetic dystrophy and compressive neuropathy remains controversial, the diffusely swollen, painful, tingling hand seems to be at risk and may benefit from early carpal tunnel release.

Tendon complications are not an infrequent occurrence following fractures of the distal radius. Involvement may include entrapment, adhesions, tenosynovitis, laceration, and rupture.

Although entrapment between fracture fragments is rare, if present it will block fracture reduction and prevent tendon excursion. The presence of a tenodesis effect in the setting of an irreducible fracture should alert the clinician to this complication. In addition, with disruption of the distal radioulnar joint, extensor carpi ulnaris, and extensor digiti minimi entrapment may occur. Entrapment requires exploration to release the tendon and achieve anatomic reduction.

Peritendinous and intertendinous adhesions may form in the post-fracture period, causing pain and limited motion. Careful attention to edema control, to immobilization that allows for full motion of the metacarpophalangeal joint, and to early active and active assisted range of motion will minimize this complication. Aggressive occupational therapy, splinting, and pain control can effectively treat adhesions if they occur, and surgical release is rarely needed.

Tenosynovitis has been reported both in the first and third dorsal compartments after distal radius fracture. DeQuervain tenosynovitis may be treated effectively with splinting, oral nonsteroidal anti-inflammatory drugs, and steroid injection. Surgical release is indicated only in refractory cases. In contrast, pain and swelling in the region of Lister's tubercle often heralds extensor pollicis longus rupture, and surgical release is indicated in this setting.

Tendon laceration is rare in these injuries; however, in open fractures or in high-energy, widely displaced fractures, lacerations may occur and should be treated by primary repair. Late tendon rupture may occur months to years after injury; however, it is most common in the first 8 to 12 weeks after injury. The extensor pollicis longus is the tendon most often involved. Both mechanical (secondary to fracture callus, prominent hardware, or displaced fragments) and vascular etiologies contribute to rupture.[56] In the case of the extensor pollicis longus, vascular injection studies have shown a 5-mm region of tendon in the area of Lister's tubercle that is devoid of intrinsic circulation. When extensor compartmental pressure is increased by a mechanical factor, such as fracture callus or edema, the extrinsic blood supply to the tendon decreases and ischemic rupture may occur. This mechanism may explain the frequency of tendon rupture seen in minimally displaced fractures in which the extensor retinaculum remains well attached to the dorsal radial surface. Treatment of late rupture is through tendon transfer, with the extensor indicis proprius being used most frequently to replace the thumb long extensor.

Acute vascular complications following distal radius fractures are rare; however, in high-energy, widely displaced fractures or open fractures, arterial laceration or entrapment may occur. Management includes exploration and microsurgical repair, if indicated. Acute forearm or hand compartment syndrome is also rare following these injuries, with a prevalence of less than 1%. As with arterial injury, compartment syndrome is more common in high-energy or crushing injuries. Because of its devastating complications, however, all patients with these significant injuries or with closed head trauma must be closely examined for compartment syndrome. Pain refractory to standard narcotic pain medication, tensely swollen and tender compartments, and pain with passive muscle-tendon stretch are hallmarks of impending compartment syndrome. Paresthesias also may be present within the distribution of nerves passing through the involved compartments. Intracompartmental pressure measures confirm the clinical diagnosis, and continuous pressure monitoring may be useful in the patient with head trauma. Because peripheral pulses are rarely decreased and motor function is retained until late in the syndrome, these criteria should not be used for diagnosis.

Elevation, expedient fracture reduction, and the avoidance of constrictive forms of immobilization are thought to help diminish the incidence of postfracture compartment syndrome. Once an impending compartment syndrome is recognized, however, emergent fasciotomy is mandatory. Myonecrosis and permanent neuropathy will result unless rapid release of intracompartmental pressure is achieved. Forearm compartment syndrome typically involves the volar compartment, which is released through an extensile incision from the antecubital fossa to the carpal canal. If dorsal compartment pressure elevation is also present, it may be released as well through the same incision. In the hand, fasciotomy involves release of the dorsal and volar interosseous compartments though dorsal longitudinal incisions over the second and fourth web spaces with separate thenar and hypothenar incisions to release their respective compartments as well as the carpal canal.

The syndrome of reflex sympathetic dystrophy is a troublesome complication of distal radius fractures. It encompasses a wide spectrum of symptoms, including pain and stiffness of the hand, vasomotor instability, skin changes, and shoulder dysfunction. The incidence of reflex sympathetic dystrophy varies depending on how it is defined and on how closely it is screened for. Using broad diagnostic criteria, the incidence of reflex sympathetic dystrophy has been reported to be 25%, with two thirds still affected 6 months after fracture.[57] Treatment should begin at the first sign of the syndrome. Pain, hyperesthesia, swelling, and poor finger motion soon after fracture treatment herald the onset of the syndrome. Aggressive treatment involving edema control, active and passive mobilization of uninvolved joints, and adequate pain control are thought to help limit progression of the syndrome. After fracture union has been achieved, scar management, therapist-supervised motion exercises, and splinting can further help restore function. In recalcitrant cases, sympathetic block may be required. The role of median nerve release in the setting of reflex sympathetic dystrophy syndrome, yet in the *absence* of neuropathy, is unclear. It is apparent, however, that in patients with reflex sympathetic dystrophy in whom objective evidence of peripheral nerve dysfunction is found, significant symptomatic improvement may be expected after decompression.[58]

Open injuries are most frequent in the polytrauma patient in association with high-energy injuries. Aggressive management of these injuries with appropriate antibiotic therapy, tetanus toxoid administration, and timely surgical debridement is mandatory in these injuries. After debridement, fracture stabilization is most commonly performed through the application of an external fixator. Close monitoring for compartment syndrome, median neuropathy, and infection are vital in the postoperative period. For the comminuted, displaced articular injury, definitive reduction and fixation may be deferred until after the patient and the local soft tissues are stabilized, while the fixator maintains length and sagittal alignment in the intervening time.

Distal Radioulnar Joint

The distal radioulnar joint and its supporting soft-tissue structures are important to normal wrist function. Distal radioulnar joint problems after distal radius fractures often are more frequent than radiocarpal complications. Ulnar styloid fracture, distal radioulnar disruption or instability, ulnar-carpal impaction, and painful arthrosis are among the most common problems.

The importance of an associated ulnar styloid fracture lies in its reflection of a higher degree of initial fracture displacement as well as in possible disruption of ulnar-carpal ligaments and the triangular fibrocartilage complex (TFCC). Fractures through the base of the styloid are often associated with rupture of the TFCC, which may cause distal ulnar instability as well as chronic ulnar wrist pain. The role of TFCC repair in these injuries, however, is unclear. Painful hypertrophic nonunion of styloid fractures in the absence of associated radioulnar instability has been reported and successfully managed by fragment excision.[59]

Although classically radioulnar disruption is more often associated with the diaphyseal Galeazzi fracture, it may occur as well in distal radius fractures. This may be recognized radiographically by gross fracture displacement and radioulnar dissociation or through clinical assessment of radioulnar stability. Radioulnar disruption is treated through anatomic reduction of the joint and maintenance of this reduction in a position of maximum stability (typically supination). Studies of cadaveric specimens have clearly documented that fixation of an ulnar styloid base fracture restores stability to the disrupted radioulnar joint. Some authors now recommend fixation of these injuries in the setting of acute instability associated with styloid fracture.[60] Chronic radioulnar instability is difficult to manage; however, recent success in reducible congruent joints utilizing soft-tissue reconstruction has been reported.[61] Alternatively, if an ulnar styloid nonunion exists, repair may restore stability in some patients. In the setting of both chronic instability and radioulnar arthrosis, a modified Suave-Kapandji procedure with distal radioulnar fusion and creation of a proximal pseudarthrosis has been recommended.[62]

Posttraumatic positive ulnar variance may result in ulnar-sided wrist pain caused by ulnar carpal impaction. If this is caused solely by radial shortening, without other significant sagittal or coronal radial deformity, management through ulnar shortening will improve symptoms, provided a congruent articulation exists between the sigmoid notch and ulna. If other radial deformity exists, radial corrective osteotomy is indicated.

Arthrosis and associated pain, decreased grip strength, and limited forearm rotation are the most common radioulnar complications following distal radius fractures. Both extra-articular and intra-articular radiocarpal injuries may involve the sigmoid fossa. Anatomic reduction of the joint surface and, most importantly, of radial length are vital in preventing this complication. Results after late treatment by distal ulnar (Darrach) resection have been unpredictable and complicated by weakness, loss of ulnar carpal support, and distal ulnar instability, leading to a variety of surgical variations in an attempt to limit these problems.

Radiocarpal Arthrosis

The incidence of both symptomatic and radiographic radiocarpal arthrosis varies greatly in the literature. Rates as low as 1% to 2% or as high as 30% have been reported, depending on fracture pattern, reduction, and length of follow-up. It has become evident, however, that failure to achieve anatomic reduction (articular step-off less than 1 to 2 mm) of intra-articular fragments will result in radiographic evidence of arthrosis in most, if not all, patients. In young adults, more than 90% of these patients have been shown to be symptomatic.[18] With anatomic reduction of the articular surface, the rate of radiocarpal arthrosis may be reduced to between 5% and 10%, even in highly comminuted injuries.[39,51] The effect of extra-articular malunion on the development of radiocarpal arthrosis has been debated, although studies of cadavers have clearly shown alterations in joint-loading patterns, which may be detrimental to long-term outcome. Associated carpal fracture, intercarpal ligament disruption, and chondral damage at time of injury also play a role in the development of degenerative radiocarpal changes.

Once established, treatment options for radiocarpal arthrosis that has failed nonsurgical management include partial and complete wrist fusion or arthroplasty.[62] In patients with a well maintained midcarpal joint space and normal midcarpal alignment, radioscapholunate fusion is a good salvage option, especially in the nondominant extremity of a low-demand individual. In younger individuals or when higher functional loading is anticipated, total wrist fusion remains the treatment of choice. Total wrist arthroplasty is best reserved for low-demand patients who are unwilling to accept a fusion.

Distal Radial Malunion and Nonunion

Distal radial malunion may be associated with significant functional limitations, including pain, deformity, carpal instability, decreased motion, and weakness. Corrective osteotomy is indicated in symptomatic patients and has been recommended by some authors in asymptomatic patients with prearthritic deformities, such as articular step-off greater than 1 to 2 mm, dorsal radial tilt greater than 30°, shortening with distal radioulnar incongruity, and secondary dynamic carpal deformity. Comparative radiographs to provide a guide to restoration of normal anatomy, CT to define clearly the triplanar deformity and assess the radiocarpal and radioulnar joints for arthrosis, and complete preoperative planning of corrective osteotomy are mandatory. Because of the difficulty in restoring palmar tilt, radial inclination and length, and rotational alignment, some authors now use computer-generated images to assist in planning the osteotomy.

Extra-articular malunion may be managed by an opening wedge osteotomy with bone grafting and rigid fixation.[62-65] Early intra-articular malunion (less than 6 weeks after injury) may be corrected by taking down the malunion at the fracture line. Late intra-articular malunion (greater than 6 weeks after injury) is difficult to manage. Simple articular malunion patterns, such as isolated lunate fossa depressions or radial styloid fractures, may be osteotomized; however, more-complex articular malunions are best managed by nonsurgical treatment with salvage procedure if symptoms become debilitating.

Good to excellent results have been reported in approximately 80% of patients treated by corrective osteotomy. Patients with limited motion, fixed carpal malalignment, or degenerative radiocarpal/radioulnar changes have a poorer prognosis. A high reoperation rate for persistent ulnar-sided wrist pain and limited forearm rotation has been reported in patients with preoperative CT evidence of early radioulnar arthrosis, suggesting that some form of distal ulnar resection is recommended in these patients at the time of radial osteotomy. If radial osteotomy fails to restore radial length adequately, concomitant ulnar shortening should be considered.

Nonunion is exceedingly rare in distal radial fractures. Continued pain at the fracture site as well as loss of reduction have been reported as late as 7 months after injury, however, and require open reduction with bone grafting and rigid internal fixation.

Associated Carpal Injury

The scaphoid is the carpal bone most commonly fractured in association with a distal radius fracture.[9] These carpal injuries usually occur in young adults as a result of high-energy trauma with significant associated injuries. Recent literature has favored fixation of both displaced and undisplaced scaphoid fractures when they occur in association with unstable distal radius fractures. Improved immobilization position, avoidance of distraction forces on the scaphoid (if an external fixator will be used), and ability to begin early rehabilitation are advantages over closed treatment. One review reported 6 patients in whom a scaphoid fracture associated with an unstable distal radius fracture was treated surgically with bone grafting combined with Herbert screw and pin fixation.[66] All fractures healed after an average of 13 weeks. Wrist and forearm motion were started as soon as the injury to the distal radius allowed.

Ligament injury and carpal instability may occur after distal radius fracture. Scapholunate disruption is most common and must be carefully evaluated for, especially in high-energy injuries.[67] Treatment is through pinning of the scaphoid to the lunate if the diastasis may be reduced by closed means. If an increased scapholunate gap cannot be reduced closed, open reduction and ligament repair is indicated. Both volar and dorsal radiocarpal ligament injury may occur as well during distal radial injuries and may result in carpal instability patterns. Extra-articular malunion is also a cause of carpal instability; however, successful treatment depends on restoring anatomic radial alignment rather than attempts at carpal stabilization.

Annotated References

1. Alffram PA, Bauer GCH: Epidemiology of fractures of the forearm: A biomechanical investigation of bone strength. *J Bone Joint Surg* 1962;44A:105-114.

2. Colles A: On the fracture of the carpal extremity of the radius. *Edinburgh Med Surg J* 1814;10:182-186.

3. Fernandez DL: Fractures of the distal radius: Operative treatment, in Heckman JD (ed): *Instructional Course Lectures 42*. Rosemont, IL, American Academy of Orthopaedic Surgeons, 1993, pp 73-88.

4. McMurtry RY, Jupiter JB: Fractures of the distal radius, in Browner BD, Jupiter JB, Levine AM, et al (eds): *Skeletal Trauma: Fractures, Dislocations, Ligamentous Injuries*. Philadelphia, PA, WB Saunders, 1992, pp 1063-1094.

5. Trumble TE, Schmitt SR, Vedder NB: Factors affecting functional outcome of displaced intra-articular distal radius fractures. *J Hand Surg* 1994;19A:325-340.

   Trumble reviews his results after surgical treatment of a variety of intra-articular fractures. He presents a treatment algorithm-related classification based on the presence of metaphyseal and/or intra-articular comminution. Regression analysis is used to determine which factors are prognostic for poor outcome.

6. Melone CP Jr: Distal radius fractures: Patterns of articular fragmentation. *Orthop Clin North Am* 1993;24:239-253.

7. Müller ME, Nazarian S, Koch P (eds): *Classification AO des Fractures: Les Os Longs*. Berlin, Germany, Springer-Verlag, 1987.

8. Cooney WP III, Dobyns JH, Linscheid RL, et al: Complications of Colles' fractures. *J Bone Joint Surg* 1980;62A:613-619.

9. Pogue DJ, Viegas SF, Patterson RM, et al: Effects of distal radius fracture malunion on wrist joint mechanics. *J Hand Surg* 1990;15A:721-727.

    Utilizing Fuji pressure-sensitive film, alterations in radiocarpal contact areas and pressures are correlated with altered palmar tilt, radial length, and radial inclination.

10. Adams BD: Effects of radial deformity on distal radioulnar joint mechanics. *J Hand Surg* 1993;18A:492-498.

11. Short WH, Palmer AK, Werner FW, et al: A biomechanical study of distal radial fractures. *J Hand Surg* 1987;12A:529-534.

12. Jenkins NH, Mintowt-Czyz WJ: Mal-union and dysfunction in Colles' fracture. *J Hand Surg* 1988;13B:291-293.

    Malunion is significantly correlated with decreased grip strength, limited range of motion and pain in this review of patients at one and three years post fracture.

13. Aro HT, Koivunen T: Minor axial shortening of the radius affects outcome of Colles' fracture treatment. *J Hand Surg* 1991;16A:392-398.

14. McQueen M, Caspers J: Colles' fracture: Does the anatomical result affect the final function? *J Bone Joint Surg* 1988;70B:649-651.

15. Kopylov P, Johnel O, Redlund-Johnell I, et al: Fractures of the distal end of the radius in young adults: A 30-year follow-up. *J Hand Surg* 1993;18B:45-49.

16. Taleisnik J, Watson HK: Midcarpal instability caused by malunited fractures of the distal radius. *J Hand Surg* 1984;9A:350-357.

    The mechanism and treatment of dynamic midcarpal instability in the setting of distal radial malunion is reviewed.

17. Bickerstaff DR, Bell MJ: Carpal malalignment in Colles' fractures. *J Hand Surg* 1989;14B:155-160.

18. Knirk JL, Jupiter JB: Intra-articular fractures of the distal end of the radius in young adults. *J Bone Joint Surg* 1986;68A:647-659.

19. McQueen MM, MacLaren A, Chalmers J: The value of remanipulating Colles' fractures. *J Bone Joint Surg* 1986;68B:232-233.

20. Abbaszadegan H, Jonsson U, von Sivers K: Prediction of instability of Colles' fractures. *Acta Orthop Scand* 1989;60:646-650.

    The results of this retrospective review indicated that the tendency for redisplacement to occur during closed treatment is significantly correlated with initial radial shortening, age of the patient, and Lidstrom class.

21. Jenkins NH: The unstable Colles' fracture. *J Hand Surg* 1989;14B:149-154.

22. Gupta A: The treatment of Colles' fracture: Immobilisation with the wrist dorsiflexed. *J Bone Joint Surg* 1991;73B:312-315.

    In this prospective study of distal radius fractures early functional results and tendency toward redisplacement are improved in the study group treated by cast immobilization with the wrist in dorsiflexion as compared to two control groups.

23. Sarmiento A, Zagorski JB, Sinclair WF: Functional bracing of Colles' fractures: A prospective study of immobilization in supination vs pronation. *Clin Orthop* 1980;146:175-183.

24. Van der Linden W, Ericson R: Colles' fracture: How should its displacement be measured and how should it be immobilized? *J Bone Joint Surg* 1981;63A:1285-1288.

25. Ledingham WM, Wytch R, Goring CC, et al: On immediate functional bracing of Colles' fracture. *Injury* 1991;22:197-201.

26. Stewart HD, Innes AR, Burke FD: Functional cast-bracing for Colles' fractures: A comparison between cast-bracing and conventional plaster casts. *J Bone Joint Surg* 1984;66B:749-753.

27. Carrozzella J; Stern PJ: Treatment of comminuted distal radius fractures with pins and plaster. *Hand Clin* 1988;4:391-397.

28. Shankar NS, Craxford AD: Comminuted Colles' fractures: A prospective trial of management. *J Roy Coll Surg Edinb* 1992;37:199-202.

29. Mah ET, Atkinson RN: Percutaneous Kirschner wire stabilisation following closed reduction of Colles' fractures. *J Hand Surg* 1992;17B:55-62.

30. Clancey GJ: Percutaneous Kirschner-wire fixation of Colles' fractures: A prospective study of thirty cases. *J Bone Joint Surg* 1984;66A:1008-1014.

31. Rayhack JM, Langworthy JN, Belsole RJ: Transulnar percutaneous pinning of displaced distal radial fractures: A preliminary report. *J Orthop Trauma* 1989;3:107-114.

32. Greatting MD, Bishop AT: Intrafocal (Kapandji) pinning of unstable fractures of the distal radius. *Orthop Clin North Am* 1993;24:301-307.

33. Abbaszadegan H, Jonsson U: External fixation or plaster cast for severely displaced Colles' fractures? Prospective 1-year study of 46 patients. *Acta Orthop Scand* 1990;61:528-530.

34. Jenkins NH, Jones DG, Johnson SR, et al: External fixation of Colles' fractures: An anatomical study. *J Bone Joint Surg* 1987;69B:207-211.

35. Howard PW, Stewart HD, Hind RE, et al: External fixation or plaster for severely displaced comminuted Colles' fractures? A prospective study of anatomical and functional results. *J Bone Joint Surg* 1989;71B:68-73.

    This prospective review compared external fixation using the early Hoffman fixator with cast immobilization for comminuted intra-articular fractures. Anatomic and functional results were improved in the fixator group at a 6-month follow-up.

36. Bartosh RA, Saldana MJ: Intraarticular fractures of the distal radius: A cadaveric study to determine if ligamentotaxis restores radiopalmar tilt. *J Hand Surg* 1990;15A:18-21.

    The authors demonstrate that in a cadaveric model, the palmar radiocarpal ligaments, if intact, prevent restoration of normal radial palmar tilt utilizing axial ligamentotaxis alone.

37. Agee JM: External fixation: Technical advances based upon multiplanar ligamentotaxis. *Orthop Clin North Am* 1993;24:265-274.

    Agee reviews the theory and biomechanics of ligamentotaxis and its limitations in restoring palmar tilt. Based on this discussion, the principles of multiplanar ligamentotaxis and the clinical results of the Agee Wrist Jack external fixator are reviewed.

38. Axelrod T, Paley M, Green J, et al: Limited open reduction of the lunate facet in comminuted intra-articular fractures of the distal radius. *J Hand Surg* 1988;13A:372-377.

    The technical aspects and clinical results of limited open, radiographically assisted reduction of intra-articular fractures involving the lunate facet is reviewed in a limited number of patients.

39. Geissler WB, Fernandez DL: Percutaneous and limited open reduction of the articular surface of the distal radius. *J Orthop Trauma* 1991;5:255-264.

    This is an excellent review of limited open reduction and internal fixation combined with external fixation or pinning and bone grafting. Loss of reduction was observed in the pinning group when dorsal comminution was present. No such loss occurred in the externally fixed group.

40. Kaempffe FA, Wheeler DR, Peimer CA, et al: Severe fractures of the distal radius: Effect of amount and duration of external fixator distraction on outcome. *J Hand Surg* 1993;18A:33-41.

    Carpal height index and duration of external fixation are evaluated for correlation with a variety of functional criteria. Decreased motion and strength are significantly associated with greater duration and magnitude of distraction, respectively.

41. Biyani A: Over-distraction of the radio-carpal and mid-carpal joints following external fixation of comminuted distal radial fractures. *J Hand Surg* 1993;18B:506-510.

42. Leung KS, Shen WY, Tsang HK, et al: An effective treatment of comminuted fractures of the distal radius. *J Hand Surg* 1990;15A:11-17.

    The authors review their results after bone grafting, external fixation, and early mobilization of comminuted distal radial fractures.

43. Seitz WH Jr, Putnam MD, Dick HM: Limited open surgical approach for external fixation of distal radius fractures. *J Hand Surg* 1990;15A:288-293.

    The authors provide an excellent review of the techniques and pitfalls in the application of a wrist external fixation device.

44. Sommerkamp TG, Seeman M, Silliman J, et al: Dynamic external fixation of unstable fractures of the distal part of the radius: A prospective, randomized comparison with static external fixation. *J Bone Joint Surg* 1994;76A:1149-1161.

45. Edwards GS Jr: Intra-articular fractures of the distal part of the radius treated with the small AO external fixator. *J Bone Joint Surg* 1991;73A:1241-1250.

46. Jakim I, Pieterse HS, Sweet MB: External fixation for intra-articular fractures of the distal radius. *J Bone Joint Surg* 1991;73B:302-306.

47. Sprenger TR: Anterior margin articular fractures of the distal radius. *J Orthop Trauma* 1993;7:6-10.

    Sprenger reviews the use of a T plate for volar lip fractures and correlates fragment size with functional outcome in a group of 20 patients.

48. Pattee GA, Thompson GH: Anterior and posterior marginal fracture: Dislocations of the distal radius. An analysis of the results of treatment. *Clin Orthop* 1988;231:183-195.

49. Axelrod TS, McMurtry RY: Open reduction and internal fixation of comminuted, intraarticular fractures of the distal radius. *J Hand Surg* 1990;15A:1-11.

    Axelrod and McMurtry review their results with open reduction and internal fixation of 20 comminuted intra-articular fractures. Functional and radiographic results are excellent; however, a significant complication rate is noted and recommendations of ways to avoid these complications are given.

50. Porter ML, Tillman RM: Pilon fractures of the wrist: Displaced intra-articular fractures of the distal radius. *J Hand Surg* 1992;17B:63-68.

51. Jupiter JB, Lipton H: The operative treatment of intraarticular fractures of the distal radius. *Clin Orthop* 1993;292:48-61.

    The authors update the management of comminuted articular injuries with marked improvement in radiographic and functional results using open reduction and internal fixation when compared to Jupiter's 1986 review of similar injuries.

52. Bradway JK, Amadio PC, Cooney WP: Open reduction and internal fixation of displaced, comminuted intra-articular fractures of the distal end of the radius. *J Bone Joint Surg* 1989;71A:839-847.

53. Cooney WP, Berger RA: Treatment of complex fractures of the distal radius: Combined use of internal and external fixation and arthroscopic reduction. *Hand Clin* 1993;9:603-612.

    The Cooney treatment algorithm for distal radius fractures is reviewed, including the use of open reduction and internal fixation in combination with external fixation and bone grafting for intra-articular injuries. The technical considerations and advantages of arthroscopic assistance during fracture reduction are also cited.

54. Aro H, Koivunen T, Katevuo K, et al: Late compression neuropathies after Colles' fractures. *Clin Orthop* 1988;233:217-225.

55. McCarroll HR Jr: Nerve injuries associated with wrist trauma. *Orthop Clin North Am* 1984;15:279-287.

56. Hirasawa Y, Katsumi Y, Akiyoshi T, et al: Clinical and microangiographic studies on rupture of the EPL tendon after distal radial fractures. *J Hand Surg* 1990;15B:51-57.

57. Atkins RM, Duckworth T, Kanis JA: Algodystrophy following Colles' fracture. *J Hand Surg* 1989;14B:161-164.

    Utilizing broad diagnostic criteria, the incidence and clinical features of reflex sympathetic dystrophy at 9 weeks and 6 months after distal radius fracture are reviewed. All cases of reflex sympathetic dystrophy developed during the first 9 weeks of treatment.

58. Jupiter JB, Seiler JG III, Zienowicz R: Sympathetic maintained pain (causalgia) associated with a demonstrable peripheral-nerve lesion: Operative treatment. *J Bone Joint Surg* 1994;76A:1376-1384.

59. Burgess RC, Watson HK: Hypertrophic ulnar styloid nonunions. *Clin Orthop* 1988;228:215-217.

60. Shaw JA, Bruno A, Paul EM: Ulnar styloid fixation in the treatment of posttraumatic instability of the radioulnar joint: A biomechanical study with clinical correlation. *J Hand Surg* 1990;15A:712-720.

    The biomechanical effect of ulnar styloid fracture/TFCC disruption on distal radioulnar stability is tested in a cadaveric model. Clinical data reviewing the use of ulnar styloid fracture fixation are provided.

61. Leung PC, Hung LK: An effective method of reconstructing posttraumatic dorsal dislocated distal radioulnar joints. *J Hand Surg* 1990;15A:925-928.

62. Fernandez DL: Reconstructive procedures for malunion and traumatic arthritis. *Orthop Clin North Am* 1993;24:341-363.

    This is an excellent review of treatment options for malunion and posttraumatic arthritis after distal radial fracture.

63. Fernandez DL: Radial osteotomy and Bowers arthroplasty for malunited fractures of the distal end of the radius. *J Bone Joint Surg* 1988;70A:1538-1551.

    Fernandez reviews the techniques, indications, and results of radial osteotomy combined with hemiresection of the distal radioulnar joint for symptomatic radial malunion.

64. Jupiter JB, Masem M: Reconstruction of post-traumatic deformity of the distal radius and ulna. *Hand Clin* 1988;4:377-390.

65. Watson HK, Castle TH Jr: Trapezoidal osteotomy of the distal radius for unacceptable articular angulation after Colles' fracture. *J Hand Surg* 1988;13A:837-843.

66. Trumble TE, Benirschke SK, Vedder NB: Ipsilateral fractures of the scaphoid and radius. *J Hand Surg* 1993;18A:8-14.

67. Mudgal C, Hastings H: Scapho-lunate diastasis in fractures of the distal radius: Pathomechanics and treatment options. *J Hand Surg* 1993;18B:725-729.

    The authors review the history, mechanism, and treatment of scapholunate ligament disruption in association with distal radius fracture.

8
Carpal Fractures and Dislocations

Introduction

Our understanding of injuries to the hand and wrist has been aided by advances made in normal and abnormal kinematic studies and by direct articular and ligamentous arthroscopic evaluation. Normal motion, carpal kinematic studies, ligamentous disruptions and their effects on carpal motion, and intercarpal arthrodesis have improved our appreciation of injuries and subsequent treatment. Force transmission both in the static, aligned wrist and in displaced, angulated states allows determination of acceptable limits in our daily treatment of wrist and hand injuries. Direct arthroscopic evaluation of wrist and hand injuries aids in the evaluation of these injuries and in the treatment decision-making process.

Hyperextension injuries of the wrist and subsequent intercarpal disruptions or fracture dislocations continue to be examined with the basic understanding of the perilunar sequence of injuries. The patterns of injuries have been correlated to demonstrate various ligamentous injuries resulting in certain instability patterns. Scapholunate joint disruptions may lead to scaphoid rotatory instability and subsequent arthritic changes. Lunotriquetral and triquetral hamate injuries may result in midcarpal instability patterns. Evaluation of these injuries has been aided by wrist arthrograms using injections of the distal radial ulnar, radiocarpal, and midcarpal joints. Magnetic resonance imaging (MRI) may also be used in the evaluation of wrist injuries, but direct visualization arthroscopically is proving to be more effective.

More rapid diagnosis of these injuries has allowed direct repair of ligaments and joint stabilization, with results better than those seen following salvage or reconstructive procedures.

Anatomy

The interrelationship of the osseous and ligamentous structures of the wrist maintains a delicate balance, allowing not only flexion and extension but also radial-ulnar deviation, pronation, and supination. The extrinsic (radius to carpus) and intrinsic (carpal bone to carpal bone) ligaments maintain the overall alignment (Figs. 1 and 2). The obliquely oriented major extrinsic ligaments (radioscapholunate and

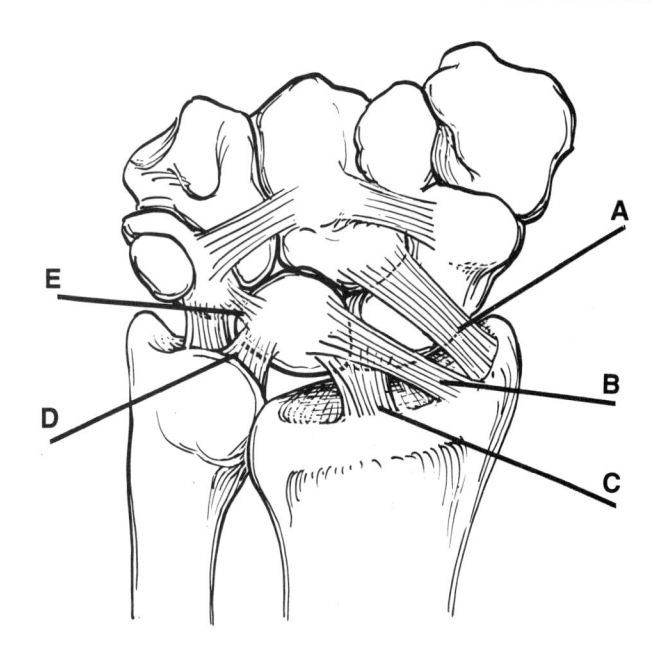

Fig. 1 Palmar view of the extrinsic radiocarpal and interosseous ligaments. **A**, Radioscaphocapitate ligament. **B**, Radiolunate ligament. **C**, Radioscapholunate ligament. **D**, Ulnocarpal ligaments. **E**, Lunotriquetral ligament.

radiolunotriquetral) and the dorsal radiotriquetral ligament resist the tendency of the carpus to migrate ulnarly and palmarly. The radioscapholunate ligament has been found to be more of a mesentery for vessels and nerves, and it does not have much structural importance.[1]

The intrinsic scapholunate and lunotriquetral ligaments support the lunate in a balanced position. The scapholunate ligament can be divided into three different zones: the dorsal and palmar ligamentous zone and the proximal membranous fibrocartilaginous zone, with the dorsal component being structurally the most important. Division of the scapholunate ligament allows the lunate to follow the triquetrum's unrestrained position of extension, radiographically seen as the dorsal intercalated segmental instability pattern (DISI). Lunotriquetral ligament disruption allows the lunate to follow the scaphoid into its position of unrestrained

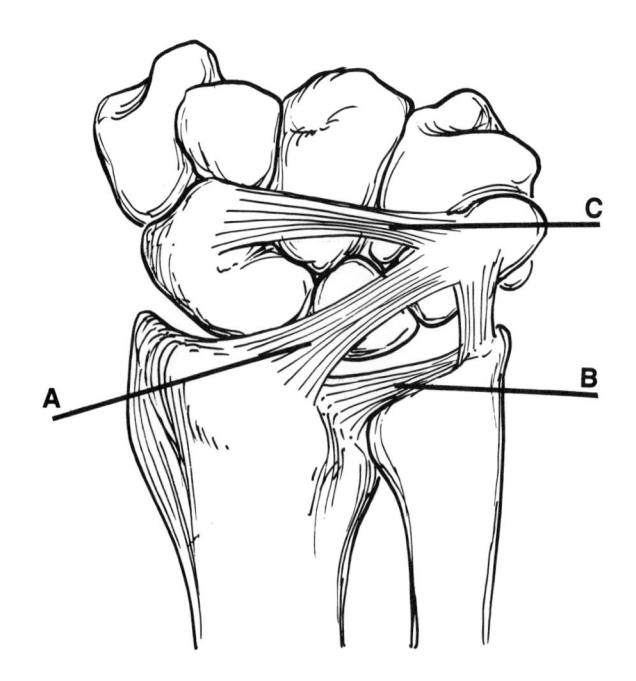

Fig. 2 Dorsal view of the extrinsic radiocarpal and interosseous ligaments. **A**, Dorsal radiotriquetral ligament. **B**, Dorsal radioulnar ligament. **C**, Triquetroscaphoid ligament.

flexion, or the volar intercalated segmental instability pattern (VISI).

Dislocations and Ligamentous Injuries

Classification

The work of Johnson[2] and Mayfield and associates[3] on perilunate injury patterns continues to be the mainstay in our understanding of hyperextension injuries. As the hand is forced into hyperextension, ulnar deviation, and intercarpal supination, the ligamentous disruption allows scapholunate dissociation followed by capitolunate dissociation and then lunotriquetral joint dissociation (Fig. 3).[3,4] The injury involves not only the interosseous ligaments, specifically the scapholunate and lunotriquetral ligaments, but also the radioscaphocapitate, radiolunotriquetral, and dorsal radiotriquetral ligaments. The final pathway of these injuries may be either a dorsal perilunate injury with a carpus dorsal to the lunate, which remains in the lunate fossa, or a lunate dislocation palmarly with the capitate residing in the lunate fossa. Recently the patterns have been referred to as stage I, with the lunate resting in the lunate fossa of the radius, or stage II, with lunate dislocation (Fig. 4).[5]

The injury scheme may involve periligamentous disruption, referred to as a lesser arc injury.[2] Dislocations involving fractures, which can include the radial styloid, scaphoid, capitate, and triquetrum, are termed greater arc injuries

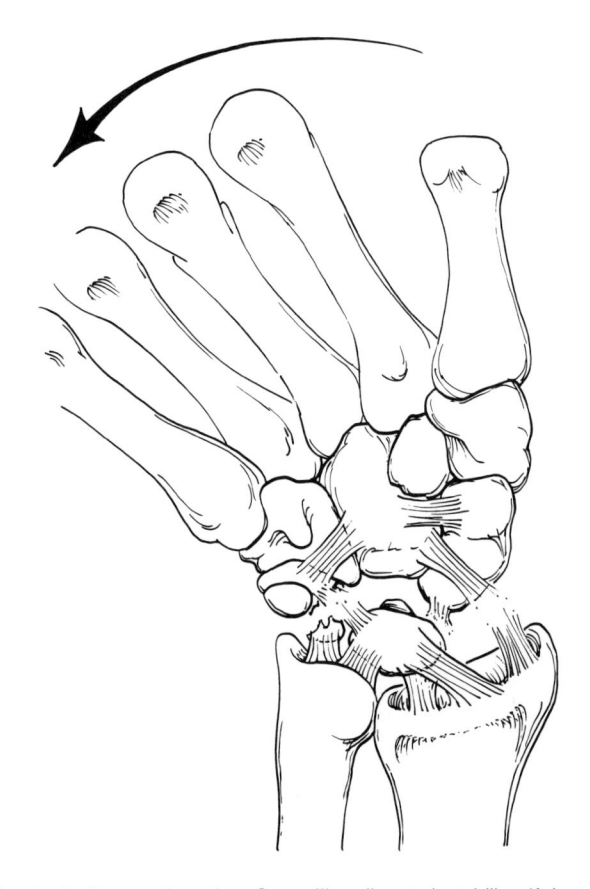

Fig. 3 Perilunate disruption. Stage III perilunate instability. (Adapted with permission from Mayfield JK, Johnson RP, Kilcoyne RF: Carpal dislocations: Pathomechanics and progressive perilunate instability. *J Hand Surg* 1980;5:226–241.)

(Fig. 5).[2] Combinations of both may occur, the most common of which is the transscaphoid perilunate dorsal fracture dislocation.

The carpus may also be disrupted in a longitudinal fashion, as opposed to the perilunate transverse pattern[6,7] (Fig. 6). Traumatic axial longitudinal dislocations separate the carpus into four patterns of injury. The first split is ulnarly. The long finger metacarpal and radial structures remain stable and the ring and small metacarpals with the hamate and triquetrum fracture and dislocate ulnarly. The axial-radial group carries the radial column with the thumb and/or index metacarpal along with the trapezium and/or trapezoid radially. The third group, axial-radial-ulnar, leaves the long metacarpal stable and the ulnar and radial columns split and dislocated. Norbeck and associates[7] have added a case that complements the three variations presented by Garcia-Elias and associates[6] with a fourth category: disruption through the lunotriquetral joint and ulnar dislocation of the triquetrum with the ulnar column.

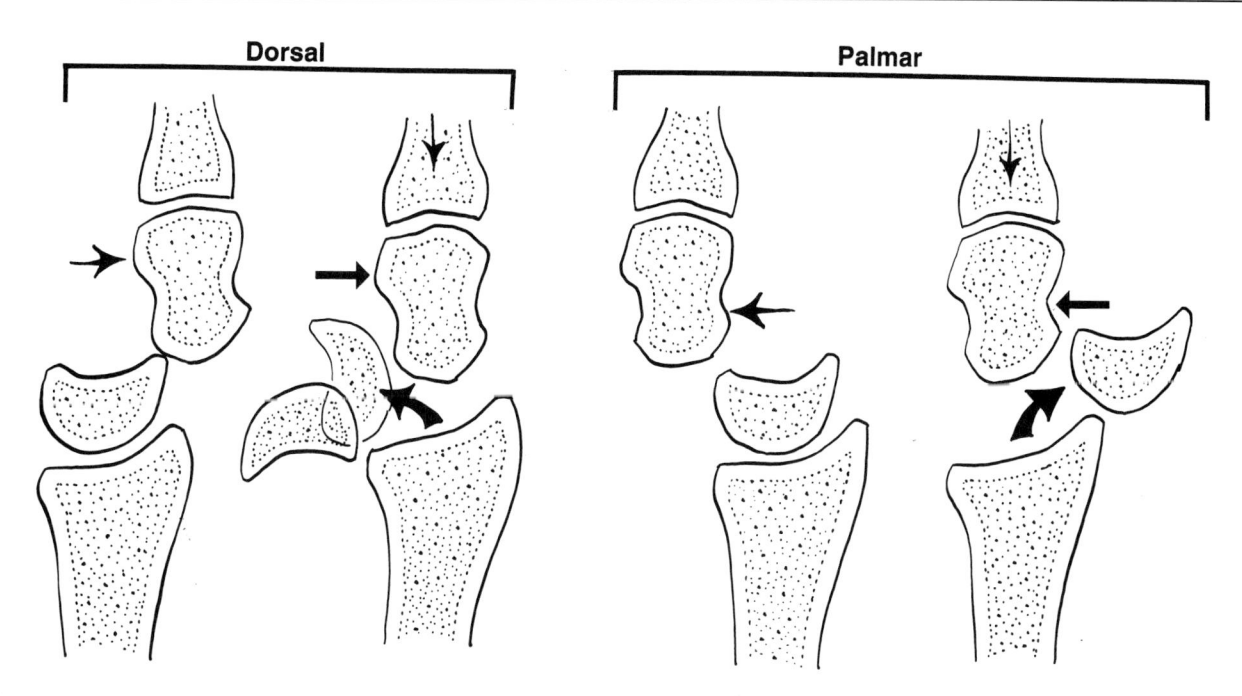

Fig. 4 Staging of perilunate dislocations. **Left,** Stage I, dorsal perilunate dislocation. **Center left,** Stage II, palmar lunate dislocation. **Center right,** Stage I, palmar perilunate dislocation. **Right,** Stage II, dorsal lunate dislocation. (Adapted with permission from Herzberg G, Comtet JJ, Linscheid RL, et al: Perilunate dislocations and fracture-dislocations: A multicenter study. J Hand Surg 1993;18A:768–779.)

Radiographic and Physical Examination

Plain radiographs with attention to the lateral projection remain the mainstay of evaluation of these injuries (Fig. 7). The lateral radiograph must demonstrate colinear alignment of the radius, lunate, capitate, and metacarpals. The posteroanterior radiograph should demonstrate a gentle continuous curve along the proximal and distal carpal bones at the radiocarpal and midcarpal articulation. Any disruption in the colinear alignment on the lateral radiograph or of the curve on the posteroanterior radiograph should raise the suspicion of carpal subluxation or dislocation. Delay in diagnosis is still common; in one large series, 25% of the perilunate injuries were missed initially.[5] Perilunate injuries may be better evaluated acutely with distraction traction radiographs to examine unappreciated, eg, capitate fractures. Chronic intercarpal injuries may be evaluated using stress radiographs, cineradiography, and triple injection arthrograms. Compared to isolated radiocarpal injections, triple injection has been shown to increase the yield of ligament injuries.[8] MRI is beneficial in diagnosing avascular carpal fracture fragments, and improving MRI technology may make ligament and vascular evaluation simpler and more accurate. The evaluation of longitudinal axial carpal injuries may be aided by computed tomography (CT).[7]

Traumatic axial longitudinal dislocation of the carpus has been found to be associated with substantial skin and soft-tissue injuries. Crush or blast injuries are common causes and are associated with massive soft-tissue disruption of the transverse arch. In one study,[6] 15 of 16 injuries were open; in another,[9] five of eight axial-ulnar type injuries were open. Neurologic injury has been documented, and the ulnar nerve is at greatest risk. The flexor retinaculum was injured in all cases, which may account for the infrequent association of carpal tunnel syndrome. Intrinsic muscle damage is also frequent. Prophylactic arteriographic evaluation has been recommended.[9]

Treatment

The treatment for perilunate injuries spans the spectrum of closed reduction, closed reduction with percutaneous Kirschner wire (K-wire) fixation, open reduction with internal fixation (ORIF) with K-wires, ORIF of the scaphoid with Herbert screws, ORIF of the scaphoid with percutaneous K-wires of the lunotriquetral joint, and augmentation of ORIF with external fixation.[4,10–12] There is a high failure rate in perilunate fracture dislocations and perilunate dislocations that had been initially successfully treated with closed reduction; one report indicated approximately 60% had loss of reduction.[10] On the other hand, ORIF maintained reduction in 75% of those cases.[10] In general, the surgical approach to perilunate dislocations depends on the direction and type of dislocation. For pure dorsal ligamentous dislocations, a palmar approach is used to repair the palmar rent and a dorsal approach is used to repair the scapholunate and lunotriquetral ligaments.[11–13] K-wire fixation is also

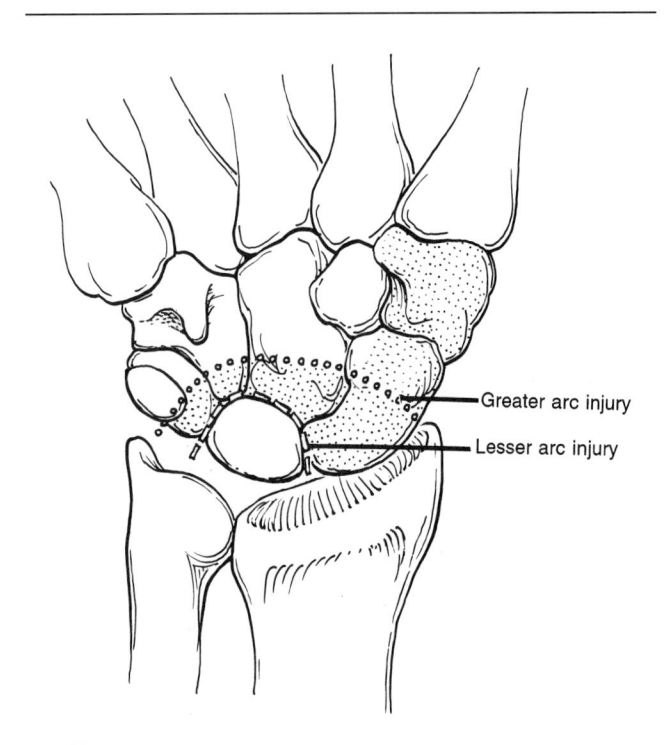

Fig. 5 Greater and lesser arc perilunate injury scheme. (Adapted with permission from Johnson RP: The acutely impaired wrist and its residuals. *Clin Orthop* 1980;149:33–34.)

required. Transscaphoid perilunate fracture dislocations may be approached in a number of directions. Screws for the scaphoid, employing a palmar approach, and appropriate K-wire fixation on the other joints have been advocated. A recent large study on perilunate injuries did not clearly define surgical approaches but indicated that, despite well-healed scaphoids, ligamentous problems persisted.[5] Use of combined approaches for direct repair of ligaments and stabilization has been supported.

Longitudinal axial disruptions require aggressive debridement and attention to neurovascular injury.[6,7,9] Intrinsic muscles (interossei, hypothenar, and thenar muscles) frequently require debridement along with attention to the ulnar nerve injury, which may cause substantial functional limitations. Because the majority of these injuries have associated fractures that may be open, direct visualization will allow reduction and K-wire fixation. Screws and Herbert screws have also been used. Closed reduction and percutaneous K-wire fixation may be undertaken in axial-radial closed injuries. Postoperative immobilization has been recommended for 4 to 8 weeks. In combined radius and intercarpal injuries, attention must be directed first to the distal radius treatment and then to appropriate scaphoid or ligamentous repair.[14]

Complications

In one study,[5] even with early treatment and satisfactory clinical results, 50% of patients with perilunate injuries developed arthritis.[5] In another study, the nerve injury, regardless of the type of disruption (axial-ulnar or axial-radial), was the major determining factor in outcome (of six patients with major nerve injuries, only one had a good result).[6] In another study, it was noted that, in a group of patients with axial-ulnar injuries, recognition of the injury within 2 weeks gave better results according to evaluation by grip strength, while the group treated after 1 month had poor results.[9] Patients tended to recover range of motion, but pinch and grip strength appeared to be limiting factors in preventing them from returning to their previous occupations. The decrease in strength is probably related to loss of intrinsic muscle disruption of the flexor retinaculum, and sensory loss. Multiple reconstructive procedures, including tenolysis, neurolysis, capsulectomies, web space releases, and delayed carpal tunnel release, are required to treat these complications.

Carpal Fractures

Classification

Scaphoid fractures have been classified based on the level, direction, and chronicity of the fracture: type A, acute, stable fractures; type B, acute, unstable fractures; type C, delayed union; and type D, nonunion (Fig. 8).[15]

A review was made of lunate fractures to develop a fracture classification system and to delineate lunate fractures at risk for the development of Kienböck's disease.[16] Seventeen lunate fractures were divided into five groups, correlating them to the vascularity patterns as described by Gelberman and associates[17] (Figs. 9 and 10).

Trapezium fractures associated with other carpal injuries and isolated trapezoid injuries are rare. The trapezium most commonly dislocates palmarly but may also dislocate dorsoradially, as described by Sherlock.[18] Fractures of the trapezium body, trapezium fractures with carpometacarpal dislocations, and Bennett fractures combined with trapezium fractures have been reported.[19] Fractures of the trapezium have six patterns (Fig. 11).[19] Various mechanisms for these injuries have been described; recently support has been given to the commissural shearing mechanism[19] (Fig. 12).

Capitate fractures are most frequently associated with perilunate fracture patterns. Isolated capitate fractures occur less commonly. Milch[20] initially classified hamate fractures as sagitally split body fractures, and hook of the hamate fractures. A third group has been added that involves coronal split of the hamate (Fig. 13).[21] The injury occurs by axial load to the ring and small metacarpals and a flexion moment to the metacarpal head. Dorsal and ulnar flake fractures are probably a variant of the ring and small metacarpal fracture dislocation group.[22]

Dorsal fractures of the triquetrum have been associated with avulsion due to flexion of the wrist. One theory suggests the concept of compression causing a chipping of the dorsal triquetrum by a prominent ulnar styloid.[23] Wrist extension therefore would be associated with this injury.

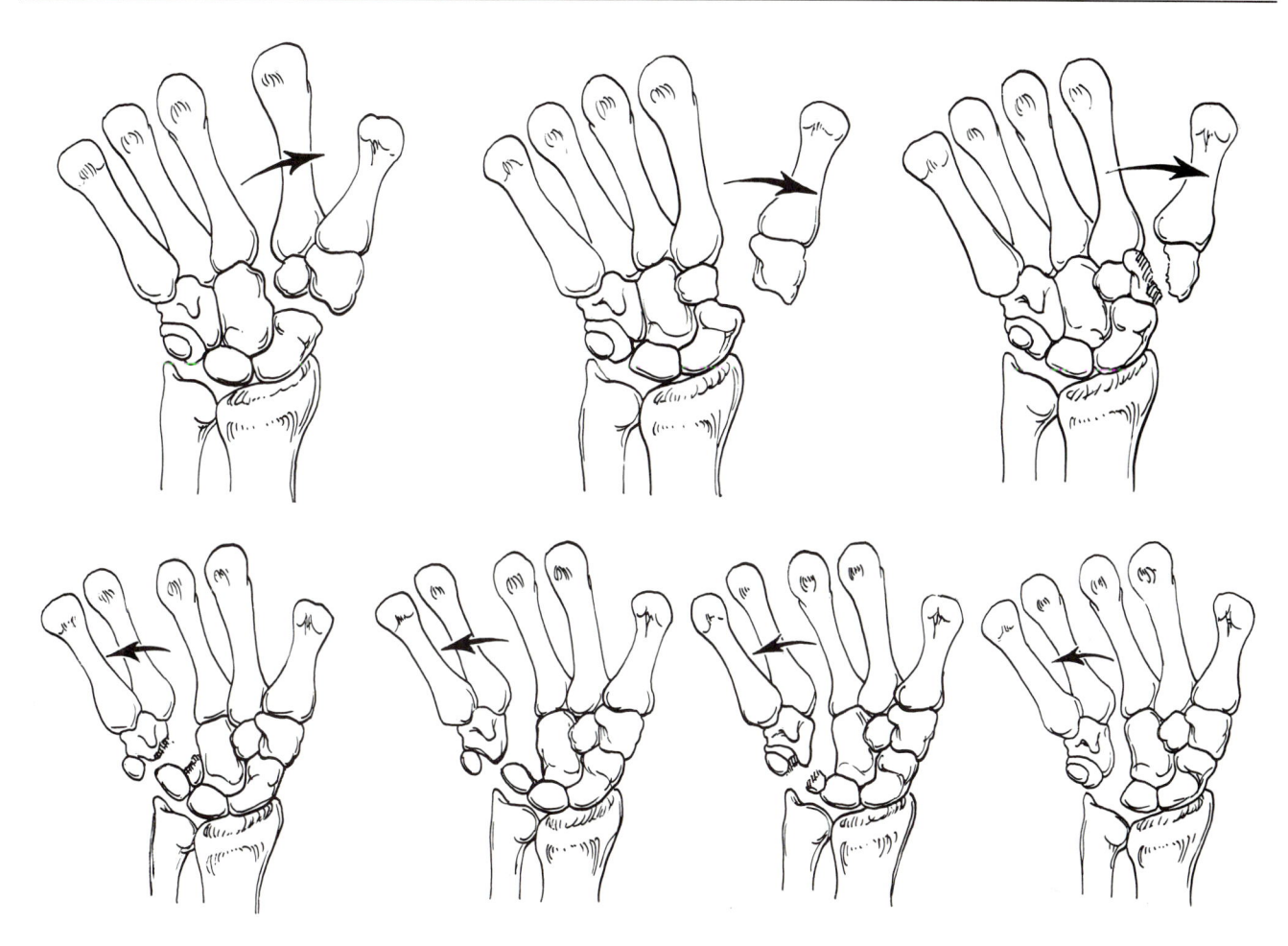

Fig. 6 Longitudinal carpus disruption. **Top,** Axial-radial disruption. **Bottom,** Axial-ulnar disruption. Arrows indicate direction of force. (Adapted with permission from Garcia-Elias M, Dobyns JH, Cooney WP, et al: Traumatic axial dislocations of the carpus. *J Hand Surg* 1989;14A:446–457.)

Avulsion fractures are probably due to the dorsal radiotriquetral ligament, which is in tension with wrist flexion.

Radiographic and Physical Examination

Scaphoid instability on plain radiographs has been defined as displacement of the fracture by more than 1 mm, any scaphoid angulation, or scapholunate angulation greater than 45°.[24] Values greater than these have been associated with nonunion and carpal collapse. The radiographic evaluation of scaphoid fractures traditionally correlated the level of fracture with potential union: distal, good; proximal, poor. Some clinicians believe that the presence of a sclerotic proximal scaphoid pole indicates an avascular fragment with poor healing potential. Poor correlation has been demonstrated between histologic viability, proximal pole sclerosis radiographically, and the absence of punctate bleeding, which was associated with a poor prognosis for healing.[25] MRI has also been used to evaluate acute scaphoid fractures and scaphoid nonunions.[26] Decreased signal content tends to be consistent with osteonecrosis in the chronic setting. Plain radiographs were found to document only approximately half of these findings. Another study correlated bone viability and osteonecrosis in scaphoid nonunions.[27] There was poor correlation between predictions based on plain radiographs and on tomograms. Radiographic confirmation of scaphoid fracture union may be difficult. Trispiral tomography and CT in the longitudinal axis of the scaphoid have been found to be helpful.[28] CT aids in the determination of scaphoid nonunion and potential humpback deformities. The study must be performed along the longitudinal axis of the scaphoid. Using trispiral tomography, lateral intrascaphoid angle has also been examined, with an intrascaphoid angle of less than 45° being associated with better radiographic and clinical findings.[28] Another evaluation found that 45° of intrascaphoid angle was not necessarily correlated with statistically significant decreased range of motion or symptoms.[29]

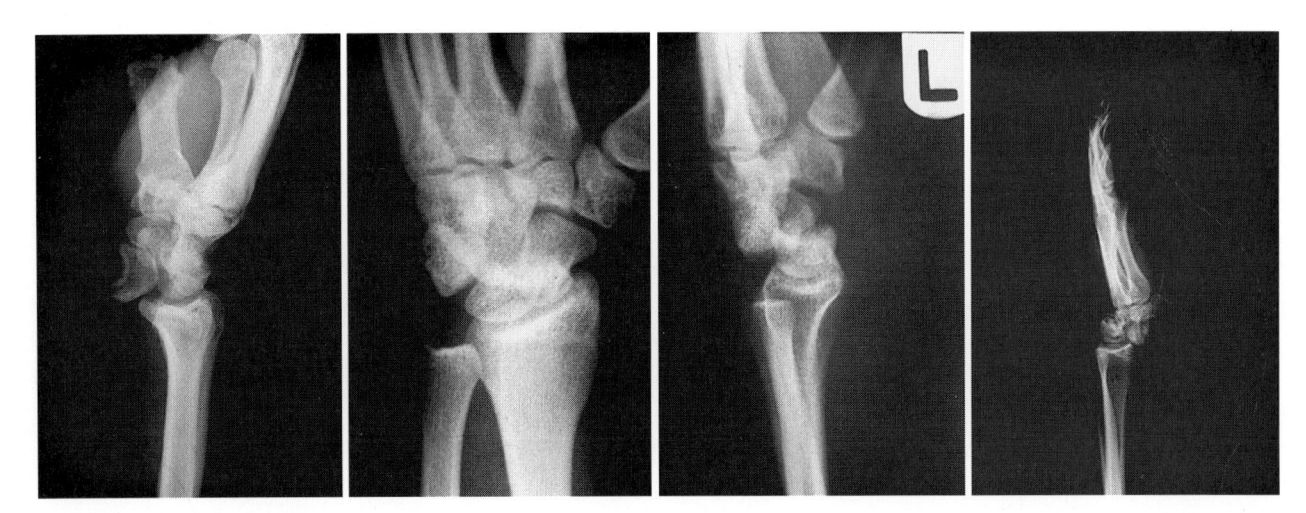

Fig. 7 **Left,** Lateral radiograph of palmar lunate dislocation. **Left center,** Posterior/anterior radiograph of dorsal transscaphoid perilunate fracture dislocation. **Right center,** Lateral radiograph of dorsal transscaphoid perilunate fracture dislocation. **Right,** Lateral radiograph of palmar transscaphoid perilunate fracture dislocation.

Trapezium fractures may require a modified Bett view, that is, an anterior oblique projection with ulnar deviation of the hand, because of problems with the trapezium trapezoid overlap.[30] Hook of the hamate fractures may sometimes elude standard radiographs; in addition to trispiral tomography and CT, three signs on a posterior anterior radiographs have been described as diagnostic aids: the absence of the hook of the hamate, the presence of sclerosis, and the absence of cortical density.[31] Carpal tunnel views, oblique projections, and trispiral tomography may also aid in fracture evaluation.[32]

Treatment

The advent of wrist arthroscopy and more aggressive ORIF has revealed a combination of injuries once thought to be mutually exclusive. Intra-articular distal radius fractures requiring ORIF may have either concomitant scaphoid or scapholunate ligament injuries.[14,33] Arthroscopically assisted distal radius fracture fixation likewise has shown a marked incidence of associated intercarpal ligament injuries and triangular fibrocartilage complex tears. The association of scaphoid fractures and scapholunate ligament tears within the perilunar sequence has also been documented.[34]

Most clinicians agree that the initial treatment of nondisplaced stable scaphoid fractures is external immobilization; however, early internal fixation and limited postoperative immobilization is an option. The spectrum of recommendations for immobilization ranges from wrapping with an elastic bandage to the long arm-thumb spica cast, including the index and long fingers. Inclusion of the thumb continues to be controversial. A study comparing short arm cast versus a short arm-thumb spica cast revealed a 10% incidence of nonunion in each group.[35] When the effects of a long arm-thumb and short arm-thumb spica cast on nondisplaced fractures were compared, all 28 fractures treated with a long arm-thumb spica cast united, whereas two of the 23 fractures with short arm-thumb spica casts failed to unite.[24] The recommendation for proximal and mid-third fractures was treatment with a long arm-thumb spica cast for 6 weeks, followed by a short arm-thumb spica cast. A distal fracture could be treated using short arm-thumb spica cast. With regard to the effect of delay in treatment, a review of 285 fractures revealed that a delay in mobilization up to 4 weeks did not increase the nonunion rate.[36] Displacement of the fracture was found to cause a three-fold increase in the incidence of nonunion and a prolongation of time to union of 2 weeks in displaced waist fractures.[36]

Internal fixation of scaphoid fractures that are unstable, displaced, nonunited, or associated with intercarpal instabilities may successfully be treated with a variety of devices such as K-wires, lag screws, and Herbert screws.[37,38] Nonunion may be treated by a number of modalities, as reviewed in Table 1.

A number of biomechanical studies have demonstrated that the Herbert screw may generate the least compression in cadaver models. Screws with a head tended to have better force compression.[51-53]

Historical reviews indicate that these fractures, if untreated, may progress to Kienböck's disease. In one long-term study of 11 patients, fractures were diagnosed early and treated with immobilization and none of the patients developed this disease. The authors believed that their evaluations of sagittal and transverse fractures were inconclusive and that these two patterns should be followed radiographically.

Nonsurgical treatment of trapezial fractures associated with other fractures has been shown to result in approxi-

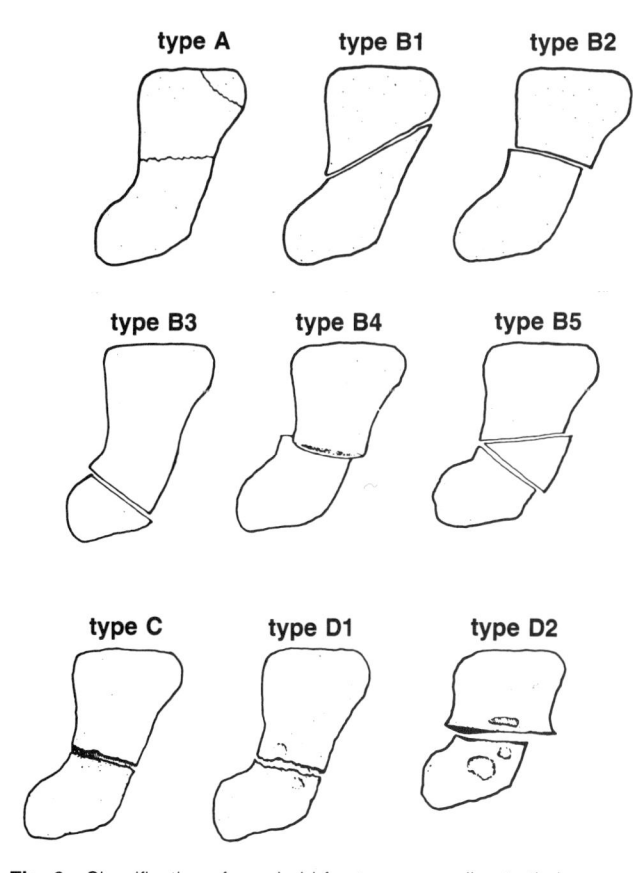

Fig. 8 Classification of scaphoid fractures according to their radiographic appearance. (Reproduced with permission from Herbert TJ, Fisher WE: Management of the fractured scaphoid using a new bone screw. *J Bone Joint Surg* 1984;66B:114–123.)

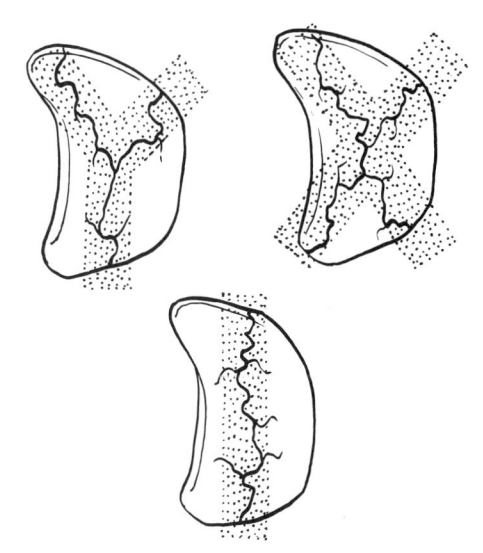

Fig. 9 Lunate vascularity patterns: Y, X, I. (Reproduced with permission from Gelberman RH, Bauman TD, Menon J, et al: The vascularity of the lunate bone and Kienbock's disease. *J Hand Surg* 1980;5A:272–278.)

Table 1 Treatment methods for scaphoid nonunions

Method/study	Unions/nonunions	% Unions
Herbert screw and bone graft		
Inoue and Miura[39]	66/70	94
Radford et al[40] (only 52% bone grafted)	52/50	84
DeMaagd et al[41] (proximal pole via retrograde)	8/9	89
Cooney et al[42]	17/21	81*
Lag screws and bone graft		
Fernandez[43]	19/20	95
Percutaneous pinning		
Cosio et al[44]	10/13	77
Iliac crest bone graft/K-wires		
Stark et al[45]	147/151	97
Ender compression blade plate and bone graft		
Huene et al[46]	19/20	95
Compression staple and bone graft		
Korkala et al[47]	19/23	83
Casting, pulsed electromagnetic field		
Adams et al[48]	37/54	69
proximal third	5/10	50
medial/distal	32/44	73
Vascularized bone graft		
Zaidemberg et al[49]	11/11	100
Scaphoid allograft		
Carter et al[50]	7/7	100

*Two required repeat ORIF

mately a 50% loss of range of motion and grip strength. In one study, ORIF and K-wires produced better results in isolated trapezial injuries than in those associated with other hand injuries.[19] Radiographic irregularities, including residual step-off and joint space narrowing, did not necessarily preclude an asymptomatic thumb or hand. Capitate fractures have the potential to develop nonunions because of a dominate palmar retrograde blood supply.[54] Internal fixation using screws has been advocated. Capitate fractures that have a coronal split require ORIF with a combination of screws and K-wires.[55] Hook of the hamate fractures diagnosed early (within 7 days) will achieve union when immobilized for 6 weeks.[56,57] Symptomatic hook of the hamate nonunions have been treated by excision.[58] In one study, the authors demonstrated only 33% asymptomatic patients and, based on this finding, recommended ORIF because they believed that removal of the hamate hook caused decreased tendon excursion and loss of strength.[59]

Complications

The natural history of the 5% to 10% of scaphoids that do not unite on initial treatment has recently been elaborated.[60,61] Mild to moderate symptoms did not correlate with radiographic signs or duration[59] and instability, location of fracture, and time since injury did not correlate with wrist pain.[61]

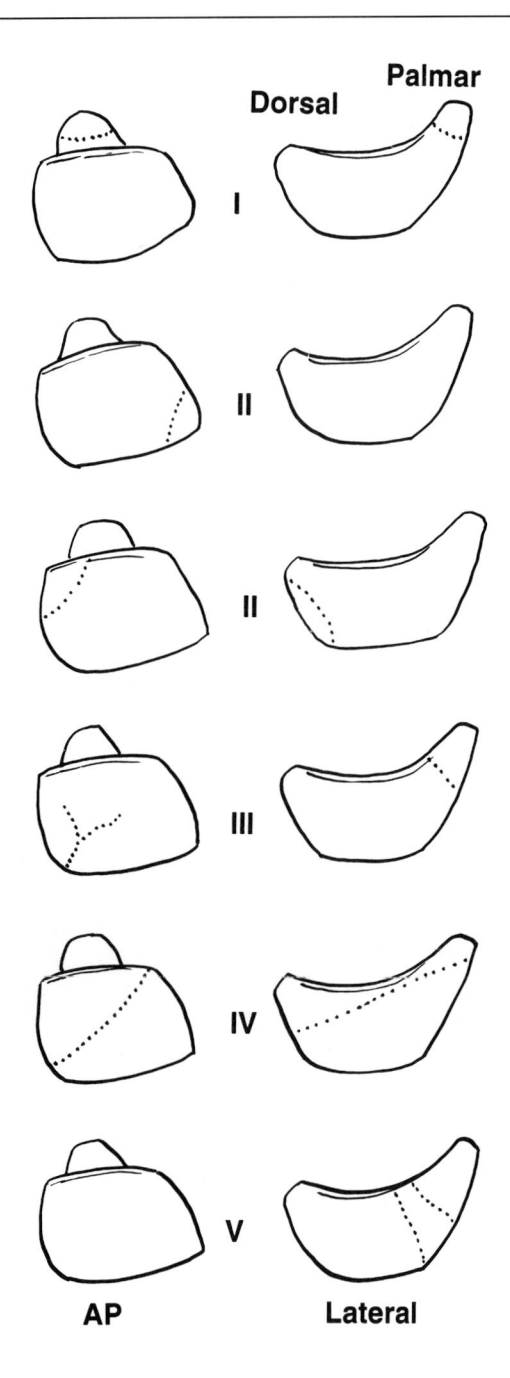

Fig. 10 Lunate fracture pattern. Group I, Fracture of the palmar pole of the lunate, possibly affecting the palmar nutrient artery. Group II, Chip fracture that does not affect the main blood supply. Group III, Fracture of the dorsal pole of the lunate, possibly affecting the dorsal nutrient artery. Group IV, Sagittal fracture through the body of the lunate. Group V, Transverse fracture through the body of the lunate. (Reproduced with permission from Teisen H, Hjarbaek J: Classification of fresh fractures of the lunate. *J Hand Surg* 1988;13B:458–462.)

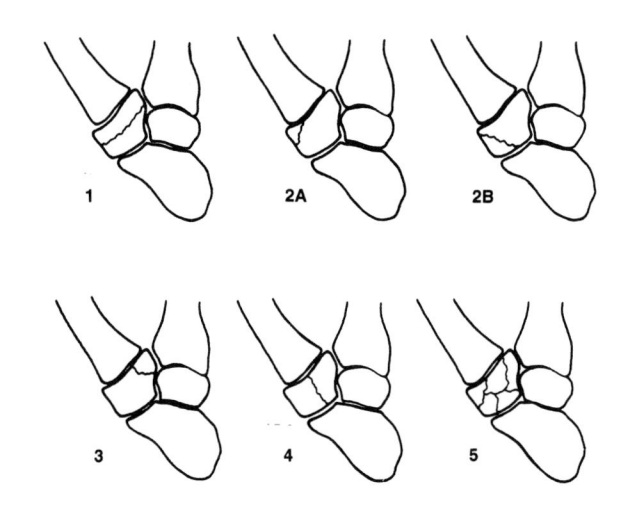

Fig. 11 Trapezial body fractures. (Reproduced with permission from Walker JL, Greene TL, Lunseth PA: Fractures of the body of the trapezium. *J Orthop Trauma* 1988;2:22–28.)

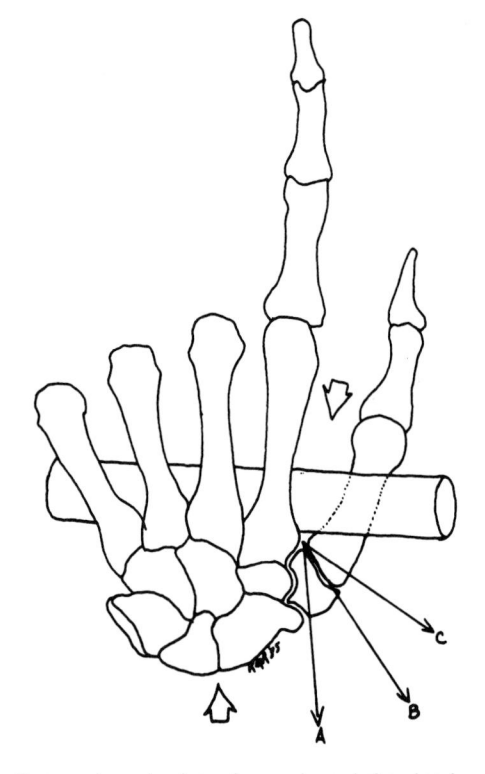

Fig. 12 Proposed mechanism of commissural shearing forces. By altering the directions of the force vector, **A** would result in a fracture of the trapezium, **B** would result in carpometacarpal dislocation, and **C** would result in a Bennett's fracture of the first metacarpal. (Reproduced with permission from Walker JL, Greene TL, Lunseth PA: Fractures of the body of the trapezium. *J Orthop Trauma* 1988;2:22–28.)

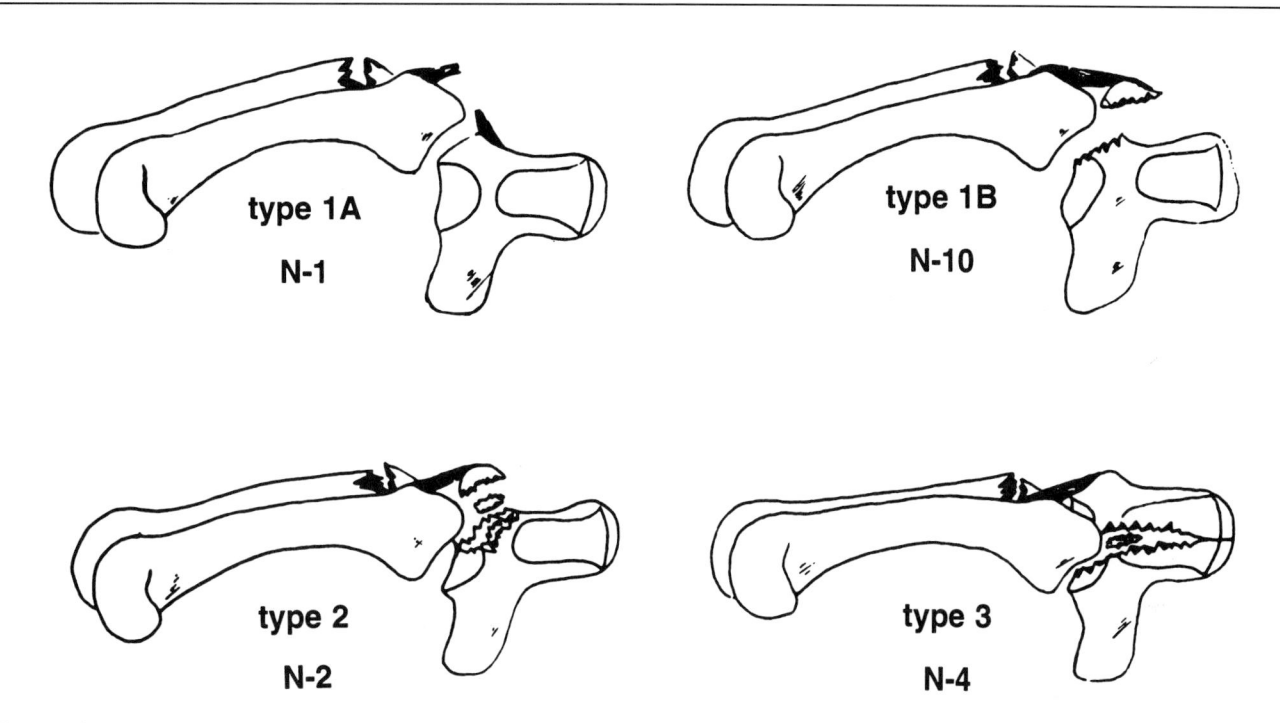

Fig. 13 Classification of ring metacarpal fractures and fifth carpometacarpal joint subluxation/dislocation. (Reproduced with permission from Cain JE Jr, Shepler TR, Wilson MR: Hamatometacarpal fracture-dislocation: Classification and treatment. *J Hand Surg* 1987;12A:762–767.)

The "second injury" cause of presentation also has been addressed in the literature. When the duration of nonunion is more than 10 years, the frequency of instability (ie, DISI deformity) increased.[62] Instability also has been associated with patterns of advanced arthritis.[63–65] Yet to be clarified in the literature, however, is the ability to alter the progression of both radiologic and symptomatic degenerative changes in treating scaphoid nonunions.[66]

Although the fate of the stable, or nondisplaced, asymptomatic fibrous nonunion is not known, the studies discussed above still allow improved counseling for the symptomatic patients with scaphoid nonunions.

Complications associated with hook of the hamate fractures have recently been evaluated. The ulnar flexor tendons course around the hook of the hamate and nonunion increases the potential for attrition of the tendon. A 14% incidence of flexor tendon problems, including fraying and rupture, has been reported.[67] A 3% treatment complication rate was found in a multicenter questionnaire.[68] The complications included flexor tendon adhesions, deep motor branch of the ulnar nerve injury, superficial arch division, and median nerve paresis secondary to retraction during surgical explorations.

Annotated References

1. Berger RA, Kauer JM, Landsmeer JM: Radioscapholunate ligament: A gross anatomic and histologic study of fetal and adult wrists. *J Hand Surg* 1991;16A:350–355.

2. Johnson RP: The acutely impaired wrist and its residuals. *Clin Orthop* 1980;149:33–44.

3. Mayfield JK, Johnson RP, Kilcoyne RK: Carpal dislocations: Pathomechanics and progressive perilunar instability. *J Hand Surg* 1980;5A:226–241.

4. Panting AL, Lamb DW, Noble J, et al: Dislocations of the lunate with and without fracture of the scaphoid. *J Bone Joint Surg* 1984;66B:391–395.

5. Herzberg G, Comtet JJ, Linscheid RL, et al: Perilunate dislocations and fracture-dislocations: A multicenter study. *J Hand Surg* 1993;18A:768–779.

The authors found that perilunate fracture dislocations occurred twice as often as pure ligamentous injuries. They reported that 95% of the perilunate fracture dislocations were transscaphoid and that 3% had palmar dislocation of the carpus. Arthritis developed in 50% of their patients despite early treatment and satisfactory clinical results. Patients treated greater than 7 days after injury and patients with open injuries, regardless of the direction of the dislocation or the pattern, had poorer results.

6. Garcia-Elias M, Dobyns JH, Cooney WP III, et al: Traumatic axial dislocations of the carpus. *J Hand Surg* 1989;14A:446–457.

7. Norbeck DE Jr, Larson B, Blair SJ, et al: Traumatic longitudinal disruption of the carpus. *J Hand Surg* 1987;12A:509–514.

8. Zinberg EM, Palmer AK, Coren AB, et al: The triple-injection wrist arthrogram. *J Hand Surg* 1988;13A:803–809.

9. Inoue G, Miura T: Traumatic axial-ulnar disruption of the carpus. *Orthop Rev* 1991;20:867–872.

10. Adkison JW, Chapman MW: Treatment of acute lunate and perilunate dislocations. *Clin Orthop* 1982;164:199–207.

11. Inoue G, Tanaka Y, Nakamura R: Treatment of trans-scaphoid perilunate dislocations by internal fixation with the Herbert screw. *J Hand Surg* 1990;15B:449–454.

12. Fernandez DL, Ghillani R: External fixation of complex carpal dislocations: A preliminary report. *J Hand Surg* 1987;12A:335–347.

13. Moneim MS, Hofammann KE III, Omer GE: Transscaphoid perilunate fracture-dislocation: Result of open reduction and pin fixation. *Clin Orthop* 1984;190:227–235.

14. Mudgal C, Hastings H: Scapho-lunate diastasis in fractures of the distal radius: Pathomechanics and treatment options. *J Hand Surg* 1993;18B:725–729.

The authors proposed that distal radial fractures with concurrent scapholunate diastasis occurred when the hand in ulnar deviation was subjected to a combination of tension forces, producing radial styloid avulsion, perilunate ligament tears, and compression and resulting in lunate fossa depression.

15. Herbert TJ, Fisher WE: Management of the fractured scaphoid using a new bone screw. *J Bone Joint Surg* 1984;66B:114–123.

16. Teisen H, Hjarbaek J: Classification of fresh fractures of the lunate. *J Hand Surg* 1988;13B:458–462.

17. Gelberman RH, Bauman TD, Menon J, et al: The vascularity of the lunate bone and Kienbock's disease. *J Hand Surg* 1980;5A:272–278.

18. Sherlock DA: Traumatic dorsoradial dislocation of the trapezium. *J Hand Surg* 1987;12A:262–265.

19. Walker JL, Greene TL, Lunseth PA: Fractures of the body of the trapezium. *J Orthop Trauma* 1988;2:22–28.

20. Milch H: Fracture of the hamate bone. *J Bone Joint Surg* 1934;16:459–462.

21. Cain JE Jr, Shepler TR, Wilson MR: Hamatometacarpal fracture-dislocation: Classification and treatment. *J Hand Surg* 1987;12A:762–767.

22. Zoltie N: Fractures of the body of the hamate. *Injury* 1991;22:459–462.

23. Garcia-Elias M: Dorsal fractures of the triquetrum-avulsion or compression fractures? *J Hand Surg* 1987;12A:266–268.

24. Gellman H, Caputo RJ, Carter V, et al: Comparison of short and long thumb-spica casts for non-displaced fractures of the carpal scaphoid. *J Bone Joint Surg* 1989;71A:354–357.

25. Green DP: The effect of avascular necrosis on Russe bone grafting for scaphoid nonunion. *J Hand Surg* 1985;10A:597–605.

The authors reviewed anterior cancellous grating using the Russe technique. Union in proximal pole scaphoid fractures occurred in greater than 92% of those with good vascularity, in 71% of those with scattered areas of bleeding, and in none of those that were avascular.

26. Trumble TE: Avascular necrosis after scaphoid fracture: A correlation of magnetic resonance imaging and histology. *J Hand Surg* 1990;15A:557–564.

Of 12 patients reviewed, six had findings that demonstrated decreased signal content consistent with osteonecrosis. Plain radiographs correctly documented only three of the six cases. Three of the six patients with MRI findings of osteonecrosis developed nonunion despite ORIF and developed radial migration of the capitate.

27. Perlik PC, Guilford WB: Magnetic resonance imaging to assess vascularity of scaphoid nonunions. *J Hand Surg* 1991;16A:479–484.

28. Amadio PC, Berquist TH, Smith DK, et al: Scaphoid malunion. *J Hand Surg* 1989;14A:679–687.

29. Jiranek WA, Ruby LK, Millender LB, et al: Long-term results after Russe bone-grafting: The effect of malunion of the scaphoid. *J Bone Joint Surg* 1992;74A:1217–1228.

The authors defined malunion as an intrascaphoid angle of 45°. Objectively, there was a difference between malunion and the normal side, but there was no difference subjectively. Grip strength of the involved side was 90% and 76% of that of the uninvolved side in patients with intrascaphoid angles of less than 45° and greater than 45°, respectively. Flexion and extension of the involved side was 90% and 76% of that of the uninvolved side in patients with intrascaphoid angles of less than 45° and greater than 45°, respectively. The differences between the groups were not statistically significant. Ninety-two percent of the patients returned to full-time employment and 88% returned to sports. The authors deemed osteotomy of the malunited scaphoids unnecessary.

30. Ahmad MH, Midha VP: Dislocation of the trapezium: Open reduction by the dorsal approach. *Injury* 1991;22:410–411.

31. Norman A, Nelson J, Green S: Fractures of the hook of hamate: Radiographic signs. *Radiology* 1985;154:49–53.

32. Bishop AT, Beckenbaugh RD: Fracture of the hamate hook. *J Hand Surg* 1988;13A:135–139.

33. Trumble TE, Benirschke SK, Vedder NB: Ipsilateral fractures of the scaphoid and radius. *J Hand Surg* 1993;18A:8–14.

34. Vender MI, Watson HK, Black DM, et al: Acute scaphoid fracture with scapholunate gap. *J Hand Surg* 1989;14A:1004–1007.

35. Clay NR, Dias JJ, Costigan PS, et al: Need the thumb be immobilised in scaphoid fractures? A randomised prospective trial. *J Bone Joint Surg* 1991;73B:828–832.

36. Langhoff O, Andersen JL: Consequences of late immobilization of scaphoid fractures. *J Hand Surg* 1988;13B:77–79.

37. Warren-Smith CD, Barton NJ: Non-union of the scaphoid: Russe graft vs Herbert screw. *J Hand Surg* 1988;13B:83–86.

38. Botte MJ, Mortensen WW, Gelberman RH, et al: Internal vascularity of the scaphoid in cadavers after insertion of the Herbert screw. *J Hand Surg* 1988;13A:216–220.

   The palmar approach does not disrupt the vascularity of the proximal 70% to 80% of the scaphoid. Disruption of the palmar vessels in the distal 20% to 30% of the scaphoid did occur in approximately one third of the cases.

39. Inoue G, Miura T: Treatment of ununited fractures of the carpal scaphoid by iliac bone grafts and Herbert screw fixation. *Int Orthop* 1991;15:279–282.

40. Radford PJ, Matthewson MH, Meggitt BF: The Herbert screw for delayed and non-union of scaphoid fractures: A review of fifty cases. *J Hand Surg* 1990;15B:455–459.

41. DeMaagd RL, Engber WD: Retrograde Herbert screw fixation for treatment of proximal pole scaphoid nonunions. *J Hand Surg* 1989;14A:996–1003.

42. Cooney WP, Linscheid RL, Dobyns JH, Wood MB: Scaphoid nonunion: Role of anterior interpositional bone grafts. *J Hand Surg* 1988;13A:635–650.

43. Fernandez DL: Anterior bone grafting and conventional lag screw fixation to treat scaphoid nonunions. *J Hand Surg* 1990;15A:140–147.

44. Cosio MQ, Camp RA: Percutaneous pinning of symptomatic scaphoid nonunions. *J Hand Surg* 1986;11A:350–355.

45. Stark HH, Rickard TA, Zemel NP, et al: Treatment of ununited fractures of the scaphoid by iliac bone grafts and Kirschner-wire fixation. *J Bone Joint Surg* 1988;70A:982–991.

46. Huene DR, Huene DS: Treatment of nonunions of the scaphoid with the Ender compression blade plate system. *J Hand Surg* 1991;16A:913–922.

47. Korkala OL, Kuokkanen HO, Eerola MS: Compression-staple fixation for fractures, non-unions, and delayed unions of the carpal scaphoid. *J Bone Joint Surg* 1992;74A:423–426.

48. Adams BD, Frykman GK, Taleisnik J: Treatment of scaphoid nonunion with casting and pulsed electromagnetic fields: A study continuation. *J Hand Surg* 1992;17A:910–914.

49. Zaidemberg C, Siebert JW, Angrigiani C: A new vascularized bone graft for scaphoid nonunion. *J Hand Surg* 1991;16A:474–478.

50. Carter PR, Malinin TI, Abbey PA, et al: The scaphoid allograft: A new operation for treatment of the very proximal scaphoid nonunion or for the necrotic, fragmented scaphoid proximal pole. *J Hand Surg* 1989;14A:1–12.

51. Shaw JA: A biomechanical comparison of scaphoid screws. *J Hand Surg* 1987;12A:347–353.

   The authors compared the biomechanical properties of the Herbert screw, the ASIF 3.5- and 4.0-mm cancellous screws, the Heune screw, the scaphoid screw, the Richards' navicular screw, and the ASIF 2.7-mm cortical screw. The Herbert screw, which generates compressive forces via a trailing set of threads that are set at different pitches, was found to provide the least compression in cadaver models and simulated scaphoids.

52. Rankin G, Kuschner SH, Orlando C, et al: A biomechanical evaluation of a cannulated compressive screw for use in fractures of the scaphoid. *J Hand Surg* 1991;16A:1002–1010.

   Evaluation of the compressive forces provided by various screws showed that the 2.7- or 3.5-mm cortical screw provided the greatest compression, followed by the 3.5-mm cannulated screw and the Herbert screw.

53. Carter FM II, Zimmerman MC, DiPaola DM, et al: Biomechanical comparison of fixation devices in experimental scaphoid osteotomies. *J Hand Surg* 1991;16A:907–912.

54. Vander Grend R, Dell PC, Glowczewski F, et al: Intraosseous blood supply of the capitate and its correlation with aseptic necrosis. *J Hand Surg* 1984;9A:677–683.

55. Richards RR, Paitich CB, Bell RS: Internal fixation of a capitate fracture with Herbert screws. *J Hand Surg* 1990;15A:885–887.

56. Whalen JL, Bishop AT, Linscheid RL: Nonoperative treatment of acute hamate hook fractures. *J Hand Surg* 1992;17A:507–511.

57. Carroll RE, Lakin JF: Fracture of the hook of the hamate: Acute treatment. *J Trauma* 1993;34:803–805.

58. Stark HH, Chao EK, Zemel NP, et al: Fracture of the hook of the hamate. *J Bone Joint Surg* 1989;71A:1202–1207.

59. Watson HK, Rogers WD: Nonunion of the hook of the hamate: An argument for bone grafting the nonunion. *J Hand Surg* 1989;14A:486–490.

60. Mack GR, Bosse MJ, Gelberman RH, et al: The natural history of scaphoid non-union. *J Bone Joint Surg* 1984;66A:504–509.

   The authors presented a large group of symptomatic patients, defining three radiologic groups: group I had a duration of nonunion of 8.2 years and changes of sclerosis, cyst formation, or resorptive changes of the scaphoid; group II averaged 17 years of nonunion and had radiocarpal arthritis; group III averaged 31.6 years of nonunion and had generalized arthritis. Mild to moderate symptoms, present in 76% of the patients, did not correlate with radiographic changes or duration. Patients with more severe symptoms had displaced nonunions and instability patterns.

61. Ruby LK, Stinson J, Belsky MR: The natural history of scaphoid non-union: A review of fifty-five cases. *J Bone Joint Surg* 1985;67A:428–432.

   The authors studied 56 scaphoid nonunions in 56 patients, of whom 22 (40%) were asymptomatic until a second injury precipitated pain and evaluation.[60] Of the patients who had been injured at least 5 years before presentation, 97% had evidence of osteoarthritis. Instability, location of the fracture, or time since injury did not correlate with wrist pain.

62. Milliez PY, Courandier JM, Thomine JM, et al: The natural history of scaphoid non-union: A review of fifty-two cases. *Ann Chir Main* 1987;6:195–202.

63. Vender MI, Watson HK, Wiener BD, et al: Degenerative change in symptomatic scaphoid nonunion. *J Hand Surg* 1987;12A:514–519.

64. Lindstrom G, Nystrom A: Natural history of scaphoid non-union, with special reference to "asymptomatic cases." *J Hand Surg* 1992;17B:697–700.

   Of the patients with primary scaphoid union 5.2% developed radiocarpal arthrosis and 10.5% had long-term wrist complaints. Although 50% of 33 patients with scaphoid nonunions were asymptomatic on presentation, radiographs taken between 10 and 17 years after presentation demonstrated arthritis in 100%. Only 5 of the patients were asymptomatic on initial follow-up. Long-term follow-up of more than 17 years for these 5 revealed that, of the surviving three, one was essentially asymptomatic and the other two had developed substantial wrist problems.

65. Duppe H, Johnell O, Lundborg G, et al: Long-term results of fracture of the scaphoid: A follow-up study of more than thirty years. *J Bone Joint Surg* 1994;76A:249–252.

    The authors obtained a lengthy follow-up (average, 36 years) on 56 of 75 patients with scaphoid fractures. Of those 56 patients, 52 had had acute scaphoid fractures and four had had nonunion at the time of presentation. Five of the 52 eventually went on to nonunion, resulting in a total of nine nonunions in this group. Radiocarpal arthritis developed in five of the nine nonunions and in only one of the healed group. Comparing the patients with united fractures to those with pseudoarthrosis, 6 (13%) of 47 and 4 (44%) of 9 respectively, had symptoms.

66. Hooning van Duyvenbode JFF, Keijser LCM, Hauet EJ, et al: Pseudoarthrosis of the scaphoid treated by the Matti-Russe operation: A long-term review of 77 cases. *J Bone Joint Surg* 1991;73B:603–606.

    The authors found that osteoarthritic changes occurred in a group of 77 patients with scaphoid pseudoarthroses. The arthritic changes, which occurred despite Matti-Russe bone grafting, appeared to be less advanced than those occurring in patients with persistent nonunions. They reported that 58/77 patients had pain preoperatively and that 44/58 patients (76%) were free of pain postoperatively. Symptoms and radiographs did not correlate.

67. Boulas HJ, Milek MA: Hook of the hamate fractures: Diagnosis, treatment, and complications. *Orthop Rev* 1990;19:518–529.

68. Smith P III, Wright TW, Wallace PF, et al: Excision of the hook of the hamate: A retrospective survey and review of the literature. *J Hand Surg* 1988;13A:612–615.

9

Fractures of the Hand

Introduction

There is an intricate and finely balanced relationship between the phalanges, the metacarpals, their articulations, and the flexor and extensor mechanisms. Fractures of the hand require precise restoration of normal anatomy and attention to soft-tissue injuries to avoid altering the functional unit. Treatment of metacarpal and phalangeal fractures is aimed at eliminating bony obstructions and skeletal deformity while allowing early joint motion and tendon gliding.

Recent advances in the use of miniscrews, microscrews, and miniature plates have broadened the indications for open, accurate reduction and rigid internal fixation of hand fractures. They have enabled more rapid mobilization of injured joints, thereby reducing the incidence of tendon adhesions and joint contractures. New static and dynamic external fixation devices have been introduced in recent years to better address highly comminuted or unstable intra-articular fractures of the hand. Biomechanical studies now have determined the rigidity of various internal fixation constructs and clinical studies of hand fractures have identified the significant prognostic indicators of outcome.

Assessment of Fractures

Important in the evaluation of any fracture of the hand is a thorough history and physical examination. A careful history will elucidate the age and cause of the fracture and alert the physician to the likelihood of other injuries. Treatment choices may be affected by the patient's occupation, handedness, and needs for use, and desired cosmesis.

Examination of the hand should identify the area of maximal tenderness, the location of any open wounds, the condition of all flexor and extensor tendons, and the neurovascular status. Evaluation of the digits for radial/ulnar deviation, volar/dorsal angulation, and length should be made both clinically and radiographically. Rotational alignment, although suggested by radiographs, must be assessed clinically. If the clinical examination is difficult because of pain, digital or wrist block anesthesia can be effective in allowing for full active and passive examination.

Radiographs should always include at least true anteroposterior (AP) and lateral views of the involved digit or metacarpal. For metacarpal fractures, 10° pronated and supinated views can help to visualize the index and fifth metacarpals, respectively. For intra-articular fractures, Breuerton views may help in evaluating the articular surface. Occasionally, computed tomography (CT) or tomograms may be necessary to visualize the articular surface.

The optimal treatment for a given fracture depends on many factors, including location, geometry, deformity, angulation, and associated soft-tissue injuries. It is through an assessment of all of these variables that the best treatment for metacarpal and phalangeal fractures can be chosen.

Phalangeal Fractures

Fractures of the Phalangeal Shaft

Fractures of the proximal phalangeal shaft typically exhibit an apex palmar angulation as a result of an imbalance of forces generated by the flexor and extensor tendons. The axis of rotation of proximal phalangeal fractures lies palmarly along the fibro-osseous tunnel of the flexor tendons.[1] The moment arm from the rotational axis of the fracture site to the extensor tendon, therefore, is greater than that between the axis and the flexor tendons, causing apex palmar angulation. In addition, the proximal fragment is flexed by the force exerted by the interossei insertions. Progressive palmar angulation of the proximal phalanx effectively shortens the skeletal length, more marked dorsally, resulting in an incompetent extensor mechanism and an extensor lag at the proximal interphalangeal (PIP) joint.

Angulation of middle phalangeal fractures is dependent on the location of the fracture. Fractures at the proximal one fourth of the phalanx angulate apex dorsal as a result of the unbalanced pull of the central slip. Midshaft fractures can angulate dorsally or palmarly. Fractures of the distal one fourth angulate apex palmar as a result of the strong flexion force of the superficialis on the proximal fragment. If the fixed distance between the insertions of the central slip and the lateral bands is shortened by middle phalangeal angulation, distal joint extension may be lost. Hyperextension of the PIP joint may then result from the overpull of the central slip relative to the weakened lateral bands, causing a swan neck deformity of the digit. Reduction of fractures should, therefore, be aimed at restoring the bony anatomy to recreate the normal tendon balance.

It is important to distinguish stable from unstable fracture patterns in the initial management of a phalangeal fracture. No more than 10° of angulation in any plane of a proximal or middle phalangeal shaft fracture or any rotational malalignment should be accepted. Fifteen percent of displaced fractures become functionally stable after closed reduction.[2] Stable fractures have good functional outcome with closed reduction and early active mobilization but need to be followed very closely because many will displace again.

Phalangeal fractures can be associated with soft-tissue injuries such as tendon lacerations, digital nerve injuries, and large skin defects requiring reconstruction. In one prospective study of 284 digital fractures, all of these associated injuries adversely affected the outcome as measured by total active motion of the digit.[2] The bone involved (metacarpal, proximal or middle phalanx) or the anatomic site (metaphyseal, diaphyseal, intra-articular) of the fractures, however, was not significantly related to outcome.

Closed Management of Phalangeal Fractures Critical to deciding between surgical and nonsurgical treatment of a phalangeal fracture is the stability of the fracture. Nondisplaced fractures tend to be stable and usually can be immobilized for only 3 weeks, after which range of motion exercises are started. Because the fracture will slip occasionally, radiographs should be repeated after several days and at weekly intervals to assure that alignment is maintained.

Displaced fractures can be reduced under digital block anesthesia. Volar/dorsal angulation and radial/ulnar deviation are fairly easy to correct and maintain with a well-formed splint. When radial/ulnar deviation is present, buddy taping to the adjacent digit opposite the direction of displacement will help maintain reduction. Serial radiographs should be taken, initially several days after reduction and then weekly to confirm maintenance of reduction. A comminuted fracture is more likely to displace again. If this occurs, surgical intervention may be necessary. Rotationally displaced fractures are more difficult to manage nonsurgically, because rotational control of a digit is difficult with a splint.

Closed reduction of phalangeal fractures can be performed under digital block anesthesia. Stable fractures can be immobilized in malleable finger splints, gutter splints, or buddy taped to the adjacent finger if early motion can be safely initiated. Immobilization should hold the metacarpophalangeal (MCP) joints in full flexion and the interphalangeal (IP) joints in extension to avoid capsular and collateral ligament contractures. Active motion should begin no later than 4 weeks after injury and preferably at 3 weeks if clinical stability and healing permit.[3] Radiographic signs of union will lag behind clinical healing and should not be awaited before beginning motion. One author advocates a short arm cast that holds the wrist in 30° of extension and the MCP joints in 90° of flexion, allowing relaxation of the intrinsics and enabling the extensor mechanism to act as a tension band over the proximal phalanx, and immediate active flexion of the PIP and distal interphalangeal (DIP) joints in the cast.[4]

When treated nonsurgically, stable phalangeal fractures will usually have a good outcome. Stable, extra-articular, noncomminuted fractures treated nonsurgically with reduction and either a finger splint or buddy taping to the adjacent finger have been shown to result in excellent outcomes with regard to pain, deformity, motion, and function.[5]

Extra-articular distal phalangeal fractures are usually treated closed. Although the treatment of distal phalangeal fractures is straightforward, the problems associated with these fractures result from the associated soft-tissue injuries, such as nail bed injuries, loss of tissue and neuromas.[6] These fractures can result in significant morbidity. In one study, more than 70% of patients at 6 months' follow-up continued to have functional impairment, pain, numbness, nail abnormalities, or less than 45° of active DIP flexion.[7]

Closed Reduction and Percutaneous Pinning The treatment of choice for unstable phalangeal fractures is often fixation with smooth pins. Kirschner wires (K-wires) should be placed percutaneously. If dissection is necessary to reduce the fracture, more rigid internal fixation should be used to allow for early motion. K-wires can be used in a variety of configurations and ideally should be placed perpendicular to the fracture site. Drawbacks of percutaneous pinning include transfixion of tendons, pin site infections, and loss of fixation. However, good results have been reported in proximal phalanx fractures treated with percutaneous K-wire fixation when evaluated for pain, deformity, and total active motion.[8]

Internal Fixation of Phalangeal Fractures If open reduction is necessary for the reduction of a fracture, then rigid internal fixation is the treatment of choice. After open reduction, rigid internal fixation facilitates early active motion and improves the functional result. Internal fixation of hand fractures using lag screws, tension banding, or plate and screws reduces the incidence of joint stiffness and tendon adhesions.[9]

The mechanical strength of common fixation techniques for spiral fractures of the phalanges has been tested in cadaveric specimens.[10–12] In both torsional and bending tests, a single compression screw, either alone or in combination with plating, provided significantly better fixation than any of the other fixation methods, including crossed K-wires, interosseous loops, dorsal mini-plates, single compression screws, and K-wire plus cerclage.

In clinical testing, screws have been shown to provide rigid fracture fixation and little interference with tendon gliding.[13] Screws alone are used in unstable, long oblique or spiral fractures of the phalanges or in intra-articular fractures involving more than 25% of the articular surface. Plates are seldom used at this level but may be necessary in transverse fractures with soft-tissue injury or unstable fractures with bone loss. Plates in addition to screws should be considered in transverse fractures or oblique fractures with fracture lines less than twice the diameter of the bone.[14] Neither the surgical dissection nor the bulk of the hardware seems to interfere with digital motion.[14]

Certain principles should be adhered to when using screws in the phalanges and metacarpals.[15] Screw fixation requires a fragment greater than three times the thread diameter of the screw to prevent splintering of the fragment. Oblique or spiral fractures should be of adequate size to accept at least two screws. Fractures with bony defects or extensive comminution are not amenable to lag screws. Grades I and II open injuries are not contraindications to screw fixation, provided proper wound management is undertaken. More recently, 1.0-mm and 1.2-mm titanium screws have been introduced, further broadening the indications and options for open reduction and internal fixation of phalangeal fractures (Fig. 1). A technique that requires less exposure and is less prominent than plates and screws is 90°–90° interosseous wiring, which yields excellent results when used for replantation, fusions, and transverse fractures.[16]

Transverse proximal phalangeal fractures, particularly distal periarticular fractures, when not amenable to percutaneous pins may best be treated using the laterally applied minicondylar plates. A study comparing dorsally applied H plates, straight plates, and minicondylar plates on these transverse fractures of the proximal phalanx in cadaveric specimens revealed that the minicondylar plate created less reduction of simulated PIP motion and provided greater strength to simulated loads.[17] Presumably, the laterally applied minicondylar plate creates less irritation of the extensor aponeurosis and better resists the primarily apex volar angulatory forces. The clinical results of the minicondylar plate in both phalangeal and metacarpal periarticular fractures have been excellent. In one study, there were no nonunions in spite of the institution of range of motion exercises as early as the first postoperative day.[18]

The use of absorbable implants for fracture fixation has attracted much attention recently. In the hand, as in other sites, biodegradable implants have obvious advantages, including the fact that they need not be removed. The use of polyglycolide implants for the intramedullary fixation of extra-articular hand fractures has been compared with K-wire fixation in a prospective, randomized trial.[19] Because the 1.5-mm polyglycolide rods were found in animal testing to lose all mechanical strength in 3 weeks, the intramedullary absorbable rods were augmented with wire loop. There were no allergic reactions to the implants. At 6 months there were no differences between the two groups in terms of time to bony union, deformity, stiffness, and return to normal activities.

The rapid loss of strength of the absorbable implants limits its use as the sole method of fixation. Larger diameter rods should retain their strength proportionately longer. When not used as an intramedullary device, passing the implant through a predrilled track across a fracture site is technically demanding.

External Fixation of Phalangeal Fractures Static external fixation offers certain advantages in the treatment of phalangeal fractures. Indications for external fixation of phalangeal fractures include severely contaminated hand trauma, gunshot wounds, severe intra-articular fractures, segmental bone loss, and highly comminuted fractures.[20] The development of miniaturized Hoffmann fixators allows fixation of phalangeal fractures while allowing adjacent digits uninhibited range of motion. Threaded half pins of 1.6- to 2.0-mm diameter are recommended for adequate stability. Midlateral insertions are preferred, except in the proximal aspect of the proximal phalanx where a dorsolateral insertion is used due to space constraints. There should be a minimum of two pins on either side of the fracture. Both cortices should be engaged by each pin.

In both phalangeal and metacarpal fractures, anatomic reduction can be achieved with a minifixator in more than three quarters of cases. An overall nonunion rate of 5% can be expected, although nonunion rates in closed fractures are significantly less.[21] The final functional results are most influenced by the severity of the initial injury. The results using the Hoffman miniexternal fixator in severe hand trauma have been reported.[22] The 8-week union rate was 85.7%. At a follow-up of 2.2 years, mean total active motion was 70% of the contralateral digit. The overall complication rate was 25%, including nonunion, infected nonunion, pin tract infection, and malunion.

The advantages of the miniexternal fixator in finger fractures include minimal or no surgical exposure of the fracture site, adequate stability, and the ability to manipulate an inadequately reduced or secondarily displaced fracture. Because transfixion of part of the extensor mechanism is often unavoidable in the proximal phalanx, functional results of external fixation at the phalangeal level are consistently worse than at the metacarpal level.

Intra-articular Fractures

Mallet Fractures The majority of mallet fractures should be treated nonsurgically. Conventionally, surgical treatment is reserved for those mallet fractures that demonstrate subluxation of the DIP joint. However, good results with conservative treatment have been reported regardless of joint subluxation or the size and amount of displacement of the bone fragment.[23] Bone remodeling and joint reconstitution occurred in all cases. There was occasionally a painless bony prominence on the dorsum of the distal interphalangeal (DIP) and a slightly higher incidence of extension lag and restricted arc of motion compared with surgical treatment. Fractures with dorsal fragments greater than two thirds of the articular surface more frequently had aching pain and radiographic evidence of arthritis. There are patients who require a more perfect functional or cosmetic result and who should be considered for surgical correction of the subluxation or displacement.

Surgical treatment of mallet fractures has been generally disappointing. Various techniques have been examined to ascertain the best surgical treatment of these injuries. A biomechanical study was conducted of cadaver hands to determine the strength of four fixation techniques currently used for mallet fractures.[24] The techniques tested included K-

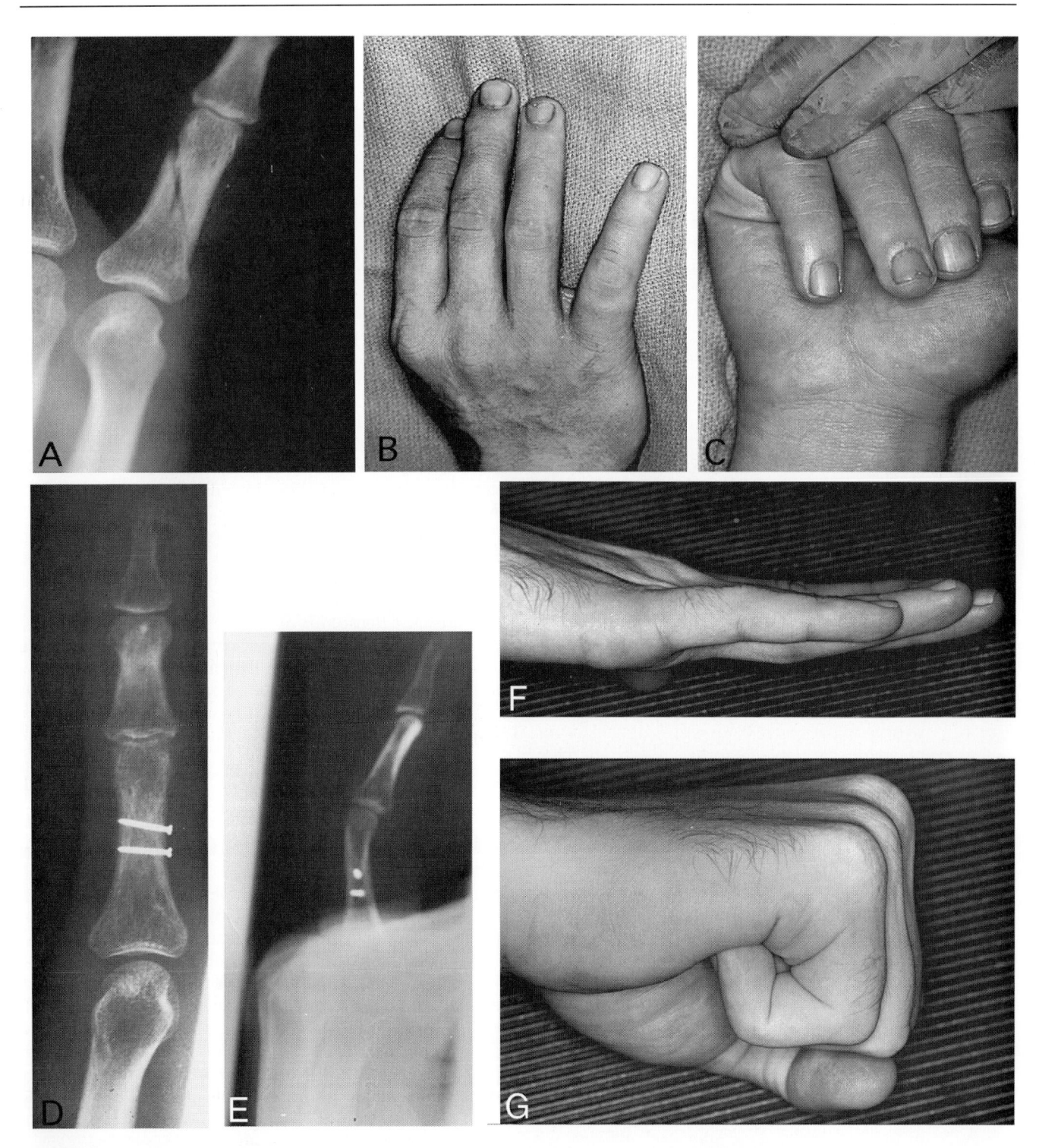

Fig. 1 **A,** Radiograph demonstrating a minimally displaced spiral fracture of the proximal phalanx. **B** and **C,** There was a significant rotational deformity to the fifth finger. **D** and **E,** Open reduction and internal fixation with two 1.0-mm AO microscrews was performed with immediate active and passive range of motion. **F** and **G,** Full range of motion was restored without rotatory deformity.

wire, figure-of-eight wire, pull-through wire, and pull-through suture tied over a button. Significantly greater energy absorbed to failure and a trend toward greater peak loads to failure were seen in the figure-of-eight wire and pull-through suture techniques. Irreversible loss of reduction occurred in all the K-wire fixed fractures, in 60% of the pull-through wire group, 50% of the figure-of-eight group, but in none of the pull-through suture group. In a subsequent clinical study that examined the results of the pull-through tension band suture technique, almost 90% had no clinical mallet deformity, pain, or functional deformity.[25] All fractures healed with a congruent articular surface.

Intra-articular Injuries of the PIP Joint Intra-articular fractures and dislocations of the PIP joint are common injuries, because this small joint has a limited single plane of motion and a proportionately long lever arm in the middle and distal phalanges. A joint injury at this level can be classified as a pure dislocation, a fracture-dislocation, an avulsion fracture, a shaft fracture that extends into the joint, a unicondylar or bicondylar fracture, or a comminuted pilon fracture.

Dislocations and Fracture-Dislocations at the PIP Joint
Pure dorsal dislocations of the PIP joint are the most common articular injury in the hand. The collateral ligaments are partially injured and the volar plate is avulsed off the base of the middle phalanx. Interposition of the volar plate may infrequently necessitate open reduction. Once reduced, the PIP joint is usually stable and can be immediately mobilized with buddy taping to the adjacent digit. Development of a flexion contracture is the most common long-term sequela.

Palmar dislocations represent a more rare and severe injury, sometimes including collateral ligament ruptures proximally and disruption of the central tendon. The lateral bands or central tendon often become interposed in the joint, blocking reduction. Closed reduction should be attempted first with the MCP and PIP joints flexed to relax the lateral bands. After reduction, if full active extension of the PIP joint can be achieved, then early motion can be started. If the patient cannot perform full active extension, the central slip must have ruptured, and the PIP should be immobilized in full extension and treated as a closed boutonniere injury. If closed reduction fails, open reduction should be performed through a midaxial incision on the side of the major ligament disruption.

Fracture-subluxations and fracture-dislocations at the PIP joint occur either dorsally with volar lip fractures or volarly with dorsal avulsion fractures at the insertion of the central slip. True lateral radiographs are essential in confirming these diagnoses. Dorsal fracture-dislocations are usually axial compression injuries and can be comminuted, often involving a substantial portion of the volar articular surface. Reduction and extension block splinting in moderate flexion can usually maintain a reduced joint when less than 40% of the articular surface is fractured. However, when a congruent reduction cannot be maintained, volar plate arthroplasty, as described by Eaton and Malerich, or internal fixation of the fragment, if it is large enough, should be considered.[26,27] The volar fragment provides a restraint to dorsal subluxation and resurfaces an irregular and deficient volar articular surface.

When displaced intra-articular fragments in the PIP joint are of sufficient size, internal fixation with K-wires or screws offers the most stable fixation (Fig. 2). Although closed reduction and percutaneous fixation is often possible, open reduction and internal fixation offers the best chance for exact anatomic reduction.[28] The surgical approach must be as unobtrusive as possible because the surgical incision will increase scar formation in an already traumatized joint. Either midaxial or dorsal incisions are applicable.

Often a fracture at this level is caused by axial impaction and can result in comminution and articular surface depression, making treatment quite difficult. Treatment methods for these pilon fractures of the middle phalanx base have included splint immobilization, mini-skeletal traction, and open fixation.[29] Patients treated with traction tend to have the best results when measured by active range of motion, grip strength, radiographic appearance, and pain. Immobilization produced the worst results. Regardless of treatment, patients were left with limitations in PIP and DIP motion.

Volar fracture-dislocations with central slip avulsions should be treated as a pure volar dislocation with static splinting in full extension for the boutonniere component. Surgical treatment should only be considered when a congruent joint reduction cannot be acheived or maintained.

Condylar Fractures of the PIP Joint Both unicondylar and bicondylar fractures are amenable to either K-wire fixation or mini- and microscrew fixation. The minicondylar plate has also been used for intra-articular fractures. In a study in which patients treated for distal unicondylar fractures of the proximal phalanx using a number of different fixation techniques, fractures treated with multiple K-wires and those fixed with miniscrews alone resulted in the best final joint motion.[30]

External Fixation of PIP Joint Fractures Dynamic external fixation for PIP joint fractures and dislocations is gaining popularity. Because the PIP joint is a ginglymoid joint with a single axis of rotation, it lends itself well to hinged dynamic external fixation. These devices allow maintenance of congruent joint reduction, distraction as necessary to reduce complex fracture fragments, protection of the joint from excessive loading forces during healing, and immediate range of active and passive motion. Complex fracture-dislocations, pilon fractures, and late fracture dislocations are potential indications for dynamic external fixation. Several devices are available, but most devices have in common adjustable control for distraction, lateral angulation, and dorsal-palmar translation. All require accurate identification of the axis of rotation.

The initial results of one device used in unstable or irreducible PIP fracture-dislocations are encouraging.[31] The fractures had an average of 48% articular involvement. After an average fixator duration of 31 days and 12 weeks of follow-up, final PIP motion averaged 2° to 100° and all

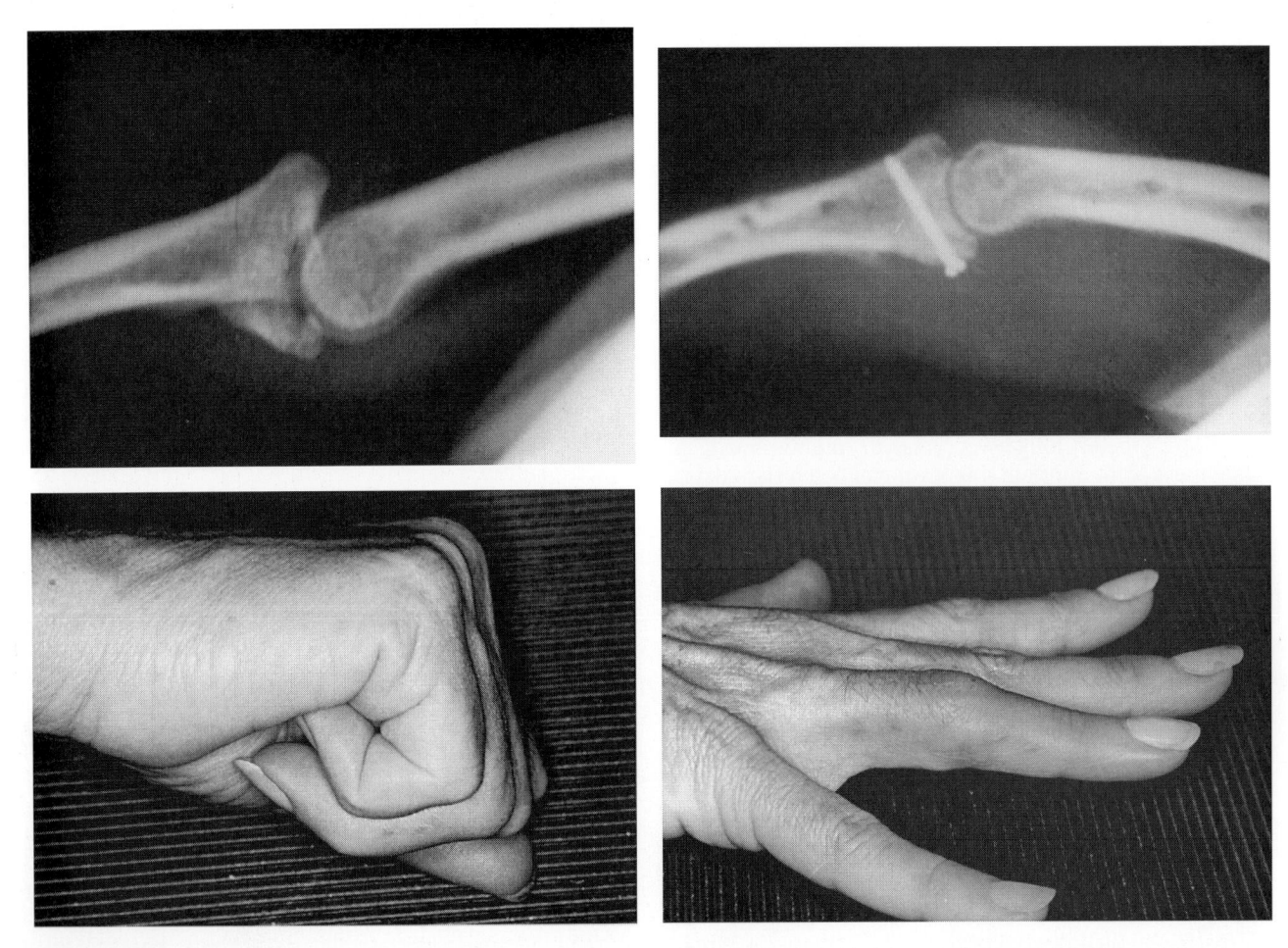

Fig. 2 Top left, Dorsal fracture dislocation. **Top right,** Open reduction and internal fixation with 1.0-mm microscrew and hinged external fixation for restoration of the articular surface and immediate range of motion. **Bottom left,** and **bottom right,** Functional range of motion is restored.

patients were free of pain and crepitus with normal alignment and stability. Another fixator design incorporates a spring mechanism that exerts a constant distraction force distally and palmarly to the middle phalanx.[32] Used in both acute injuries and old malunited fracture-dislocations for 8 weeks, the fixator resulted in a mean active range of motion of 3° to 88° with no pin tract infections or nonunions. Acute injuries had superior results. Dynamic hinged external fixation in patients with dorsal fracture-dislocations and posttraumatic stiff PIP joints have also been used with good results.

Immediate Salvage Procedures for the PIP Joint Treatment alternatives other than volar plate arthroplasty for unsalvageable PIP joints are generally unattractive. Arthrodesis, Silastic arthroplasty, and interpositional arthroplasty all restore length and stability with very little mobility. Swanson hinged implants used acutely for unsalvageable intra-articular fractures only obtained an average active range of motion of 29° in the PIP joint.[33]

Metacarpal Fractures

Metacarpal Neck Fractures

Metacarpal neck fractures are the result of an axial load against a clenched fist and most commonly involve the ring and little finger. Most authors would agree that any rotational or lateral deviation deformity of the metacarpal should be corrected. However, the amount of apex dorsal angulation (secondary to the pull of the interossei) that can be accepted varies. Less than 15° should be accepted in the index and long finger metacarpals because of their more rigid carpometacarpal (CMC) joints. In the more mobile ring and little fingers, up to 35° and 45° of dorsal angulation, respectively, can be accepted. The reduction

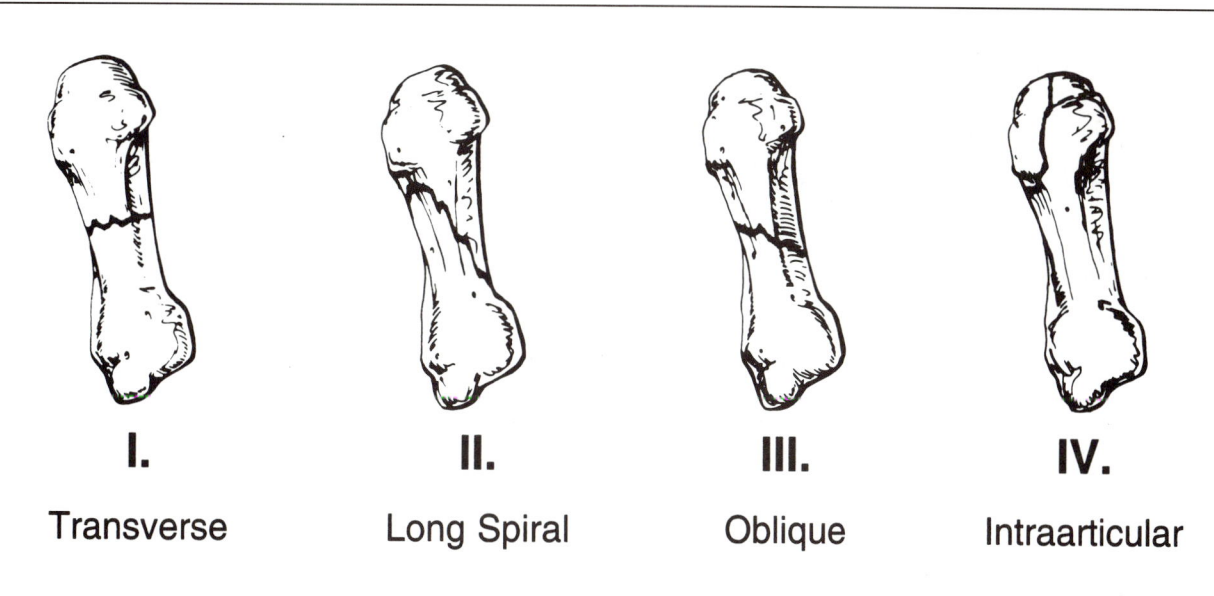

I. Transverse   II. Long Spiral   III. Oblique   IV. Intraarticular

Fig. 3 Metacarpal fracture patterns. (Reproduced with permission from Dabezies EJ, Schutte JP: Fixation of metacarpal and phalangeal fractures with miniature plates and screws. J Hand Surg 1986;11A:283–288.)

technique of PIP and MCP flexion to 90° described by Jahss is effective.[34] Treatment recommendations vary from immediate mobilization without splinting to open reduction and internal fixation.

For treatment of fifth metacarpal neck fractures, some advocate immediate mobilization without regard to degree of angulation. In a review of patients treated with immediate mobilization, there was no demonstrable correlation between the degree of residual angulation and persistent symptoms of pain, range of motion, disability, grip strength, or clinical deformity.[35] Even angular deformities up to 70° were not associated with functional loss. In a comparison of closed treatment and surgical repair of fifth metacarpal neck fractures, good results were found in both groups of patients.[36] There was no difference in injury severity between the two groups as determined by comminution and initial degree of angulation. There were no statistical differences between the groups in terms of final joint motion, grip strength, long-term pain, or subjective dissatisfaction with the functional or cosmetic result. There was less residual dorsal angulation in the surgically treated group. Surgical treatment is recommended only for open fractures, fractures with rotational or lateral malalignment, and fractures angulated sufficiently to produce a dorsal prominence and knuckle deformity in patients who demand perfect cosmesis. Otherwise, initial splinting for comfort followed in 5 to 7 days with early mobilization is advised.

Fractures of the Metacarpal Shaft

Metacarpal shaft fractures can be classified by fracture pattern: transverse, oblique, spiral, and comminuted (Fig. 3). Axial loading forces generally result in transverse fractures. Torsional forces create either spiral or oblique patterns. Direct impact often causes comminuted and shortened fractures. Apex dorsal angulation of the shaft is typical because of the pull of the interossei. The border metacarpals (of the index and little fingers) are more likely to shorten because they do not have the suspensory effect of the adjacent metacarpals acting as a support through the intermetacarpal ligaments. As with metacarpal head fractures, radiographs in the lateral plane are difficult to interpret because there is overlap of adjacent metacarpals. Adequate oblique films are helpful.

Nonsurgical Treatment of Metacarpal Shaft Fractures

The majority of metacarpal shaft fractures can be treated effectively with closed reduction and external splinting.[37] Although angulation of metacarpal shaft fractures is generally well tolerated, reduction should be considered in fractures angulated in excess of 30° in the small finger, 20° in the ring finger, and any angulation in the middle and index fingers.[38] Shortening of up to 0.5 cm in comminuted fractures does not affect function.[39] Any rotational malalignment is not well tolerated. Only 5° of rotation causes 1.5 cm of finger overlap.[40]

Closed Reduction and Immobilization of Metacarpal Fractures Traditional treatment methods have always involved immobilization of the wrist and fingers or, as in phalangeal fractures, dorsal extension blocking splints holding the wrist in extension and the MCP joints in flexion. In one study, functional cast immobilization of the fracture allowed free motion of the wrist, MCP, and PIP joints, resulting in a superior outcome.[41] When compared with conventional casting that included the wrist and fingers, patients treated with the functional cast maintained the fracture reduction while allowing earlier return to work, earlier resumption of normal grip strength, and greater range of motion at the wrist and digits at the time of cast removal.

In one functional brace design that applies the principles of three-point fixation to metacarpal fractures,[42] one pad is placed dorsally over the apex of the fracture and two others are placed volarly, one proximal and one distal to the fracture. Subsequent reports, however, have demonstrated dorsal skin necrosis with the use of the functional splint. Design modifications may be necessary to address this problem.

Closed Reduction and Percutaneous Pinning of Metacarpal Shaft Fractures Open or closed fixation of metacarpal shaft fractures is indicated for unstable fractures, displaced intra-articular fractures, displaced open fractures, multiple fractures, and fractures with segmental bone loss or concomitant soft-tissue injury. The standard for fixation of metacarpal shaft fractures has been percutaneous fixation with K-wires. Little has been written in the literature recently on this method, except in comparison to new AO internal fixation systems.[11,12] Its best application is probably in the stabilization of closed transverse fractures.

Open Reduction and Internal Fixation of Metacarpal Shaft Fractures Indications for open reduction and internal fixation include unstable fractures not amenable to percutaneous pins, open fractures with soft-tissue injury and bone loss, and multiple fractures. Approximately 10% of metacarpal (as well as phalangeal) fractures are either irreducible by closed manipulation or unsuitable for percutaneous pinning and require open treatment.[43]

Composite wiring of metacarpal fractures using various configurations of K-wiring in conjunction with monofilament stainless steel tension banding was reviewed and found to yield good results.[44] Active motion was begun within 1 week. The mean final total active motion for all metacarpal fractures was 256°. There were no nonunions, malunions, or losses of reduction.

With new techniques of internal fixation of metacarpal fractures with AO miniscrews and microscrews and plates, rigid fixation and early mobilization of the digit is possible (Fig. 4). Recent studies have centered on comparable fatigue strengths of various fixation techniques. Biomechanical studies using cadavaric specimens to compare the stability of commonly used fixation techniques employed in metacarpal fractures have been conducted.[45–47] Cyclic testing of the metacarpals was performed in bending, torsion, and axial loading after osteotomies fixed with different methods (dorsal plate with lag screw, two dorsal lag screws, crossed K-wire tension banding, and intramedullary K-wire fixation). The dorsal plate with lag screw was superior in all testing modes. Dorsal plating with or without lag screws provided significantly more stability than wiring techniques. The use of AO miniscrews alone in the fixation

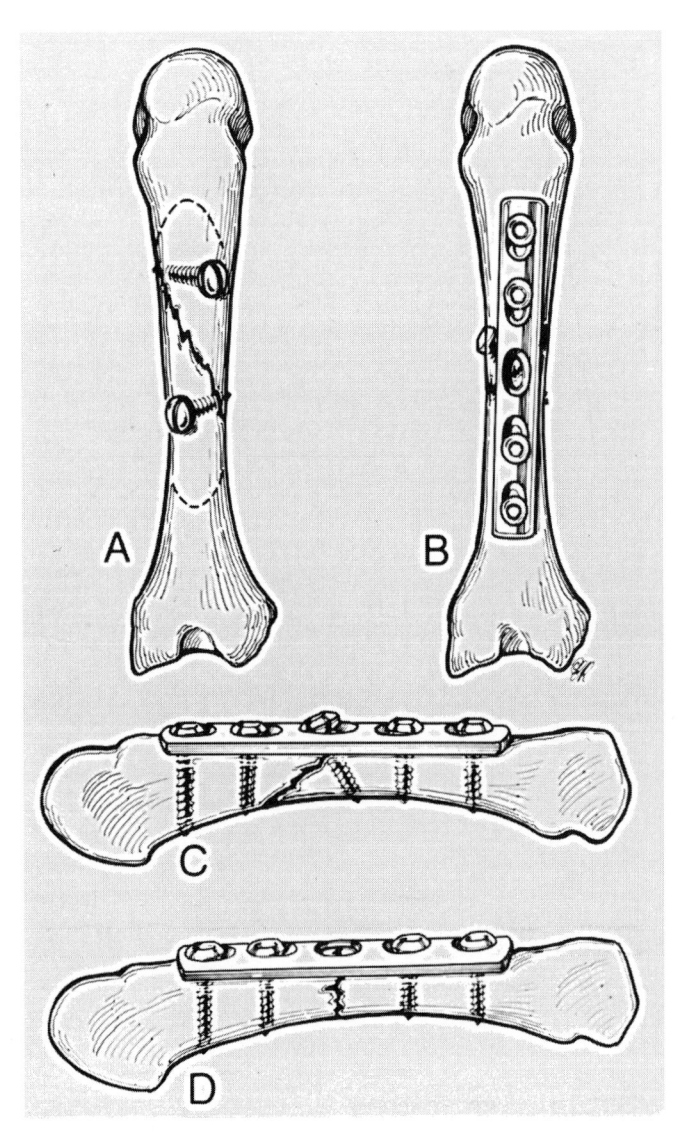

Fig. 4 Plate and screw fixation for metacarpal shaft fractures. **A,** Lag screw fixation of a spiral shaft fracture. **B,** Plate fixation of an oblique metacarpal shaft fracture with a separate lag screw across the fracture. **C,** Plate fixation of an oblique metacarpal shaft fracture with a lag screw across the fracture inserted through the plate. **D,** Plate fixation of a transverse metacarpal shaft fracture. (Reproduced with permission from O'Brien ET: Fractures of the metacarpals and phalanges, in Green DP (ed): *Operative Hand Surgery*, ed 2. New York, NY, Churchill Livingstone, 1988, pp 709–775.)

of metacarpal fractures was compared to K-wire fixation in a clinical review of 40 metacarpal fractures (and 50 proximal phalanx fractures).[48] Superior results were obtained with screw fixation when graded for deformity, range of motion, and grip strength.

In a clinical study of 26 fractured metacarpals treated by internal fixation using AO minifragment plates and screws, all fractures united without deformity.[49] The mean duration of postoperative immobilization was 7 days. In

75% of fractures total active movement exceeded 220°; 81% had greater than 180° of movement. The primary advantage of rigid internal fixation with plates and screws is precise anatomic reduction and the ability to begin early active motion to reduce extrinsic and intrinsic adhesions.

In a prospective study examining the use of AO minifragment screws and plates on 31 metacarpal and seven phalangeal fractures, more than 90% had an excellent recovery, described as total active motion greater than 220°.[50] Either screws alone or screws and plates were used for oblique and spiral metacarpal fractures; screws and plates were used for transverse metacarpal fractures. Fractures were immobilized for 3 weeks, after which motion was allowed. There were no nonunions or malunions. This technique allows for superior rigid anatomic fixation of metacarpal fractures but demands meticulous care in avoiding unnecessary soft-tissue trauma and excessive periosteal stripping.

External Fixation of Metacarpal Shaft Fractures External fixation of metacarpals is indicated for open fractures, severely comminuted fractures, and fractures with soft-tissue injury or bone loss. The advantages and disadvantages are similar to those mentioned for external fixation of phalangeal fractures, however, the functional results are generally better than in phalangeal fractures. In a study of external fixation of 19 metacarpal and 11 phalangeal fractures, the metacarpal fractures had a mean percentage return of assisted range of motion of 96%, while phalangeal fractures had a mean of 84% compared with the opposite hand.[51] There were no pin tract infections or loss of reduction. Another similar study had good and excellent functional results in 94% of metacarpal fractures and in 85% of phalangeal fractures treated with external fixation.[52] Good and excellent results were those that at follow-up had no pain, minimal or no deformity, total active motion greater than 180°, and PIP flexion greater than 80°.

Metacarpal Base Fractures

Fractures at the base of the metacarpal are generally stable fractures; however, even minor rotational malalignment at this level will be greatly magnified at the fingertips and will interfere with function. These fractures are often missed on initial evaluation because of inadequate radiographs due to poor quality or poor positioning. Breuerton views are helpful if clinical examination suggests injury to the metacarpal base. Fractures in this region are usually the result of crush injuries, but may also result from avulsions of the extensor carpi radialis brevis or longus at the base of the middle and index metacarpals. In a report of three such cases, surgical treatment of avulsion fractures is recommended only if the avulsed fragment causes a symptomatic bony prominence.[53] The remainder of metacarpal base fractures should be treated as shaft fractures.

Intra-articular Fractures and Dislocations

Injuries to the MCP Joint of the Fingers Injuries to the metacarpophalangeal joint are less common than those to the proximal interphalangeal joint, but the consequences of loss of range of motion at this joint can have a profound effect on hand function.[54] Arthrodesis at this level is clearly extremely disabling. When evaluating injuries of the MCP joint radiographically, overlap of the metacarpal heads on the lateral view necessitates oblique films. The Breuerton view is helpful in diagnosing collateral ligament avulsion injuries. Skyline or tangential views will identify metacarpal head impaction injuries that result from closed fist injuries. For large articular fragments, open reduction and internal fixation can be achieved with K-wires, absorbable pins, interosseous wires, minifragment screws, or minicondylar plates. Ligamentous avulsions of bone, when small, can often be treated closed in the index through little finger.

Carpometacarpal Joint Injuries Fractures and dislocations of the carpometacarpal joints of the fingers are relatively rare and are often diagnosed late because of inadequate radiographs at the time of initial evaluation. They usually are the result of high-energy injuries. Swelling and local tenderness over the joints should raise the surgeon's suspicions. The motor division of the ulnar nerve may be injured in fifth carpometacarpal joint disruptions because of its close proximity to that joint.

These dislocations can often be managed with closed reduction and percutaneous pinning. Open reduction using a dorsal surgical approach may be necessary when there are interposed fracture fragments or ligamentous tissue.[55] When all four metacarpals are dislocated, it may not be necessary to fix all the joints because intact intermetacarpal ligaments will help stabilize adjacent metacarpals. Fixation should be maintained for up to 3 months because these dislocations are inherently unstable. Carpometacarpal injuries can be associated with carpal bone injuries. These most often require open reduction, repair of torn ligaments, and internal fixation. In one study of 20 patients with dislocations of the second through fifth carpometacarpal joints, 13 of 15 who were treated with open reduction and internal fixation had excellent results.[56]

Fractures and Dislocations of the Thumb

Fractures of the Thumb Metacarpal and Phalanges

Fractures of the phalanges of the thumb should be evaluated and treated in the same way as finger fractures. Fractures of the the thumb metacarpal, however, are distinct from those of other metacarpals. Shaft fractures are rare because there are no structures fixing the proximal portion of the metacarpal. Forces are transmitted through the rigid diaphysis to the softer cancellous base, where metaphyseal or intra-articular fractures occur. Angulation of extra-articular base fractures of up to 30° is well tolerated because of the large compensatory motion available at the carpometacarpal joint. Excessive angulation, however, can result in adaptive hyperextension at the MCP joint.

Articular Injuries of the Basal Joint of the Thumb

The carpometacarpal joint of the thumb is a highly specialized articulation designed to allow the considerable motion required for pinch, grasp, and opposition while resisting joint compressive forces magnified over 10-fold through the thumb metacarpal. Fractures and dislocations at the basilar joint of the thumb are caused by an axial force directed through a partially flexed metacarpal shaft. An intra-articular fracture with a small volar metacarpal fragment characterizes a Bennett's fracture. A Rolando's fracture is essentially a "T" or "Y" intra-articular fracture that is often comminuted and results from a greater injuring force. The volar fragments in both fracture configurations remain attached to the anterior oblique ligament while the base of the shaft is displaced in a dorsal and radial direction by the pull of the abductor pollicis longus and the distal metacarpal is adducted by the adductor pollicis muscle.

Disagreement on the treatment of these fractures centers around the acceptable amount of intra-articular displacement. A 10-year follow-up study of 25 Bennett's fractures found no correlation between articular incongruity and symptomatic posttraumatic osteoarthritis.[57] Precise reconstitution of the articular surface continues to be advocated, if necessary by open reduction. In another follow-up study of 41 Bennett's fractures treated variously with closed reduction and immobilization, percutaneous K-wire fixation, and open reduction and internal fixation, 83% of patients whose fractures healed in excellent position were free of symptoms, whereas only 46% with residual displacement were asymptomatic.[58] The relationship of the size of the fracture fragments to the results was not addressed. In a similar study of Rolando's fractures, no relationship could be discerned between the quality of reduction and the occurence of late symptoms or arthritis.[59] The current trend, pending further studies, is for anatomic reduction and fixation of significant intra-articular fragments.

A technique of combined external fixation with a minifixator and limited internal fixation with wire or interfragmentary screw has been described for addressing comminuted fractures at the base of the thumb.[60] The external fixator is placed between the thumb and index metacarpals in a quadrilateral configuration to apply distraction to the thumb. Good results were reported in spite of focal irregularities of the joint surface, which could still be seen on follow-up radiographs. Currently, the advent of minifragment and microfragment screw and plate devices allow rigid internal fixation of suitable fracture configurations using the AO technique.

Pure dislocations of the carpometacarpal joint are rare injuries. Although reduction of the joint is relatively simple, maintaining the reduction can be problematic. A study involving serial sectioning of the basal joint ligaments in cadaveric specimens has further elucidated the complex stabilizers of this joint.[61] There are four main ligaments of the thumb carpometacarpal joint—the anterior oblique, the posterior oblique, the intermetacarpal, and the dorsoradial ligaments. The primary restraint to dorsal dislocation was found to be the dorsoradial ligament. Although the anterior oblique ligament could stabilize the joint in extension, flexion caused the ligament to be stripped off the metacarpal attachment, allowing dorsal migration. In dislocations in which the anterior oblique ligament is intact, immobilization in extension and pronation best stabilizes this joint. For ligament reconstructions, the dorsoradial ligament as well as the anterior oblique ligament should be addressed.

Fractures of the Hand in Polytrauma Patients

Multiply injured patients with hand fractures must have their life-threatening injuries addressed first. During the initial evaluation and treatment of a polytrauma patient, however, fractures of the extremities should not be overlooked. At one trauma center, 5% of upper extremity fractures were initially missed in patients with multiple injuries.[62] When hand fractures in these patients require surgical stabilization, they should be accomplished concurrently with other early surgical interventions whenever possible to avoid additional anesthetic exposures. It is preferable to treat all hand fractures in polytrauma patients within 24 to 48 hours.[63]

Complications of Hand Fractures

Open Fractures and Infection

The classification and scheme for treating open long bone fractures does not apply to open fractures of the hand. The abundant vascularity of the hand makes open fractures less susceptible to infection, with rates varying between 6% and 11%.[64,65] Infection rates are significantly increased in the presence of gross wound contamination, extensive soft-tissue and skeletal crush injury, systemic illness, or a delay in treatment greater than 24 hours.[64] Nevertheless, delays in treatment of up to 12 hours do not increase the incidence of infection nor do they afffect outcome.[65] Infection rates are not increased by the presence of internal fixation; immediate wound closure; large wound size; or tendon, nerve, and vascular injuries. Delayed wound closure is still recommended for open injuries with gross contamination.

The functional outcome of open hand fractures was determined in 140 fractures after an average of 17 months.[66] Total active range of digital motion was highly correlated with the severity of soft-tissue injury. Metacarpal fractures had significantly better results than phalangeal fractures. Proximal phalangeal joint and PIP joint injuries had the worst outcomes.

Low-energy gunshot injuries to the hand often result in significant fracture comminution and bone loss. Soft-tissue damage, however, is generally limited, especially when compared to severe crush or high-energy bullet injuries. The wound should be irrigated and debrided immediately. Definitive osseous reconstruction should be undertaken within 1 week, depending on the condition of the wound, and early active motion should be initiated.[67] Primary closure of the wound, internal fixation, and autologous bone grafting do not increase the incidence of infection.[67]

Complications of Internal Fixation

K-wire fixation remains the most common method of fixation for hand fractures. Although the success of this method is well reported, pin fixation of hand fractures is not without complications. In a review of 422 pins used to stabilize hand and wrist fractures in 137 patients, complications occurred in 11% of the pins (45) and in 18% of the patients;[68] 69% of these complications occurred in the phalanges. Complications included infection, pin loosening, loss of reduction, symptomatic nonunion, and impaled flexor tendon. Poor initial pin placement and lack of patient compliance were most often associated with these complications. In most cases, poor pin placement was not recognized at the time of surgery and was discovered on follow-up. Careful radiographic confirmation of pin placement at the time of operation should include oblique views. A secure method of protecting the internal fixation from premature dressing or splint removal or inappropriate activities could minimize these problems in noncompliant patients. Pin loosening developed at a mean of 8 weeks while pin tract infections occurred at a mean of 10 weeks. Therefore, pins should be removed in a timely manner as soon as bony healing allows (3 to 4 weeks).

Plate fixation of fractures of metacarpals and phalanges was found in one study to be associated with a 67% complication rate for phalanges and 34% for metacarpals.[69] Stiffness was the most common complication. Soft-tissue dissection required to apply the plates and the interference of the plates with tendon excursion was thought to be the cause. Twenty-five percent of the plates were eventually removed because of discomfort or lack of motion. Alternative fixation techniques should be considered in phalangeal fractures. More recently, however, smaller, lower profile plates have become available and may improve the results of plating for these fractures.

Loss of Motion

Capsular contracture as well as extensor and flexor tendon adhesions can result in diminished motion following fractures of the hand. Joint stiffness or contracture can be the result of prolonged immobilization (greater than 3 to 4 weeks), immobilization in inappropriate positions, associated soft-tissue injuries, or an inadequate rehabilitation program. Extension contractures of the MCP joints and flexion contractures of the PIP joints are the most common patterns of stiffness. Aggressive therapy, which includes active assisted range of motion exercises and dynamic splinting, usually can overcome moderate degrees of stiffness and should be pursued for at least 6 months. Recalcitrant contractures of the MCP joint may require surgery for dorsal capsulectomy, while PIP contractures may respond to release of the volar checkrein ligaments. Dynamic miniexternal fixators for the PIP joint are now being used in the treatment of posttraumatic stiffness. Joint fusions in more functional positions should be considered in severe cases.

Tendon adhesions can best be prevented by restoring a smooth gliding surface at the time of fracture reduction and initiating early active motion exercises during the healing process. Flexor tendon adherence is identified by limited active motion in the presence of a full passive range of motion. Once full passive motion is achieved through aggressive therapy, surgical tenolysis that preserves the essential pulley system can restore active motion. Excision of the superficialis tendon is sometimes advocated. Extensor tendon adhesions typically present as an active extensor lag in the absence of a fixed joint contracture, but may also present as a block to flexion. Extensor tenolysis around the MCP joint is difficult to perform because of the broad surface area of the extensor hood, and techniques involving the excision of portions of the hood have been described. Tenolysis over the shaft of the metacarpal is more straightforward.

In a review of extensor tenolysis after phalangeal and metacarpal fractures,[70] digits requiring only tenolysis had a 54° improvement in TAM (31%) by 6 months. There was a 50% improvement in the extensor lag. Those digits that required both an extensor tenolysis and dorsal capsulotomy showed a 34° improvement in TAM (21%) after 6 months. In this group, there was no improvement of the extensor lag.

Malunion

Malunion of a metacarpal or phalanx is a troublesome complication because both rotational and angular deformities significantly impair hand function.[71,72] A rotational deformity causes deviation of the digit, particularly in flexion, and interferes with the other fingers by crossing over or scissoring. A recent review of corrective osteotomies of phalanges and metacarpals for both rotational and angular malunions using either K-wire or interosseous wiring of phalangeal osteotomies and miniplating of metacarpals revealed a 100% union rate with no loss of preoperative range of motion and full correction of preoperative deformity in 87%.[73] A step-cut osteotomy has been advocated by some to improve stability and healing of the osteotomy at the malunion site.[74]

Corrective osteotomies for rotational deformities can be performed at the site of malunion or at the metacarpal level.[75] Osteotomy at the site of the malunion has the greatest potential for correction, but at the phalangeal level, the intimate relationship of the bone to the extensor and flexor mechanisms risk adhesions and loss of motion. For this reason, proximal metacarpal osteotomies have been advocated. Studies using cadaveric specimens have shown that basal metacarpal osteotomies can correct malrotation of up to 19° in the index, long, and ring fingers and from 20°

to 30° in the small finger.[76] The deep transverse metacarpal ligament limits the maximum rotation.

Bone Loss and Shortening

Traumatic injuries of the hand involving bone loss are often associated with extensive soft-tissue injuries. Initial treatment should consist of irrigation and debridement of all nonviable tissue and temporary skeletal fixation. In 3 to 7 days, if the wound permits, delayed primary bone grafting using cancellous or corticocancellous autograft with definitive fixation is performed.[77] Skin graft and flap coverage should be performed concurrently, if necessary.

Annotated References

1. Agee J: Treatment principles for proximal and middle phalangeal fractures. *Orthop Clin North Am* 1992;23:35–40.

   This is an excellent overview and update of the functional anatomy, clinical assessment, and treatment principles of phalangeal fractures. Reduction and fixation techniques based on the countering and resisting of physiologic deforming forces on the fracture are emphasized.

2. Pun WK, Chow SP, Luk KDK, et al: A prospective study on 284 digital fractures of the hand. *J Hand Surg* 1989;14A:474–481.

   This prospective study of 284 digital fractures in 235 patients found that not all displaced fractures were unstable. The authors established the criteria that patients with functionally stable fractures could actively move the adjacent joints by more than 30% of the expected normal range while maintaining less than 10° of angulation in any plane or less than 45° in the sagittal plane in the fifth metacarpal. Stable fractures were treated with immediate mobilization. Fifteen percent of displaced fractures became functionally stable after closed reduction and their results were comparable to undisplaced fractures.

3. Strickland JW, Steichen JB, Kleinman WB, et al: Phalangeal fractures: Factors influencing digital performance. *Orthop Rev* 1982;11:39–50.

   The authors present a retrospective review of 415 phalangeal fractures to assess factors that influence the outcome of treatment of these fractures. Fingers should be mobilized by at least the fourth week. Concomitant injuries to tendons are poor prognostic factors, extensor injuries being worse than flexor injuries. Increasing patient age also has a significant aggravating effect on the outcome. Comminution and displacement have a lesser effect on the result.

4. Burkhalter WE: Closed treatment of hand fractures. *J Hand Surg* 1989;14A:390–393.

5. Maitra A, Burdett-Smith P: The conservative management of proximal phalangeal fractures of the hand in an accident and emergency department. *J Hand Surg* 1992:17B:332–336.

   Of 2,004 hand fractures reviewed, 242 were phalanx fractures and 147 were proximal phalanx fractures. Of the 147 fractures, 93 (63%) were extra-articular, uncomminuted, and stable, and these were treated in the emergency room with either splinting or buddy taping for a mean period of 14.1 days and 33.8 days, respectively. Only 4.3% of these fractures had significant complications; 95.7% had a successful outcome as measured on an outcome scale taking into account pain, deformity, and movement. Those fractures referred to a hand specialist were articular, oblique, or comminuted and were in most cases treated surgically.

6. Schneider LH: Fractures of the distal phalanx. *Hand Clin* 1988;4:537–547.

7. DaCruz DJ, Slade RJ, Malone W: Fractures of the distal phalanges. *J Hand Surg* 1988;13B:350–352.

8. Belsky MR, Eaton RG, Lane LB: Closed reduction and internal fixation of proximal phalangeal fractures. *J Hand Surg* 1984;9A:725–729.

9. Jabaley ME, Freeland AE: Rigid internal fixation in the hand: 104 cases. *Plast Reconstr Surg* 1986;77:288–297.

10. Black DM, Mann RJ, Constine RM, et al: The stability of internal fixation in the proximal phalanx. *J Hand Surg* 1986;11A:672–677.

11. Matloub HS, Jensen PL, Sanger JR, et al: Spiral fracture fixation techniques: A biomechanical study. *J Hand Surg* 1993;18B:515–519.

    Two hundred forty cadaver proximal phalanges and metacarpals were fractured in a spiral pattern and fixed by either crossed K-wires, interosseous loops, dorsal miniplate, single compression screw, or K-wire plus cerclage wire. Bending tests were conducted on an Instron tensiometer and torsional rigidity was measured on a materials testing system. Proximal phalanx apex-palmar bending tests demonstrated significantly more rigidity with the compression screw technique. Single compression screw was also significantly better under the torsional rigidity testing of the proximal phalanx than any of the other techniques.

12. Vanik RK, Weber RC, Matloub HS, et al: The comparative strengths of internal fixation techniques. *J Hand Surg* 1984;9A:216–221.

13. Ford DJ, El-Haddidi S, Lunn PG, et al: Fractures of the phalanges: Results of internal fixation using 1.5mm and 2mm AO screws. *J Hand Surg* 1987;12B:28–33.

    Thirty-eight phalangeal fractures were treated with 1.5- and 2-mm screws only. Mean postoperative immobilization was 9 days. After a mean follow-up of 24 months, total active motion was 220° or greater in 24 cases, 180° to 215° in eight cases, and less than 180° in only two patients. Mean time off work was 6 weeks. Results were considered satisfactory in 90% based on TAM, PIP flexion greater than 80°, and distance from fingertip to palm less than 1.5 cm.

14. Dabezies EJ, Schutte JP: Fixation of metacarpal and phalangeal fractures with miniature plates and screws. *J Hand Surg* 1986;11A:283–288.
15. Hastings H: Unstable metacarpal and phalangeal fracture treatment with screws and plates. *Clin Orthop* 1987;214:37–52.
16. Zimmerman NB, Weiland AJ: Ninety-ninety intraosseous wiring for internal fixation of the digital skeleton. *Orthopedics* 1989;2:99–104.
17. Nunley JA, Kloen P: Biomechanical and functional testing of plate fixation devices for proximal phalangeal fractures. *J Hand Surg* 1991;16A:991–998.
18. Buchler U, Fischer T: Use of a minicondylar plate for metacarpal and phalangeal periarticular injuries. *Clin Orthop* 1987;214:53–58.
19. Kumta SM, Spinner R, Leung PC: Absorbable intramedullary implants for hand fractures: Animal experiments and clinical trial. *J Bone Joint Surg* 1992;74B:563–566.
20. Nagy L: Static external fixation of finger fractures. *Hand Clin* 1993;9:651–657.
21. Schuind F, Cooney WP, Burny F, et al: Small external fixation devices for the hand and wrist. *Clin Orthop* 1993;293:77–82.
22. Seitz WH, Gomez W, Putnam MD, et al: Management of severe hand trauma with a mini external fixateur. *Orthopedics* 1987;10:601–610.
23. Wehbe MA, Schneider LH: Mallet fractures. *J Bone Joint Surg* 1984;66A:658–669.

   The authors reviewed 21 mallet fractures followed for a mean of 3.25 years. Six were treated surgically, and 15 were splinted. All but one had a good result regardless of the form of treatment. The articular surface remodelled and there was near-normal painless motion in all but one fracture. Subluxation and the size and amount of displacement of the bone fragment did not affect the outcome. Occasionally a painless bony prominence was noted on the dorsum of the DIP joint. A slightly higher incidence of extension lag was found in the nonsurgical group.

24. Damron TA, Engber WD, Lange RH, et al: Biomechanical analysis of mallet finger fracture fixation techniques. *J Hand Surg* 1993;18A:600–607.
25. Damron TA, Engber WD: Surgical treatment of mallet finger fractures by tension band technique. *Clin Orthop* 1994;300:133–139.
26. Eaton RG, Malerich MM: Volar plate arthroplasty of the proximal interphalangeal joint: A ten year review. *J Hand Surg* 1980;5B:260–268.
27. Durham-Smith G, McCarten GM: Volar plate arthroplasty for closed proximal interphalangeal joint injuries. *J Hand Surg* 1992;17B:422–428.
28. Freeland AE, Benoist LA: Open reduction and internal fixation method for fractures at the proximal interphalangeal joint. *Hand Clin* 1994;10:239–250.

   The authors provide detailed technical descriptions of the reduction and fixation methods of all patterns of intra-articular fractures of the PIP joint. These include unicondylar, bicondylar, avulsion, and pilon fractures of the PIP joint.

29. Stern PJ, Roman RJ, Kiefhaber TR, et al: Pilon fractures of the proximal interphalangeal joint. *J Hand Surg* 1991;16A:844–850.

   Twenty patients with pilon fractures of the base of the middle phalanx were treated with splint, skeletal traction through the middle phalanx, or open reduction with K-wire fixation. Perfect anatomic restoration of the joint could not be achieved using any of the techniques; regardless of treatment, some stiffness of the PIP joint ensued. Immobilization yielded the worst outcomes. Traction and open reduction showed no significant difference in outcome with regard to range of motion and radiographic evaluation.

30. Weiss AC, Hastings H: Distal unicondylar fractures of the proximal phalanx. *J Hand Surg* 1993;18A:594–599.

   The authors reviewed the results of 38 patients treated for distal unicondylar fractures of the proximal phalanx and compared the results of fragment fixation using a number of different fixation techniques: a single K-wire, multiple K-wires, a miniscrew with a K-wire, or only mini-screw fixation alone. After an average follow-up of 3 years, those fractures treated with multiple K-wires and those fixed with miniscrews alone resulted in the best final joint motion. The final range of motion was poorest in those treated with a single K-wire because there was a high incidence of secondary displacement.

31. Hastings H, Ernst JMJ: Dynamic external fixation for fractures of the proximal interphalangeal joint. *Hand Clin* 1993;9:659–674.

   This overview of the skeletal and ligamentous anatomy of the PIP joint includes the determination of the joint's axis of motion. Necessary requirements for a dynamic external fixator are summarized and a design for such a fixator is described. The clinical experience and case illustrations are presented. After an average fixation period of 31 days and 12 weeks of follow-up, final PIP motion averaged 2° to 100°, with normal alignment and stability.

32. Inanami H, Ninomiya S, Okutsu I, et al: Dynamic external finger fixator for fracture dislocation of the proximal interphalangeal joint. *J Hand Surg* 1993;18A:160–164.
33. Nagle DJ, Ekenstam FW, Lister GD: Immediate silastic arthroplasty for non-salvageable intraarticular phalangeal fractures. *Scand J Plast Reconstr Surg* 1989;23:47–50.
34. Jahss SA: Fractures of the metacarpals: A new method of reduction and immobilization. *J Bone Joint Surg* 1938;20A:178–186.
35. Ford DJ, Ali MS, Steel WM: Fractures of the fifth metacarpal neck: Is reduction or immobilisation necessary? *J Hand Surg* 1989;14B:165–167.
36. McKerrell J, Bowen V, Johnston G, et al: Boxer's fractures: Conservative or operative management? *J Trauma* 1987;27:486–490.

   Sixty-three patients with isolated, closed fifth metacarpal fractures were recalled for follow-up evaluation, of whom 25 had been treated conservatively with early motion or immobilization for 5 to 21 days and 15 had undergone surgical treatment with closed or open K-wire fixation. Patients in both groups had good results in terms of joint motion and grip strength. The surgical group had less residual dorsal angulation but no difference in functional outcome. The authors conclude that surgery should be considered only for patients demanding perfect cosmesis.

37. Ashkenaze DM, Ruby L: Metacarpal fractures and dislocations. *Orthop Clin North Am* 1992;23:19–33.

   This is a review of the current understanding of functional anatomy, fracture evaluation methods, and treatment indications for metacarpal fractures of all patterns, including thumb metacarpals and intra-articular injuries. The vast majority of metacarpal fractures and dislocations, according to the authors, can be treated nonsurgically.

38. Stern PJ: Fractures of the metacarpals and phalanges, in Green DP, Hotchkiss RN (eds): *Operative Hand Surgery*, ed 3. New York, NY, Churchill Livingstone, 1993.

39. Burkhalter WE: Hand fractures, in Greene WB (ed): *Instructional Course Lectures XXXIX*. Park Ridge, IL, American Academy of Orthopaedic Surgeons 1990, pp 249–253.

40. Freeland AE, Jabaley ME, Hughs JL (eds): *Stable Fixation of the Hand and Wrist*. New York, NY, Springer-Verlag, 1986.

41. Konradsen L, Nielsen PT, Albrecht-Beste E: Functional treatment of metacarpal fractures: 100 randomized cases with or without fixation. *Acta Orthop Scand* 1990;61:531–534.

42. Viegas SF, Tencer A, Woodard P, et al: Functional bracing of fractures of the second through fifth metacarpals. *J Hand Surg* 1987;12A:139–143.

43. Melone CP: Rigid fixation of phalangeal and metacarpal fractures. *Orthop Clin North Am* 1986;17:421–435.

44. Greene TL, Noellert RC, Belsole RJ, et al: Composite wiring of metacarpal and phalangeal fractures. *J Hand Surg* 1989;14A:665–669.

45. Firoozbakhsh KK, Moneim MS, Howey T, et al: Comparative fatigue strengths and stabilities of metacarpal internal fixation techniques. *J Hand Surg* 1993;18A:1059–1068.

   One hundred five metacarpals from cadaveric specimens were cyclically tested in bending, torsion, and axial loading in a material testing system machine after oblique osteotomies and internal fixation. Dorsal plating with lag screw was superior to two dorsal lag screw, crossed K-wire tension banding, and intramedullary K-wire fixation. The fatigue strength of plate fixation was greater than the next strongest fixation (by two dorsal lag screws) by 1.5 times in bending, 1.6 times in torsion, and 2.5 times in axial loading.

46. Black DM, Mann RJ, Constine R, et al: Comparison of internal fixation techniques in metacarpal fracture. *J Hand Surg* 1985;10A:466–472.

47. Mann RJ, Black D, Constine R, et al: A quantitative comparison of metacarpal fracture stability with five different methods of internal fixation. *J Hand Surg* 1985;10A:1024–1028.

48. Diwaker HN, Stothard J: The role of internal fixation in closed fractures of the proximal phalanges and metacarpals in adults. *J Hand Surg* 1986;11B:103–108.

49. Ford DJ, El-Haddidi S, Lunn PG, et al: Fractures of the metacarpals: Treatment by AO screw and plate fixation. *J Hand Surg* 1987;12B:34–37.

50. Bosscha K, Snellen JP: Internal fixation of metacarpal and phalangeal fractures with AO minifragment screws and plates: A prospective study. *Injury* 1993;24:166–168.

   The prospective study involved 43 patients with 47 metacarpal or phalangeal fractures with significant displacement, rotation, or angulation and considered unstable. The fractures were treated with either screws alone or screws and plates through a dorsal or dorsolateral approach, depending on the fracture configuration and metacarpal involved. After a mean follow-up of 28 months, 34 patients with 38 fractures were examined. Ninety-two percent of the fractures had greater than 220° of total active motion and there were no nonunions or malunions. Two patients had superficial inflammation that resolved with antibiotics.

51. Shehadi SI: External fixation of metacarpal and phalangeal fractures. *J Hand Surg* 1991;16A:544–550.

   Twenty-six patients with 30 fractures (19 metacarpal and 11 phalangeal) were treated by closed reduction and external fixation with K-wires and methylmethacrylate rods and a palmar plaster splint and were followed for 3 to 12 months. Motion exercises were begun after 1 week. Percentage return of total range of motion in metacarpal fractures was 96% (77% to 100%) and in phalangeal fractures 84% (66% to 98%) of the opposite hand. There were no rotational deformities, losses of reduction, or pin tract infections.

52. Parsons SW, Fitzgerald JAW, Shearer JR: External fixation of unstable metacarpal and phalangeal fractures. *J Hand Surg* 1992;17B:151–155.

53. Crichlow TPKR, Hoskinson J: Avulsion fracture of the index metacarpal base: Three case reports. *J Hand Surg* 1988;13B:212–214.

54. Light TR, Bednar MS: Management of intra-articular fractures of the metacarpophalangeal joint. *Hand Clin* 1994;10:303–314.

55. Gurland M: Carpometacarpal joint injuries of the fingers. *Hand Clin* 1992;8:733–744.

56. Lawlis JF, Gunther SF: Carpometacarpal dislocations: Long-term follow-up. *J Bone Joint Surg* 1991;73A:52–58.

57. Cannon SR, Dowd GSE, Williams DH, et al: A long-term study following Bennett's fracture. *J Hand Surg* 1986;11B:426–431.

58. Kjaer-Petersen K, Langhoff O, Andersen K: Bennett's fracture. *J Hand Surg* 1990;15B:58–61.

   Forty-one patients with Bennett's fractures were followed up and evaluated for arthritic changes, symptoms, and disability. Patients were treated with either closed reduction and immobilization, percutaneous K-wire fixation, or open reduction and fixation. After a median follow-up of 7.3 years, 15 of 18 patients with healing and excellent reduction were free of symptoms, while only six of 13 patients with residual displacement were asymptomatic. Radiographic signs of arthritis were found in only three of 14 patients with excellent reduction and seven of 10 with residual displacement. Therefore, the authors advocate exact reduction of these fractures by surgery, if necessary.

59. Langhoff O, Andersen K, Kjaer-Petersen K: Rolando's fracture. *J Hand Surg* 1991;16B:454–459.

60. Buchler U, McCollam M, Oppikofer C: Comminuted fractures of the basilar joint of the thumb: Combined treatment by external fixation, limited internal fixation, and bone grafting. *J Hand Surg* 1991;16A:556–560.

61. Strauch RJ, Behrman MJ, Rosenwasser MP: Acute dislocation of the carpometacarpal joint of the thumb: An anatomic and cadaver study. *J Hand Surg* 1994;19A:93–98.

   Thirty-eight thumbs of cadaver specimens were subjected to a dorsal dislocating force and the ligaments were serially sectioned. The ligaments examined included the dorsoradial, anterior oblique, posterior oblique, and intermetacarpal. The primary restraint to dorsal dislocation was the dorsoradial ligament. After reduction, the joint was most stable in pronation and extension, which tightened the anterior oblique ligament.

62. Laasonen EM, Kivioja A: Delayed diagnosis of extremity injuries in patients with multiple injuries. *J Trauma* 1991;31:257–260.

63. Bone L, Bucholz R: The management of fractures in the patient with multiple trauma. *J Bone Joint Surg* 1986;68A:945–949.

64. Swanson TV, Szabo RM, Anderson DD: Open hand fractures: Prognosis and classification. *J Hand Surg* 1991;16A:101–107.

65. McLain RF, Steyers C, Stoddard M: Infections in open fractures of the hand. *J Hand Surg* 1991;16A:109–112.

66. Duncan RW, Freeland AE, Jabaley ME, et al: Open hand fractures: An analysis of the recovery of active motion and of complications. *J Hand Surg* 1993;18A:387–394.

    One hundred forty open hand fractures in 104 patients were treated surgically and were followed up at an average of 17 months and assessed for total active motion. Results correlated highly with severity of soft-tissue injury. Surgical extension of the wound to achieve reduction and stabilization resulted in worse outcomes. Metacarpal fractures had significantly better outcomes than phalangeal fractures.

67. Gonzalez MH, McKay W, Hall RF: Low-velocity gunshot wounds of the metacarpal: Treatment by early stable fixation and bone grafting. *J Hand Surg* 1993;18A:267–270.

68. Botte MJ, Davis JLW, Rose BA, et al: Complications of smooth pin fixation of fractures and dislocations in the hand and wrist. *Clin Orthop* 1992;276:194–201.

69. Stern PJ, Wieser MJ, Reilly DG: Complications of plate fixation in the hand skeleton. *Clin Orthop* 1987;214:59–65.

70. Creighton JJ, Steichen JB: Complications in phalangeal and metacarpal fracture management: Results of tenolysis. *Hand Clin* 1994;10:111–116.

71. Royle SG: Rotational deformity following metacarpal fracture. *J Hand Surg* 1990;15B:124–125.

72. Seitz WH, Fromison AI: Management of malunited fractures of the metacarpal and phalangeal shafts. *Hand Clin* 1988;4:529–536.

    The authors review the most common patterns of malunion of the phalangeal and metacarpal bones. They also describe techniques of secondary reconstruction to address these deformities. Transverse osteotomies for rotational deformities and closing wedge and oblique osteotomies and bone grafting for angular deformities are presented. Osteotomies at the site of deformity and distant from the deformity are discussed for phalangeal and metacarpal malunions.

73. van der Lei B, de Jonge J, Robinson PH, et al: Correction osteotomies of phalanges and metacarpals for rotational and angular malunion: A long-term follow-up and a review of the literature. *J Trauma* 1993;35:902–908.

74. Pichora DR, Meyer R, Masear VR: Rotational step-cut osteotomy for treatment of metacarpal and phalangeal malunion. *J Hand Surg* 1991;16A:551–555.

75. Green DP: Complications of phalangeal and metacarpal fractures. *Hand Clin* 1986;2:307–328.

    The author reviews and discusses the major complications of the treatment of phalangeal and metacarpal fractures, including malunion, nonunion, tendon adherence, joint stiffness, and the problems of internal fixation. Methods of addressing these complications are described.

76. Gross MS, Gelberman RH: Metacarpal rotational osteotomy. *J Hand Surg* 1985;10A:105–108.

77. Freeland AE, Jabaley ME: Stabilization of fractures in the hand and wrist with traumatic soft tissue and bone loss. *Hand Clin* 1988;4:425–436.

II
Lower Extremity

Robert J. Brumback, MD
Section Editor

10
Intracapsular Hip Fractures

Introduction

As the average age and life expectancy of the population has increased, so has the prevalence of fractures of the proximal end of the femur, including intracapsular hip fractures. The absolute number of these fractures has doubled in the 30 years since the mid 1960s, and this trend will probably continue into the next century. It is estimated that management of proximal femoral fractures costs more than $8 billion annually.[1] It has been suggested that the best way to optimize the cost-benefit ratio was through surgical fixation of these fractures.[2]

In general, intracapsular hip fractures occur more often in women than in men and, more often in whites than in blacks; in addition, intracapsular fractures occur more frequently and in younger individuals than do intertrochanteric fractures.[3,4] Those sustaining intracapsular hip fractures can be divided into two groups: the elderly and young adults. In the elderly population, the fracture usually occurs as a result of low-energy trauma, such as a fall. Etiologic factors for this group include neurologic impairment, poor balance, impaired vision, malnutrition, malignancy, and decreased physical activity.[5] It should be noted that although patients with femoral neck fractures are at risk for osteoporosis, this condition occurs no more frequently in patients with fracture than in age-matched patients without fracture,[6] disproving the common belief that elderly patients with a fracture are more likely to be porotic than those without fracture. In addition, there is no association between osteoarthritis and femoral neck fractures. In young, healthy patients, fractures of the proximal part of the femur are the result of high-energy trauma, such as a motor vehicle accident; more than half are associated with multiple injuries.

Anatomy

The key to understanding the intracapsular hip fracture lies in knowing the anatomy and physiology of the proximal femur.

Normal Anatomy

At skeletal maturity (age 16, male or female), the proximal femoral epiphysis is fused and the neck shaft angle is approximately 130° ± 7° with anteversion of 10° ± 7°. The calcar femorale, a dense portion of cortex of the proximal femur, extends from the posteromedial portion of the shaft and radiates superiorly toward the greater trochanter, fusing with the posterior portion of the femoral neck; it is not the medial cortical portion of the femoral neck.

The vascular supply to the proximal femur, including the femoral head, originates from the medial and lateral femoral circumflex arteries. These form an extracapsular arterial ring at the base of the femoral neck. The lateral epiphyseal artery (the terminal branch of the medial femoral circumflex) pierces the capsule and proceeds superiorly as the retinacular (the retinaculum of Weitbrecht) arteries. The lateral epiphyseal artery and the artery of the ligamentum teres supply the major portion of the femoral head and, in most cases, the terminal branch of the ascending portion of the lateral femoral circumflex artery supplies the anterior and inferior portion of the femoral head.[7]

Pathologic Anatomy

A femoral neck fracture disrupts the blood supply to the femoral head in direct proportion to the amount of fracture displacement. In studies of femoral neck fractures, almost all femoral head specimens studied show signs of cellular death and varying degrees of necrosis.[8] In the adult miniature swine, a minimally displaced fracture of the femoral neck was shown to cause a 60% diminution in blood flow to the femoral head.[9] If not all of the arteries are disrupted, reduction of femoral neck fractures has been shown to lower the rate of osteonecrosis of the femoral head. The major problem secondary to this decreased blood flow and subsequent necrosis is late segmental collapse of the femoral head. This collapse occurs as the femoral head is revascularized and the osteoclastic remodeling of the necrotic bone weakens the support of the articular cartilage.

A markedly displaced fracture of the femoral neck will usually tear the posterior portion of the hip capsule. A less displaced fracture, can however, decrease blood flow to the femoral head and increase the likelihood of osteonecrosis because maintaining capsule integrity confines an expanding hematoma and may increase the intracapsular pressure, occluding the venous drainage from the capsule and impeding arteriole inflow. However, the clinical significance of the role of the intracapsular hematoma is unproven. In cases where the capsule remains intact, the hip position can also increase the intracapsular pressure. Because capsular volume is greatest in the position of flexion and external rotation, the limb should be maintained in this position before surgery.

Diagnosis

Clinical Signs and Symptoms

The clinical signs and symptoms of a patient presenting with a fracture of the femoral neck may vary. The symptoms may be mild in patients with impacted, incomplete, or nondisplaced fractures. Such patients may complain of hip and/or groin pain with weightbearing or with internal rotation of the limb. Patients with displaced femoral neck fractures have shortening and external rotation of the extremity with mild abduction. The clinician should rule out fractures of the pubic ramus. Patients suspected of having femoral neck fractures will be more comfortable placed at rest with a pillow under the knee and with the knee and hip in slight flexion, a position that allows maximum capsular volume.

In the polytrauma patient, these signs and symptoms may be masked by many factors, such as head injury. Because of the catastrophic sequelae of the unrecognized displaced fracture, or possibly the late displacement of an originally undisplaced fracture, the polytrauma patient must be examined carefully, both clinically and radiographically, with special attention to the identification of the femoral neck fracture.

Imaging

Standard anteroposterior (AP) and cross-table lateral radiographs of the hip are required for evaluating fractures of the femoral neck. Any discontinuity in the cortex or trabecular pattern should raise suspicion for a femoral neck fracture. In the patient with pelvic trauma, the computed tomography (CT) scan should be carefully examined for evidence of fracture. Therefore, the orthopaedist should ensure that there are a sufficient number of CT slices through the femoral neck region. CT can also provide valuable information about the amount and location of comminution in high-energy fractures.

The orthopaedic surgeon has several options for determining the presence of a fracture in a patient with a suspected fracture, but one that is not evident on plain film. A T1-weighted MRI study will confirm or deny the presence of a fracture in 100% of the cases.[10] If such imaging is unavailable, a bone scan performed 3 days after injury will be definitive. In a study of 179 bone scans taken at various stages after injury, bone scans, even within 24 hours of injury, were shown to have a high sensitivity and specificity for fracture.[11] However, these results do not match the accuracy of magnetic resonance imaging (MRI).

Some reports in the literature address the use of MRI and bone scans to evaluate osteonecrosis after fracture of the femoral neck. Enhanced MRI has been shown to be very sensitive in identifying osteonecrosis of the femoral head,[12] whereas the two-dimensional Fourier transform spin-echo technique has not.[13] Titanium used for implant causes less interference on MRI evaluation than does stainless steel. Bone scans can be used to evaluate blood flow to the femoral head; however, the overlying acetabulum and difficulty in comparing both femoral heads makes this method less reliable.

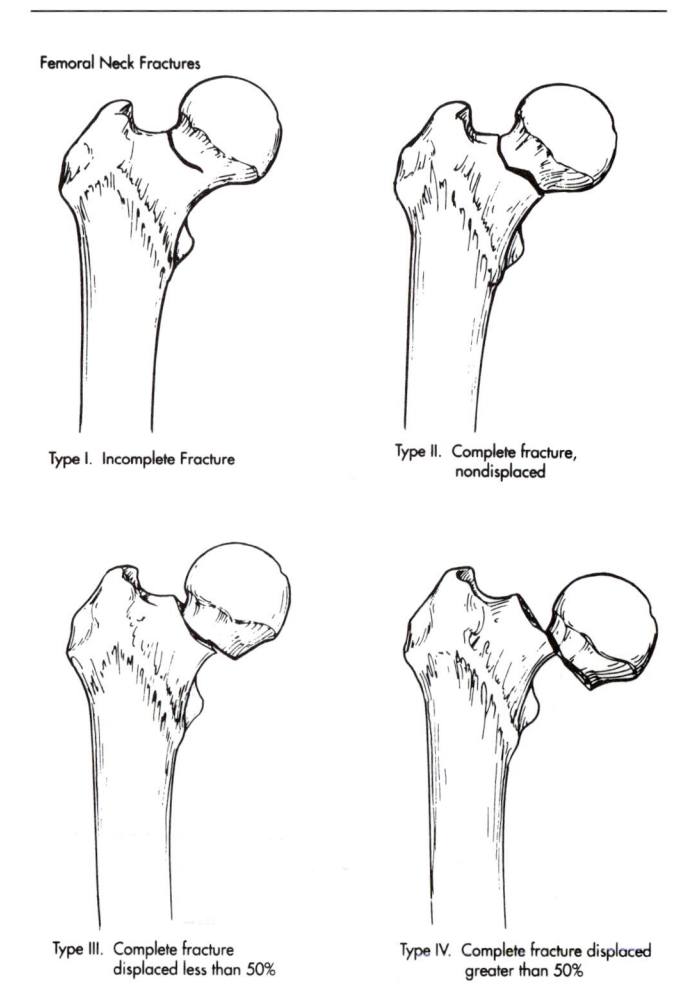

Fig. 1 Garden's classification. (Reproduced with permission from Kyle RF: Fractures of the hip, in Gustilo RB, Kyle RF, Templeman DC (eds): *Fractures and Dislocations*. St. Louis, MO, Mosby-Year Book, 1993, vol 2, p 795.)

Classification

Garden's[14] classification scheme for femoral neck fractures is the most commonly accepted system (Fig. 1). It is based on the degree of displacement shown on the AP radiograph of the hip. Types I and II are nondisplaced and have a better prognosis for healing and a lower rate of osteonecrosis than do displaced fracture types III and IV. Interobserver disagreement exists in classifying these fractures, most

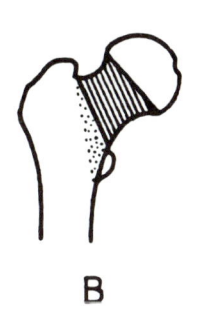

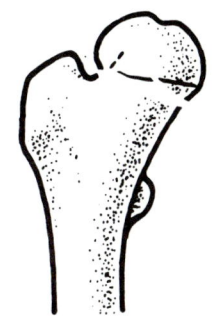

B1 Neck fracture, subcapital with slight displacement
.1 impacted in valgus > 15°
.2 impacted in valgus < 15°
.3 non-impacted

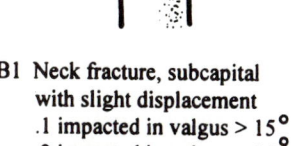

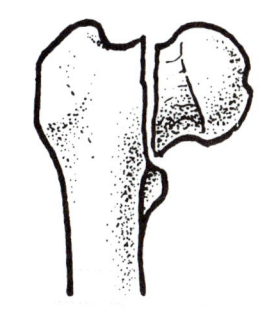

B2 Neck fracture, transcervical
.1 basicervical
.2 midcervical
.3 midcervical shear

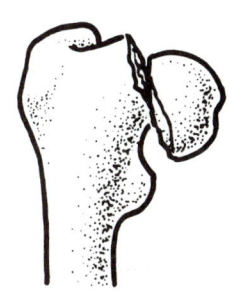

B3 Neck fracture, subcapital non-impacted, displaced
.1 moderate displacement in varus and external rotation
.2 moderate displacement with vertical translation and external rotation
.3 marked displacement

Fig. 2 AO classification. (Reproduced with permission from Müller ME, Nazarian S, Koch P (eds): *Classification AO Des Fractures*. Berlin, Germany, Springer-Verlag, 1987, pp 48–49.)

evident in differentiating Garden types III and IV; however, variations in classification by a single observer are minimal. Pauwel's classification is used less frequently. Based on the angle formed by the fracture line and the horizontal plane, it calls attention to the importance of the vertical fracture, which results from higher shear forces and is associated with a poorer prognosis, most often seen in the patient with high-energy injury.

In an effort to eliminate interobserver variations and facilitate standardized classification of fracture types, The Orthopaedic Trauma Association is developing a database incorporating modifications of existing classification systems such as the AO system (Fig. 2). Coding for fractures of the femoral neck in the AO system range from 31.B.1.1 to 31.B.3.3. In this system, "31" identifies the proximal femur, the "B" subgroup localizes the fracture to the femoral neck, and the subsequent designations further categorize the fracture type and location.

Treatment

Although no current literature advocates nonsurgical treatment for these fractures, the surgical treatment of femoral neck fractures depends on the physiologic age of the patient and the degree of displacement of the fracture. All patients, however, whether young or old, should be fully evaluated and stabilized before being taken to the operating room. The goal of treatment is to return the patient to preinjury function.

The patient with a nondisplaced or minimally displaced fracture is at low risk (less than 10%) for osteonecrosis and nonunion, assuming no subsequent displacement occurs, and therefore should be managed with stable internal fixation. Because these essentially nondisplaced fractures may occur in an intact capsule, which can increase intracapsular pressure and lead to decreased blood flow to the femoral head, an anterior capsulotomy may be indicated. This procedure, however, does not have universal support.

The displaced femoral neck fracture places the patient at high risk for osteonecrosis and nonunion. A nonunion rate of 19% and a late segmental collapse rate of 12% were reported in a series of more than 1,500 patients.[15] These results were echoed in another large series.[16] The rate of osteonecrosis may be higher than 12% because this condition also occurs in patients without segmental collapse. Several large studies, for example, showed an average rate of 25% (range, 10% to 45%).

In young adults, the mechanism of injury for these fractures is usually high-energy trauma, resulting in multiple injuries. In this age group, 20% of the femoral neck fractures have an associated fracture of the femoral shaft. Because the femoral shaft fracture is so obvious and is most often in the midshaft, the femoral neck fracture is missed up to 30% of the time.[17]

Young adults seem to be at high risk for osteonecrosis and nonunion. Although a recent study[18] reported an 18% incidence of osteonecrosis and no nonunions (all healed within 16 weeks), in a group of 27 patients younger than 50 years of age with femoral neck fractures, very high rates of such complications have been reported with these fractures.[18] Therefore, every effort should be made in this population to retain the femoral head with closed or open reduction and internal fixation of the fracture.

In the older patient, treatment again depends on the physiologic age and activity level of the patient. Although the literature does not define the most appropriate age at which to replace the proximal femur, prosthetic replacement is indicated for more debilitated patients, eg, those physiologically older or with concurrent chronic disease, because it will obviate a second surgery should internal fixation fail.

In any patient with a fracture of the femoral neck, the quality of the reduction is the greatest determinant of outcome in terms of mechanical stability and the reestablishment of blood supply to the femoral head. More than 20° of valgus is associated with an increased rate of osteonecrosis, as is a varus reduction. Garden[20] commented that increased posterior comminution led to decreased stability of reduction and that angulation of greater than 10° in the AP plane should not be accepted.

There are numerous devices for fixation of the femoral neck fracture. A device that maintains alignment of the two fragments and provides stability so that the fracture may heal is ideal. Fixation with multiple pins or screws is recommended. The critical element in the stability of the fixation is the density of the bone.[21] Stability is maximized by the use of three pins in a triangular configuration; using more than three pins has no mechanical advantage.[22] Screws should be inserted at an angle of 130° to 135° to the femoral shaft because starting points in the lateral cortex at or below the lesser trochanter have been associated with a 20% incidence of subtrochanteric fracture. The use of large hip compression screws placed in the posterior and superior portion of the femoral head can cause compromise of the blood flow to that portion.[23] Therefore, if a large compression screw is used, a pin should be placed superiorly and left in place to supply the rotational control lacking in the screw.

As mentioned earlier, prosthetic replacement is indicated for the elderly, more-debilitated patient. A cemented unipolar hemiarthroplasty is indicated for a patient who is confined to bed or requires transfer from bed to chair because thigh pain and acetabular protrusion are not issues. Recently, bipolar protheses have been designed with the same considerations given to total hip stems. To date, the reports show no conclusive evidence that the results of bipolar protheses are superior to those provided by the unipolar prosthesis, although dislocations are less frequent with bipolar prostheses, as is protrusion. Certainly, a total hip replacement is indicated in a patient with severe pre-existing hip disease.

Figure 3 provides a treatment algorithm.

Special Considerations

Ipsilateral Femoral Neck and Shaft Fractures

Fewer than 3% of femoral shaft fractures occur in conjunction with ipsilateral fractures of the femoral neck. For as many as 30% of these injuries, the diagnosis may be missed.[17] Surgical stabilization is indicated for this injury, with reduction and fixation of the femoral neck having the highest priority. Several options for fixation exist.

If the femoral neck is not displaced, it may be stabilized with anteriorly placed screws, after which a standard first-generation locking nail or second-generation reconstruction nail may be used. Alternatively, the neck may be stabilized in the standard fashion and the shaft fracture may be stabilized by retrograde nailing. Plate fixation of the shaft component is also an option.

A displaced femoral neck fracture requires reduction and fixation. Reduction may be obtained in several ways: (1) open reduction, (2) closed reduction using a Schanz pin to manipulate the shaft component, and (3) rapid stabilization of the shaft fracture followed by closed reduction of the femoral neck.

If the femoral neck fracture will be treated with prosthetic replacement, one may choose either a long-stem prosthesis, plate fixation of the shaft component and prosthetic replacement for the neck, or retrograde nailing of the shaft component and prosthetic replacement for the neck fracture, depending on the location of the shaft fracture.

Patients with Renal Failure, Parkinson's Disease, or Arthritis

In patients with renal failure there is an increased incidence of failure of fixation because of the bone demineralization that accompanies the disease. In these situations, prosthetic replacement is indicated because fixation failure is very common.

Parkinsonism poses a different problem. Because of the increased incidence of contractures and the advanced age of patients with this disease, prosthetic replacements are common. The common belief that the posterior approach is associated with higher rates of dislocation is a misconception.[24]

Patients with rheumatoid and advanced osteoarthritis are best served with prosthetic total hip replacement.

Complications

Osteonecrosis, nonunion, and failure of fixation are the most common complications of femoral neck fracture and its treatment. The incidence of osteonecrosis ranges from 10% to 45% in various reports. As stated earlier, adequate reduction remains the most important factor in preventing the development of this complication. Garden's study showed that approximately one third of patients with this complication will require further surgery. In the young patient with involvement of less than 50% of the femoral head, an osteotomy may be an alternative; otherwise, a noncemented arthroplasty may be indicated. A hip arthrodesis remains a good alternative in the young patient who will make high demands on the hip (eg, a laborer).

Most clinicians agree that there should be evidence of healing within 6 to 12 months after fracture of the femoral

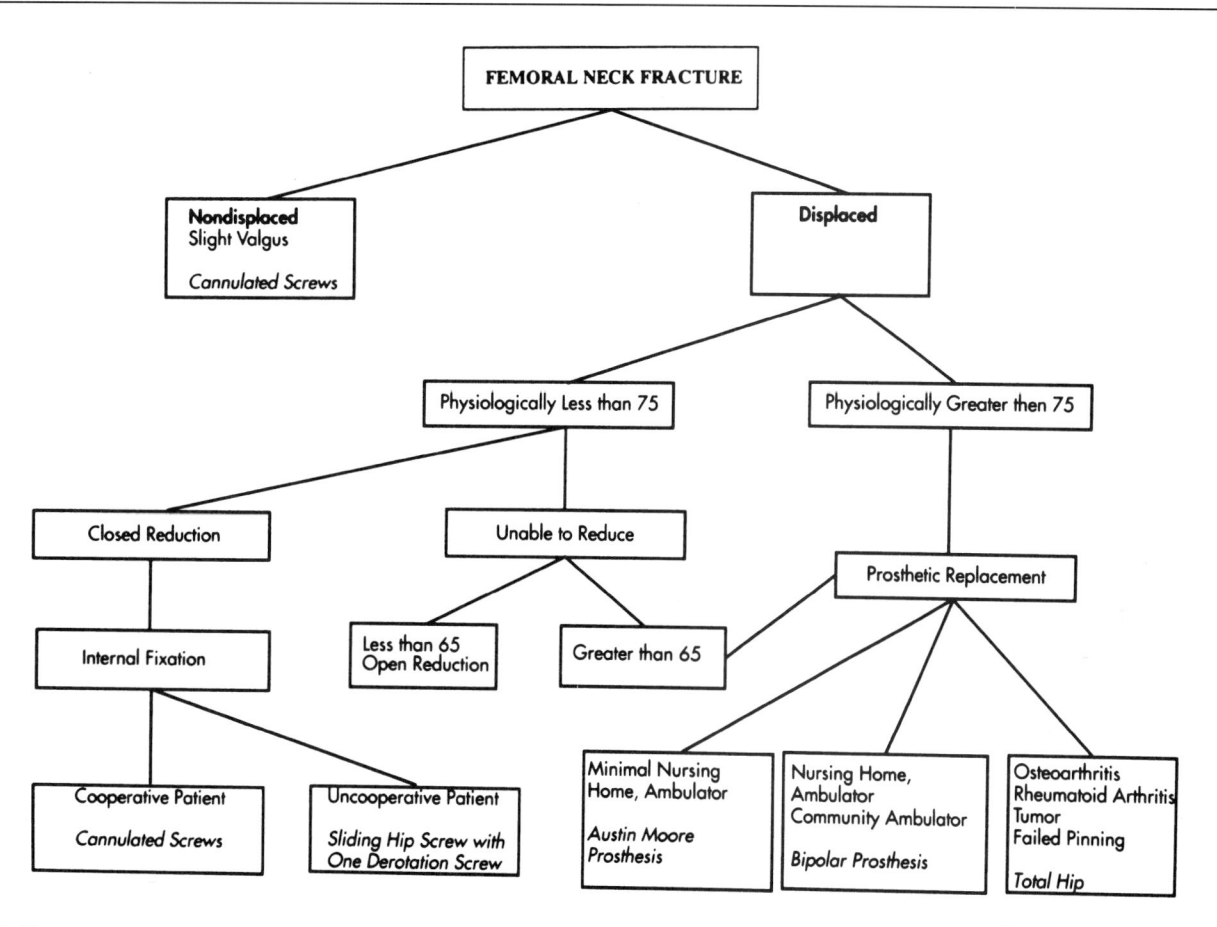

Fig. 3 Treatment algorithm for fractures of the femoral neck. (Reproduced with permission from Kyle RF: Fractures of the hip, in Gustilo RB, Kyle RF, Templeman DC (eds): *Fractures and Dislocations*. St. Louis, MO, Mosby-Year Book, 1993, vol 2, p 800.)

neck. Therefore, nonunion of the femoral neck can be defined as a fracture that has not healed within the first year after injury and the reported incidence ranges from 10% to 30%. In the fracture with a nonunion, MRI is indicated to assess the viability of the head. For the young patient with a viable femoral head, an osteotomy is indicated; if the femoral head is not viable, total hip arthroplasty is an option.

Failure of fixation usually manifests itself by pain in the groin and buttock. There may be lucency about the hardware, backing out of implants, and often a resultant neck shaft angle in varus. Traumatic arthrosis may occur with joint penetration. If the patient is young, one alternative is to replace the implants with or without osteotomy; otherwise, prosthetic replacement may be indicated.

A recent report utilizing meta-analysis observed that the mortality rate associated with the displaced fractures of the femoral neck at 30 days was higher for those treated with primary hemiarthroplasty than those treated with internal fixation.[25] However, this difference was not statistically significant and did not persist beyond 3 months. This observation is not unexpected because internal fixation is reserved for generally healthier individuals.

Conclusion

The treatment of femoral neck fractures in the adult remains "the unsolved fracture" and, although many modalities have been explored, the optimal method of fixation and reduction remains to be identified. Future investigations should focus on the following questions: Should capsulotomies be performed? Is there an optimal time for performing arthroplasty versus internal fixation? What form of internal fixation is best? How can the complications of osteonecrosis and nonunion be avoided? If osteonecrosis occurs, what is the best way to manage it? What is the best treatment for nonunion of the femoral neck with and without an avascular femoral head?

Annotated References

1. Praemer A, Furner S, Rice DP: *Musculoskeletal Conditions in the United States*. Park Ridge, IL, American Academy of Orthopaedic Surgeons, 1992.

2. Parker MJ, Myles JW, Anand JK, et al: Cost-benefit analysis of hip fracture treatment. *J Bone Joint Surg* 1992;74B:261–264.

3. Hinton RY, Smith GS: The association of age, race, and sex with the location of proximal femoral fractures in the elderly. *J Bone Joint Surg* 1993;75A:752–759.

   The authors retrospectively reviewed the records of 27,370 patients (at least 65 years old) discharged with a diagnosis of fracture of the proximal part of the femur. The ratio of intertrochanteric fractures to femoral neck fractures increased with age in women but remained relatively stable in men. Fracture occurrence was highest in white women, followed, in order, by white men, black women, and black men.

4. Griffin MR, Ray WA, Fought RL, et al: Black-white differences in fracture rates. *Am J Epidemiol* 1992;136:1378–1385.

   This epidemiologic study showed a decreased rate of fracture in blacks as compared with whites in patients older than 65 years old.

5. Astrom J, Ahnqvist S, Beertema J, et al: Physical activity in women sustaining fracture of the neck of the femur. *J Bone Joint Surg* 1987;69B:381–383.

   The authors compared the activity level among 49 women 15 to 49 years of age who sustained fractures of the femoral neck to that of a control group without fracture. The adolescents with fractures were found to have been less active than those without fractures.

6. Aitken JM: Relevance of osteoporosis in women with fracture of the femoral neck. *Br Med J* 1984;288:597–601.

7. Trueta J, Harrison MHM: The normal vascular anatomy of the femoral head in adult man. *J Bone Joint Surg* 1953;35B:442–461.

   This is a classic description of vascular anatomy of the femoral head using injection techniques.

8. Catto M: A histological study of avascular necrosis of the femoral head after transcervical fracture. *J Bone Joint Surg* 1965;47B:749–776.

9. Swiontkowski MF, Tepic S, Rahn BA, et al: The effect of femoral neck fracture on femoral head blood flow, in Arlet J, Mazieres B (eds): *Bone Circulation and Bone Necrosis: Proceedings of the IVth International Symposium on Bone Circulation*. Berlin, Germany, Springer-Verlag, 1990, pp 150–153.

10. Quinn SF, McCarthy JL: Prospective evaluation of patients with suspected hip fracture and indeterminate radiographs: Use of T1-weighted MR images. *Radiology* 1993;187:469–471.

    Twenty patients with suspected hip fracture and indeterminate plain radiographs were prospectively evaluated. MRI was found to be 100% predictive. In addition, the cost of the study was less than that for CT or bone scan.

11. Holder LE, Schwarz C, Wernicke PG, et al: Radionuclide bone imaging in the early detection of fractures of the proximal femur (hip): Multifactorial analysis. *Radiology* 1990;174:509–515.

    The authors discuss the use of bone scan in the detection of fractures about the proximal femur, in 179 bone scans, 105 gathered retrospectively and 74, prospectively. Approximately half of the bone scans were performed at less than 72 hours after injury; 17.5% were obtained less than 24 hours after injury. The results showed a high sensitivity (93.3%) and specificity (95.0%) for the identification of fractures: the positive predictive value was 91.8%; the negative predictive value was 96.0%. In patients with equivocal radiographs, the sensitivity and specificity was 97.8% and 95.0%, respectively.

12. Lang P, Mauz M, Schorner W, et al: Acute fracture of the femoral neck: Assessment of femoral head perfusion with gadopentetate dimeglumine-enhanced MR imaging. *AJR* 1993;160:335–341.

    Contrast-enhanced MRI scans were compared with unenhanced MRI scans and digital subtraction angiography with good results for diagnosing perfusion abnormalities and viability of the femoral head postinjury.

13. Walters R, Simon SR: Joint destruction: A sequel of unrecognized pin penetration in patients with slipped capital femoral epiphyses, in Riley LH Jr (ed): *The Hip: Proceedings of the Eighth Scientific Meeting of the Hip Society*. St. Louis, MO, CV Mosby, 1980, pp 145–164.

    A two-dimensional Fourier transform spin-echo technique was not adequate in determining viability of the femoral head within 48 hours after fracture of the femoral neck.

14. Garden RS: Low-angle fixation in fractures of the femoral neck. *J Bone Joint Surg* 1961;43B:647–663.

15. Barnes R, Brown JT, Garden RS, et al: Subcapital fractures of the femur: A prospective review. *J Bone Joint Surg* 1976;58B:2–24.

16. Arnold WD, Lyden JP, Minkoff J: Treatment of intracapsular fractures of the femoral neck: With special reference to percutaneous Knowles pinning. *J Bone Joint Surg* 1974;56A:254–262.

17. Riemer BL, Butterfield SL, Ray RL, et al: Clandestine femoral neck fractures with ipsilateral diaphyseal fractures. *J Orthop Trauma* 1993;7:443–449.

18. Swiontkowski MF, Winquist RA, Hansen ST Jr: Fractures of the femoral neck in patients between the ages of twelve and forty-nine years. *J Bone Joint Surg* 1984;66A:837–846.

    The authors reported on 27 patients (12 to 49 years old) with femoral neck fractures. Twenty of those injuries had been caused by high-energy trauma. Only 18% of the 27 had signs of osteonecrosis.

19. Protzman RR, Burkhalter WE: Femoral-neck fractures in young adults. *J Bone Joint Surg* 1976;58A:689–695.

    Twenty-two patients sustained high-energy trauma resulting in femoral neck fractures. The rate of nonunion was 59% and the rate of osteonecrosis was 86%.

20. Garden RS: Malreduction and avascular necrosis in subcapital fractures of the femur. *J Bone Joint Surg* 1971;53B:183–197.

21. Smith MD, Cody DD, Goldstein SA, et al: Proximal femoral bone density and its correlation to fracture load and hip-screw penetration load. *Clin Orthop* 1992;283:244–251.

22. Swiontkowski MF, Harrington RM, Keller TS, et al: Torsion and bending analysis of internal fixation techniques for femoral neck fractures: The role of implant design and bone density. *J Orthop Res* 1987;5:433–444.

   The authors evaluated bone density and pin screw and plate fixation for the management of femoral neck fractures. Results showed three 6.5-mm screws in a triangular pattern was the most biomechanically sound. Bone density was found to correlate with fracture stability.

23. Brodetti A: The blood supply of the femoral neck and head in relation to the damaging effects of nails and screws. *J Bone Joint Surg* 1960;42B:794–801.

24. Staeheli JW, Frassica FJ, Sim FH: Prosthetic replacement of the femoral head for fracture of the femoral neck in patients who have Parkinson disease. *J Bone Joint Surg* 1988;70A:565–568.

   A retrospective review of 49 patients with Parkinson's disease showed there was only one dislocation. An anterolateral approach had been used for that patient. Stability at the time of surgery was shown to be important to outcome. Tenotomy was required in 5 patients.

25. Lu-Yao GL, Keller RB, Littenberg B, et al: Outcomes after displaced fractures of the femoral neck: A meta-analysis of one hundred and six published reports. *J Bone Joint Surg* 1994;76A:15–25.

11

Intertrochanteric Femur Fractures

Introduction

As our population ages, intertrochanteric femur fractures are occurring more frequently. They account for approximately 200,000 hip fractures yearly in the United States and represent half of all hospital days for fracture care. This growing problem is the focus of many cost-containment programs. Although this problem impacts many aspects of the health care delivery system, the orthopaedic surgeon has a central role in the treatment of these patients.

Prevention

Several risk factors have been identified for hip fractures. The effect of most individual factors is moderate, but together their impact can be substantial. Some are predetermined. The risk for fracture is doubled if there is a history of maternal hip fracture. A woman may be able to minimize her risk of hip fracture by walking for exercise, avoiding sedatives, reducing caffeine intake, quitting smoking, treating impaired vision, and taking measures that maintain bone density.[1] There is compelling evidence that hormonal supplementation in postmenopausal women, coupled with an adequate calcium intake, can reduce the incidence of hip fractures.[2] Education and evaluation of the home environment can help eliminate hazards (throw rugs, electrical cords, and stairs) that contribute to the trip and fall scenario.

Evaluation of the Injury

In the geriatric population, the intertrochanteric femur fracture generally results from a low-energy fall. If loss of consciousness contributes to the fall, the underlying medical condition needs appropriate evaluation and treatment. High-energy trauma is usually the cause of these fractures in younger patients. Physical examination of a patient with a displaced intertrochanteric fracture typically reveals a painful, shortened, and externally rotated lower extremity.

Minimally displaced fractures are difficult to diagnose based on a clinical or radiographic evaluation. Patients may report hip pain with weightbearing or certain movements. Occasionally, a fracture is suspected clinically, but is not evident on the standard anteroposterior (AP) and lateral

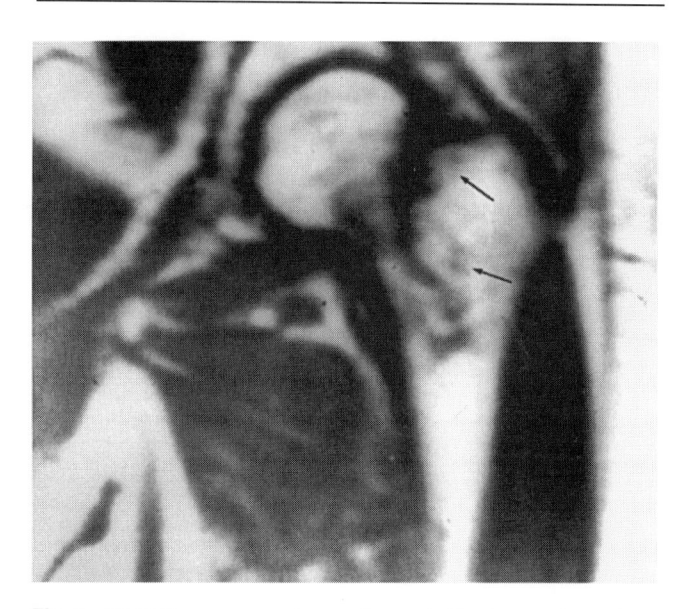

Fig. 1 Magnetic resonance image demonstrating intertrochanteric fracture. (Reproduced with permission from Foley P, Gould E, Lyden J: Diagnosis of occult fractures about the hip. *J Bone Joint Surg* 1993;75A:396.)

views of the proximal femur, which are usually used to determine treatment. Repeating AP radiographs in traction or with internal rotation may demonstrate the fracture line. Further diagnostic testing for an occult fracture may include a technetium (Tc 99m) bone scan, limited magnetic resonance imaging (MRI), or a tomogram. The Tc 99m bone scan is most reliable at 72 hours. A report of similar accuracy within 24 hours with short (15 minutes), limited (T1-weighted only) MRI (Figs. 1 and 2) promises to expedite definitive treatment.[3]

Classification

Several authors have classified intertrochanteric fractures. Jensen and associates[4] found the modified Evans classification (Fig. 3, Table 1) to be the most predictive of anatomic

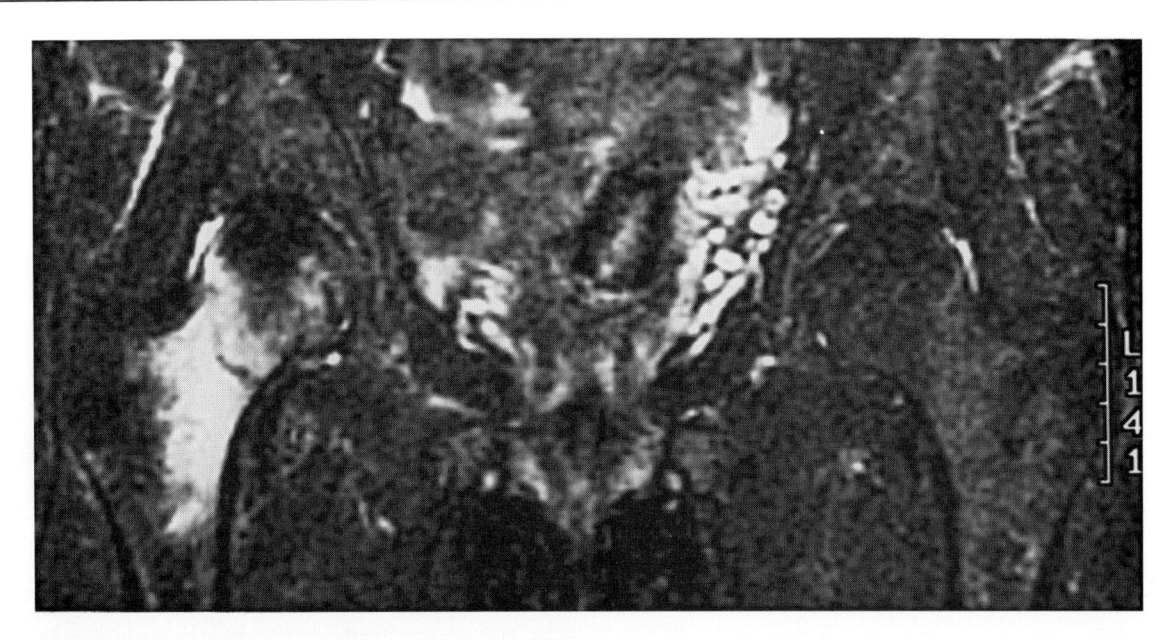

Fig. 2 Magnetic resonance image demonstrating proximal femoral fracture.

Table 1 Evans-Jensen classification system for intertrochanteric fractures

Type I Stable (two-part) fracture	Type II Unstable (three-part) fractures	Type III Very unstable (four-part) fractures
Undisplaced Displaced	Lesser trochanter comminution Greater trochanter comminution	Both trochanter comminution

(Reproduced with permission from Naidu SH, Reilly TM, Hoppenstall RB: Intertrochanteric fracture fixation with sliding hip compression-screw. *Oper Tech Orthop* 1994;4:67.)

reducibility and postfixation stability for a given fracture. The classification by Evans[5] addresses the stability of the fracture pattern. Unstable fracture patterns include those that have comminution of the posterior medial cortex or a reverse obliquity pattern. An unstable pattern can be made more stable by reduction of the medial cortex.

Treatment

Isolated, avulsion-type fractures of the greater or lesser trochanter usually can be managed with protected weight-bearing (Fig. 4). There is concern that this may represent or progress to a complete intertrochanteric disruption.

Surgical stabilization is the treatment of choice for intertrochanteric femur fractures. The goal is to mobilize the patient by obtaining and maintaining a stable fracture reduction. Several factors play a role in a successful outcome: the quality of the bone, the alignment and stability of the reduction, and the fixation device.

Another factor contributing to a successful outcome is the timing of surgery. Recent studies have come to conflicting conclusions regarding this issue. Kenzora and associates,[6] in a retrospective study, found that patients who had been managed surgically within 1 day after admission had a significantly greater 1-year mortality rate than those who underwent the operation between the second and fifth days after admission. This relationship was even stronger in relatively healthy patients (three or fewer preexisting medical conditions).

In contrast, Sexson and Lehner[7] reported an increased 1-year mortality rate for relatively healthy patients when surgery occurred more than 24 hours after admission. For patients who had at least three preexisting medical conditions, such a delay was associated with a reduced mortality rate. White and associates[8] found an increased 1-year mortality rate when surgery was delayed for more than 24 hours.

In a prospective unrandomized study, Zuckerman and associates[9] found that a delay of 3 calendar days or more from the time of admission to the time of the surgery almost doubled the risk of mortality within the first year after the fracture. This remained true even when the age and sex of the patient and the number of preexisting medical

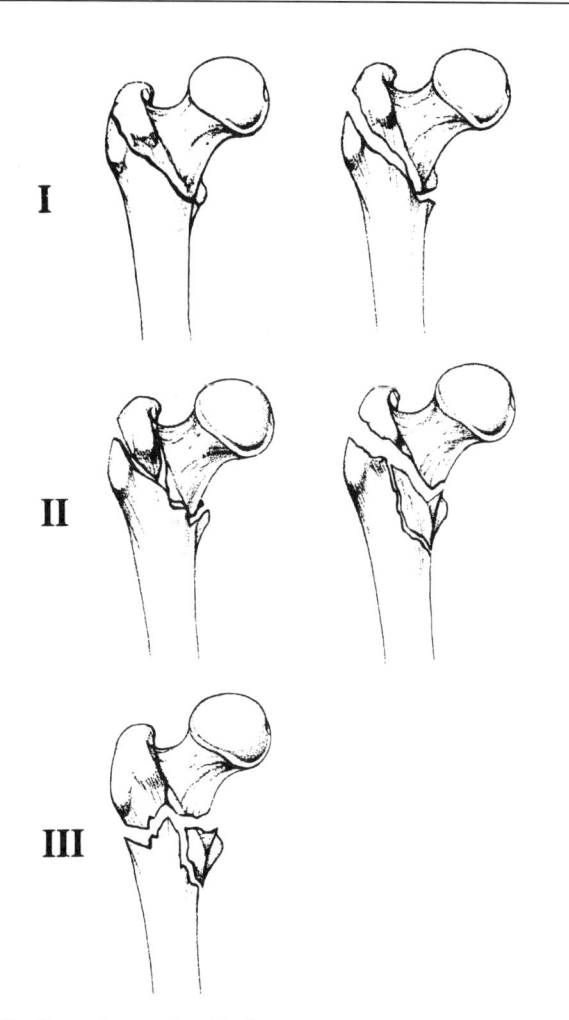

Fig. 3 Evans-Jensen classification.

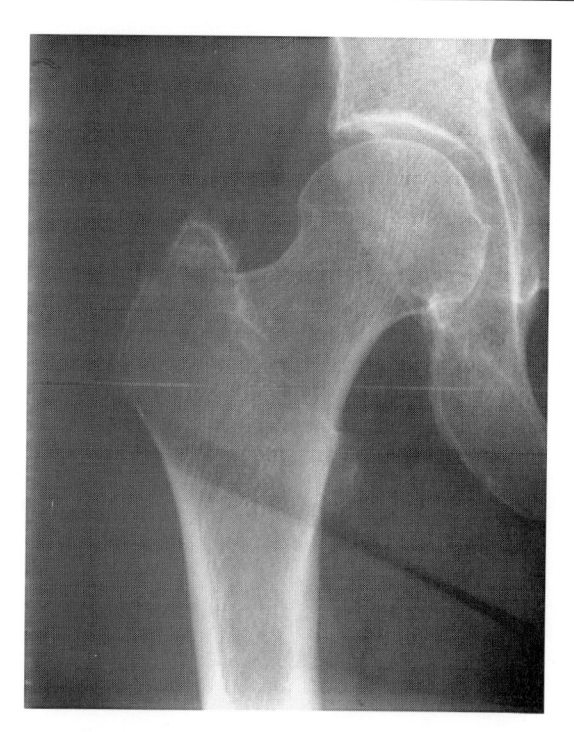

Fig. 4 Greater trochanter avulsion fracture.

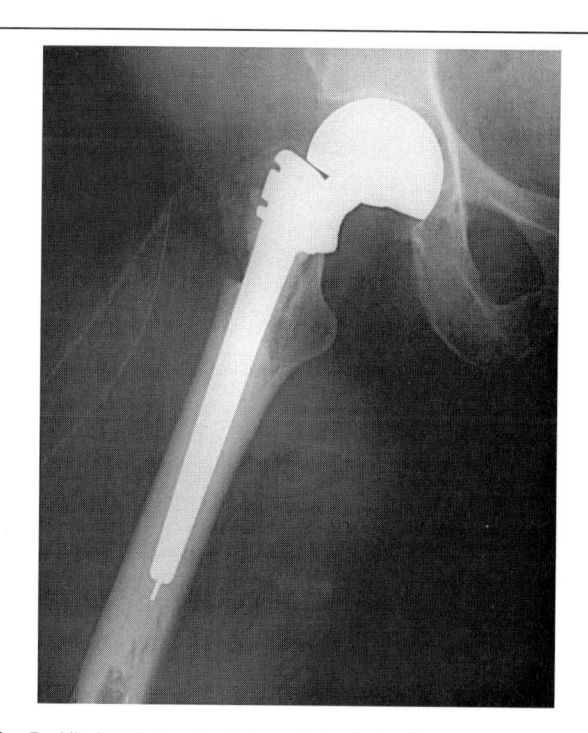

Fig. 5 Hip hemiarthroplasty for pathologic fracture.

conditions were controlled. This association was not conditional on the number or severity of the medical conditions. No association was found between a delay in surgery and postoperative complication during hospitalization. This study was limited to patients at least 65 years of age who were cognitively intact, living at home, and able to walk before the fracture. They recommended that those patients should have surgery within 2 calendar days after admission to the hospital.

The vast majority of intertrochanteric fractures occur in the osteoporotic bone of the geriatric population. The bone is rarely ideal for fixation. There is no reliable method of accurately assessing the quality of the bone preoperatively. In rare cases, methylmethacrylate can augment bone fixation.[10] A better option may be the development of an injectable calcium phosphate paste that quickly hardens in situ, with mechanical properties similar to bone and potential for incorporation and remodeling.[11] Prosthetic replacement is an alternative in the treatment of comminuted,

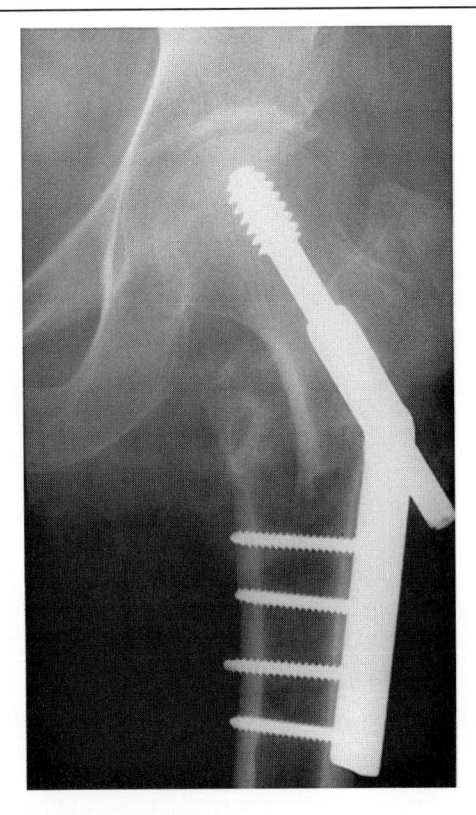

Fig. 6 Medial displacement.

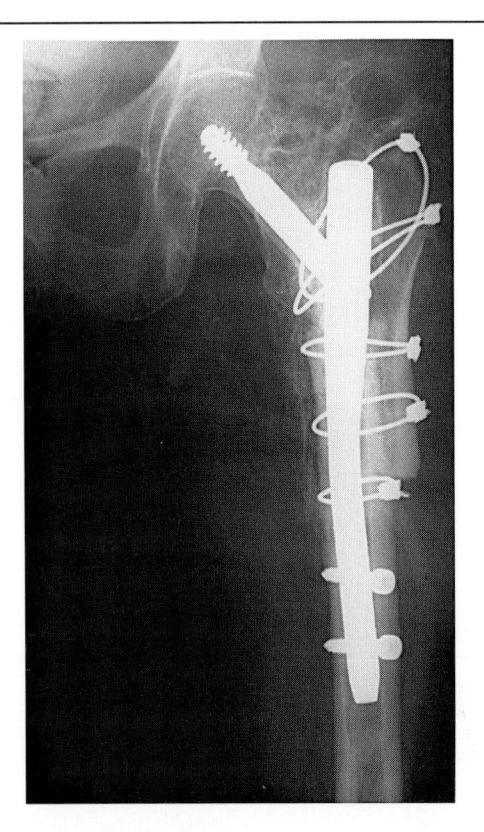

Fig. 7 Intramedullary hip screw.

severely osteoporotic or pathologic fractures, but this method does introduce the risk of dislocation[12] (Fig. 5). Use of a primary bipolar hemiarthroplasty in elderly patients with unstable intertrochanteric fractures allows early full weightbearing, an advantage in comparison to use of internal fixation. Haentjens and associates[13] reported better rehabilitation and a lower incidence of decubiti and pulmonary complications in these patients.

The goal of surgery is to achieve an anatomic and stable reduction. The larger the posterior medial fragment is, the greater its reduction and fixation contribute to load resistance.[14] Medial displacement osteotomies offer no benefit over anatomic reduction when using a compression screw device.[15] Well-aligned unstable fractures fixed with a compression hip screw often collapse to a stable medial displacement alignment. Performing an osteotomy to achieve medial displacement results in more inherent shortening of the extremity (Fig. 6).

Compression hip screws are the most commonly used devices for fixation of these fractures. Hip screw fixation is strongest when central in the femoral head on both AP and lateral views and within 1 cm of the subchondral bone.[16] The angle of the sideplate is less important. A fracture with a reverse obliquity pattern does not benefit from the sliding properties of the "compression" hip screw. Other devices may be more appropriate to counteract the medial displacement forces also seen with subtrochanteric fractures. Although there is no consensus in the literature, these fractures have been successfully treated with interlocked rods, intramedullary hip screws, and right-angle blade plates, or condylar screws (Figs. 7 through 9).

Intertrochanteric femur fractures have been managed with several other devices. Rigid and flexible intramedullary condylocephalic nails have had some success (Fig. 10), but they have higher complication rates, especially in unstable fractures.[17] Short interlocked intramedullary hip screws (eg, gamma nails) provide several theoretical biomechanical advantages in management of peritrochanteric fractures. Its intramedullary position shifts the mass moment of inertia medially, permitting more effective calcar load sharing. The shorter lever arm decreases its bending moment. Its sliding screw allows for controlled impaction of the fracture. The surgical technique for insertion requires less exposure of the fracture site. Recent clinical studies[18] have proven no significant difference in terms of surgical time, blood loss, and fluoroscopy exposure. Short interlocked medullary screws have produced outcome results comparable to the compression hip screw and sideplate experience; however, there have been infrequent, but troublesome, "secondary" femoral shaft fractures at the distal end of the device.[19]

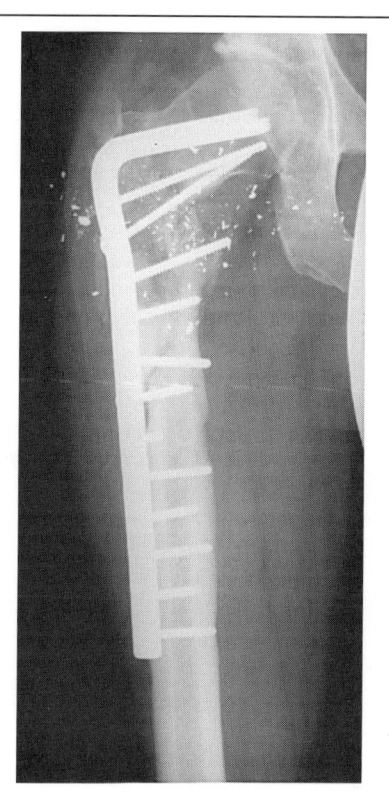

Fig. 8 Right-angled blade plate.

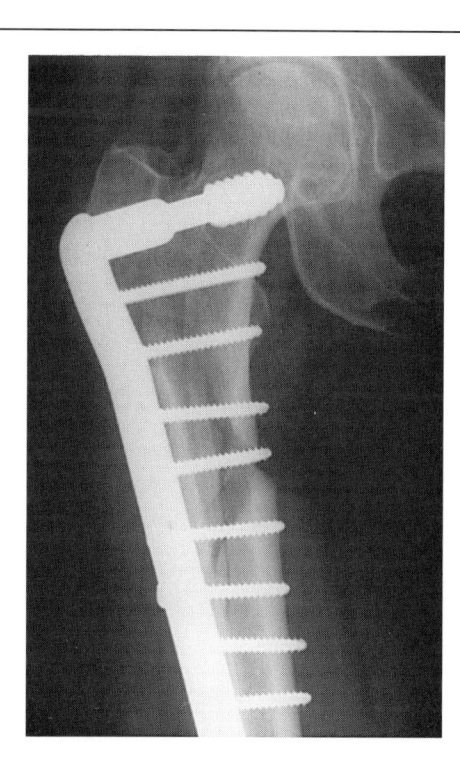

Fig. 9 Condylar screw.

Complications

The major complications in the treatment of intertrochanteric femur fractures are loss of reduction and loss of fixation. Davis and associates[20] reported a 16% mechanical failure rate in 203 intertrochanteric femur fractures treated with internal fixation. Screw cutout accounted for 12% of these failures. Implants placed posteriorly in the femoral head cut out more often (27%) than those placed centrally (7%). The cutout rate was also related to the stability of the fracture reduction, but not to age, ambulatory status, or bone density. The resulting varus malunion may be acceptable in debilitated patients.

If a symptomatic nonunion develops, valgus osteotomy, bone grafting, and stabilization can be considered. In elderly patients or in patients in whom screw cutout has occurred, a calcar-replacing prosthetic arthroplasty is indicated.[21] Femoral length and version are more difficult to judge intraoperatively, resulting in higher dislocation rates than arthroplasties for femoral neck fractures. Clinically significant malrotation, osteonecrosis, and hardware failure are rare. Subcapital fractures have been reported when the screw has not been set deeply in the femoral head.[22] Patients with rheumatoid arthritis have higher complication rates following fixation of intertrochanteric fractures. Bogoch and associates[23] reported a 10% rate of osteonecrosis, a 10% rate of infection, and a 28% rate of revision to total hip arthroplasty, although only one had preexisting hip involvement. Total hip replacement may be the treatment of choice for rheumatoid patients with intertrochanteric fractures with or without preexisting hip arthritis.

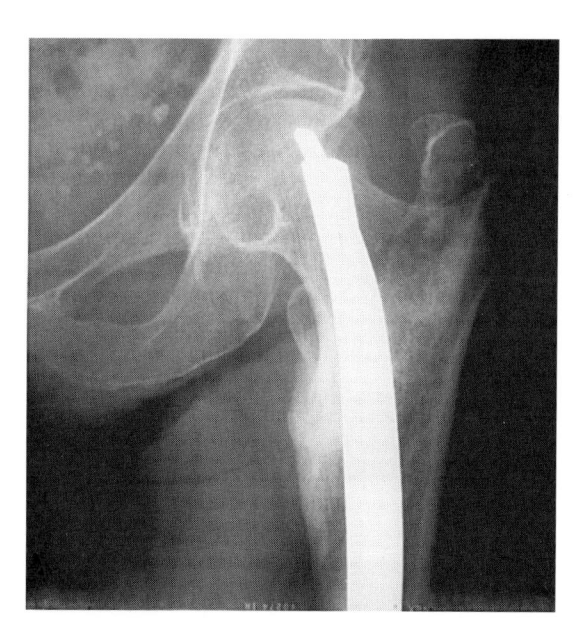

Fig. 10 Healed intertrochanteric fracture.

References

1. Cummings SR, Nevitt MC, Brown WS, et al: Risk factors for hip fracture in white women. *N Engl J Med* 1995;332:767-773.
2. Cauley JA, Seeley DG, Ensrud K, et al: Estrogen replacement therapy and fractures in older women. *Ann Intern Med* 1995;122:9-16.
3. Rizzo PF, Gould ES, Lyden JP, et al: Diagnosis of occult fractures about the hip: Magnetic resonance imaging compared with bone-scanning. *J Bone Joint Surg* 1993;75A:395-401.
4. Jensen JS, Sonne-Holm S, Tondeuold E: Unstable trochanteric fractures: A comparative analysis of four methods of internal fixation. *Acta Orthop Scand* 1980;51:949-962.
5. Evans EM: The treatment of trochanteric fractures of the femur. *J Bone Joint Surg* 1949;31B:190-203.
6. Kenzora JE, McCarthy RE, Lowell JD, et al: Hip fracture mortality: Relation to age, treatment, preoperative illness, time of surgery, and complications. *Clin Orthop* 1984;186:45-56.
7. Sexson SB, Lehner JT: Factors affecting hip fracture mortality. *J Orthop Trauma* 1987;1:298-305.
8. White BL, Fisher WD, Laurin CA: Rate of mortality for elderly patients after fracture of the hip in the 1980's. *J Bone Joint Surg* 1987;69A:335-340.
9. Zuckerman JD, Skovron ML, Koval KJ, et al: Postoperative complications and mortality associated with operative delay in older patients who have a fracture of the hip. *J Bone Joint Surg* 1995;77A:1551-1556.
10. Bartucci EJ, Gonzalez MH, Cooperman DR, et al: The effect of adjunctive methylmethacrylate on failures of fixation and function in patients with intertrochanteric fractures and osteoporosis. *J Bone Joint Surg* 1985;67A:1094-1107.
11. Constantz BR, Ison IC, Fulmer MT, et al: Skeletal repair by in situ formation of the mineral phase of bone. *Science* 1995;267:1796-1799.
12. Stern MB, Angerman A: Comminuted intertrochanteric fractures treated with a Leinbach prosthesis. *Clin Orthop* 1987;218:75-80.
13. Haentjens P, Casteleyn P, DeBoeck H, et al: Treatment of unstable intertrochanteric and subtrochanteric fractures in elderly patients. *J Bone Joint Surg* 1989;71A:1214-1225.
14. Apel DM, Patwardhan A, Pinzur MS, et al: Axial loading studies of unstable intertrochanteric fractures of the femur. *Clin Orthop* 1989;246:156-164.
15. Desjardins AL, Roy A, Paiement G, et al: Unstable intertrochanteric fracture of the femur: A prospective randomised study comparing anatomical reduction and medial displacement osteotomy. *J Bone Joint Surg* 1993;75B:445-447.
16. Den Hartog BD, Bartal E, Cooke F: Treatment of the unstable intertrochanteric fracture: Effect of the placement of the screw, its angle of insertion, and osteotomy. *J Bone Joint Surg* 1991;73A:726-733.
17. Sernbo I, Johnell O, Gentz CF, et al: Unstable intertrochanteric fractures of the hip: Treatment with Ender pins compared with a compression hip screw. *J Bone Joint Surg* 1988;70A:1297-1303.
18. Goldhagen PR, O'Connor DR, Schwarze E: A prospective comparative study of the compression hip screw and the gamma nail. *J Orthop Trauma* 1994;5:367-372.
19. Bridle SH, Patel AD, Bircher M, et al: Fixation of intertrochanteric fractures of the femur: A randomised prospective comparison of the Gamma nail and the Dynamic Hip Screw. *J Bone Joint Surg* 1991;73B:330-334.
20. Davis T, Sher JL, Horsman A, et al: Intertrochanteric femoral fractures. *J Bone Joint Surg* 1990;72B:26-31.
21. Mehlhoff T, Landon GC, Tullos HS: Total hip arthroplasty following failed internal fixation of hip fractures. *Clin Orthop* 1991;269:32-37.
22. Mariani EM, Rand JA: Subcapital fractures after open reduction and internal fixation of intertrochanteric fractures of the hip. *Clin Orthop* 1989;245:165-168.
23. Bogoch ER, Ouellette G, Hastings DE: Intertrochanteric fracture of the femur in rheumatoid arthritis patients. *Clin Orthop* 1993;294:181-186.

12

Fractures of the Femoral Diaphysis, Including the Subtrochanteric Region

Prior to the advent of modern treatment techniques, fractures of the femur were disabling and frequently fatal injuries. Treatment of femoral shaft fractures has evolved over the past century from simple splinting or traction of the limb to refined techniques of internal fixation. This has greatly lessened both the morbidity and mortality of this injury.

Evaluation

The diagnosis of acute traumatic fracture of the femoral shaft is in general not subtle. Shortening of the thigh, swelling, deformity, and severe pain call immediate attention to this condition. Because of the magnitude of forces required to create these fractures, serious associated injuries are common. Initial physical examination should focus on identification of life-threatening injuries following advanced trauma life support (ATLS) guidelines, which should be accompanied by a detailed history from the patient, if possible, and prehospital personnel. This should be followed by a complete, sequential head-to-toe examination of the entire patient. Examination of the involved extremity includes palpation of the pelvis, hip, and knee; circumferential examination of the integument for evidence of soft-tissue injury; and assessment of distal neurologic and vascular integrity. Gross malalignment should be reduced, open wounds should be dressed with a sterile dressing, and traction or longitudinal splinting should be applied to minimize further soft-tissue injury, muscle spasm, and discomfort.

Initial radiographs should include anteroposterior and lateral views of the entire femur, the hip, and the knee, as well as an anteroposterior view of the pelvis. Careful inspection of the femoral neck is important to avoid overlooking subtle fracture of the femoral neck.

Fractures of the femoral diaphysis are most commonly described by the location and geometry of the fracture, the degree of comminution, and the severity of the soft-tissue injury. The classification of Winquist and Hansen[1] is useful to grade the degree of comminution (Fig. 1). The OTA (AO) classification combines all of these elements in an organized, integrated system (Fig. 2).

Treatment

Traction

Treatment of femoral fractures with traction or the combination of traction and cast bracing results in predictable healing but has the disadvantages of prolonged hospitalization and immobilization and has been associated with common complications such as shortening, rotational malunion, and knee stiffness.[2,3] Traction treatment of femoral shaft fractures in adults is now reserved for patients who cannot undergo surgical treatment or who are treated in centers not equipped to perform intramedullary nailing.

External Fixation

External fixation of the femur is hindered by the envelope of muscle that surrounds it. External fixation pins that traverse the quadriceps frequently cause pin tract complications, scarring, and knee stiffness.[4] Because of the superior clinical results reported using intramedullary nailing, external fixation is currently reserved for severe open fractures of the femur. In the unstable patient who cannot tolerate prolonged anesthesia, or in fractures with associated vascular injury, external fixation may provide rapid, minimally invasive stabilization of the femur. In these cases, external fixation may be used as definitive stabilization of the fracture, or as temporary stabilization, with removal and conversion to internal fixation. The potential for infection with this technique, however, is at least theoretically of concern.

Plating

Open reduction and plate fixation of femoral fractures offers the potential advantages of anatomic reduction and rigid stabilization, allowing early functional rehabilitation. This technique requires extensive exposure of the lateral aspect of the femur, which may further devitalize fracture fragments, delay healing, and increase the likelihood of infection. Ruedi and Luscher[5] reported a series of 126

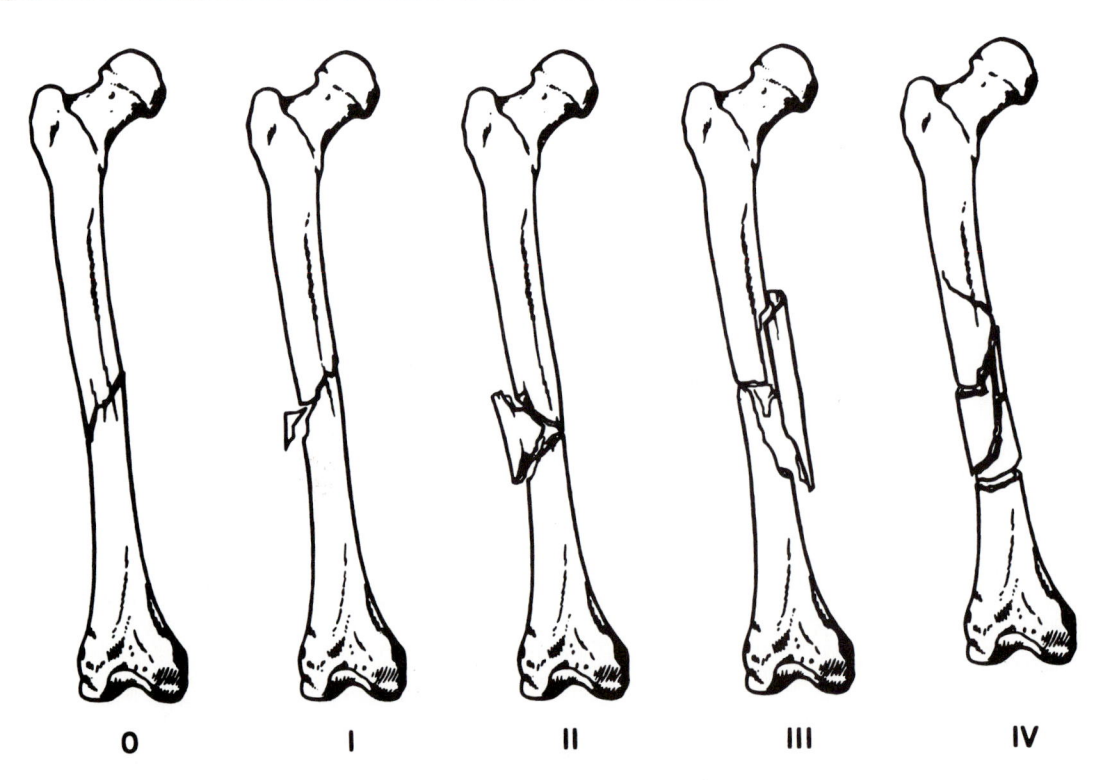

Fig. 1 Winquist classification of femoral shaft fractures. (Reproduced with permission from Poss R (ed): *Orthopaedic Knowledge Update 3*. Park Ridge, IL, American Academy of Orthopaedic Surgeons, 1990, pp 513-527.)

fractures of the femur treated with open reduction and internal fixation, with 92% good or excellent results. Complications, however, included loss of fixation in 9% secondary to nonunion, delayed union requiring bone grafting in 9%, and infection in 6%. Because of the superior results of intramedullary nailing, open reduction and plating of femoral shaft fractures is limited to special situations, such as ipsilateral shaft and articular fractures, in most trauma centers. If open reduction and plating are performed, more recent techniques of "indirect reduction" that minimize soft-tissue dissection should be used.

Intramedullary Nailing

Intramedullary nailing has supplanted other methods of treatment for the vast majority of fractures of the femoral diaphysis. Nailing allows the use of closed techniques, without extensive soft-tissue dissection; affords stable alignment of the bone; and favors rapid healing with early return to function. Results of published studies indicate that intramedullary nailing of femoral shaft fractures is superior to other forms of treatment.[6,7] The largest series by Winquist and associates[7] includes 520 femoral fractures in 500 patients treated with intramedullary nailing. Union occurred in 99%, while complications were low (infection 0.9%, shortening 2%, malrotation 2.3%). Knee motion in this series averaged 130°.

Surgical Considerations

Interlocking Nails

Many refinements in intramedullary nailing have occurred since it was popularized by Küntscher following World War II. Closed nailing techniques have minimized soft-tissue dissection. Location of the starting hole in the piriformis fossa avoids increased hoop stresses associated with a more anterior placement that may lead to fracture of the proximal femur.[8] Early problems of shortening and malrotation have been avoided by the addition of locking screws.

A three-part study by Brumback and associates[9-11] clarified many of the questions that arose with widespread use of locking intramedullary nails. In the first part of the study, they retrospectively reviewed 311 femoral nailings in 296 patients (172 statically locked, 133 dynamically locked). In the 133 dynamically locked nailings, fourteen (10.5%) were complicated by shortening (13) or rotational instability (one). Errors in decision-making were attributed to inadequate preoperative analysis of the fracture pattern, failure to detect increases in comminution, and instability of the fracture, both intraoperatively and postoperatively.[9] The second phase of the study evaluated the effect of static interlocking on fracture healing in a prospective series of 100 femoral shaft fractures in 97 patients. Static inter-

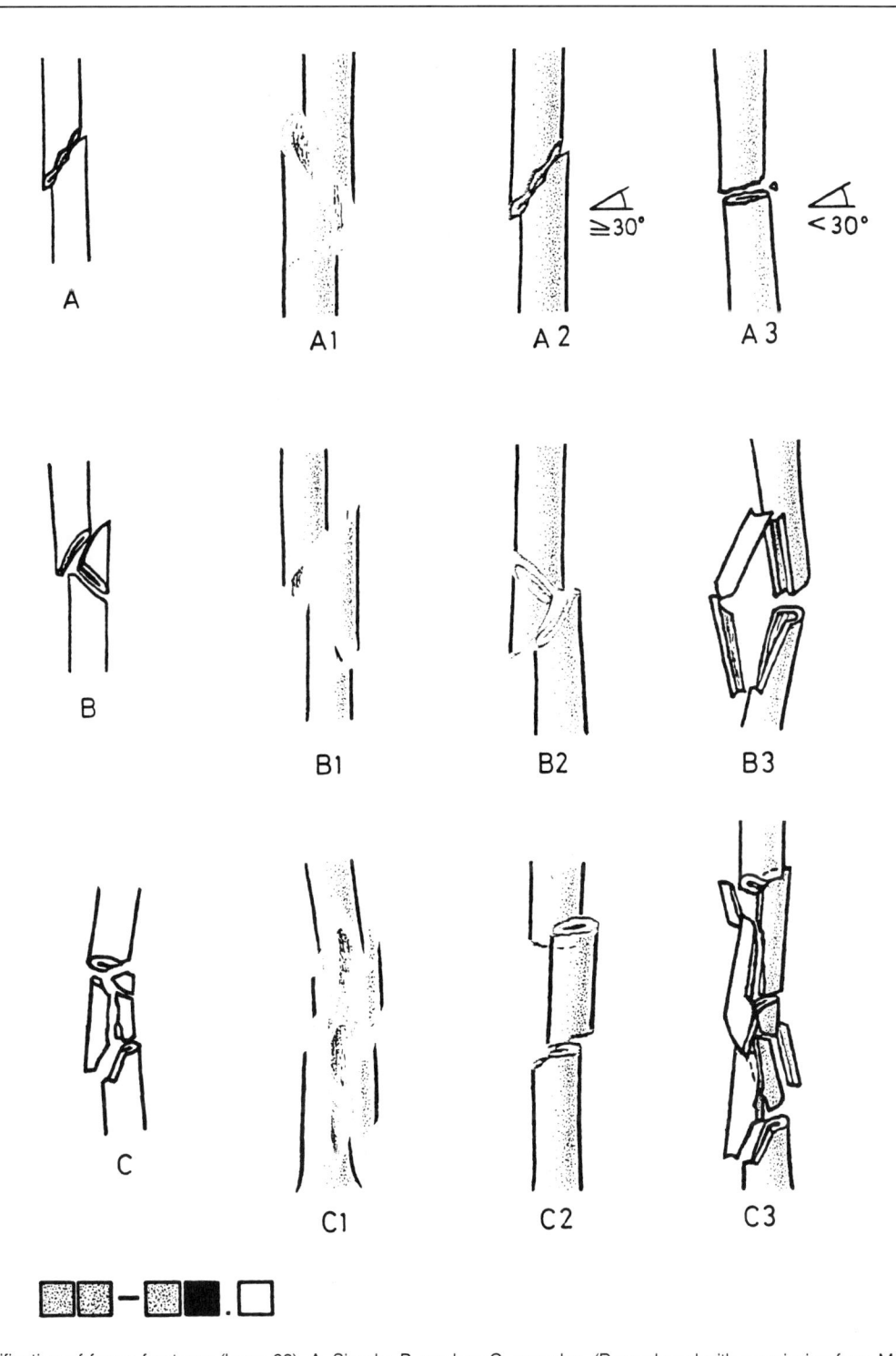

Fig. 2 OA classification of femur fractures (bone 32). A, Simple; B, wedge; C, complex. (Reproduced with permission from Müller ME, Nazarian S, Koch P, et al (eds): *The Comprehensive Classification of Fractures of Long Bones.* Berlin, Germany, Springer-Verlag, 1990.)

locking did not inhibit fracture healing, and routine conversion to dynamic fixation (dynamization) appeared to be unnecessary.[10] In the third part of this series, Brumback and associates[11] investigated the clinical importance of stress-shielding properties of static interlocking nailing. At two- to three-year follow-up of 214 fractures, there was one refracture at the original site of fracture following nail removal and no fractures through screw holes, both for patients in whom the nail had been retained and for those in whom the nail was removed without conversion to a dynamic construct. The result of these investigations is the current consensus that nearly all femoral shaft fractures should be treated with statically locked intramedullary nailing, which should not be routinely converted to a dynamic construct without evidence of delayed union.

There appears to be no biomechanical or clinical advantage in the use of one versus two distal locking screws for diaphyseal fractures treated with reamed, interlocking nailing. If one distal locking screw is used, it should be placed in the more proximal location. In fractures of the distal femur, both distal locking screws should be used.

Timing
The benefits of early stabilization of femoral fractures are well recognized. Bone and associates[12] in a prospective, randomized comparison of immediate versus delayed stabilization of femoral shaft fractures demonstrated a decrease in the incidence of pulmonary insufficiency and adult respiratory distress syndrome, fewer days in the intensive care unit and hospital, and lower costs in the subgroup of patients with multiple organ system injury (ISS > 18). No pulmonary complications or mortality occurred in isolated fractures, but the patients who underwent immediate stabilization had fewer days in the hospital and lower cost.

Effects of Reaming
Embolization of fat and marrow elements is known to occur during intramedullary nailing, particularly during intramedullary reaming. Reamer design influences the degree of pressurization of the femoral canal as well as the degree of fat embolism. Reamers with deep flutes and small shafts create lower intramedullary pressures and less fat embolism than reamers with shallow flutes and large shafts. Pape and associates[13,14] have suggested that the beneficial effects on pulmonary function of early stabilization of femoral fractures may be outweighed by the deleterious effects of reamed intramedullary nailing and concomitant fat embolism in the patient with associated pulmonary injury. However, no prospective, randomized comparison exists to demonstrate a beneficial effect of techniques that avoid intramedullary reaming, such as "unreamed" nailing or plate fixation, in patients with pulmonary injury. Currently, there is no compelling evidence that immediate, reamed intramedullary nailing should not be performed in femoral fracture patients with pulmonary injury.

Mechanical Considerations
The principal factor that alters bending stiffness of femoral intramedullary nails is nail diameter. The presence of a longitudinal slot decreases torsional stiffness by as much as 40 times, compared to nonslotted nails. Implant failure in the absence of nonunion is rare. Axial loading of diaphyseal fractures may result in failure of the locking screws, while bending forces result in fractures of the nail at the level of the fracture, particularly in the subtrochanteric region. In fractures that are located within 5 cm of the most proximal of the distal locking screws, the peak stress around the hole may exceed the endurance limit of the implant, with fracture of the nail through the locking screw hole.

Surgical Technique
Antegrade reamed interlocking nailing using a fracture table with the patient in a supine or lateral position is the accepted standard for stabilization of the vast majority of femoral shaft fractures. Careful attention to the location of the starting hole, fracture length and rotation, and static locking of essentially every fracture minimizes errors in surgical technique. Poststabilization examination of leg length, rotation, and knee stability and inspection of anteroposterior and lateral radiographs to assess reduction and identify occult femoral neck fracture helps avoid unplanned returns to surgery.

Special situations, such as multiple injuries, spine injury, vascular injuries, or ipsilateral fracture of the femoral neck or tibia have led some surgeons to develop alternative nailing techniques that avoid the need for positioning on a fracture table. Antegrade nailing using a radiolucent table and a femoral distractor or manual traction without the use of a fracture table has been used successfully. Retrograde femoral nailing using an entry point in the intercondylar notch or medial condyle may offer advantages in some situations, such as ipsilateral femoral neck or tibial fracture, but the long-term effect on knee function is unknown.

Special Situations

Open Fractures
Surgical debridement, irrigation of the wound, administration of broad-spectrum antibiotics, and delayed closure of open wounds are the basic principles of open femur fracture treatment. In 1988, Lhowe and Hansen[15] reported successful treatment of open femoral fractures with debridement, irrigation, and immediate reamed intramedullary nailing in 67 patients. Other authors have reported similar results.[16,17] Intramedullary nailing is not recommended in cases of gross contamination, or when initial treatment has been delayed. The theoretical advantages of the smaller diameter nails inserted without reaming of the fracture site are currently unproven.

Ipsilateral Neck and Shaft Fractures
Fractures of the femoral diaphysis are associated with ipsilateral femoral neck fracture in 2.5% to 5% of cases. Non-

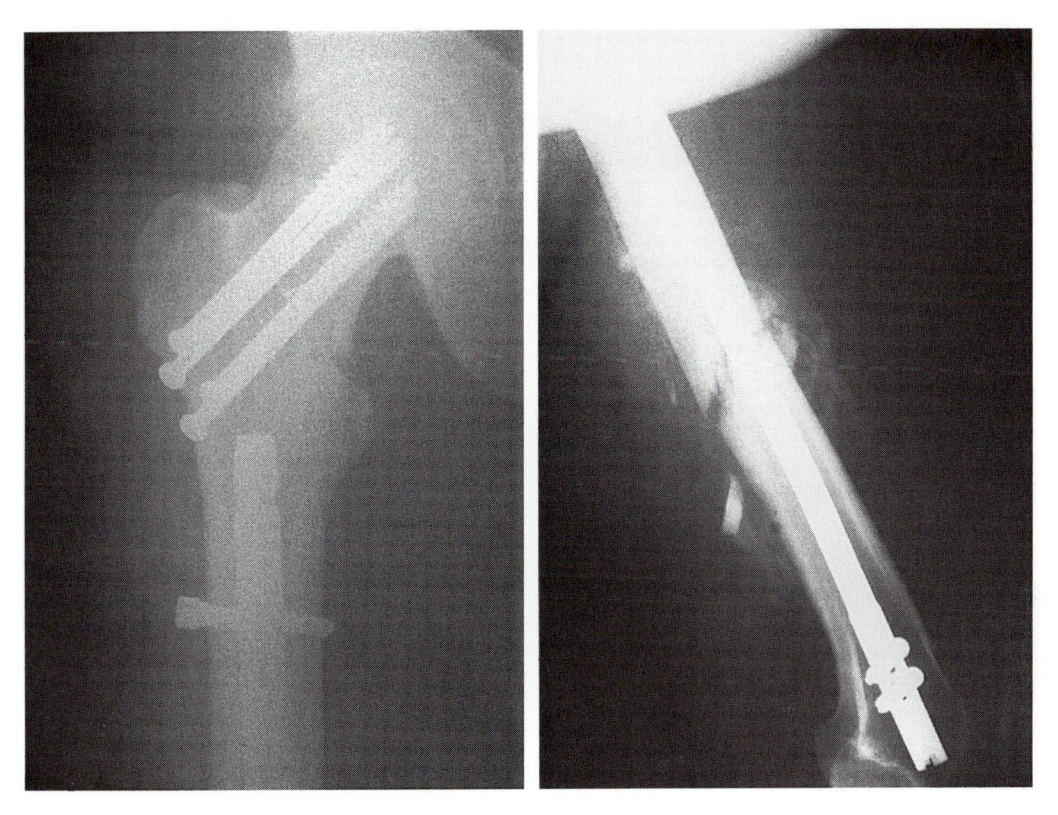

Fig. 3 **Left,** Anteroposterior view of the proximal femur. **Right,** Diaphyseal lateral of an ipsilateral neck and shaft fracture stabilized with screw fixation and retrograde intramedullary nailing.

displaced fractures of the femoral neck are easily missed initially despite careful inspection of adequate quality radiographs.[18,19] Because successful treatment of femoral neck fractures hinges on anatomic reduction and stable fixation, the femoral neck component of this injury is given first priority. A combination of techniques and devices is frequently used.

Screw fixation of nondisplaced femoral neck fractures prior to stabilization of the shaft minimizes the chance of fracture displacement but requires careful screw placement to allow standard antegrade intramedullary nailing. Alternatively, stabilization of the diaphyseal component with compression plating or retrograde nailing (Fig. 3) while avoiding the proximal femur have been used. The use of a second-generation interlocking femoral nail allows stabilization of both components of the fracture with a single device, but it is technically difficult and displacement of the femoral neck fracture may occur during nailing. Screw stabilization of the femoral neck fracture prior to second-generation nailing may minimize this risk.

Displaced fractures of the femoral neck in association with fracture of the femoral shaft demand reduction and stabilization of the femoral neck component prior to shaft stabilization. Reduction is accomplished in most cases by closed means on a fracture table but may require open reduction. Following reduction, stabilization of the femoral neck, then shaft, are accomplished as in nondisplaced fractures.

If a nondisplaced or reducible missed fracture of the femoral neck is discovered after femoral nailing, it may be treated with screw fixation anterior to the femoral nail. Nail removal may be required if reduction of the femoral neck component is prevented by the intramedullary nail.

Gunshot Fractures

Most gunshot fractures of the femur are caused by low-velocity hand gun projectiles. Following local wound care, these can be treated with intramedullary nailing with results comparable to those of closed injuries.[20-22] High-velocity gunshot injuries, and close range shotgun injuries are associated with extensive soft-tissue injury. Immediate surgical debridement and repeat debridement at frequent intervals similar to those of other severe open fractures (Gustilo grade III) is indicated.

Adolescents

The treatment of femoral shaft fractures in adolescents remains controversial. Satisfactory results may be obtained

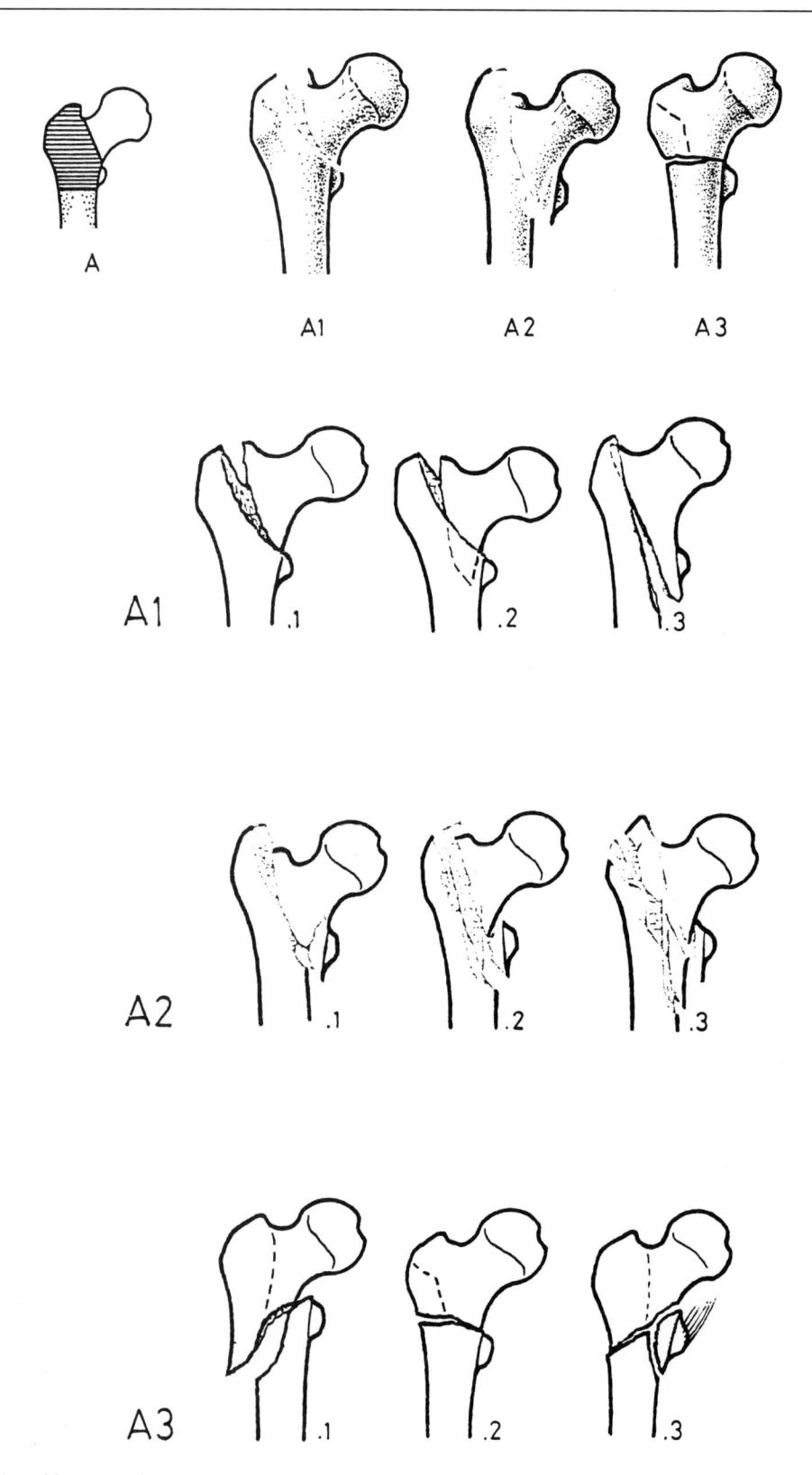

Fig. 4 OA classification of fractures of the subtrochanteric region (bone 31). **Top row,** Trochanteric area fracture: simple, multifragmentary, and intertrochanteric. **Bottom rows,** The subgroups and their qualifications. (Reproduced with permission from Müller ME, Nazarian S, Koch P, et al (eds): *The Comprehensive Classification of Fractures of Long Bones.* Berlin, Germany, Springer-Verlag, 1990.)

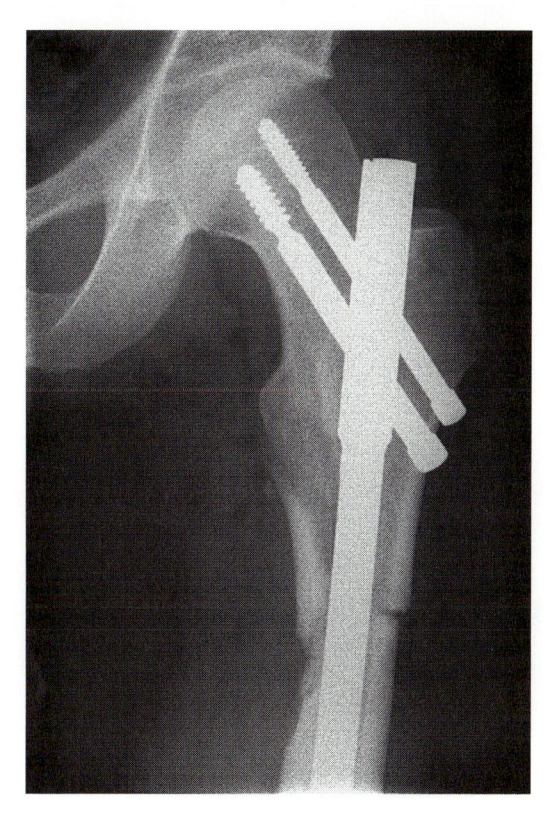

Fig. 5 Subtrochanteric fracture stabilized with second generation interlocking nail.

with traction and spica casting, which avoids the risks of infection, physeal damage, and osteonecrosis of the femoral head. However, the results of nonsurgical treatment are less satisfactory when compared with those of internal fixation.[23-25] Reeves and associates[25] compared the results of nonsurgical treatment with traction and cast bracing to internal fixation in 96 adolescent femur fractures. The group that underwent surgical treatment with either compression plating or intramedullary nailing had shorter hospital stays, lower costs, and fewer complications.

Internal fixation of femoral fractures is recommended for adolescents with associated head injury, ipsilateral tibial fracture, or multiple injuries. Optimum treatment of isolated fractures remains debatable. A safe alternative to nonsurgical treatment appears to be intramedullary nailing of the femoral shaft while avoiding the proximal and distal physes, and giving careful attention to the starting hole.

Complications

Infection
Infection following intramedullary nailing is rare, occurring in less than 1% of patients.[7] Principles of treating deep infection following intramedullary nailing include surgical debridement of all infected soft tissue and necrotic bone, administration of parenteral antibiotics, and stabilization of the fracture. If rigid fixation is maintained, the intramedullary nail can be left in place until the fracture has healed. Removal of the implant and further surgical and medical treatment may be required to eradicate infection.

Nonunion
Up to 99% of femoral fractures achieve uneventful union following intramedullary nailing.[7] Like acute fractures, delay of union or nonunion is most effectively treated with intramedullary reaming and nailing.[26] Bone grafting may be required for marked bone loss. Indolent infection may be exacerbated by reaming and intramedullary nailing but does not preclude a successful result.

Malunion
When modern concepts of statically locked intramedullary stabilization are used, symptomatic malunion rarely occurs following diaphyseal fracture of the femur.[7,9,10] Axial malalignment is uncommon but may occur, particularly in fractures of the distal one third. Shortening is effectively prevented with static interlocking. Rotation malalignment of greater than 15° may occur in up to 19% of patients; however, most do not experience symptoms. Gross malrotation, if identified in the immediate postoperative period, can be treated by removal of locking screws, correction of deformity, and reinsertion of locking screws. Rotational malalignment after healing of femoral fractures can be treated effectively with closed femoral osteotomy, correction of rotational alignment, and static intramedullary nailing.

Compartment Syndrome
Acute compartment syndrome of the thigh is rare following femoral fracture. Schwartz and associates[27] reported the largest series of 21 compartment syndromes in 17 patients. Ten occurred in patients with femoral fracture, and five followed reamed intramedullary nailing. Risk factors include vascular injury, coagulopathy, history of external compression, use of pneumatic antishock garments, and hypotension. Eight patients died; of the remaining nine, six patients became infected. Residual morbidity, including sensory and motor deficits, was common.

Nerve Injury
Nerve injuries can occur during intramedullary nailing. Most are due either to excessive traction or to improper positioning on a fracture table. Compression injuries of the pudendal nerve can occur with excessive longitudinal traction against the perineal post.[28] Sciatic nerve injuries can occur with excessive traction, particularly when shortening of the fracture is present and treatment is delayed. Most of these injuries resolve.

Heterotopic Ossification
Heterotopic bone formation occurs in as many as 20% to 26% of patients following intramedullary nailing. Compro-

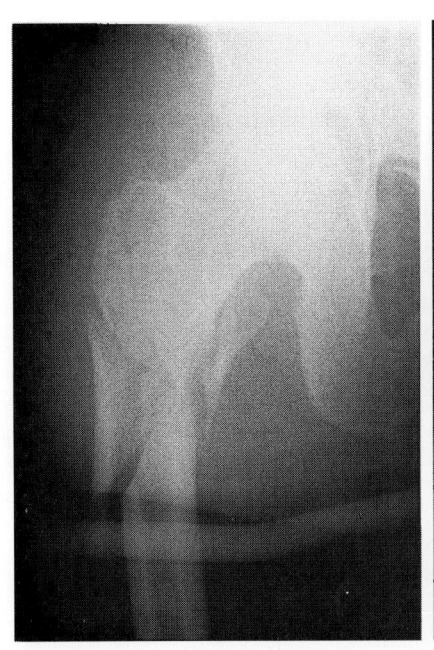

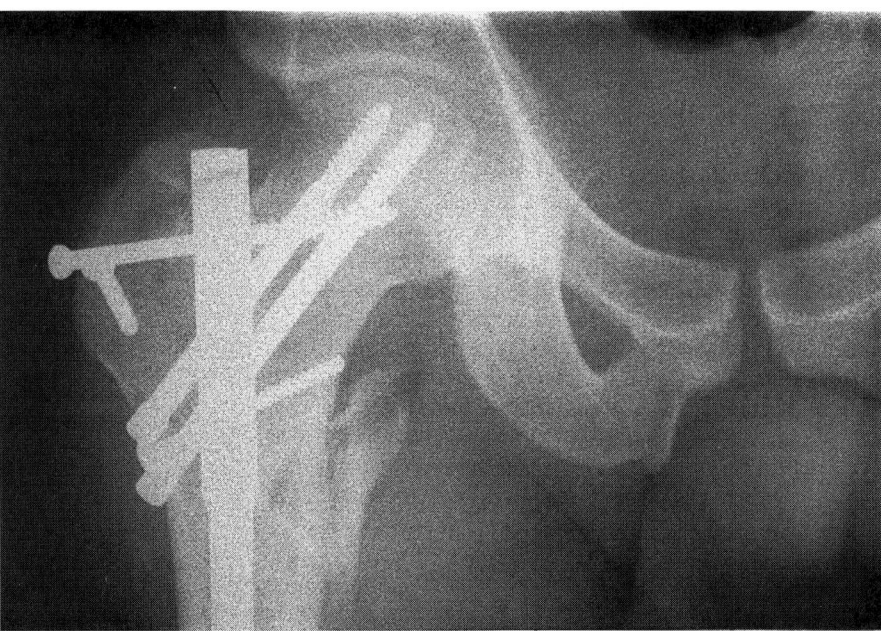

Fig. 6 Left, Comminuted subtrochanteric fracture with involvement of the greater trochanter and piriformis fossa. **Right,** Fracture stabilized with a second generation interlocking nail supplemented by additional lag screw fixation.

mised hip function is rare, however. Irrigation of the wound with pulsatile lavage does not appear to lessen the severity or frequency of ectopic bone.[29] Prophylaxis with indomethacin or irradiation is not indicated.

Subtrochanteric Fractures

Successful treatment of subtrochanteric femoral fractures is hampered by several factors peculiar to the proximal femur. The magnitude of bending forces present in this region of the femur not uncommonly leads to implant failure prior to union. The subtrochanteric region of the femur is composed primarily of cortical bone, which, although ideally designed to withstand the forces placed upon it, is slower to heal.

Most fractures of the subtrochanteric region are described by fracture location with respect to the lesser and greater trochanters, degree of comminution, and displacement. The OTA (AO) classification combines these elements in an integrated system (Fig. 4).

Fractures below the lesser trochanter can be successfully treated with standard interlocking nailing with careful attention to alignment of the short proximal fragment. Fractures at or above the level of the lesser trochanter are not adequately stabilized by standard first-generation interlocking femoral nails and require alternative methods of fixation. A variety of implants and techniques have been devised for use in these injuries. These techniques can be divided into three major groups: plate fixation combined with fixed-angle blade or compression screw fixation; intramedullary devices of various lengths combined with fixed-angle compression screws; and interlocking screws directed into the femoral neck and head.

Intramedullary fixation using second-generation intramedullary nails is technically more difficult than first-generation interlocking nailing but can be used successfully in fractures that do not involve the region of the greater trochanter and piriformis fossa (Fig. 5).[30,31] When the greater trochanter and piriformis fossa is involved in the fracture, proximal fixation of intramedullary devices is lessened and consideration should be given either to supplemental fixation to restore the structural integrity of this region (Fig. 6) or to the use of plate fixation combined with a fixed-angle screw or blade. Bone grafting is recommended when comminution of the medial cortex is present.

The use of shorter intramedullary devices, such as the gamma nail, is associated with complications related to the implant, including fractures through the distal locking screw holes.[32]

Annotated References

1. Winquist RA, Hansen ST Jr: Comminuted fractures of the femoral shaft treated by intramedullary nailing. *Orthop Clin North Am* 1980;11:633-648.

2. Carr CR, Wingo CH: Fractures of the femoral diaphysis: A retrospective study of the results and costs of treatment by intramedullary nailing and by traction and a spica cast. *J Bone Joint Surg* 1973;55A:690-700.

3. Gates DJ, Alms M, Cruz MM: Hinged cast and roller traction for fractured femur: A system of treatment for the Third World. *J Bone Joint Surg* 1985;67B:750-756.

4. Dabezies EJ, D'Ambrosia R, Shoji H, et al: Fractures of the femoral shaft treated by external fixation with the Wagner device. *J Bone Joint Surg* 1984;66A:360-364.

5. Ruedi TP, Luscher JN: Results after internal fixation of comminuted fractures of the femoral shaft with DC plates. *Clin Orthop* 1979;138:74-76.

6. Wiss DA, Fleming CH, Matta JM, et al: Comminuted and rotationally unstable fractures of the femur treated with an interlocking nail. *Clin Orthop* 1986;212:35-47.

7. Winquist RA, Hansen ST Jr, Clawson DK: Closed intramedullary nailing of femoral fractures: A report of five hundred and twenty cases. *J Bone Joint Surg* 1984;66A:529-539.

   The authors reviewed 520 femur fractures in 500 patients (86 open fractures), of which 497 were performed closed and 23 were performed open with cerclage wires. Union occurred in 99.1%; infection, in 0.9% (two in closed fractures, two in open fractures); shortening, in 2.0%; and malrotation, in 2.3%. Range of motion of the knee averaged 130°. The authors also discuss a classification system and recommend static locking of all but the simple fracture patterns.

8. Johnson KD, Tencer AF, Sherman MC: Biomechanical factors affecting fracture stability and femoral bursting in closed intramedullary nailing of femoral shaft fractures, with illustrative case presentations. *J Orthop Trauma* 1987;1:1-11.

   The authors present a biomechanical study of factors affecting proximal femoral bursting and fracture stability in femoral nailing. Measurement of hoop stresses on the proximal femur were measured during nail insertion. Hoop stresses increased most significantly with anterior displacement of the starting hole. Anterior displacement of more than 6 mm was likely to result in femoral bursting. More rigid nails produced significantly higher insertion stresses.

9. Brumback RJ, Reilly JP, Poka A, et al: Intramedullary nailing of femoral shaft fractures: Part 1. Decision-making errors with interlocking fixation. *J Bone Joint Surg* 1988;70A:1441-1452.

   The authors retrospectively reviewed 311 femoral nailings in 296 patients (172 statically locked, 139 dynamically locked). Of the 133 dynamic intramedullary nailings, 14 (10.5%) had major unanticipated loss of fixation and reduction (preoperative comminution graded as Winquist I in 7; II, in 4; and III, in 3). One cannot assume all fracture lines are evident on the preoperative radiographs. Dynamic intramedullary nailing is reserved for transverse or short oblique isthmus fractures, with no intraoperative increase in comminution.

10. Brumback RJ, Uwagie-Ero S, Lakatos RP, et al: Intramedullary nailing of femoral shaft fractures: Part II. Fracture-healing with static interlocking fixation. *J Bone Joint Surg* 1988;70A:1453-1462.

    The authors present a prospective study of 97 consecutive patients with 100 femoral shaft fractures treated with statically locked intramedullary nailing. Eighty-four patients with 87 fractures were followed to union (three patients died, three were treated with a dynamized nail by outside physicians without evidence of delayed union, six were lost to follow-up, and one became infected and required repeat nailing). Eighty-five fractures (98%) healed with static interlocking fixation. Two patients required conversion to dynamic fixation prior to union. Static interlocking nailing does not appear to inhibit femoral fracture healing. Routine conversion to dynamic fixation, unless evidence of delayed union is present, appears unnecessary.

11. Brumback RJ, Ellison TS, Poka A, et al: Intramedullary nailing of femoral shaft fractures: Part III. Long-term effects of static interlocking fixation. *J Bone Joint Surg* 1992;74A:106-112.

    The authors present a retrospective review of 204 patients with 214 femoral shaft fractures treated with interlocking femoral nailing. Patients were divided into two groups. In group I, the hardware was retained (n = III fractures). In group II, the hardware was removed without prior conversion to a dynamized nail (n = 103 fractures). There were no fractures or failure of the nail or locking screws in group I; in group II, one patient experienced refracture at the original fracture site 6 weeks after nail removal, but, in retrospect, this patient did not have circumferential healing. Routine removal of femoral nails is not recommended. Routine nail dynamization prior to nail removal appears to be unnecessary.

12. Bone LB, Johnson KD, Weigelt J, et al: Early versus delayed stabilization of femoral fractures: A prospective randomized study. *J Bone Joint Surg* 1989;71A:336-340.

    This is a prospective study of 178 patients randomized to early or delayed stabilization of femur fractures. In patients with multiple injuries (ISS > 18), there was a significant decrease in the incidence of respiratory complications in the early stabilization group. Average hospital cost was also significantly less in the group of patients with multiple trauma who were stabilized early. In patients with isolated injuries, there were no significant pulmonary complications in either group; however, the early stabilization group was less expensive.

13. Pape HC, Auf'm'Kolk M, Paffrath T, et al: Primary intramedullary femur fixation in multiple trauma patients with associated lung contusion: A cause of posttraumatic ARDS? *J Trauma* 1993;34:540-548.

14. Pape HC, Regel G, Dwenger A, et al: Influences of different methods of intramedullary femoral nailing on lung function in patients with multiple trauma. *J Trauma* 1993;35:709-716.

15. Lhowe DW, Hansen ST: Immediate nailing of open fractures of the femoral shaft. *J Bone Joint Surg* 1988;70A:812-820.

    Irrigation and debridement followed by immediate reamed intramedullary nailing was performed in 67 patients with open fractures of the femoral shaft. Nineteen patients were lost to follow-up, 42 patients were followed for an average of 23 months (15 grade I, 19 grade II, and 8 grade III). Complications included infection in two patients (one deep), loss of fixation in four patients, seroma in two patients, and one sciatic nerve palsy. Immediate reamed intramedullary nailing is an acceptable treatment for open fractures of the femoral shaft.

16. Brumback RJ, Ellison PS Jr, Poka A, et al: Intramedullary nailing of open fractures of the femoral shaft. *J Bone Joint Surg* 1989;71A:1324-1331.

   In this retrospective review of 86 open fractures of the femur treated by intramedullary nailing, 27 were grade I; 16, grade II; 46, grade III. Fifty-six were done initially, and 33 were done after a delay of 5 to 7 days after wound closure. All fractures healed at an average of 5.2 months. Three infections occurred in the 27 patients in grade IIIB (one immediate, two delayed nailing). Important recommendations include using other forms of stabilization (external fixation) in the presence of gross contamination or prolonged delay in the initial debridement.

17. Grosse A, Christie J, Tagiang G, et al: Open adult femoral shaft fracture treated by early intramedullary nailing. *J Bone Joint Surg* 1993;75:562-565.

18. Casey MJ, Chapman MW: Ipsilateral concomitant fractures of the hip and femoral shaft. *J Bone Joint Surg* 1979;61A:503-509.

19. Swiontkowski MF, Hansen ST Jr, Kellam J: Ipsilateral fractures of the femoral neck and shaft: A treatment protocol. *J Bone Joint Surg* 1984;66A:260-268.

   The authors review 15 cases of femoral neck and shaft fractures. Most were treated with multiple screws and retrograde nailing or with screws and plating. Two fractures were missed initially (review of the literature reveals approximately one third are missed initially). Recommended protocol is the femoral neck fracture is the first precedent and this should be stabilized prior to stabilization of the neck fracture, regardless of the method of stabilization.

20. Wright DG, Levin JS, Esterhai JL, et al: Immediate internal fixation of low-velocity gunshot-related femoral fractures. *J Trauma* 1993;35:678-682.

21. Bergman M, Tornetta P, Kerina M, et al: Femur fractures caused by gunshots: Treatment by immediate reamed intramedullary nailing. *J Trauma* 1993;34:783-785.

22. Nowotarski P, Brumback RJ: Immediate interlocking nailing of fractures of the femur caused by low- to mid-velocity gunshots. *J Orthop Trauma* 1994;8:134-141.

23. Mann DC, Weddington J, Davenport K: Closed Ender nailing of femoral shaft fractures in adolescents. *J Pediatr Orthop* 1986;6:651-655.

   The authors reviewed 16 fractures in 15 adolescents (9-15). Average time to independent ambulation was 7.1 days. Hospitalization averaged 11.4 days. There were no infections, nonunions, malunions, loss of range of motion, leg length discrepancies, or evidence of growth disturbance.

24. Kirby RM, Winquist RA, Hansen ST Jr: Femoral shaft fractures in adolescents: A comparison between traction plus cast treatment and closed intramedullary nailing. *J Pediatr Orthop* 1981;1:193-197.

25. Reeves RB, Ballard RI, Hughes JL: Internal fixation versus traction and casting of adolescent femoral shaft fractures. *J Pediatr Orthop* 1990;10:592-595.

   In this review of 96 femur fractures in 90 patients treated either with traction and casting, or with internal fixation (33 nails, 19 platings), mean hospital stay was 29 days for traction and casting, versus 15 days for internal fixation. Total hospital charges were less in patients treated with internal fixation, even with hardware removal included. There were four delayed unions, five malunions, and one refracture in the traction/casting group. In the internal fixation group, there were no malunions or nonunions. Complications in this group included one plate fracture, one bent rod following repeat trauma, and one transient peroneal palsy. Internal fixation of adolescent femoral shaft fractures appears to offer fewer complications, shorter hospitalization, and lower cost.

26. Webb LX, Winquist RA, Hansen ST: Intramedullary nailing and reaming for delayed union or nonunion of the femoral shaft: A report of 105 consecutive cases. *Clin Orthop* 1986;212:133-141.

   The authors reviewed 49 delayed unions and 56 nonunions of the femur treated by reamed intramedullary nailing. Bone grafting was performed in seven patients through an open wound used for hardware removal and intramedullary bone grafting was used in two. Four patients were lost to follow-up, leaving 101 for review. Ninety-eight of the 101 healed in an average of 20 weeks. Four required repeat nailing prior to healing. Of the patients with preexisting osteomyelitis, the condition was exacerbated after the procedure in four. Three healed and subsequently had removal of hardware; one patient had persistent drainage. Two patients had proximal migration of the nail, one required reoperation. Two patients were nailed in external rotation; one required reoperation. Intramedullary nailing appears to be the treatment of choice for femoral nonunion.

27. Schwartz JT Jr, Brumback RJ, Lakatos R, et al: Acute compartment syndrome of the thigh: A spectrum of injury. *J Bone Joint Surg* 1989;71A:392-400.

   Retrospective review of 21 thigh compartment syndromes, ten associated with femoral fracture, five of which were open. Five cases followed intramedullary nailing, the other 11 followed blunt trauma, compression, or ischemia. Risk factors include hypotension, history for external compression, use of MAST trouser, coagulopathy, and vascular injury. Eight patients died; of the remaining nine patients, six became infected. Residual morbidity, including sensory and motor deficits were common.

28. Brumback RJ, Ellison TS, Molligan H, et al: Pudendal nerve palsy complicating intramedullary nailing of the femur. *J Bone Joint Surg* 1992;74A:1450-1455.

29. Brumback RJ, Wells JD, Lakatos R, et al: Heterotopic ossification about the hip after intramedullary nailing for fractures of the femur. *J Bone Joint Surg* 1990;72A:1067-1073.

30. Wiss DA, Brien WW: Subtrochanteric fractures of the femur: Results of treatment by interlocking nailing. *Clin Orthop* 1992;283:231-236.

31. Brien WW, Wiss DA, Becker V Jr, et al: Subtrochanteric femur fractures: A comparison of the Zickel nail, 95 degrees blade plate, and interlocking nail. *J Orthop Trauma* 1991;5: 458-464.

32. Pagnani MJ, Lyden JP: Post-operative femoral fracture after intramedullary fixation with a gamma nail: A case report and review of the literature. *J Trauma* 1994;37:133-137.

Impacted or minimally displaced fractures without intercondylar displacement can be treated with a knee immobilizer or cast and later converted to a fracture brace or cast brace once the pain and swelling have subsided. The patient should be mobilized with partial weightbearing ambulation on the involved extremity. Fracture alignment must be monitored until union to detect fracture displacement.

Displaced fractures in patients with other contraindications to surgery should be treated with either one- or two-pin skeletal traction. The goal of skeletal traction is restoration of the overall limb length and alignment, not anatomic fracture reduction. Apex posterior fracture angulation can be corrected by adjusting the traction, increasing the amount of knee flexion, or placing a soft pad underneath the distal thigh. The patient should be encouraged to move the knee. A fracture brace can be applied at 3 to 6 weeks, when callus formation permits. The brace is worn for approximately 4 to 5 months, until fracture union.

Displaced supracondylar and intercondylar distal femur fractures are optimally treated with open reduction and internal fixation.[7,8] Displaced intra-articular fractures should undergo anatomic articular restoration, stable fixation, and early range of knee motion. Anatomic reduction of displaced intra-articular fractures cannot be performed using closed techniques. There are three emergent surgical indications. (1) All open fractures require surgical debridement. At the initial debridement, limited internal fixation of the articular surface should be performed. The timing of definitive fracture stabilization is controversial. (2) In fractures with associated vascular compromise, the sequence of revascularization and osseous stabilization is dependent on the ischemic time and limb vascularity.[9] (3) Fractures with associated compartment syndrome require emergent surgical intervention.

The principles of surgical treatment include: (1) appropriate surgical timing, (2) preoperative planning, (3) careful soft-tissue dissection, (4) anatomic restoration of the distal femoral articular surface, (5) restoration of the limb axial alignment, rotation, and length, (6) stable internal fixation, (7) bone grafting of osseous defects, particularly if vascularity to that area has been impaired, and (8) early patient mobilization with range of knee motion.

The timing of surgical reconstruction should be as early as possible after the necessary equipment and surgical assistants are available. Surgeon experience also must be considered. Early stabilization of femur fractures in polytrauma patients, particularly femoral shaft fractures in patients with a high injury severity score, has been shown to decrease the mortality rate.[10] However, surgical management should not be undertaken without adequate preoperative evaluation. Open fractures and fractures with an associated vascular injury or compartment syndrome require emergent treatment. Delay of definitive stabilization for 3 or more weeks markedly increases the amount of difficulty encountered at surgery. The fracture is often malreduced and shortened; with early callus formation, the fracture lines lose their clear demarcation, particularly in cancellous bone.

The exact nature of the fracture, with identification of all major fracture fragments, should be determined before definitive surgical intervention is attempted.[11] Identification of the individual fragments is often facilitated with traction radiographs. Radiographs of the opposite, normal extremity serve as templates for preoperative planning; the individual fracture fragments, chosen implant, and surgical tactic can be drawn on the intact femoral template. This forces the surgeon to understand the "personality of the fracture" and to prepare mentally for the surgical procedure.

Most distal femur fractures can be approached through a single lateral incision. If additional exposure of the condylar surface is required, an osteotomy of the tibial tubercle or a Z-plasty of the patella tendon can be performed. A medial exposure of the distal femur is occasionally needed and involves elevation of the vastus medialis. The distal femoral articular surface must be anatomically reduced and stabilized. Definitive stabilization of intercondylar fractures involves use of large cancellous screws with washers. Screw location is dependent on the chosen fixation device for shaft stabilization.

Implants available for stabilization of the supracondylar fracture are (1) 95° fixed angle condylar blade-plates or screws, (2) condylar buttress plates, (3) interlocking intramedullary nails, placed either antegrade or retrograde, (4) flexible intramedullary nails, and (5) external fixators.

There is a large body of literature documenting success with the 95° condylar blade-plate for supracondylar and intercondylar distal femur fractures.[12,13] Correct use of this device restores femoral alignment and provides stable fixation. However, placement of the 95° condylar blade plate is a technically demanding procedure, requiring exact three planar insertion.[14] Incorrect use of both this device and the 95° dynamic condylar screw may lead to angular malalignment and lateralization of the femoral shaft. The path for the condylar blade plate must be precut with a seating chisel. Hammering this device into hard cancellous bone in a young patient may require significant force and can displace a previously reduced condylar fracture. It is not always feasible to use the condylar blade plate in fractures with severe intra-articular comminution.

The 95° dynamic condylar screw is a two-piece device; it has basically the same design as the 95° condylar blade plate with the blade replaced with a compression screw. Several authors have reported good results using this device for both supracondylar and intercondylar distal femur fractures.[15,16] Technically, the 95° dynamic condylar screw is easier to insert than the blade-plate;[17] the compression screw is cannulated and is inserted over a guide wire after its channel is reamed and tapped. Varus/valgus malalignment of the guide wire is easily corrected; flexion/extension can be adjusted by compression screw rotation. The lag screw can be used to apply interfragmentary compression across the femoral condyles. This device may provide better purchase in osteoporotic bone than the condylar blade plate. Use of the 95° dynamic condylar screw requires a minimum of 4 cm of distal femoral because of the large

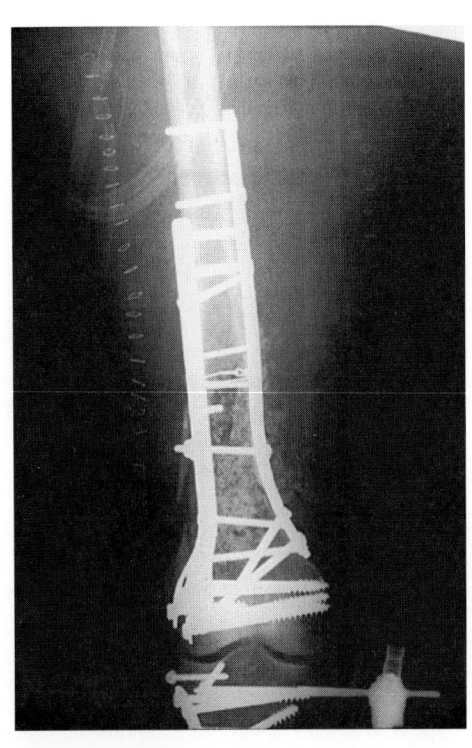

Fig. 3 Severely comminuted distal femur fracture stabilized with a lateral condylar buttress plate, supplemental medial plate, and bone graft.

diameter of the lag screw. It does not provide as much control of the distal fragment as does the 95° blade plate and requires insertion of an additional screw through the plate into the distal fragment for rotational stability.

The condylar buttress plate, precontoured for the lateral distal femur, consists of a dynamic compression side plate and a thin distal portion through which six cancellous screws can be inserted. Mechanically, the implant is weaker than a 95° condylar blade plate or screw. The distal screw holes lack a locking mechanism for the screwheads to prevent shifting at the screw-plate junction. If there is an inadequate medial buttress, the distal fragment can collapse. Therefore, use of this device necessitates a stable medial buttress.[18] Methods of creating this buttress include anatomic reduction or use of a medial plate or external fixator (Fig. 3). Indications for use of the condylar buttress plate include (1) low transcondylar fractures where a 95° condylar blade plate or screw is not possible and (2) coronal or comminuted fractures where lag placement precludes insertion of a 95° condylar blade plate or screw.

Success with both antegrade and retrograde inserted interlocked medullary nails has been reported for the treatment of supracondylar and intercondylar distal femur fractures.[19,20] Intramedullary nails are biomechanically superior to plates, particularly in fractures with an osseous gap. Because the intramedullary canal is closer to the femur's bending axis than the usual plate position on the external surface of the bone, intramedullary nails are subjected to smaller bending moments than plates and thus are less likely to fail by fatigue. In addition, intramedullary nails can act as load-sharing devices in those instances where there is sufficient cortical contact to prevent loss of reduction.

With the use of antegrade inserted interlocked nails, two interlocking screws should be used in the distal fragment in order to control flexion and extension. The distal tip of the nail may need to be cut in order to allow more distal placement of the screws. Fracture alignment must be assessed carefully during nail insertion, because there is a greater risk of angular fracture malalignment than with femoral shaft fractures. The knee must be flexed and/or the distal thigh supported during nail insertion to prevent residual hyperextension deformity. Prior to nail insertion, the distal femoral articular surface must be anatomically reduced; lag screw location must be planned so that they do not interfere with nail insertion.[21] Careful evaluation of the intercondylar area is mandatory during nail insertion in order to detect any loss of reduction of the articular surface. The presence of a coronal fracture of the femoral condyle is a relative contraindication to intramedullary nailing.

Interlocked intramedullary nails are at increased risk of implant breakage, particularly through the more proximal of the two distal locking screw holes, when used to stabilize distal femur fractures. Fatigue fracture of the intramedullary nail is possible when this screw is inserted within 5 cm of the fracture site.[22]

The supracondylar intramedullary nail has been successful in the treatment of supracondylar and intercondylar femur fractures (Fig. 4).[23,24] This cannulated interlocked nail is inserted retrograde through the femoral notch and has multiple holes for locking screw placement. Among the concerns with use of an intramedullary nail inserted through an intra-articular portal are septic arthritis and synovial metallosis.[25] The intra-articular portal allows direct access for infection or metal debris to pass into the knee joint. This device must be used cautiously in younger patients because removal requires a repeat knee arthrotomy.

Flexible intramedullary nails available for treatment of distal femur fractures include the Zickel nail, Rush pin, and Ender nail. Although there are reports of success using these devices,[26,27] their use has fallen out of favor because they cannot be statically locked. Use of these devices may require supplemental fixation, including cerclage wire, unicortical plate, or limb immobilization.

External fixation is indicated in fractures with significant soft-tissue injury, including those in patients with burns, other life-threatening injuries that preclude more definitive fracture stabilization, and sepsis. Use of a temporary external fixator across the knee allows limb access, soft-tissue management, and patient mobilization (Fig. 5). Care must be taken that the pins are sufficiently proximal and distal so that they will not compromise later surgical exposure of the distal femur. There has been recent interest in the use of uniplanar half-pin fixators and circular fixators with small-diameter tensioned wires for the definitive treatment of distal femur fractures. Problems associated with long-term external fixator use include pin tract infection, loss of knee motion secondary to quadriceps binding, delayed union, nonunion, and loss of reduction following device removal.

In one paper that reported good results with primary total knee arthroplasty after distal femur fracture, the authors advocated its use in elderly patients with significant medical comorbidities, severe osteoporosis, or significant degenerative knee disease.[28] However, this was a small series (13 patients) with short-term follow-up. Prosthetic replacement requires use of a modular or custom-designed constrained implant in order to compensate for the loss of bone stock and ligamentous support. The indications for primary prosthetic replacement in the treatment of acute distal femur fractures have not been defined and require further study.

Displaced unicondylar fractures require anatomic reduction and internal fixation to restore joint congruity and allow early range of knee motion.[29] Coronal fractures of either the medial or lateral condyle (Hoffa fractures) should be stabilized with cancellous lag screws countersunk below the articular surface. Medial and lateral sagittal unicondylar fractures should be stabilized using cancellous lag screws with washers and supplemented with an antiglide plate dependent on bone quality.

A bone graft should be used whenever there is medial fracture comminution or soft-tissue stripping, particularly when the fracture is stabilized with a lateral plate. Recent studies, however, have suggested that bone grafting may be unnecessary if the medial aspect of the distal femur and its soft-tissue attachments are left undisturbed through use of indirect reduction techniques.

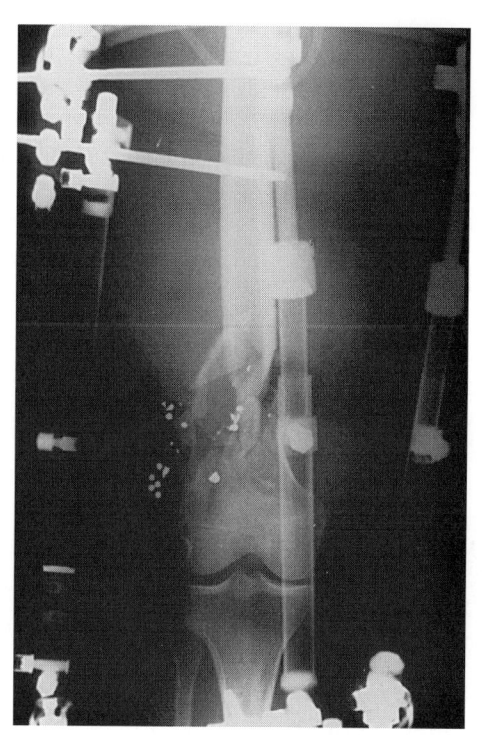

Fig. 5 Use of a temporary external fixator that crosses the knee after debridement of a shotgun wound to the distal thigh.

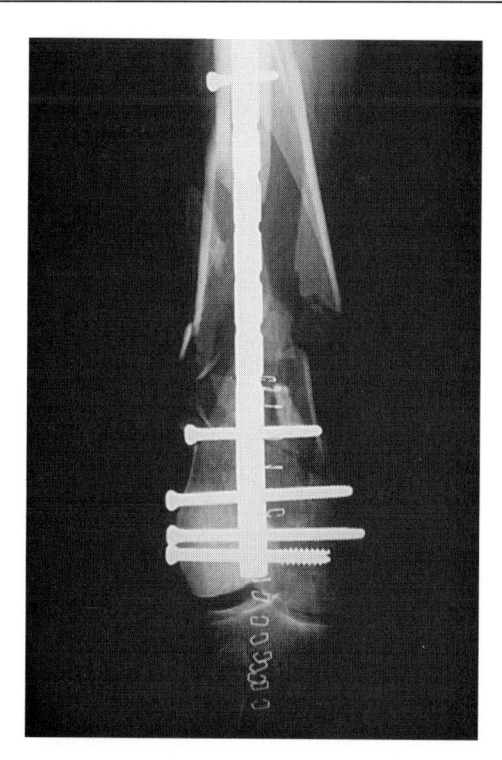

Fig. 4 Severely comminuted distal femur fracture stabilized with a retrograde inserted reamed interlocked nail.

Results

The results of both surgical and nonsurgical treatment are dependent on the severity of the initial injury and the quality and stability of the fracture reduction. The mechanism of injury, degree of comminution, and articular damage all affect the long-term clinical result.[30] An important factor is the ability of the surgeon to reconstruct the articular surface and apply stable fixation to allow early range of knee motion.

A good to excellent result can be expected with nonsurgical treatment of minimally displaced and impacted distal femur fractures. It is difficult to evaluate the results of treatment of displaced distal femur fractures because there is no universally accepted classification scheme, indications for surgery, or grading system for follow-up results. In one study of 71 fractures of the distal femur, 32 of which were treated surgically with anatomic open reduction, stable internal fixation, and early range of knee motion, good to excellent results were achieved in 75% of patients treated surgically, compared to 32% of those treated nonsurgically.[8] The results of many studies[12,17,31] underscore the importance of strict adherence to the above noted surgical principles. In a series of 35 distal femur fractures, good to excellent results were achieved in 71% of the cases treated surgically and which followed the principles of anatomic reduction, stable fixation, and early knee motion, but only 21% good to excellent results in patients in whom these principles were not followed.[31] In a series of 30 distal femur fractures stabilized with a 95° condylar blade plate, 80% had good to excellent functional results at an average follow-up of 28 months after using the criteria of Schatzker.[12] In a series of 35 distal femur fractures stabilized with a 95° dynamic condylar screw, there were 71% good to excellent functional results at an average follow-up of 28 months, using the same grading criteria.[17] In a study of interlocked medullary nailing of supracondylar and intercondylar femur fractures, all fractures united at an average follow up of 21 months.[32]

Complications

The most frequent complications after distal femur fracture are infection, nonunion, malunion, loss of fixation, and loss of knee motion. According to the most recent literature, the infection rate after surgical stabilization of distal femur fractures ranges from 0% to 6%. Factors that predispose to infection include (1) high-energy injuries, especially those with significant osseous devascularization, (2) open fractures, (3) extensive surgical dissection that compromises osseous vascularity, (4) an operating team with limited experience leading to prolonged open wound time, and (5) inadequate fixation.

The incidence of nonunion after open reduction and internal fixation ranges from 0% to 6%. The nonunion invariably occurs in the supracondylar region. Factors predisposing to nonunion include (1) bone loss or defect, (2) high-energy injuries with significant soft-tissue stripping and loss of osseous vascularity, (3) inability to achieve adequate osseous stabilization, (4) failure to bone graft, and (5) infection.

Nonunions of the distal femur are uncommon but difficult to manage.[33,34] The short distal fragment often has poor bone stock from disuse osteopenia and prior implants. The proximity to the knee joint frequently results in limited knee motion, which increases the stresses on the pseudoarthrosis and fixation device. Successful treatment of these nonunions requires adherence to the proven principles for the treatment of metaphyseal nonunions: mobilization of the adjacent joint, debridement of infected tissue, realignment of the mechanical axis, mechanical stabilization, pseudarthrosis compression, bone grafting of avascular fragments, early range of motion, and late full weightbearing.

Malunion following distal femur fracture is more common with nonsurgical than surgical management. The usual deformity associated with distal femoral malunion is varus and recurvatum. Varus results from medial loading of the femoral shaft through the femoral head; recurvatum results from the deforming forces of the gastrocnemius muscle. Malunion treatment must be directed at restoring the normal mechanical axis. Correction of the malunion involves supracondylar osteotomy and placement of stable fixation with early range of knee motion.

Factors predisposing to loss of fixation include (1) fracture comminution, (2) increased patient age and osteopenia, (3) low transcondylar and intracondylar fractures in which distal fixation may be compromised, (4) poor patient compliance with premature loading and weightbearing, and (5) infection. Once loss of fixation occurs, infection should be ruled out as a possible etiology. If nonunion or malunion has developed, treatment consists of removal of hardware, with placement of stable fixation and bone graft.

Because distal femur fractures are in close proximity to the knee, they often result in limited knee motion. Possible etiologies for the loss of knee motion include protruding intra-articular hardware, articular malreduction, intra-articular adhesions, ligamentous or capsular contractures, quadriceps or hamstring scarring, and posttraumatic arthritis.

Treatment of the restricted motion is dependent on the etiology. Protruding hardware must be removed; articular malreduction should be repositioned if significant posttraumatic changes do not already exist. Closed knee manipulations are rarely successful and may result in an iatrogenic tibial plateau or femur fracture. An arthrotomy should be performed with lysis of adhesions followed by progressive capsular and ligamentous releases. A short medial incision may be needed to fully release the patella. The vastus lateralis is freed from the linea aspera and the vastus intermedius is elevated off the femur. If needed, the vastus lateralis can be released from the greater trochanter and rectus femoris can be released from its origins.[35] A quadriceps V-Y advancement should be considered if significant intramuscular contracture/scarring exists. Postoperatively, the extremity should receive continuous passive motion and the patient should be started on early aggressive physical therapy.

Annotated References

1. Kolmert L, Wulff K: Epidemiology and treatment of distal femoral fractures in adults. *Acta Orthop Scand* 1982;53:957–962.
2. Arneson TJ, Melton LJ III, Lewallen DG, et al: Epidemiology of diaphyseal and distal femoral fractures in Rochester, Minnesota, 1965–1984. *Clin Orthop* 1988;234:188–194.
3. Scinshcimcr F: Fractures of the distal femur. *Clin Orthop* 1980;153:169–179.
4. Müller ME, Nazarian S, Koch P, et al: *The Comprehensive Classification of Fractures of Long Bones.* Berlin, Germany, Springer-Verlag, 1990, pp 116–147.
5. Connolly JF, Dehne E, Lafollette B: Closed reduction and early cast-brace ambulation in the treatment of femoral fractures: II. Results in one hundred and forty-three fractures. *J Bone Joint Surg* 1973;55A:1581–1599.
6. Neer CS II, Grantham SA, Shelton ML: Supracondylar fracture of the adult femur: A study of one hundred and ten cases. *J Bone Joint Surg* 1967:49A:591–613.
7. Healy WL, Brooker AF Jr: Distal femoral fractures: Comparison of open and closed methods of treatment. *Clin Orthop* 1983;174:166–171.
8. Schatzker J, Horne G, Waddell J: The Toronto experience with the supracondylar fracture of the femur, 1966–1972. *Injury* 1975;6:113–128.
9. Johansen K, Bandyk D, Thiele B, et al: Temporary intraluminal shunts: Resolution of a management dilemma in complex vascular injuries. *J Trauma* 1982;22:395–402.
10. Bone LT, Bucholz R: The management of fractures in the patient with multiple trauma. *J Bone Joint Surg* 1986;68A:945–949.
11. Mast J, Jakob R, Ganz R (eds): *Planning and Reduction Techniques in Fracture Surgery.* Berlin, Germany, Springer-Verlag, 1989.
12. Mize RD, Bucholz RW, Grogan DP: Surgical treatment of displaced, comminuted fractures of the distal end of the femur. *J Bone Joint Surg* 1982;64A:871–879.
13. Olerud S: Surgical treatment of supracondylar-condylar fractures of the femur: Technique and results in fifteen cases. *J Bone Joint Surg* 1972;54A:1015-1032.
14. Zehntner MK, Marchesi DG, Burch H, et al: Alignment of supracondylar/intercondylar fractures of the femur after internal fixation by AO/ASIF technique. *J Orthop Trauma* 1992;6:318–326.

    Fifty-nine supracondylar/intercondylar fractures of the femur were evaluated at a mean follow-up of 67 months. Axial alignment was compared to the uninjured side using radiographic evaluation. Identical values for varus/valgus were noted in 24%, ante/recurvatum in 72%, and rotation in 61% of patients. Differences in varus/valgus of up to 5° were noted in 74%, ante/recurvatum in 78%, and rotation in 83% of patients. The authors concluded that restoration of the distal femoral angle is more difficult than restoration of the sagittal plane and rotation. However, a satisfactory functional result was compatible with angulation differences up to 5° in any plane.

15. Giles JB, DeLee JC, Heckman JD, et al: Supracondylar-intercondylar fractures of the femur treated with a supracondylar plate and lag screw. *J Bone Joint Surg* 1982;64A:864-870.
16. Pritchett JW: Supracondylar fractures of the femur. *Clin Orthop* 1984;184:173–177.
17. Sanders R, Regazzoni P, Ruedi TP: Treatment of supracondylar-intercondylar fractures of the femur using the dynamic condylar screw. *J Orthop Trauma* 1989;3:214–222.
18. Sanders R, Swiontkowski M, Rosen H, et al: Double-plating of comminuted, unstable fractures of the distal part of the femur. *J Bone Joint Surg* 1991;73A:341–346.

    Nine patients who had a complex fracture of the distal femur and deficient medial cortical buttress were reviewed. Stabilization required use of a lateral condylar buttress plate and an additional medial plate. At an average follow-up of 26 months, all fractures had united. Functional evaluation revealed five good and four fair results.

19. Wu CC, Shih CH: Treatment of femoral supracondylar unstable comminuted fractures: Comparisons between plating and Grosse-Kemph interlocking nailing techniques. *Arch Orthop Trauma Surg* 1992;111:232–236.

    A prospective study was performed of 66 supracondylar femur fractures stabilized with either an intramedullary nail (38) or plate (28). Displaced intercondylar fractures were excluded. Those fractures stabilized with intramedullary nails had a higher union rate (90% vs 79%) and better knee motion.

20. Lucas SE, Seligson D, Henry SL: Intramedullary supracondylar nailing of femoral fractures: A preliminary report of the GSH supracondylar nail. *Clin Orthop* 1993;296:200–206.
21. Butler MS, Brumback RJ, Ellison TS, et al: Interlocking intramedullary nailing for ipsilateral fractures of the femoral shaft and distal part of the femur. *J Bone Joint Surg* 1991;73A:1492–1502.

    Twenty-three ipsilateral femoral shaft and distal femur fractures were stabilized with an interlocking intramedullary nail. If there was an intercondylar fracture component (11 patients), reduction and stabilization of the articular surface was performed through an open (nine) or closed (two) technique prior to nailing. All fractures united; the average knee flexion was greater than 115°. Three patients had an angular malunion of the supracondylar area. Four fractures had greater than 1 mm displacement of the articular surface. Three patients needed additional surgery because of missed coronal fractures of the femoral condyle.

22. Bucholz RW, Ross SE, Lawrence KL: Fatigue fracture of the interlocking nail in the treatment of fractures of the distal part of the femoral shaft. *J Bone Joint Surg* 1987;69A:1391–1399.

    The clinical and mechanical factors predisposing to nail fatigue fracture were studied in seven patients who had a distal femur fracture stabilized with an interlocking nail. In all seven patients, the fracture occurred within 5 cm of the more proximal of the distal screw holes. A finite element analysis confirmed that the stress on this screw hole exceeded its fatigue endurance limit when this screw hole was located within 5 cm of the fracture. The femur would have to regain 50% of its original stiffness in order to accommodate weightbearing without risk of fatigue failure.

23. Henry SL, Trager S, Green S, et al: Management of supracondylar fractures of the femur with the GSH

intramedullary nail: Preliminary report. *Contemp Orthop* 1991;22:631–640.

24. Iannacone WM, Bennett FS, DeLong WG, et al: Initial experience with the treatment of supracondylar femoral fractures using the supracondylar intramedullary nail: A preliminary report. *J Orthop Trauma* 1994;8:322–327.

    Forty-one distal femur fractures (22 open, 19 closed fractures) were stabilized using the supracondylar intramedullary nail. Thirty-two fractures healed within 4 months. There were five delayed unions and four nonunions. Two of the five delayed unions required revision internal fixation; two required screw removal and dynamization. The four nonunions united after revision internal fixation and bone grafting. Four patients had fatigue failure of the rod; all occurred in rods that had 6.4-mm locking screws. Thirty-five of 41 knees achieved at least 90° of knee motion.

25. Johnson EE, Marroquin CE, Kossovsky N: Synovial metallosis resulting from intraarticular intramedullary nailing of a distal femoral nonunion. *J Orthop Trauma* 1993;7:320–326.

26. Zickel RE, Fietti VG Jr, Lawsing JF, et al: A new intramedullary fixation device for the distal third of the femur. *Clin Orthop* 1977;125:185–191.

27. Zickel RE, Hobeika P, Robbins DS: Zickel supracondylar nails for fractures of the distal end of the femur. *Clin Orthop* 1986;212:79–88.

28. Bell KM, Johnstone AJ, Court-Brown CM, et al: Primary knee arthroplasty for distal femoral fractures in elderly patients. *J Bone Joint Surg* 1992;74B:400–402.

29. Ostermann PA, Neumann K, Ekkernkamp A, et al: Long-term results of unicondylar fractures of the femur. *J Orthop Trauma* 1994;8:142–146.

    Twenty-four unicondylar fractures of the distal femur underwent open reduction and lag screw fixation. At mean follow-up of 62 months, 20 patients had an excellent result, three had a satisfactory result, and one had an unsatisfactory result based on Neer rating system. The four patients who did not have an excellent result had accompanying injuries. The authors concluded that open reduction and screw fixation of unicondylar distal femur fractures provides overall excellent long-term results.

30. Siliski JM, Mahring M, Hofer HP: Supracondylar-intercondylar fractures of the femur: Treatment by internal fixation. *J Bone Joint Surg* 1989;71A:95–104.

    The results of surgical treatment of 52 intercondylar distal femur fractures were reviewed at 20 to 120 month follow-up. All fractures were stabilized using the following protocol: a single lateral incision, interfragmentary screws and plates, and bone grafting of comminuted metaphyseal segments. Early active range of knee motion was encouraged. The final arc of knee motion averaged 107°. Simple supracondylar fractures that had a single intercondylar fracture extension had a better outcome (92% good and excellent results using the Neer rating scale) than those that had either supracondylar or intra-articular comminution (77% good and excellent results).

31. Schatzker J, Lambert DC: Supracondylar fractures of the femur. *Clin Orthop* 1979;138:77–83.

32. Leung KS, Shen WY, So WS, et al: Interlocking intramedullary nailing for supracondylar and intercondylar fractures of the distal part of the femur. *J Bone Joint Surg* 1991;73A:332–340.

    The authors reported the results of interlocked intramedullary nailing in a series of 37 supracondylar and intercondylar femur fractures. All fractures underwent closed antegrade intramedullary nailing after closed reduction and percutaneous fixation of the articular surface. At an average follow-up of 21 months, all fractures had united; there were no malunions nor instances of nail breakage. Thirty-one patients (94%) had a good or excellent functional result using the Hospital for Special Surgery knee rating scale.

33. Moore TJ, Watson T, Green SA, et al: Complications of surgically treated supracondylar fractures of the femur. *J Trauma* 1987;27:402–406.

34. Wu CC, Shih CH: Distal femoral nonunion treated with interlocking nailing. *J Trauma* 1991;31:1659–1662.

    Twenty-eight distal femoral nonunions were stabilized using an antegrade inserted interlocking nail. Seven of 28 nonunions (25%) were located in the supracondylar region. All were bone grafted. All nails were locked distally with either one or two bolts. Twenty-four patients were available for follow-up at an average of 32 months. The union rate was 91.7% with an average time to union of 4.5 months. The range of knee motion was not reported. Two nails fractured, both occurring in nails used to stabilize supracondylar nonunions.

35. Ebraheim NA, DeTroye RJ, Saddemi SR: Results of Judet quadricepsplasty. *J Orthop Trauma* 1993;7:327–330.

    This study reported the results of Judet quadricepsplasty (a technique involving disinsertion and sliding of the quadriceps muscle) in 12 patients with a knee extension contracture after distal femur fracture. At an average follow-up of 25 months, the average improvement in knee motion was 53°; the average loss of knee flexion was 14° from the maximum intraoperative correction.

14
Knee Dislocation

Definition and Classification

Knee dislocation, as described by Kennedy,[1] in 1963, is the displacement of the tibia with respect to the femur. There are five major types of dislocation: anterior, posterior, medial, lateral, and rotatory. There are four types of rotational dislocation, each representing an anatomic quadrant: anteromedial, anterolateral, posteromedial, and posterolateral (Fig. 1). Anterior and posterior are the most frequently reported types of dislocations and posterolateral is the most common direction of rotational dislocation.

The mechanism of injury can be correlated with the direction of dislocation. Anterior dislocations occur most commonly from hyperextension, with a posteriorly directed force acting on a fixed extremity. Posterior dislocations often occur when the proximal tibia strikes the dashboard during a car accident, forcing the tibia posteriorly on the femur. Coincident femur fractures, tibia fractures, hip dislocations, and extensor mechanism disruptions have all been reported in association with this mechanism.[2,3] Medial and lateral dislocations are caused by a valgus or varus force, respectively. Rotational dislocations are usually indirect and include a rotational component. The mechanism of posterolateral dislocation, for example, has been described as an abduction and internal rotation force acting on a flexed, nonweightbearing extremity.

A significant number of dislocations in all reported series are of unknown direction. They represent spontaneous reductions or those that were reduced at the scene. Patients with global instability should also be included in this category. The definition of severe ligamentous disruption include recurvatum greater than 30°, anteroposterior (AP) instability greater than 1 cm, a lateral capsular sign, and a large hemarthrosis. Patients with global instability should be treated as dislocations because they have a similar incidence of ligamentous, vascular, and neurologic injuries.[4]

In addition to the direction of dislocation, knee dislocations have been divided into high-energy and low-energy, based on the kinematics of the trauma.[5] High-energy injuries tend to result from direct trauma, such as from motor vehicle accidents, falls from a height, and crush injuries. Low-energy injuries are usually caused by indirect trauma and include falls, twisting injuries, and athletic injuries.

Evaluation and Treatment

Associated Injuries

It is necessary to know what injuries are commonly associated with a knee dislocation in order to direct the physical examination of the patient. The reported incidences of associated injuries are: vascular injury, 30% (range, 5% to 45%); neurologic injury, 23% (range, 10% to 40%); open injury, 5% (range, 0% to 20%); and fractures, 10% (range, 0% to 60%). Vascular injury is more common in anterior and posterior dislocations and has been reported in as many as 53% of cases. This high incidence is due to the tethering of the popliteal artery between the adductor hiatus proximally and the origin of the soleus distally. Low-energy dislocations have a slightly lower incidence of vascular injury, but should be examined in the same way as high-energy dislocations. Neurologic injury usually occurs to the peroneal nerve as it is stretched over the femoral condyle during posterolateral dislocation[6] or as it is injured with the lateral ligaments following an adduction stress. Meniscal injury is common (up to 40%), but not easily discernible by physical examination. Compartment syndrome occurs rarely.

Fracture-dislocations should be considered a separate entity from pure dislocations. Most types of fracture-dislocation have a lower rate of vascular injury than pure dislocations.[4,7] In addition, the treatment of these combined injuries differs from that of a pure dislocation.[7]

Initial Examination

Before the knee is reduced, the examiner must first assess the vascular status of the extremity.[8] Dorsalis pedis and posterior tibial pulses should be sought. Motor and sensory neurologic function should be documented. A stocking glove pattern of hypesthesia or anesthesia, particularly if it is evolving, may indicate ischemia from vascular insufficiency or compartment syndrome. Decreased capillary refill and a temperature lower than the contralateral extremity also indicate ischemia. Because peroneal nerve injury can be partial or complete, differentiation from ischemia can be difficult.

The entire extremity should be examined for coincident fractures and dislocations as noted above. The skin about the knee must be carefully examined to rule out open

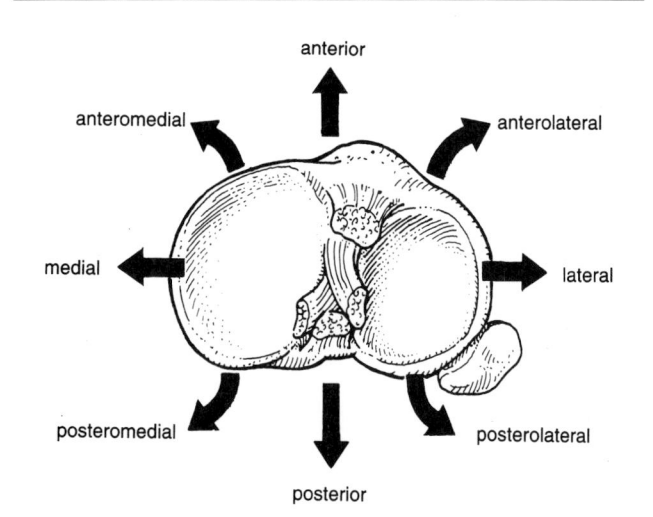

Fig. 1 The possible directions of knee dislocation as seen looking down on the tibia.

wounds. The typical medial skin furrow, or puckering,[9] as originally described by Quinlan and Sharrard[10] (Fig. 1) indicates a posterolateral dislocation with the medial femoral condyle buttonholed through the capsule or extensor mechanism and the medial capsule and/or collateral ligament caught in the joint. Because this furrow is usually irreducible, open reduction should be performed if closed reduction is not easily accomplished.[11] Attempts at closed reduction often will deepen the furrow, indicating that open reduction is needed.

Radiography

Standard AP and lateral radiographs will clearly show the presence and direction of a knee dislocation. Oblique views, however, can help detect associated fractures about the knee. These views are particularly helpful if they are obtained after the knee is reduced. Radiographs of the hip, femur, tibia, and ankle should be standard for high-energy dislocation.

Reduction

After radiographic confirmation of the dislocation, the knee must be reduced. Closed reduction is usually not difficult and is performed by stabilizing the femur, applying traction to the tibia, and reversing the direction of dislocation. It is prudent to avoid applying direct pressure to the popliteal fossa. After reduction, the knee should be immobilized in the position of most stability; 15° to 20° of flexion is usually a safe position.

Vascular Injury

Examination of the knee after it is reduced begins with a reassessment of the vascular and neurologic status. Pulses that were initially absent may now be present; however, this does not rule out vascular injury. Many authors have reported cases of major vascular injury in the presence of pulses.[12,13]

Vascular injury can be present with or without obvious signs of ischemia. Absent pulses, clear signs of vascular injury (active bleeding, expanding hematoma, bruit or thrill), or obvious signs of ischemia require emergent surgical repair of the vascular injury. Arteriography is usually unnecessary in this situation unless more than one level of injury is suspected. In this case, arteriography should be performed in the operating room because the average delay for formal arteriography is 3 hours.[14] Some vascular surgeons elect to perform a one-shot arteriogram on the operating table before they proceed with the exploration.

Many studies have demonstrated increased rates of amputation with delays in vascular repair. In one study, amputation was not needed if repair was done within 6 hours of injury,[15] compared with an amputation rate of 30% if repair was done between 7 and 12 hours after injury. Amputation has also been correlated with popliteal vein injury, nerve injury, and significant soft-tissue damage.

Currently, reverse saphenous interposition graft is the favored method of repair. The liberal use of four-compartment fasciotomy for significant ischemia times (usually more than 4 hours) is recommended.[16,17] Several authors have also discussed the importance of popliteal vein repair when possible. Of nine patients who had vascular repair, intraoperative arteriograms after repair effected changes in the management in seven.[18] All of the extremities were salvaged.

The knee should be immobilized in a reduced position until further treatment decisions are made. External fixation may be helpful in maintaining the knee reduced after fasciotomy or if the vascular repair is tenuous.

Presentation without hard signs of injury *does not* rule out injury. Many authors have reported major vascular injury in the presence of distal pulses. These patients either have a completely normal history and examination or have a history (sometimes pre-reduction) of ischemia, a history of pulse deficit, or some physical sign of injury.

Physical signs of injury include diminished but palpable pulses, decreased capillary refill, neurologic deficit, hypotension, nonexpansile hematoma, decreased temperature of the extremity, and decreased ankle pressure index (API). Vascular injury correlates well with diminished pulse and diminished capillary refill.[19,20] Pulse differential had a sensitivity of 85% for presence of vascular injury.[14] Only 17% of their patients with an abnormal pulse had a normal arteriogram.

Thus, arteriography is currently indicated for all patients with knee dislocation or severe ligamentous instability and a history of ischemia or pulse deficit. It is also indicated if there are any physical signs of vascular injury, especially a pulse differential. Arteriographically defined occlusive lesions require emergent repair as discussed above.

The vascular management of a patient with a knee dislocation who has normal pulses but no history of ischemia is more controversial. There have been numerous reports of patients with initially intact pulses who later develop complete thrombosis; the incidence has been reported to be as high as 15%.[21] This has been observed to occur as late as 12 days after injury.[6] The overall incidence of vascular injury in the presence of normal pulses ranges from 0% to 35%, however, many of these injuries are nonocclusive.

The natural history of nonocclusive lesions has been defined more clearly and the treatment has evolved. Several authors have advocated nonsurgical management of minor arterial injuries.[22,23] The indications for nonsurgical management include small, nonocclusive, low-energy injuries with intact distal circulation and no active extravasation. Segmental narrowing, as well as intimal defects, flaps, and pseudoaneurysms smaller than 5 mm have been treated with repeat arteriography and/or close clinical observation. Approximately 10% of intimal injuries and 20% of pseudoaneurysms will progress. Ninety percent of these minor injuries never require surgery, however, most of the patients in these studies sustained penetrating rather than blunt trauma.

This strategy in the vascular management of nonocclusive lesions has raised questions about the need for arteriography in cases of knee dislocation with no history of ischemia and normal pulses. This issue was addressed in studies in which patients having "normal" pulses did not have occlusive vascular injuries.[14,24] Patients were managed with arteriography and observation or observation alone. The incidence of nonocclusive vascular injury in the group treated with arteriography was 10% to 35%. Only one patient progressed from having normal pulses to ischemia, and this occurred within 8 hours. Patients with "abnormal" pulses had a high rate of occlusive vascular injury requiring repair (59% to 100%). However, the assessment of normalcy was made by the vascular surgeon without any objective measurements.

An attempt has been made to use reproducible objective measures to correlate a diminished arterial systolic pressure index (API) of the injured extremity/uninjured arm with arterial injury.[25] Using an API ≥ 0.9 as normal, the negative predictive value of this simple test as compared with vascular injury requiring repair was 99%. The sensitivity and specificity compared with arteriographic findings were 87% and 97%, respectively. This method may be helpful in determining which patients have "normal" pulses and which would benefit from arteriography.

These studies indicate that a more selective approach to arteriography in patients with no history of ischemia and normal pulses is possible, but *only if a nonsurgical approach to nonocclusive vascular lesions is chosen*. This requires close observation of the patient's status by a vascular surgeon or other experienced personnel and the ability to perform an emergent repair if any change in status is detected. Although this may be possible in trauma centers, it could be extremely difficult to manage in smaller institutions. If these criteria of close monitoring and easy availability of the operating room are not met, these patients should undergo arteriography and possibly repair at the discretion of the vascular surgeon.

The management of the ligament injuries must also be factored into the decision. The natural history of nonocclusive lesions that are exposed to tourniquet ischemia has not been clearly defined. Tourniquet stasis combined with exposed subintimal tissue may lead to thrombosis and even amputation.[26] Until the true risk of tourniquet stasis on nonocclusive lesions is better delineated, arteriography should be performed prior to tourniquet use.

The result of tourniquet use after vascular repair is also poorly documented. Just 1 hour of tourniquet ischemia has been shown to increase the risk of thrombosis in an animal model.[27] However, anecdotal reports of patients who had ligament reconstructions after vascular repair and under tourniquet stasis have revealed no vascular complications.[27] Despite this, because of the poorly defined risks, ligament surgery after vascular repair should be delayed by several weeks or should be performed without tourniquet if possible. If a tourniquet is to be used, the vascular surgeon should be available if thrombosis should occur.

Ligament Injury

After the full neurovascular examination, the extent of ligamentous damage must be determined. In the large majority of cases, both the anterior cruciate ligament (ACL) and the posterior cruciate ligament (PCL) are ruptured. However, the common belief that both cruciate ligaments must be disrupted to allow the knee to dislocate has been disproved.[28,29] Complete dislocations have been reported with either the PCL or the ACL intact. In all cases with an intact PCL, dislocations have been either anterior or anterolateral. A possible mechanism for this injury has been proposed on the basis of several cadaveric studies,[30] which demonstrated that the ACL ruptures before the PCL in hyperextension and that marked hyperextension occurs after sectioning the ACL but not after sectioning the PCL.[31] Thus, it is possible that the knee is hyperextended until the ACL ruptures and then the tibia is dislocated anteriorly, allowing the PCL to remain intact. This same mechanism may work in reverse, allowing complete dislocation without rupture of the ACL.

Physical Examination

It is important to remember several key relationships while performing the examination. Posterior translation is prevented by the lateral collateral ligament (LCL) and posterolateral corner (arcuate ligament, popliteus tendon, popliteofibular ligament, fabellofibular ligament, and the capsule) at 30° and by the PCL at all positions of flexion. Anterior translation is primarily resisted by the ACL. The LCL is the primary restraint to varus stress in all positions, but can be tested in isolation at 30°. Varus instability in extension indicates LCL and cruciate incompetence (usually ACL). The medial collateral ligament (MCL) and medial capsule are the initial restraints to valgus stress and can be tested in isolation at 30°. Instability in extension again indicates cruciate incompetence (usually PCL). Several coupled motions also exist: anterior translation is coupled to internal rotation via the ACL and posterior translation is coupled to external rotation via the PCL. Thus, if the PCL is ruptured, there will be a loss of coupled external rotation with posterior translation.

All patients should undergo a systematic examination of the knee for ligamentous instability. Many authors recommend that this be done under regional or general anesthesia, particularly if surgical treatment is contemplated.

The examination should begin with visual inspection. A posterior sag is a sign of PCL injury. The knee should be tested for anterior and posterior translation and for varus and valgus instability in extension and at 30° and 90° of flexion. The posterior drawer test at 90° is useful for evaluating PCL injury. PCL rupture allows 15 to 20 mm of posterior translation with 100 N of force.

The Lachman and pivot shift tests can be helpful in defining ACL injury. However, the lack of a firm endpoint is paramount in the diagnosis because anterior movement from a posterior position to a reduced position in a PCL deficient knee can mimic ACL injury. The normal position of the proximal tibia is 1 cm anterior to the femoral condyles with the knee in 90° of flexion.

Valgus instability at 30° of knee flexion indicates MCL rupture. If instability is also present in extension, PCL rupture is likely.

The LCL and posterolateral corner must be carefully examined. In the face of a PCL injury (which is most commonly the case) the LCL and posterolateral structures can be tested by varus stress at 30° and extension and external rotation in 30° and 90° of flexion. LCL and posterolateral injury are present in addition to cruciate injury if there is an increase in external rotation at both 30° and 90° and gross instability to varus stress in 30° and in extension. Posterolateral injury also can be tested by the external recurvatum and posterolateral drawer tests.

Before deciding on a treatment course, several authors have recommended MRI. This is not needed for all knee dislocations, however, it can help in determining the status of a ligament (such as the PCL) when the results of the physical examination are not definitive. Midsubstance tears can sometimes be differentiated from avulsions, and the menisci can be fully evaluated.

Treatment and Results

Regardless of the type of treatment undertaken, few patients who have suffered a knee dislocation will have normal knee function. This attests to the significance of this injury. Significant rates of stiffness, pain, and instability are the rule rather than the exception. In general, stiffness is a bigger problem for patients than instability. Despite this, most patients will be able to return to work and continue their normal activities of daily living. Paralleling other extremity injuries, patients with low-energy dislocations may have a better prognosis than those with high-energy injuries.

There are three treatment approaches: nonsurgical, acute repair, and delayed reconstruction. Each has its proponents, advantages, and disadvantages. Treatment must also be tailored to the individual patient. Age, activity level, job requirements, and individual goals play a large part in the decision.

Nonsurgical Management

Only one large study has focused on nonsurgical treatment,[32] in which 43 cases of mostly high-energy dislocations were reviewed. Of 26 patients treated using immobilization for an average of 5.5 weeks, 24 had satisfactory results. However, the criteria used for evaluation were not stringent and most patients had significant stiffness. No more than 6 weeks of immobilization was recommended.

Acute Repair

Most authors have recommended surgical repair of all torn ligaments within several weeks of injury to avoid instability. Two studies that demonstrated high rates of cruciate ligament avulsions rather than midsubstance tears favor surgical repair (Table 1).[7,21] Primary repair of cruciate ligament avulsions back to bone is more successful than the repair of intrasubstance tears. Only four recent reports focused on primary repair of all ligaments after knee dislocation; in all, each of the injured knees had bicruciate injuries.[6,18,33,34]

These reports share several findings. Instability is rare, but pain and stiffness are common. The large majority of patients resume normal activities and a minority return to athletics at their previous level. Shorter periods of immobilization have been suggested by all authors. Manipulation should be considered at 3 months if motion is unsatisfactory.

Delayed Reconstruction

Because of the high incidence of stiffness and lack of complaints from minor instabilities whether the patient is treated nonsurgically or surgically, some authors have directed treatment toward regaining motion first and reconstructing instabilities second. A treatment protocol based on regaining motion and strength followed by delayed PCL reconstruction has been presented.[29] This technique was used in only a few patients with low-energy dislocations, but yielded stable knees with excellent motion. The applicability of this regimen for high-energy dislocations has not been demonstrated.

Augmentation

The long-term results after primary repair of isolated midsubstance cruciate tears has been improved by augmentation procedures. Several authors have advised using these techniques for knee dislocations. If the surgeon chooses to treat the cruciate injuries with acute repair, augmentation of midsubstance tears may help to provide long-term stability. This is not necessary when repairing an avulsion, unless severe intrasubstance injury is present. Autograft is gener-

Table 1. Percentage of avulsions identified at surgery

Study	ACL			PCL		
	Femur	Tibia	Total	Femur	Tibia	Total
Frassica et al[18]	5 (38%)	1 (8%)	6 (46%)	10 (77%)	0 (0%)	10 (77%)
Sisto and Warren[6]	5 (31%)	5 (31%)	10 (62%)	12 (75%)	2 (13%)	14 (88%)
Total	10 (34%)	6 (21%)	18 (55%)	22 (76%)	2 (7%)	24 (83%)

ally recommended, but allograft also has been used. Allograft is particularly advantageous when the number of ligamentous injuries limits the availability of autologous tissue.

Collateral Ligaments

Excellent healing of the medial collateral ligament (MCL) has been reported with bracing, even after cruciate repair or reconstruction. Thus, the brace used after repair or before reconstruction is sufficient for the treatment of the MCL.

This is not the case for the LCL and posterolateral corner. Acute repairs have demonstrated better results than late repair or reconstruction.[35,36] Retraction of these structures makes late repair difficult. Early repair of these structures is a necessary prerequisite to early motion. Thus, if LCL and posterolateral instability are detected, early repair is recommended in order to allow early motion. These suggestions must be balanced with the fact that posterolateral instability has not been reported to be a major problem after nonsurgical treatment. This is probably related to long periods of immobilization, however. With rehabilitation protocols, including early motion, repair of the LCL and posterolateral corner is likely to improve results.

Incomplete Cruciate Injury

As described earlier, dislocation can occur without rupturing both cruciate ligaments. If the PCL is competent, then treatment should be directed at the other ligament injuries. This pattern more closely resembles an ACL or combined ACL/collateral ligament injury. Several authors recommend treating this by reconstruction of the ACL only, or the ACL and LCL if both are ruptured. MRI can be useful in determining the status of the PCL if it is in question.

Complications

Stiffness is the most common complication after knee dislocation. Aggressive rehabilitation is recommended after the initial period of immobilization. If adequate range of motion is not obtained within 3 months of injury, manipulation should be considered.

Although minor objective instability occurs with some frequency, it is rarely symptomatic. If symptoms exist and do not resolve with rehabilitation, appropriate ligament reconstruction should be performed. A further question exists regarding the long-term effects of minor instability on the development of degenerative arthritis.

Peroneal nerve injury occurs in approximately 10% to 40% of knee dislocations. Incomplete lesions have a high rate of recovery, but complete lesions can be permanent. In two separate reports, three of four complete lesions were noted to be permanent[34] and four of six complete lesions did not resolve without treatment.[6] Many treatments have been recommended for complete palsy. In one study, exploration and release of the peroneal nerve in 2 patients with complete palsies resulted in one complete and one partial recovery.[6] Acute exploration has been recommended if ligamentous surgery is indicated, and delayed exploration (after 3 to 6 months) with possible repair if no acute ligament surgery is planned.[38]

Early work regarding nerve repair for peroneal traction palsies yielded poor recovery. This resulted in the almost universal recommendation for tendon transfer (posterior tibial) to enable patients to walk without a brace. However, because the posterior tibial tendon is an antagonist, transfer does have a tenodesis effect. Active plantarflexion is decreased by an average of 15°. Ninkovik and associates[39] described a new procedure consisting of lateral gastrocnemius transfer and neurotization with the motor branch of the peroneal nerve. This provides an active protagonist for dorsiflexion of the foot, and preliminary results in 6 patients were excellent.

Nerve exploration with release or repair is also an option. The indication for this is a complete palsy with no electromyographic or clinical evidence of recovery for at least 3 months after injury. Plantarflexion contracture of the ankle is a contraindication. Two recent series used multiple sural nerve cable grafts spanning 4 to 20 cm with good results: 30% had complete recovery, 40% had partial recovery, and 28% had no recovery.[40,41] This is a good option and can be salvaged with tendon transfer if no recovery occurs.

Summary

There are several options for the treatment of ligamentous injuries after knee dislocations. The goals of each are a stable, painless knee with good motion and strength. The goals of stability and mobility are diametrically opposed. Long-term immobilization will predictably produce a stable joint, but sacrifice motion. Early motion without ligament repair will result in an excellent arc of motion, but at the expense of stability. The orthopaedist must weigh the treatment options and the patient's goals in order to decide on the most suitable treatment for each case.

If surgical treatment is chosen for a particular patient, the orthopaedist must decide between acute repair and

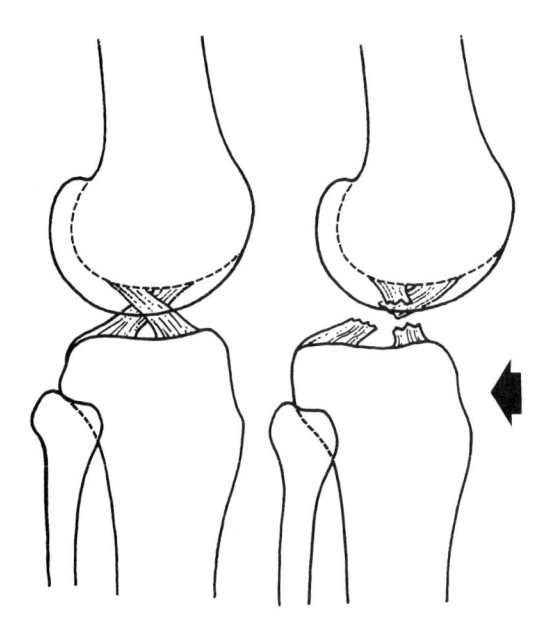

Fig. 2 Left, A lateral view of the knee showing the tibia in its normal position relative to the femur. **Right,** With both cruciate ligaments ruptured after dislocation, the tibia subluxes posteriorly.

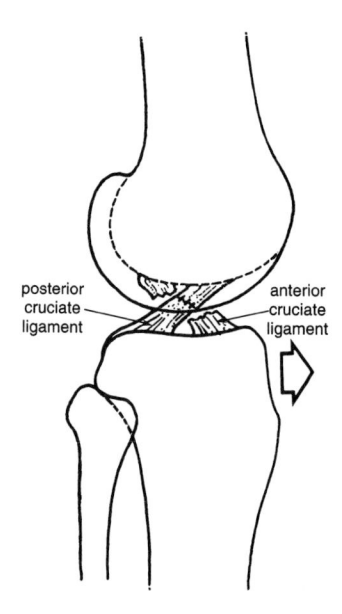

Fig. 3 Restoration of the posterior cruciate ligament holds the tibia in its normal anatomic position. Other ligamentous repairs may be done with the knee in its normal position.

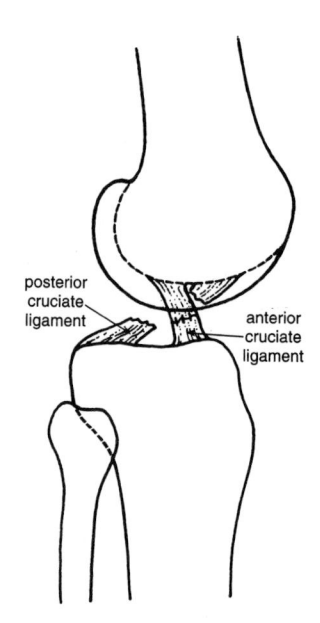

Fig. 4 Because of its posterior origin on the femur and anterior insertion on the tibia, a tight repair of the anterior cruciate ligament will force a posterior subluxation of the tibia. This will lead to a flexion contracture.

reconstruction. Because results for the repair of avulsions are superior to that of midsubstance tears, primary repair may be preferred in this circumstance. Radiographs can diagnose avulsions if a bony fragment is involved. If not, MRI may establish the type of ligament injury present. This may be particularly helpful given that physical examination of complex ligament injuries has been shown to be inconsistent, even among experienced examiners. This is particularly true for the diagnosis of rotational instability.[42]

In all cases, the joint must be reduced and maintained in that position to decrease incongruity and the risk of arthritis. The tibia tends to rest in a posteriorly displaced position relative to the femur after dislocation (Fig. 2). This has implications for both surgical and nonsurgical management.

The tibia can be reduced by external immobilization (casts or external fixators) or by restoring the function of the PCL via repair or reconstruction. The normal function of the PCL maintains the tibia in its appropriate position. For this reason, if primary ligament repair or delayed reconstruction is planned, it must address the PCL first. If primary repair is undertaken, the PCL should be tied before the ACL to maintain the correct position of the joint (Fig. 3). If the ACL is tied first, the tibia will sublux posteriorly and a flexion contracture will result (Fig. 4).

If delayed reconstruction is planned, it must be centered around the PCL. Adequate strength and range of motion should be obtained before reconstruction. If both the ACL and PCL are to be reconstructed, the PCL should be done before the ACL. If only one reconstruction is planned, it should be the PCL in order to maintain a reduction of the joint.

After stability is obtained, treatment should emphasize restoration of motion and strength. Most authors recommend immobilization for less than 6 weeks to decrease stiffness. More aggressive rehabilitation protocols following acute repair or reconstruction are also being advocated and include earlier range of motion exercises in a hinged brace. Extension bracing at night has also been suggested and may aid in avoiding flexion contracture.

Annotated References

1. Kennedy JC: Complete dislocation of the knee joint. *J Bone Joint Surg* 1963;45A:889-904.

2. Matthews DE, Jones GS, Hughes JL: Femur fracture with ipsilateral knee dislocation. *Orthopedics* 1993;16:917-919.

3. Kreibich DN, Moran CG, Pinder IM: Ipsilateral hip and knee dislocation: A case report. *Acta Orthop Scand* 1990;61:90-91.

4. Varnell RM, Coldwell DM, Sangeorzan BJ, et al: Arterial injury complicating knee disruption. *Am Surg* 1989;55:699-704.

5. Shelbourne KD, Porter DA, Clingman JA, et al: Low velocity knee dislocation. *Orthop Rev* 1991;20:995-1004.

   Low-energy dislocations may have better results than high velocity. Aggressive early rehabilitation yields improved motion. An excellent discussion of a PCL based treatment protocol is presented.

6. Sisto DJ, Warren RF: Complete knee dislocation: A follow-up study of operative treatment. *Clin Orthop* 1985;198:94-101.

   The authors followed 13 patients treated by primary ligamentous repair without augmentation. In addition to the cruciate injuries, there were nine MCL ruptures, four LCL ruptures, and three combined MCL and LCL ruptures. The medial meniscus was injured in five knees. Patients were immobilized for 6 weeks after surgery. No patient had posterior instability and one had some anterior instability with a positive pivot shift. The average ROM was −2° to 118°, including six patients who required nine manipulations. Pain was a complaint in 46%. Eight patients returned to their previous level of athletic competition, including one professional athlete.

7. Moore TM: Fracture-dislocation of the knee. *Clin Orthop* 1981;156:128-140.

   A complete review and classification of fracture-dislocation is presented. Neurovascular injury was common in rim avulsion and four part types. Surgery is indicated based on instability defined on stress radiographs. Long-term results correlated with the severity of neurologic and ligamentous injury.

8. Kaufman SL, Martin LG: Arterial injuries associated with complete dislocation of the knee. *Radiology* 1992;184:153-155.

9. Wand JS: A physical sign denoting irreducibility of a dislocated knee. *J Bone Joint Surg* 1989;71B:862.

10. Quinlan AG, Sharrard WJW: Postero-lateral dislocation of the knee with capsular interposition. *J Bone Joint Surg* 1958;40B:660-663.

11. Nystrom M, Samimi S, Ha'Eri GB: Two cases of irreducible knee dislocation occurring simultaneously in two patients and a review of the literature. *Clin Orthop* 1992;277:197-200.

12. McCoy GF, Hannon DG, Barr RJ, et al: Vascular injury associated with low-velocity dislocations of the knee. *J Bone Joint Surg* 1987;69B:285-287.

13. McCutchan JD, Gillham NR: Injury to the popliteal artery associated with dislocation of the knee: Palpable distal pulses do not negate the requirement for arteriography. *Injury* 1989;20:307-310.

14. Treiman GS, Yellin AE, Weaver FA, et al: Examination of the patient with a knee dislocation: The case for selective arteriography. *Arch Surg* 1992;127:1056-1062.

    The authors studied 115 patients with knee dislocations. Ninety percent of those with normal pulses had a normal arteriogram and 59% of those with abnormal pulses required vascular repair.

15. Downs AR, MacDonald P: Popliteal artery injuries: Civilian experience with sixty-three patients during a twenty-four year period (1960 through 1984). *J Vasc Surg* 1986;4:55-62.

16. Bryan T, Merritt P, Hack B: Popliteal arterial injuries associated with fractures or dislocations about the knee as a result of blunt trauma. *Orthop Rev* 1991;20:525-530.

17. Peck JJ, Eastman AB, Bergan JJ, et al: Popliteal vascular trauma: A community experience. *Arch Surg* 1990;125:1339-1344.

    In a series of 108 patients from 5 regional centers, amputation correlated with nerve, vein, and soft-tissue injury.

18. Frassica FJ, Sim FH, Staeheli JW, et al: Dislocation of the knee. *Clin Orthop* 1991;263:200-205.

    The authors reported on 13 patients repaired within 5 days. Avulsions were reattached to bone and midsubstance tears were repaired. In three patients with midsubstance PCL ruptures, PCL repair augmented. Immobilization averaged 8 weeks. Two patients regained full motion. The average flexion was 112° (75° to 140°) and three patients had a flexion contracture of 10° or more. Four patients had minimal amounts of instability. Eleven (91%) of the 12 patients available for follow-up had good or excellent results.

19. Applebaum R, Yellin AE, Weaver FA, et al: Role of routine arteriography in blunt lower-extremity trauma. *Am J Surg* 1990;160:221-225.

20. Rose SC, Moore EE: Trauma angiography: The use of clinical findings to improve patient selection and case preparation. *J Trauma* 1988;28:240-245.

    In 173 patients with normal pulses and various injuries (blunt and penetrating), 15 (9%) had vascular injury. In 74 patients with a fracture and a clinical sign (usually a diminished pulse), 51% had a vascular injury. On the basis of 7 patients, it was concluded that knee dislocation is a separate indication for arteriogram.

21. Kendall RW, Taylor DC, Salvian AJ, et al: The role of arteriography in assessing vascular injuries associated with dislocations or the knee. *J Trauma* 1993;35:875–878.
22. Meek AC, Robbs JV: Vascular injury with associated bone and joint trauma. *Br J Surg* 1984;71:341–344.
23. Frykberg ER, Crump JM, Dennis JW, et al: Nonoperative observation of clinically occult arterial injuries: A prospective evaluation. *Surgery* 1991;109:85–96.

    Excellent review of nonoperative treatment for nonocclusive vascular injuries.

24. Stain SC, Yellin AE, Weaver FA, et al: Selective management of nonocclusive arterial injuries. *Arch Surg* 1989;124:1136–1141.

    Excellent review of arteriographic findings that may be treated expectantly.

25. Dennis JW, Jagger C, Butcher JL, et al: Reassessing the role of arteriograms in the management of posterior knee dislocations. *J Trauma* 1993;35:692–697.

    The authors reviewed 38 cases of posterior dislocation. Only those with hard signs of ischemia required surgery. 35% incidence of nonocclusive vascular injury in patients with normal pulses.

26. Lynch K, Johansen K: Can Doppler pressure measurement replace "exclusion" arteriography in the diagnosis of occult extremity arterial trauma? *Ann Surg* 1991;214:737–741.
27. Lohmann M, Lauridsen K, Vedel P: Arterial lesions in major knee trauma: Pedal pulse a false sign of security? *Arch Orthop Trauma Surg* 1990;109:238–239.
28. Fernandez EJ, Nadal RD, Gonzalez SM, et al: The effect of stasis on a microvascular anastomosis. *Microsurgery* 1983;4:176–177.
29. Cooper DE, Speer KP, Wickiewicz TL, et al: Complete knee dislocation without posterior cruciate ligament disruption: A report of four cases and review of the literature. *Clin Orthop* 1992;284:228–233.

    Four cases of anterior or anterolateral dislocation with competent PCL. The PCL was partially torn (avg 25%) in 3/4.

30. Shelbourne KD, Pritchard J, Rettig AC, et al: Knee dislocations with intact PCL. *Orthop Rev* 1992;21:607–611.

    The authors present a treatment approach based on regaining motion and strength, followed by delayed PCL reconstruction. Two of 3 patients returned to their previous athletic level. The results for all methods of treatment in this group of patients were betteer than those reported for high-energy injuries; flexion averaged 125° with a minimum of 110°; 77% of patients returned to athletics; pain and stiffness, not instability, were the predominant complaints. The applicability to high-energy dislocations has yet to be determined.

31. Bratt HD, Newman AP: Complete dislocation of the knee without disruption of both cruciate ligaments. *J Trauma* 1993;34:383–389.
32. Girgis FG, Marshall JL, Monajem A: The cruciate ligaments of the knee joint: Anatomical, functional, and experimental analysis. *Clin Orthop* 1975;106:216–231.
33. Taylor AR, Arden GP, Rainey HA: Traumatic dislocation of the knee: A report of forty-three cases with special reference to conservative treatment. *J Bone Joint Surg* 1972;54B:96–102.
34. Roman PD, Hopson CN, Zenni EJ Jr: Traumatic dislocation of the knee: A report of 30 cases and literature review. *Orthop Rev* 1987;16:917–924.

    The authors presented 14 patients treated with complete ligamentous repair. At final follow-up, 86% had no laxity but motion was poor. Six patients (43%) lacked 90° of motion and had flexion contractures of 8° to 20°. All but one of these patients had transarticular Steinmann pins for 8 weeks. Patients immobilized without the use of pins had better motion.

35. Thomsen PB, Rud B, Jensen UH: Stability and motion after traumatic dislocation of the knee. *Acta Orthop Scand* 1984;55:278–283.

    The authors studied five patients treated with primary repair. One patient had gross instability and two of the five complained of pain. Immobilization was for a shorter time and range of motion was greater than 100° in all five.

36. DeLee JC, Riley MB, Rockwood CA Jr: Acute posterolateral rotatory instability of the knee. *Am J Sports Med* 1983;11:199–207.
37. Hughston JC, Jacobson KE: Chronic posterolateral rotatory instability of the knee. *J Bone Joint Surg* 1985;67A:351–359.
38. Terranova WA, McLaughlin RE, Morgan RF: An algorithm for the management of ligamentous injuries of the knee associated with common peroneal nerve palsy. *Orthopedics* 1986;9:1135–1140.
39. Ninkovic M, Sucur D, Starovic B, et al: A new approach to persistent traumatic peroneal nerve palsy. *Br J Plastic Surg* 1994;47:185–189.
40. Sedel L, Nizard RS: Nerve grafting for traction injuries of the common peroneal nerve: A report of 17 cases. *J Bone Joint Surg* 1993;75B:772–774.

    Seventeen patients had multiple sural nerve cable grafts of 7 to 20 cm for peroneal n. repair with complete recovery in 38%, partial recovery in 41%, and no recovery in 31%.

41. Wood MB: Peroneal nerve repair: Surgical results. *Clin Orthop* 1991;267:206–210.

    Good results were obtained in 55% of patients.

42. Noyes FR, Cummings JF, Grood ES, et al: The diagnosis of knee motion limits, subluxations, and ligament injury. *Am J Sports Med* 1991;19:163–171.

    Even for experienced examiners, physical examination of complex knee ligament injuries is difficult. Combined ACL/MCL injuries were misdiagnosed as posterolateral instability by seven of 11 examiners.

15
Injuries to the Patella and Extensor Mechanism

Introduction

Patellar fractures and extensor mechanism injuries account for more than 1% of the fractures diagnosed and treated every year.[1] These injuries are caused by many diverse forces: direct blows, falls, dashboard impacts, and longitudinal forces from powerful quadriceps contractions. While direct primary repair of patellar tendon and quadriceps tendon ruptures is standard, no consensus has been reached concerning treatment for displaced patellar fractures. Treatment has included closed extension casting/splinting, external fixation, internal fixation, and patellar excision with primary soft-tissue repairs. Pauwel's method of anterior tension band wiring[2] and Weber's[3] subsequent modification have been the basis for most fracture treatment procedures. The current trend is to make every effort to save some if not all of the patella, even if the fracture is very comminuted.

Anatomy

The patella is the largest sesamoid bone. It is pear-shaped with the broadest aspect oriented proximally and with a gradual taper distally to a nonarticular apex, which serves as the origin for the patellar tendon. The articular surface is divided into three facets: medial, lateral, and odd. The lateral is the largest of the three facets, occupying more than 50% of the total articular surface. In the normal patella, the thickness of the articular cartilage is greater than 1 cm. The patella is firmly invested in a strong fascial structure—formed by a coalition of the quadriceps tendon, the fascia lata, and the iliotibial band—to form the joint capsule and the strong expansions known as the medial and lateral retinaculi. The discrete patellar tendon originates at the apex of the patella and inserts into the tibial tubercle. The quadriceps tendon, the patella and its investing soft tissues, and the patellar tendon are collectively called the extensor mechanism. The primary blood supply is based on a dorsal ring formed by the geniculate arteries, however, a significant secondary supply enters via the nonarticular posterior surface of the apex.[4]

Evaluation

The chief complaint of patients with a patellar fracture or an extensor mechanism injury is acute knee pain and swelling after trauma. A secondary complaint is commonly the inability to extend or straighten the knee. Knee effusions are dependent on an intact joint capsule; if the soft tissues are disrupted, the effusion is replaced by diffuse periarticular swelling. A complete physical examination should be performed from hip to ankle to identify associated injuries. Close attention should be paid to the skin to identify small puncture wounds. These skin breaks portend an open fracture unless proven by surgical exploration not to be communicated with the fracture site, fracture hematoma, or joint. Open fractures of the patella are treated like all open fractures: a surgical urgency with irrigation, debridement, and antibiotics.

Palpation will identify soft-tissue defects associated with quadriceps tendon or patella tendon ruptures as well as fracture displacement. All patients should be asked to do an active straight leg lift. The inability to actively raise the leg indicates an injury to the extensor mechanism that requires surgical consideration. Patients must not internally or externally rotate the leg in order to use secondary extensors in the iliotibial band and adductor muscle groups. Intra-articular injection of a local anesthetic may make this exercise more tolerable to the patient.

Patients in whom a patellar fracture or an extensor mechanism injury is suspected are evaluated with anteroposterior (AP), lateral, and "sunrise" radiographs. The lateral view is scrutinized for fracture lines, fracture displacement, and patellar position. The sunrise view is most helpful with vertical fracture lines and displacement. A confusing finding is the congenital bipartite or tripartite patella. This abnormality has one or two fragments in the superior lateral corner that are irregular in shape with smooth edges. The bipartite patella has an incidence of 8% and is routinely bilateral. If there is doubt as to the presence of a fracture, a comparison view will usually differentiate between fracture and bipartite patella. In addition to visible signs of fracture, the radiograph should be scrutinized for the position of the patella. A baja, or low-riding, patella is indicative of a quadriceps tendon rupture. An alta, or high-riding, patella is a sign of a patella tendon rupture.

Other imaging studies used to evaluate the patella and extensor mechanism include plain radiographs, tomography, computed tomography, bone scans, and magnetic resonance imaging (MRI). All but MRI have little clinical efficacy. MRI has been used to identify ruptures of both quadriceps and patellar tendons, which is clinically useful because quadriceps tendon ruptures are difficult to diagnose and can be easily missed.

Mechanism of Injury

The geometric pattern of the fracture is determined by the direction of the injuring force on the patella and extensor mechanism. Most patellar fractures are transverse at any point in the body of the patella. Transverse fractures are caused by excessive longitudinal forces and are best identified on the anteroposterior radiograph. Polar fractures are avulsion fractures of either the base or apex. In both transverse and polar fractures, the amount of displacement is correlated, if present, with the injury to the soft tissues. Wide displacement is associated with disruption of the retinaculum as well as extensor mechanism. Occasionally, the base or apex fractures are so small as to best represent disruptions of the quadriceps or patella tendons rather than true fractures. Vertical fractures are caused by a direct blow in a partially flexed knee and are rarely displaced.[5] These fractures can easily be missed and are best identified on the sunrise view.

Stellate fractures are caused by a high-energy direct blow to the patella. Because energy is transmitted, there is commonly an associated injury to the femoral condyles. Since this is a direct blow, the soft-tissue envelope is usually intact and the fracture is not displaced. If displaced, however, as with the transverse fractures, the amount of displacement is directly related to the integrity of the extensor mechanism soft tissues.

Fracture Classification

Most fracture classifications are simple descriptive terms of the fracture pattern or location. No classification system has been widely accepted. The literature comparisons are based not on type of fracture, but type of treatment. A simple treatment-directed classification is nondisplaced and displaced.[6] Displacement is defined as a fracture separation of more than 3 mm and an articular incongruity of 2 mm. Displaced fractures can be subdivided by the descriptive geometric terms of vertical, transverse, polar, or stellate. Nondisplaced fractures can be similarly described, but such description is unnecessary because it does not help with planning treatment or predicting outcome.

Treatment

Nondisplaced Fractures
Nondisplaced patella fractures are treated nonsurgically. Treatment consists of a cylinder cast for 6 to 8 weeks

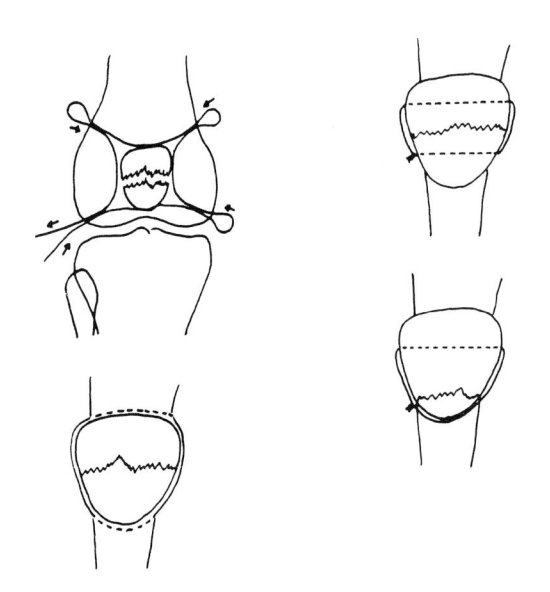

Fig. 1 Ma technique for percutaneous suture treatment of patellar fractures. (Reproduced with permission from Ma Y-Z, Thang YF: Treatment of fractures of the patella with percutaneous suture. *Clin Orthop* 1984;191:235-241.)

and then active rather than passive motion is begun. This treatment has had excellent and good results in more than 95% of the cases.[1] Functional bracing using progressive active range of motion has been used with equal results. The reported results are based on subjective functional outcome as opposed to objective measurement of range of motion, knee stability, or strength.

Displaced Fractures

Vertical Displaced vertical fractures are rare. Anatomic open reduction and internal fixation (ORIF) using the classic lag screw technique is the treatment of choice. Both 4-mm partially threaded cancellous and 3.5-mm cortical screw have been used successfully. A functional knee brace with early motion is used postoperatively. The knee is held in full extension until the wound heals sufficiently to allow motion, usually 10 days. The brace is continued for 6 weeks. Disruption of the extensor mechanism in a displaced vertical fracture is extremely rare. If the patient is unable to perform a straight leg lift, the extensor mechanism should be explored and repaired at the time of fracture fixation.

Transverse Fractures The classic midpatella displaced transverse fracture with loss of the extensor mechanisms has been treated using many methods and has been subjected to intense study. Closed treatment of these injuries has been abandoned because of poor results secondary to pain, nonunion, and loss of extension and strength. External fixation, initially described by Malgaine and abandoned with the advent of newer techniques, has recently been revisited by Quan-Yi and Ha-Wen.[7] Transverse percutaneous pins were connected to an external compression device after open reduction. This method produced good and excellent results in 26 of 27 patients when judged using a functional evaluation for pain, limp, and job performance.

The current treatment of choice is anatomic ORIF using the modified tension band technique. This method involves the use of parallel vertical K-wires at the midpatella with either a figure-of-eight or box-type anterior tension band. The box-type is recommended over the classic figure-of-eight tension band due to a decrease in anterior knee discomfort. The box technique does not change the need for hardware removal. A modification using 3.5-mm cannulated lag screws in place of vertical K-wires and an intrascrew (wire passed through the screw guide wire hole) "tension band" has shown excellent results.[8] (Although the wire through the screws does meet the classic description of a tension band, it is not accepted as such by many authors.) Postoperative care involves a period of immobilization in full extension and then controlled active therapy to regain range of motion. In those with excellent fixation of the fracture, early (10 days to 2 weeks) active range of motion in either a functional knee brace or in a controlled therapy environment has been advocated. If fixation stability is questionable at the time of wound closure, however, the patient should remain in extension casting or splinting for the first 4 weeks and then should begin controlled motion. Total time of bracing is 6 to 8 weeks and total recovery of motion and strength takes a minimum of 1 full year and many times longer.

The long-term outcome of this type of treatment has uniformly produced excellent results in 30% to 40%, good results in 30% to 40%, and poor results in 25%.[9,10] Absorbable (2 Vicryl) suture has been used in place of wire in an attempt to reduce the need for hardware removal. Results have equaled those of wire.[11] In all reports, the retinacular defect, if present, was primarily repaired along with patellar fracture fixation. This was thought to be a critical step. A percutaneous cerclage wiring technique (Fig. 1) reported in 1984 involved closed reduction of the fracture and no retinacular repair. The results of late follow-up of 81 of 107 fractures paralleled those of ORIF[12] with soft tissue repair.

Vertical comminution of a proximal or distal section of a transverse fracture by secondary fracture lines is treated using transverse lag screw(s) to convert a three-part fracture into a classic transverse fracture pattern, which is then treated as outlined above. Severe comminution of a segment in which the joint surface is not reconstructable is best treated by either a distal or proximal pole patellectomy, as indicated. The quadriceps tendon or patellar tendon should then be reattached with a modified Krakow suture and passed through drill holes in the patella. The tendon must be repaired to the midsubstance of the patella to prevent the remaining patella from impinging on the femoral condyles during motion. Distal pole patellectomies should be protected by McLaughlin (box-type) or AO (figure-of-eight type) wires or nonabsorbable sutures. In either case, the suture should pass as close as possible to the superior border of the patella or to a transverse drill hole in the patella.

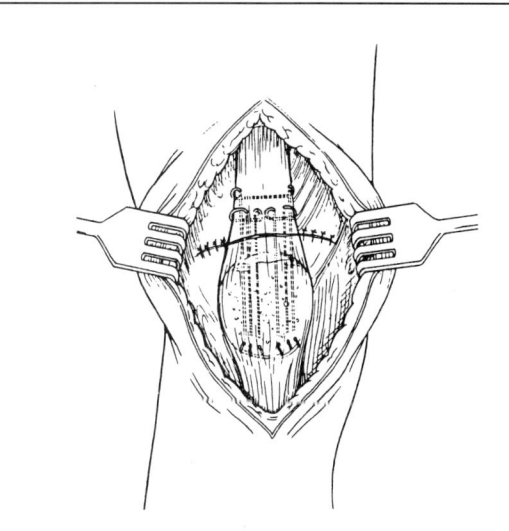

Fig. 2 Haas method for repair of quadriceps tendon rupture. (Reproduced with permission from Haas SB, Callaway H: Disruptions of the extensor mechanism. *Orthop Clin North Am* 1992;23:687-695.)

Initial postoperative treatment of a partial patellectomy and repair of the extensor mechanism is full extension for 6 weeks and then active extension. A study in 1988 recommended that a load-sharing cable be added to the treatment of transverse fractures of the patella because it improved the stability of the fracture fixation, avoided the need for casting, and allowed earlier motion. While no long-term clinical trials have shown the benefit of this treatment method, 13 of 14 patellae treated in this manner healed without complication.[13]

Historical results from partial patellectomies are similar in most series, with excellent results in 20% to 30%, good results in 40% to 50%, and poor results in 20% to 25%.[14,15] Saltzman and associates[16] were able to correlate subjective functional outcomes of a partial patellectomy directly to isokinetic strength.

Stellate Fractures

Stellate fractures are a heterogeneous group and present a difficult decision for all surgeons. The basic treatment philosophy has been to retain the largest possible congruous piece or pieces of the patella using multiple techniques, including K-wires, lag screws, tension bands, and cerclage wires. An aggressive attempt at fixation should be made to produce and retain at least one section of patella. No critical or minimum size has been determined, however, the data clearly show that a smooth articular surface is necessary if any part of the patella is to be retained. If an articular surface reduction of less than 2 mm of step-off cannot be obtained and maintained, a total patellectomy should be performed. The remaining retinacular soft tissues are then repaired. Postoperatively, the patellectomy patient is braced in full extension for 4 weeks and then allowed 30° of active flexion for 4 weeks. The brace is removed at 8 weeks and the patient is begun on full active assist motion.

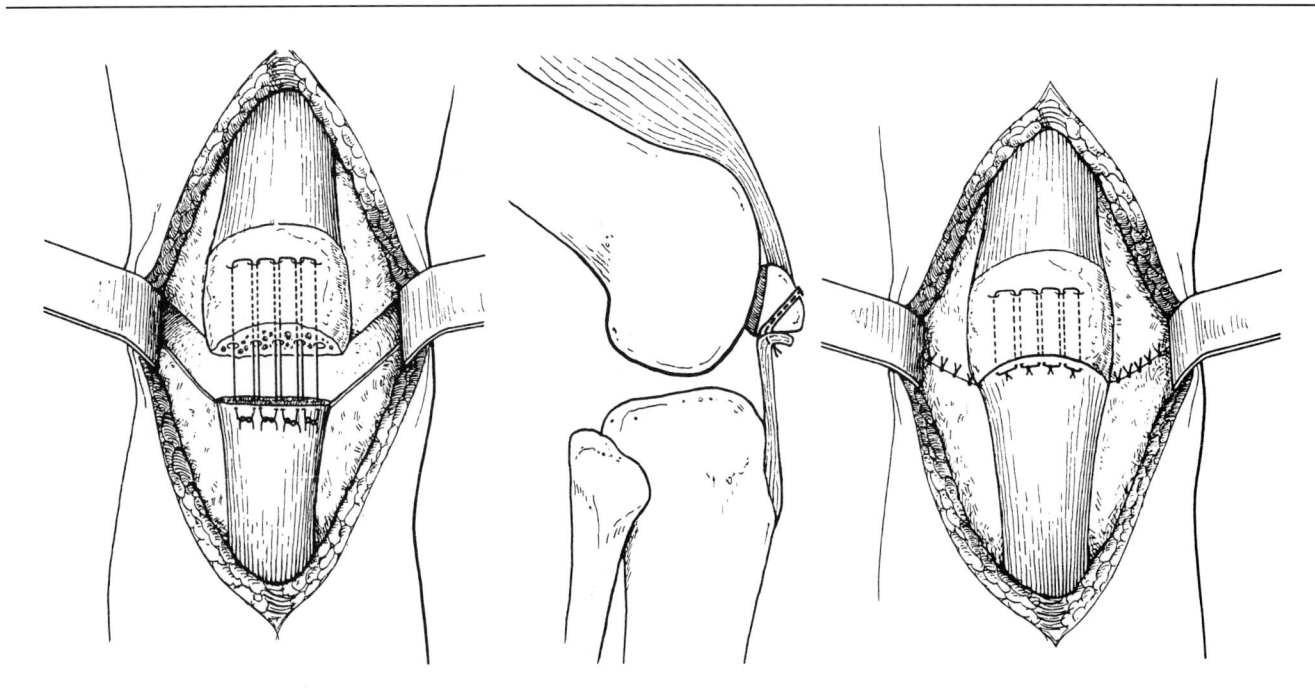

Fig. 3 Saltzman method for patellar tendon repair. **Left,** The retained fragment is approximated to the tendon with large, nonabsorbable sutures. **Center,** Drill holes are oriented to reattach the tendon close to the articular surface. **Right,** Quadriceps expansions are completely repaired. (Reproduced with permission from Saltzman CL, Goulet JA, McClellan RT, et al: Results of treatment of displaced patellar fractures by partial patellectomy. *J Bone Joint Surg* 1990;72A:1279-1285.)

Most results from total patellectomy parallel very closely the results from partial patellectomies.[17] However, a recent study of 17 patients showed excellent results in 88% at 12 years. This may be related to the fact that Wilkinson[18] showed that maximum recovery may require 3 years and the usual follow-up is done at 2 years. Further long-term follow-up of this issue is indicated because recent results have varied widely.

Nonunion

Nonunions of patellar fractures are rare and no large study exists. Nonunions are treated as indicated by the fracture type and displacement. In all cases, the remaining patella should have minimal chondromalacia, and the reduction should have less than 2 mm of step-off. Satku and Kumar[19] described three patients with patellar nonunions that were treated with classic modified tension band technique with excellent results.

Patellar Dislocations

True acute traumatic patellar dislocations are extremely rare. Acute traumatic lateral dislocations should be reduced with full extension of the knee and gentle downward pressure on the lateral surface of the patella. The knee and the postreduction radiographs are then carefully re-examined.

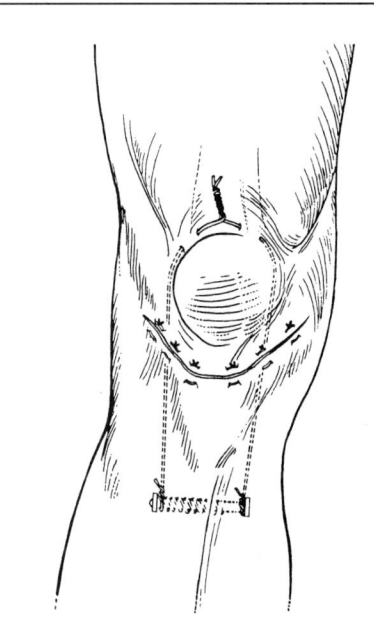

Fig. 4 Classic McLaughlin wire technique. (Reproduced with permission from Haas SB, Callaway H: Disruptions of the extensor mechanism. *Orthop Clin North Am* 1992;23:687-695.)

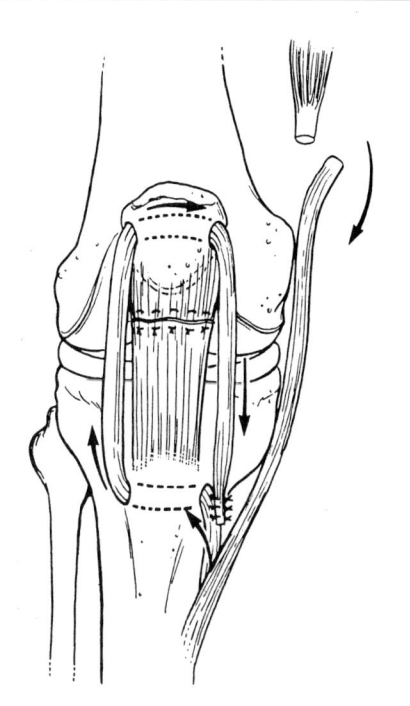

Fig. 5 Kelikian technique for augmentation of patellar tendon repair. (Reproduced with permission from Haas SB, Callaway H: Disruptions of the extensor mechanism. *Orthop Clin North Am* 1992;23:687-695.)

The examiner must be careful not to lift the patella back into the groove because this can change a simple lateral dislocation into an intra-articular vertical dislocation.[20] Iatrogenic and traumatic vertical dislocation are extremely rare and reduction requires direct mechanical forces, such as a Schanz screw or towel clip.[21] After reduction, the leg is placed in a cylinder cast in full extension for 6 weeks and then an aggressive quadriceps rehabilitation program is begun.

Examination under anesthesia and arthroscopy are helpful to identify osteochondral fractures, retinacular tears, and vastus medialis obliquus (VMO) avulsions. A simple retinacular tear can be treated nonsurgically with extension bracing for 6 weeks. A VMO torn from the superior medial patella should be surgically repaired. The leg then should be treated with a full extension brace or cast for 6 weeks. Isometric quadriceps exercises in the brace should begin as soon as pain permits.

Rupture of the Quadriceps Tendon

Rupture of the quadriceps tendon is rare and is commonly missed on initial presentation. More than 80% of the patients are older than 40 years of age and many have preexisting medical conditions, such as renal failure. The tendon usually ruptures in an area of preexisting tendonosis. Only one third are diagnosed correctly at the first visit.[22] Most patients are able to straighten the knee using secondary extensors, but are unable to do a voluntary straight leg lift. Young patients usually give a history similar to that of an Achilles tendon rupture in that they feel like they were struck or kicked at the time of tendon failure. A recent study by Kaneko and associates[22] gave four radiographic signs of rupture: patella baja, obliteration of quadriceps tendon shadow, suprapatellar calcification, and suprapatellar mass. In a retrospective review, three of the four signs were present in all missed cases. Berlin and associates[23] have described an MRI finding of corrugated patellar tendon suggestive of rupture of the quadriceps tendon.

Treatment of quadriceps tendon rupture is early primary surgical repair. One recommended method is to use three Bunnel sutures in the quadriceps tendon, passing the suture through the patella after a cancellous trough has been made to accept the tendon (Fig. 2). The leg is immobilized in full extension for 6 to 8 weeks and then active assist-only flexion is begun. No passive knee flexion is done because it risks loss of repair. Quadriceps strengthening is not done until after the cast is removed. Results from early repair are uniformly good in more than 90% of the cases. It is important to do an early repair to prevent the retraction of the quadriceps muscle, which can lead to difficult reconstruction. Late surgical repair using quadriceps tendon turndown procedures led to poorer results in almost all cases.[24] A high index of suspicion, careful review of the initial radiographs, and early repair can avoid this complication.

Patellar Tendon Rupture

Patellar tendon ruptures are rare. In contrast to the quadriceps rupture, these injuries occur in patients younger than 40 years old who are athletically active. Steroid injections in and around the patellar tendon have been implicated in patellar tendon ruptures. Early diagnosis via history, physical examination, and radiographs is important. Delayed diagnosis will lead to contraction of the quadriceps muscle and retraction of the patella.

Early repair can be accomplished easily with direct repair using Krakow or modified Kessler sutures anchored into the patella via drill holes (Fig. 3). The repair should be protected via a rectangular (McLaughlin) (Fig. 4) or figure-of-eight (AO) wire. Timing of wire removal has varied between 8 weeks and 6 months; the most common recommendation is 10 to 12 weeks. Postoperative care and rehabilitation is accomplished as in a quadriceps tendon rupture. Late repair is accomplished with preoperative skeletal traction through the patella until the patella is at the normal position. A direct repair is accomplished and augmented in the way of Kelikian with semitendinous and/or gracilis (Fig. 5). The leg is again treated in full extension for 6 to 8 weeks and then active-assist flexion rehabilitation is started. Long-term results are much better for early primary repair than for late repair and augmentation.

Annotated References

1. Bostrom A: Fractures of the patella: A study of 422 fractures. *Acta Orthop Scand* 1972;143(suppl):1-80.

    The authors present an exceptional review of more than 400 patellar fractures treated surgically (203) and nonsurgically (219). This paper is the basis of the current view of surgically treated outcomes of patellar fractures.

2. Mueller M, et al: Fractures of the patella, in *Manual of Internal Fixation*, ed 3. Berlin, Germany, Springer-Verlag, 1991.

3. Weber MJ, Janecki CJ, McLeod P, et al: Efficacy of various forms of fixation of transverse fractures of the patella. *J Bone Joint Surg* 1980;62A:215-220.

    This is the classic article on the modified tension band. This paper compared the biomechanics and subjective stability of four forms of patella fixation: cerclage, Magnusson technique, classic tension band, and modified tension band. The authors determined that the Magnusson and modified tension band were better but almost equal and that the retinacular repair contributes to the stability of the fracture fixation.

4. Scapinelli R: Blood supply of the human patella: Its relation to ischaemic necrosis after fracture. *J Bone Joint Surg* 1967;49B:563-570.

5. Dowd GS: Marginal fractures of the patella. *Injury* 1982;14:287-291.

6. Sanders R: Patella fractures and extensor mechanism injuries, in Browner BD, Jupiter JB, Levine AM, et al (eds): *Skeletal Trauma: Fractures, Dislocations, Ligamentous Injuries*. Philadelphia, PA, WB Saunders, 1992, vol 2, pp 1685-1716.

7. Liang QY, Wu JU: Fractures of the patella treated by open reduction and external compressive skeletal fixation. *J Bone Joint Surg* 1987;69A:83-89.

8. Berg EE, Bassett T: Fixation of displaced transverse patellar fractures: Anterior wiring through cannulated screws. *South Orthop J* 1993;2:197-199.

9. Bostman O, Kivilutoto O, Santavirta S, et al: Fractures of the patella treated by operation. *Arch Orthop Trauma Surg* 1983;102:78-81.

10. Levack B, Flanagan JP, Hobbs S: Results of surgical treatment of patella fractures. *J Bone Joint Surg* 1985;67B:416-419.

11. Wissing JC, van der Werken C: Tension band osteosynthesis of resorbable material. *Unfallchirug* 1991;94:45-46.

12. Ma YZ, Zhang YF, Qu KF, et al: Treatment of fractures of the patella with percutaneous suture. *Clin Orthop* 1984;191:235-241.

13. Perry CR, McCarthy JA, Kain CC, et al: Patella fixation protected with a load sharing cable: A mechanical and clinical trial. *J Orthop Trauma* 1988;2:234-240.

14. Canton S, Larch C, Lavage P, et al: Patellectomy: Results of a long-term follow-up. *Can J Surg* 1993;36:461-463.

15. Pandey AK, Pandey S, Pandey P: Results of partial patellectomy. *Arch Orthop Trauma Surg* 1991;110:246-249.

16. Saltzman CL, Goulet JA, McClellan RT: Results of treatment of displaced patellar fractures by partial patellectomy. *J Bone Joint Surg* 1990;72A:1279-1285.

17. Mishra US: Late results of patellectomy in fractured patella. *Acta Orthop Scand* 1972;43:256-263.

18. Wilkinson J: Fracture of the patella treated by total excision: A long-term follow-up. *J Bone Joint Surg* 1977;59B:352-354.

19. Satku K, Kumar V: Surgical management of non-union of neglected fractures of the patella. *Injury* 1991;22:108-110.

20. Feneley RC: Intra-articular dislocation of the patella: A case report. *J Bone Joint Surg* 1968;50B:653-655.

21. Alioto RJ, Kates S: Intra-articular vertical dislocation of the patella: A case report of an irreducible patellar dislocation and unique surgical technique. *J Trauma* 1994;36:282-284.

22. Kaneko K, DeMouy EH, Brunet ME, et al: Radiographic diagnosis of quadriceps tendon rupture: Analysis of diagnostic failure. *J Emerg Med* 1994;12:225-229.

23. Berlin RC, Levinsohn EM, Chrisman H: The wrinkled patellar tendon: An indication of abnormality in the extensor mechanism of the knee. *Skeletal Radiol* 1991;20:181-185.

24. Haas SB, Callaway H: Disruptions of the extensor mechanism. *Orthop Clin North Am* 1992;23:687-695.

    The authors present an extensive review of both quadriceps and patella tendon disruption and methods of repair and provide an excellent discussion and description of multiple methods for early and late repairs of the disruptions. Included are both new and classic methods for protection of repairs.

16
Fractures of the Tibial Plateau

Introduction

A plateau fracture involves the articular surface of the proximal tibia that supports the opposing femoral condyle. The medial and/or lateral condyles may be involved. Biomechanical studies using cadavers have shown that the observed fracture patterns can be generated through the application of varus-valgus loading either alone or combined with axial compression.[1] Severe fractures involving both condyles are usually caused by axial forces.

The age and gender distribution of patients with this injury appear to show a bimodal pattern. The peak incidence in men occurs in the fourth decade, reflecting high-energy trauma; the peak incidence in women occurs in the seventh decade and typically involves osteopenic fractures.[2] The left knee is more often injured than the right (60% versus 40%),[2,3] which may reflect the position of the motor vehicle driver. The mechanism of injury in urban settings is nearly equally divided between falls, motor vehicle accidents, and pedestrian impacts. Sports injuries are the cause in only 5% to 10%.

Injury Assessment

General

As in all traumatic injuries, evaluation must include a general history and assessment of the patient and a search for associated visceral, spinal, and extremity injuries. In particular, the status of the leg compartments, peroneal and tibial nerves, and distal pulses must be evaluated. A general ligament examination should be performed with particular attention to varus-valgus instability in full extension. Some plateau fractures have associated ligament injuries, which are not apparent on initial radiographic evaluation and that render them functional knee dislocations; when recognized,[4] arteriography should be considered.

Imaging

Evaluation of a tibial plateau fracture involves careful imaging to classify the fracture accurately and to determine the most effective treatment plan. Degree of involvement of both medial and lateral plateaus, intercondylar eminence, and posterior aspects of the condyles is crucial in planning treatment. Amount and location of articular depression, presence and location of split fracture lines, and axial alignment of the condyles will all affect clinical decision-making.

Anteroposterior (AP), lateral, and 45° oblique views are standard. Angulation of the X-ray beam to match the 10° to 14° posterior slope of the proximal tibia constitutes the tibial plateau view and is recommended in addition to the AP view in order to obtain accurate data regarding the amount of depression of the articular surface. Error associated with using the AP radiograph to determine the amount of depression of a portion of articular surface can be substantial. In the case of a 10-mm depression, an AP radiograph will overestimate the depression by as much as 50% compared to the plateau view.

The amount of depression visible on the AP view also depends on the position of the central ray with respect to the tibial crest. The amount of posterior depression is magnified and the amount of anterior depression is underestimated if the beam is centered below the joint line. On routine AP projections, a "shadow" appears across the joint space of the medial compartment. This shadow is cast by the anterior rim of the concave medial articular surface and is not seen on a properly angled tibial plateau view. Absence of this shadow is proof that the central ray is tangent to the articular surface.[5]

Plain radiographs usually do not provide a complete picture of the injury. Lateral and AP tomography at 5-mm intervals has been the traditional adjunct to plain radiographs. The addition of tomography to plain radiographs has been shown to yield new information which affects clinical decision-making in about 75% of cases.[6] Unfortunately, tomography can be uncomfortable for the patient. Total time for AP and lateral tomograms is about 45 minutes. Patients must be placed on their side for the lateral images, and this can be painful for a patient with an unstable knee.

Computed tomography (CT) has been used increasingly to evaluate fractures of the tibial plateau.[7-9] The recommended technique is to place the patient supine on the scanner with the well leg flexed. This allows acquisition of an unobstructed scout lateral of the injured leg. The posterior slope of the tibial articular surface is determined from the lateral scout allowing accurate tilting of the gantry to obtain images that are tangent to the articular surface. Recommended slice thickness is 5 mm or less. Images obtained in this way allow the amount of depression to be calculated by subtracting the gantry position of the cut containing the depressed segment from the cut of the intact condyle. This information can also be obtained by direct measurement from images reformatted in the sagittal or coronal planes.

In studies where both plain tomography and CT were performed, CT was found to be superior in delineating the borders of depressed segments. The addition of CT imaging changed the classification of the fracture in 15% and treatment in 10%. CT is generally better tolerated by the patient in that it requires no change in position, the splints can be left on, and the total scan time is less than 20 minutes on most current machines. From a physician's perspective, CT images are easier to review than tomograms and the axial images correspond to the view seen at surgery (Fig. 1).

The possibility of simultaneously imaging the fracture as well as menisci and ligament injuries has led to increase in investigating magnetic resonance imaging (MRI) in tibial plateau fractures. A recent study compared axial CT (2-mm cuts) with coronal and sagittal MRI in 22 patients with fractures of the tibial plateau. Measurement of fracture depression from coronal or sagittal MRIs was direct and accurate. In the case of CT, measurement of fracture depression required counting of the axial images or measurement after two-dimensional reconstruction and was less precise than MRI. Accuracy was highly dependent on the thickness and interval of the CT images and quality of the two-dimensional reconstructions. In depicting fracture configuration, the two techniques were thought to be equivalent in 14 patients (64%). In 3 patients with complex and comminuted fractures, CT was found to show bone detail better than MRI. An axial fracture line missed by CT in 1 patient was readily shown in the sagittal and coronal MRI images. Complete ligament tears were noted in 8 (36%) of 22 patients with the majority being anterior cruciate ligament (ACL) and medial collateral ligament (MCL). Meniscal injuries were noted on MRI in 12 (55%) of patients in a lateral to medial ratio of 3:1. A high correlation was noted between MRI and surgical findings, with no false-negative MRI of soft-tissue injuries. The MRI was found to be more sensitive than physical examination or surgical findings in detecting associated injuries. Detecting injuries that have no clinical significance may be a problem with this technique. In most cases, MRI gives fracture information equivalent to that provided by CT. Use of MRI may obviate the need for diagnostic arthroscopy and may change treatment based on the soft-tissue information (Fig. 2).[10]

Classification

Classification of fractures of the tibial plateau is largely based on the site and direction of the fracture lines. The Schatzker classification[11] has been widely employed in reporting results and is familiar to most orthopaedic surgeons. The basic fracture types are shown in Figure 3. Three fracture types involve the lateral condyle: split fracture (type I), split-compression (type II), and compression fractures (type III). Fracture of the medial condyle, type IV, is further subdivided into type A, which is a high-energy fracture-dislocation, and type B, which is an osteoporotic compression fracture. Bicondylar fractures are divided into type V, in which the medial and lateral condyles are displaced similarly, and type VI, in which the metaphysis is separated from the diaphysis.

Except for type IVA, collateral and cruciate injuries are not intrinsically included as part of the classification, yet they can extend the severity of the injury along a spectrum from increased medial-lateral instability to fracture-dislocation with the attendant risks to neurovascular structures. Fracture-dislocations of the knee and their distinction from simple plateau fractures were described and classified by Moore in 1981.[4]

Subsequent authors have subdivided the bicondylar fractures into medially tilted, laterally tilted, and purely axially displaced, based on important differences in their natural history[12] (Fig. 4).

The AO group has recently adopted a universal alphanumeric classification system[13] that involves a systematic identification of fracture lines, displacement, and comminution. Extra-articular fractures are designated as A; partial articular fractures, as B; and fractures involving the entire articular surface, as C. Each group is divided into three groups by increasing complexity, designated 1, 2, or 3. Each of these groups is further subdivided into three subtypes (.1, .2, and .3). A total of 27 fracture types are identified, A1.1 through C3.3. The extra-articular group includes ligamentous avulsion fractures with the fibular head designated as A1.1, the tibial tuberosity as A1.2, and the intercondylar eminence as A1.3. This last classification is further subdivided, with A1.31 referring to an avulsion of the anterior cruciate insertion and A1.32 referring to an avulsion of the posterior cruciate insertion. Figure 5 displays the nine basic subtypes. Cruciate or collateral ligament injuries *not* associated with a bone avulsion are not included in this classification. Use of the universal classification system in reporting outcome studies in the future may allow better comparison of treatment methods between like fracture types than is possible with systems in current use.

Associated Injuries to the Meniscus and Ligaments

Maximal preservation of the meniscus is crucial to a lasting satisfactory outcome after a fracture of the tibial plateau. The spectrum of meniscal pathology associated with plateau fractures has been described recently.[14] Approximately 50% (17 of 36) of plateau fractures were found to have meniscal injuries that were amenable to surgical treatment. No correlation was noted between meniscal pathology and type of fracture or the presence

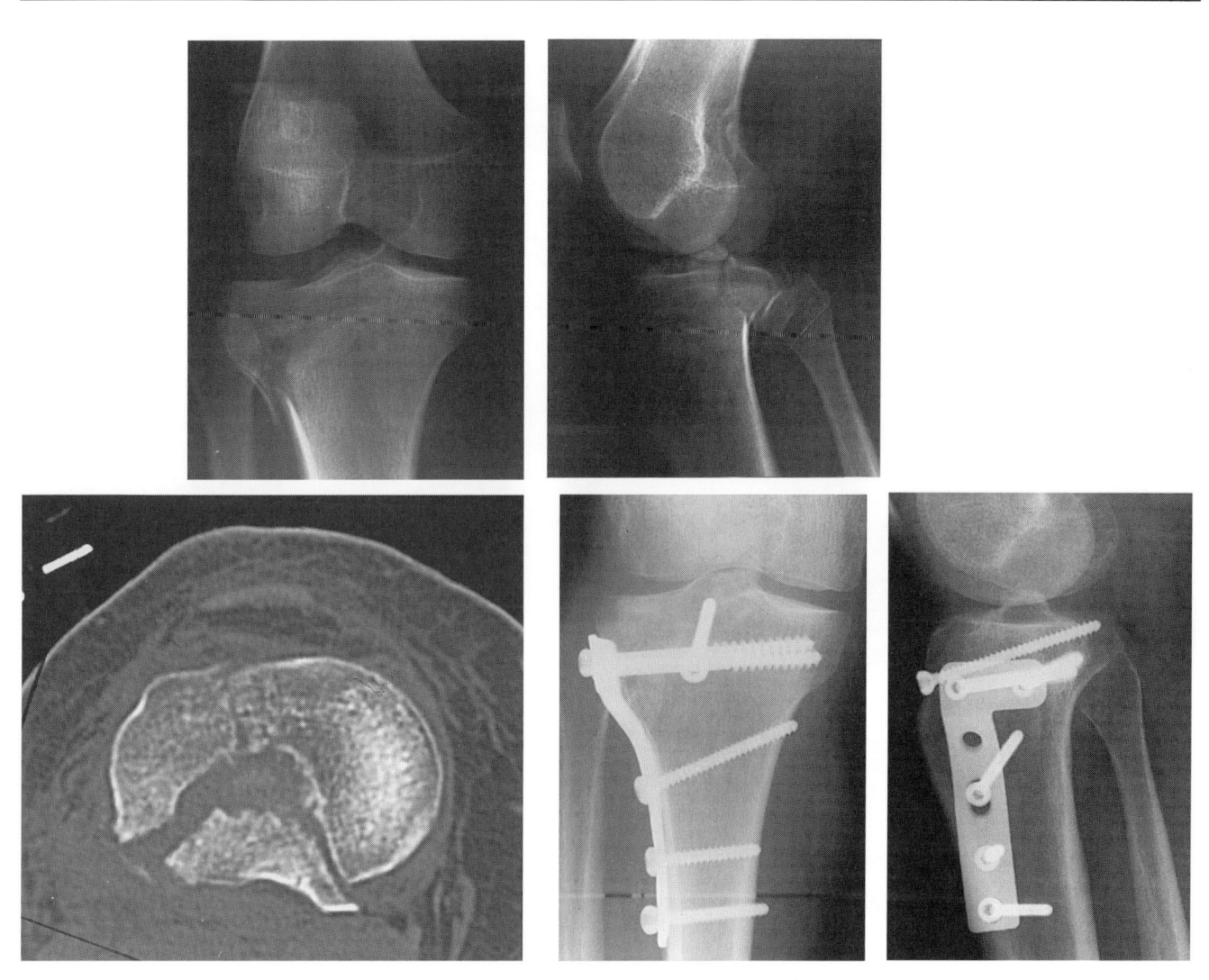

Fig. 1 Anteroposterior (**A**) and lateral (**B**) radiographs of a lateral split fracture with intercondylar extension. The axial CT scan (**C**) clearly delineates the size and location of the central posterior fragment, allowing indirect anatomic reduction and fixation of this fragment with a percutaneous lag screw (**D** and **E**) in conjunction with application of a lateral plate.

or absence of ligament injury. Most of the tears occurred in the posterior half and always on the side with the fractured condyle. The four medial tears were all complex tears associated with a medial plateau (Schatzker IV) fracture. Most tears occurred in the vascular region of the meniscus and were amenable to surgical repair. The remainder required partial resection.

The classic work of Kennedy and Bailey[1] suggests that an MCL injury concomitant with a lateral tibial plateau fracture would be very unusual. An intact collateral was thought to be necessary to act as a fulcrum to generate a compressive force on the lateral condyle. Subsequent series have shown that this injury combination may be clinically important and must be considered when a primarily varus or valgus mechanism is present.

A recent study correlated ligament injury with the type of plateau fracture.[15] In a series of 30 fractures, ten ligament injuries were recorded. The ACL injuries were associated with split depression (Schatzker II) and bicondylar fractures. Both bony avulsions and midsubstance injuries were noted. Preoperatively, four additional knees displayed a positive Lachman test, but this resolved after rigid fixation of the condyle. All of the MCL injuries occurred in either split or split depression (Schatzker I and II) fractures. The single lateral collateral ligament (LCL) injury occurred as expected in a medial plateau (Schatzker IV) fracture. Overall, the split depression and medial condyle fractures accounted for 80% of all ligament injuries in this study.

The incidence and long-term results of ligament injuries associated with fractures of the tibial plateau have recently

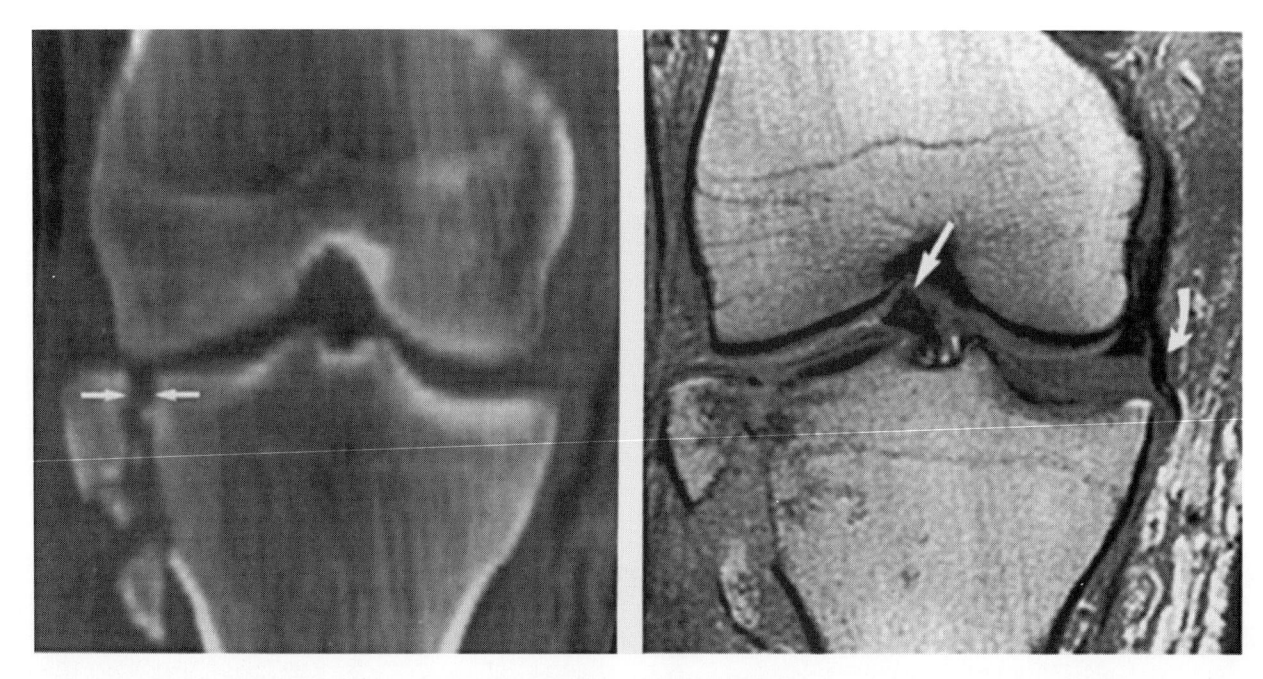

Fig. 2 A 27-year-old man with a split fracture of the lateral tibial plateau. The coronal reconstruction of an axial CT scan (**left**) shows 6-mm displacement of the fracture and bone fragments within the fracture. The coronal proton density-weighted MR image (**right**) shows a similar configuration of the fracture. In addition, a bucket-handle tear of the lateral (straight arrow) and a complete tear of the medial collateral ligament (curved arrow) were identified. Both tears were repaired at surgery. (Reproduced with permission from Kode L, Lieberman JM, Motta AO, et al: Evaluation of tibial plateau fractures: Efficacy of MR imaging compared with CT. *Am J Roentgenol* 1994;163:141–147.)

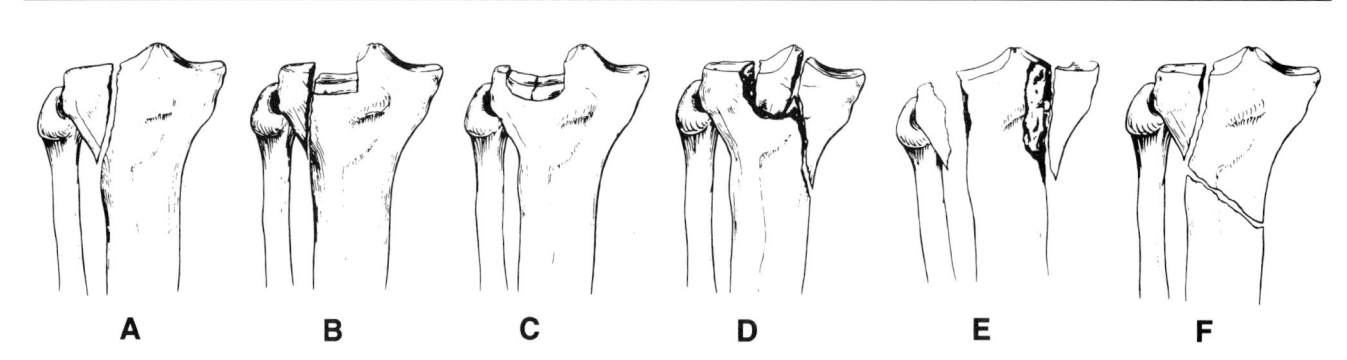

Fig. 3 Diagram of the Schatzker classification of tibial plateau fractures. **A,** Type I, cleavage of wedge fracture of the lateral tibial plateau. **B,** Type II, lateral split/depression fracture. **C,** Type III, pure central depression. **D,** Type IV, medial condyle fracture (may involve tibial spine). **E,** Type V, bicondylar fracture. **F,** Type VI, metaphyseal/diaphyseal disassociation. (Reproduced with permission from Schatzker J, McBroom R, Bruce D: The tibial plateau fracture: The Toronto experience 1968–1975. *Clin Orthop* 1979;138:94–104.)

been elucidated. In one study ligament injuries were identified in approximately 20% to 25% of tibial plateau fractures, with the MCL being the most commonly injured.[16] In a retrospective review, knees with unrepaired collateral ligaments were noted to have a poorer outcome with regard to both late instability and overall knee function compared to knees with surgical repair of their collateral ligament injuries at the time of open reduction and internal fixation of their fracture. No patient with a repaired MCL or LCL had late varus-valgus instability greater than 10°. All cruciate ligament injuries occurred as combined injuries and surgical repair of the cruciate did not improve outcome beyond repair of the collateral ligament alone. Patients with cruciate ligament injuries tended to do poorly because of late arthrosis. A poor late outcome was strongly associated with greater than 10° of instability in full extension.

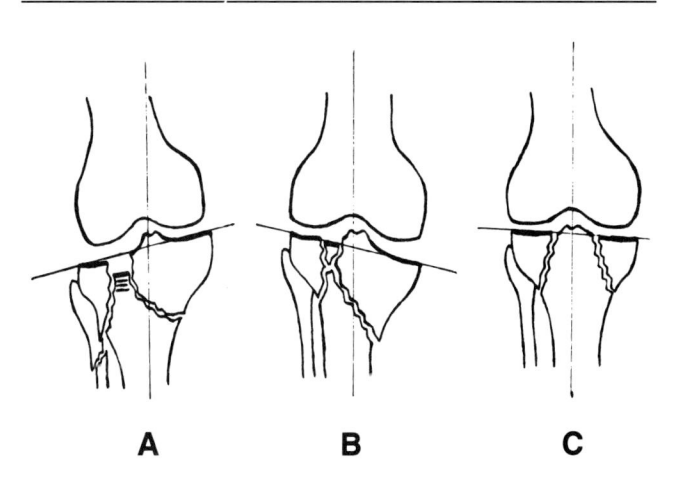

Fig. 4 Subtypes of bicondylar fractures. **A,** Laterally tilted. **B,** Medially tilted. **C,** Symmetric axial displacement. (Reproduced with permission from Honkonen SE, Jarvinen MJ: Classification of fractures of the tibial condyles. *J Bone Joint Surg* 1992;74B:840–847.)

Outline 1. Radiologic criteria for surgical treatment of fractures of the tibial condyles

Fractures of the lateral condyle
    Lateral tilting of the plateau > 5°
    Step-off > 3 mm
    Condylar widening > 5 mm

Fractures of the medial condyle
    All, except nondisplaced fissures

Laterally tilted bicondylar fracture
    When the medial condyle is undisplaced, see criteria for lateral tibial condyle
    When the medial condyle is displaced, surgery is always recommended

Medially tilted bicondylar fractures
    All

Axial bicondylar fractures
    All, except nondisplaced fissures

(Reproduced with permission from Hankonen SE: Indications for surgical treatment of tibial condyle fractures. *Clin Orthop* 1994;302:199–205.)

Treatment

Nonsurgical Treatment

Nonsurgical treatment of properly selected plateau fractures can yield excellent results as described in several recent long-term studies. In a study with a 10-year follow-up, cast-brace treatment of fractures with less than 4 mm of displacement in any plane did well with an average final Iowa knee score of 93.[17] Displaced unicondylar fractures did less well with a knee score of 68. Displaced bicondylar fractures did the poorest with a knee score of 50 and a 70% rate of radiographic osteoarthritis.

In two large studies,[18,19] stability of the knee in full extension (less than 10° varus-valgus) independent of the radiographic appearance of the fracture was used as the criterion for nonsurgical treatment. The treatment technique consisted of closed reduction using ligamentotaxis and cast bracing with delayed weightbearing.

In a 20-year follow-up study of 102 patients selected for nonsurgical treatment using the criteria described, 90% achieved a good or excellent rating by Rasmussen's criteria.[18] This included 18 patients with bicondylar and 14 with medial condylar fractures. The best results occurred in split fractures of the lateral condyle and in depressed fractures in which the depression was confined to the anterior or posterior part of the plateau.

In a smaller study, 89% of 73 fractures had a good or excellent result by Rasmussen's criteria at an average of 5.1 years.[19] In this group, 35% were bicondylar and 12% medial condylar. Residual varus malalignment was associated with a poor result. The complication rate was 12%.

The conclusion that stability of the knee in full extension is a valid criterion for nonsurgical treatment appears justified and provides guidelines for nonsurgical management.

In most series reporting the results of nonsurgical treatment, good results were obtained in nondisplaced fractures or those fractures meeting the nonsurgical criteria in Outline 1. Cast brace treatment with early range of motion and delayed weightbearing was the most commonly employed nonsurgical technique. Maintenance of the reduction and avoiding varus malalignment while healing appeared to be most important in achieving a good nonsurgical result. For displaced fractures in patients who are not candidates for surgery, traction at 5% body weight via a calcaneal pin for 4 to 6 weeks together with early motion has also been shown to yield satisfactory results.[20]

Surgical Indications

Indications for the surgical treatment of tibial plateau fractures remain controversial. Published series have employed widely differing scoring systems in the evaluation of the outcome after a plateau fracture, making it difficult to determine the effectiveness of treatment. In addition, there is significant divergence in treatment results based on functional outcome versus results based on the radiographic appearance of the knee joint. There is no general consensus on the indications for surgical treatment of tibial plateau fractures.

Based on the results of long-term functional follow-up studies, some authors recommend that instability of the extended knee of greater than 10° be used as the indication for reduction and stabilization despite the radiographic appearance of the fracture.[18] This recommendation is based on the observation that 1° of instability is associated with approximately 1 mm of joint depression in the absence of a ligament injury. Honkonen[2] attempted to determine which elements of both the fracture and treatment play a pivotal role in the long-term outcome. The radiologic criteria for surgical treatment recommended by these authors are listed in Outline 1. Biomechanical factors appear to be significant. Clinical function was found to deteriorate with any medial tilt of the plateau, but lateral tilt up to 5° was well tolerated. Lateral articular step-off up to 3 mm and condylar widening up to 5 mm were also compatible with excellent

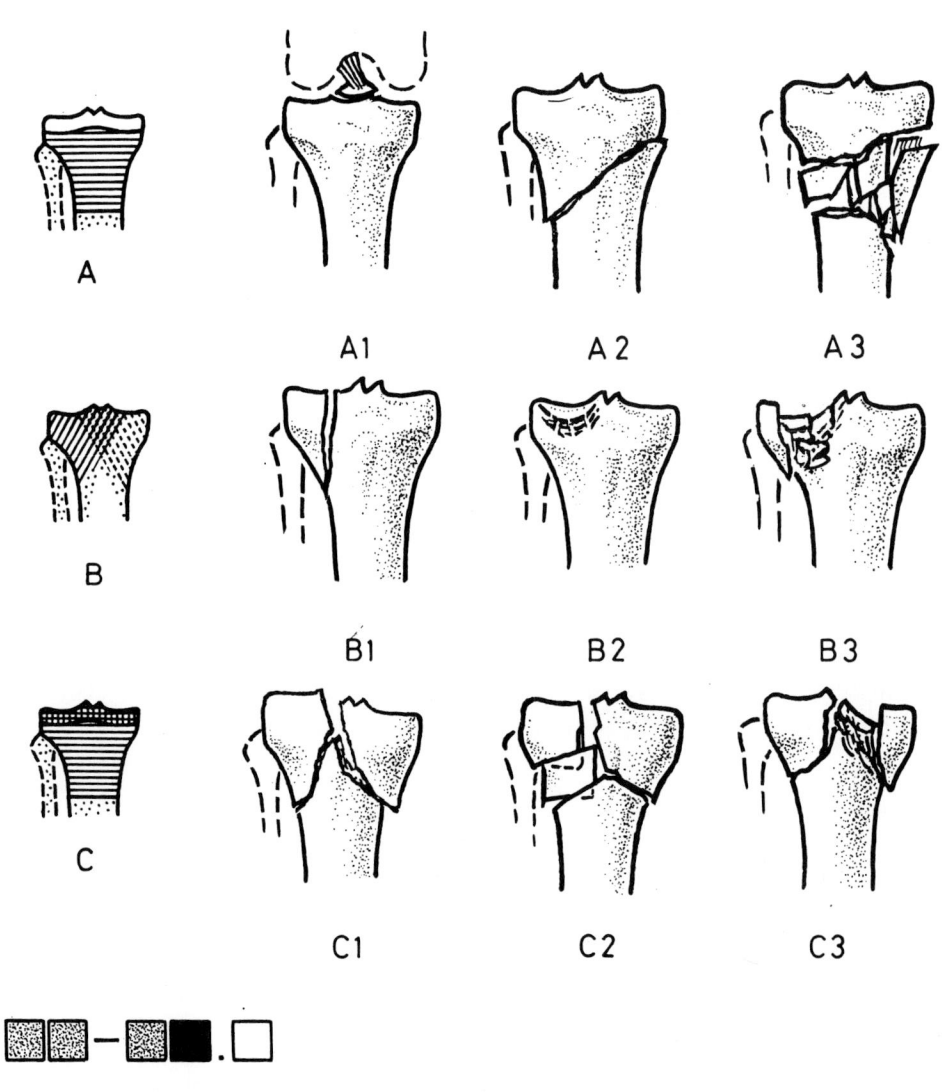

Fig. 5 AO/ASIF universal classification system for tibial plateau fractures (see text). (Reproduced with permission from Müller ME, Nazarian S, Koch P, et al (eds): *The Comprehensive Classification of Fractures of Long Bones*. Berlin, Germany, Springer-Verlag, 1990.)

results. Surgical stabilization of a medial condyle fracture (Schatzker IVA) with any displacement, medially tilted bicondylar fracture, or axially displaced bicondylar fracture is recommended. The aggressive treatment of these fracture types appears to be justified by the high rate of redisplacement and residual varus malalignment observed when these fracture patterns are treated nonsurgically. When indicated, medial stabilization to prevent varus malalignment usually requires a biomechanical buttress, either in the form of a plate or external fixation.

In general, anatomic restoration of condylar depression will yield the best results. However, because of the modifying effects of an intact meniscus, 4 mm or less of residual depression has been shown by several authors[3,21] to have little detrimental effect on the final objective or subjective knee score. Relative contraindications to surgical treatment include advanced age, systemic disease, severe osteopenia, or pre-existing osteoarthritis.[21]

Surgical Approaches When the criteria for open reduction and internal fixation (ORIF) are met, most authors prefer an extensile longitudinal skin incision deviated slightly to the side of the injury. Alternatively, the medial or lateral condyle can be exposed in a nonextensile fashion through an inverted L-shaped incision, which minimizes the skin flap that must be raised.[3] The short horizontal limb is placed 5 mm distal and parallel to the joint line. Visualization of the joint surface is usually accomplished via incision of the coronary ligament and elevation of the involved meniscus. Preservation of the meniscus is considered crucial for a satisfactory long-term outcome.

Preservation of the coronary ligament and incising the anterior horn of the lateral meniscus has also been described.[22] In this approach, the entire split fragment can be rotated on its posterior hinge, providing excellent visualization of the depressed joint surface. Healing of the repaired meniscus using this technique has been documented by arthroscopy.

Complex fractures that have a large posteromedial fragment can be stabilized via a front to back screw when the fracture is minimally displaced or nondisplaced. When displaced, use of a second posteromedial incision has been described.[23] The deep interval is between the medial head of the gastrocnemius and the semitendinosus. Indirect reduction and plate fixation of the posteromedial fragment has been accomplished through this incision.

Extensile approaches to both the medial and lateral sides of the knee have been described.[24] The approach to the medial wall utilizes an anteromedial incision that is taken down to bone and the entire fascia/periosteal layer is detached from anterior to posterior, including the insertions of the pes tendons and the MCL. The medial meniscus is kept in continuity with this layer and retracted out of the joint. The entire medial and posteromedial plateau can be visualized through this approach.

The posterolateral plateau can be approached through an osteotomy and posterior retraction of the fibular head. The peroneal nerve is at risk and must be located and protected. The fibula can be repaired with a lag screw. Alternatively, the head of the fibula can be used for bone graft and the LCL and biceps tendon repaired to the fibula.[25]

Visualization of the joint surface in bicondylar fractures can be particularly difficult and an extensile approach involving osteotomy of the tibial tubercle and detachment of the anterior horn of one or both menisci has been described in selected patients with severely displaced fractures.[26] This approach requires an intact posterior tibial cortex for repair of the tibial tubercle. Alternatively, Z-plasty of the patellar tendon may offer comparable exposure.

The ''Y'' or Mercedes incision described initially by the AO group to expose a bicondylar fracture has been associated with significant wound problems[3] and alternate approaches are recommended.

Open Reduction and Internal Fixation In addition to appropriate indications, the importance of several aspects of surgical treatment of plateau fractures has been reinforced in the recent literature. The significance of preserving the meniscus cannot be overstated. Higher rates of post-traumatic arthritis after only 70 months have been reported in those patients undergoing meniscectomy at the time of their open reduction compared to those with preserved menisci.[21] Failure to bone graft voids left after impacted articular segments have been elevated has also been noted to result in a significantly poorer outcome compared to patients with grafts.[18] Stable fixation, particularly of displaced medial condyles sufficient to allow early motion, has been stressed. Fixation of cruciate ligament injuries associated with an avulsed bone fragment and primary repair of all torn collateral ligaments, particularly when treating a fracture-dislocation, was emphasized by many authors.[24,16] Delay in full weightbearing until 12 weeks in those cases in which depressed segments were elevated was thought to be important to avoid loss of reduction.[18] Postoperative use of a cast brace to further protect surgical repair has been shown to be efficacious.[27]

Open Fractures

The treatment of the open complex fracture of the plateau is somewhat controversial. Excellent results in a small series have been reported using a protocol of debridement and antibiotic administration with immediate open reduction and rigid internal fixation.[28] Delayed primary wound closure was performed at an average of 5 days. This protocol resulted in no infections in 14 open bicondylar fractures. Good results have also been reported with immediate closed reduction and thorough debridement. Definitive fixation and wound closure/coverage was delayed until 7 to 10 days after the injury, and the limb was stabilized in the intervening period with an external fixator that spanned the knee joint.[24]

Arthroscopy and Percutaneous Fixation

Because of the complication rate of formal open reduction, less invasive methods to reduce and stabilize displaced fractures have been investigated. The results of percutaneous reduction and stabilization of selected fractures using cannulated screws coupled with either arthroscopic[29-32] or fluoroscopic monitoring[33,34] of the reduction has been recently reported. In addition to monitoring the reduction of displaced segments, arthroscopy has the added advantage of further defining the anatomy of the fracture. Ligament and meniscus pathology can also be diagnosed and treated simultaneously. Fracture patterns that appear to be most amenable to this form of treatment are those in which a split and/or a depression is present and fixation can be achieved with cannulated screws without the need for a buttress plate (Schatzker types I to III).[35] Some authors have extended the indications to the more unstable types IV to VI by the addition of medial or lateral external fixation.[31]

When arthroscopy is used, gravity distension only of the knee is recommended to avoid overdistension and extravasation of fluid into the injured soft-tissue planes that may result in a compartment syndrome. Depressed segments have been elevated using a bone impactor placed through a small cortical window in the intact metaphyseal portion of the proximal tibia. Most authors stressed the highly technical nature of arthroscopically assisted surgery but found that it only lengthened the procedure by 20 to 30 minutes in experienced hands. Complications were few with this technique and range of motion returned after an average of 6 weeks.

Fluoroscopic imaging was accurate in judging the reduction of a split fracture; however, due to the confluence of shadows, this technique was not helpful in judging the

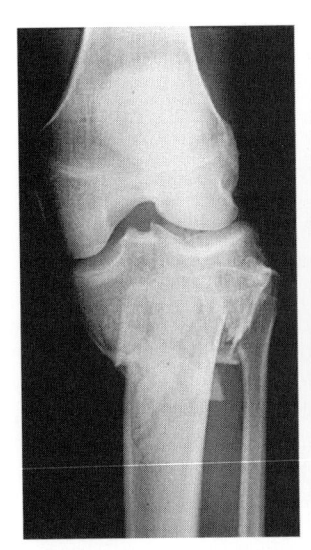

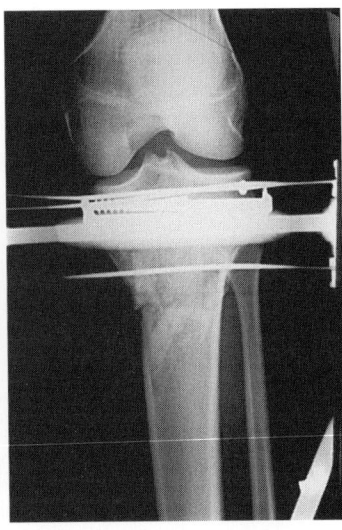

Fig. 6 Anteroposterior radiograph (**A**) of a displaced bicondylar fracture that occurred as a result of a pedestrian bumper injury. The fracture was reduced closed using indirect techniques and stabilized with percutaneous cannulated screws and a "hybrid" external frame (**B**).

reduction of depressed segments. In one study, more than 50% of the reductions were found to be nonanatomic (more than 2 mm) with this technique.[34]

External Fixation

External fixation either as a primary method of stabilization or as an adjunct to internal fixation has become more popular in recent years. The indications for its use are still evolving. The advantages include the ability to stabilize complex fractures with minimal additional soft-tissue injury such as encountered in high-energy bicondylar fractures or fractures with severe soft-tissue compromise.

Unilateral fixators have been used to prevent varus displacement of the medial side of a bicondylar fracture. Periarticular circular frames using small-diameter tensioned wires have been coupled to diaphyseal half pins to create the "hybrid fixator" and are being used increasingly in this application (Fig. 6). The basic technique involves closed or limited open reduction and application of the frame. Percutaneous interfragmentary lag screws are occasionally useful. The frame essentially allows knee motion while preventing varus-valgus displacement during the period of healing. To date, only a small series[36,37] are available for review but it appears that this technique may offer a better alternative to extensive ORIF in selected patients. A reported complication unique to this form of treatment is the progression of a periarticular pin tract infection to a septic arthritis. The mechanism by which the infection becomes intra-articular is unclear but appears to be either through displaced fracture lines or directly if the pin passes through the reflected joint capsule in route to the subchondral bone. These authors recommended that pins be kept at least 15 mm from the joint surface.[37]

Bone Grafting and Bone Graft Substitutes

Cancellous autograft has been the material traditionally used to fill metaphyseal defects after elevating depressed segments. Fresh-frozen allografts have also been used with no adverse effects.[24] Interporous hydroxyapatite has become commercially available for use as a bone graft substitute. Its use in filling metaphyseal defects of the proximal tibia has been addressed. In a randomized controlled study comparing interporous hydroxyapatite to cancellous autograft in 40 patients undergoing ORIF with AO technique, no significant differences between the two groups with respect to healing, maintenance of reduction, infection or long-term outcome (34 months) were noted.[38] Good results were also obtained when this material was packed underneath an elevated segment through a small cortical window in an arthroscopically assisted technique.[39]

Results of Surgical Treatment

It is difficult to compare series of surgically treated plateau fractures due to the lack of uniform classification systems, length of follow-up, and outcome grading scale. Despite these limitations, some general conclusions can be gleaned from the recent literature. For displaced unstable fractures, surgical treatment yields significantly better results than nonsurgical treatment, with satisfactory results ranging from 65% to 87%. This improvement, however, is at a cost of consistently higher complication rates, the most devastating of which is deep infection. Some authors believe that the quality of the reduction of the articular surface is directly related to the long-term outcome,[40] but the tolerance of the plateau to malreduction in the face of an intact meniscus is still unclear. Biomechanical factors, such as residual axial malalignment or instability secondary to persistent ligament laxity, appear to be equally important. These factors may explain the poorer results for bicondylar fractures and fracture-dislocations observed in many series.[24,40–42]

Complications

Important complications have been reported after both closed and open treatment of tibial plateau fractures. Selection of traction and early motion, while attractive for its lack of wound problems, is associated with an incidence of pneumonia, DVT, PE, peroneal nerve palsy, and skin breakdown not significantly different than after surgical treatment.[3] The overall incidence of complications from traction was 8%. The incidence of malunion also appears to be higher with nonsurgical treatment.

The number of complications associated with surgical treatment of plateau fractures appears to grow as the severity of the fracture and aggressiveness of surgical treatment increase; the surgical approach is responsible for nearly 50% of complications.[18] The risk of infection is almost negligible in split fractures treated with percutaneous screws.[33,34] Formal surgical reduction with internal fixation employing a single buttress plate using AO technique is also associated with a low rate of wound problems and infections (0% to 7%) in most series.[11,40,43,44] Application of medial and lateral plates through a single anterior incision to stabilize fractures involving both condyles has been reported to have a very high rate of wound complications and/or infections.[3,24,44] The extensive stripping through an already injured soft-tissue bed required to place the implants plays an important role. In addition, the total bulk of the implants may make wound closure difficult, increasing the likelihood of dehiscence and subsequent infection. Other factors associated with infection were longer surgical times in the more severe cases. The occurrence of deep infection of a tibial plateau fracture carried a poor prognosis and required on the average five additional surgical procedures.[44] Additional complications include peroneal nerve palsy, particularly after fracture dislocations. The incidence is similar after both closed or open treatment of the fracture. Compartment syndrome is a rare complication but may have a greater incidence after high-energy bicondylar fractures, and the onset may be delayed.[45] Nonunion of a plateau fracture is exceedingly rare but successful treatment with bone grafting and rigid internal fixation,[46,47] or custom total knee arthroplasty[48] has been reported.

Early Motion

The clinical importance of early motion in the treatment of tibial plateau fractures is controversial. The effect of timing the initiation of motion on final knee range of motion in 112 patients was investigated.[49] Undisplaced fractures and fractures treated nonsurgically regained full knee motion when immobilized for up to 6 weeks after injury. Immobilization longer than this decreased final ROM. In the displaced fractures treated surgically, knee stiffness tended to develop after only 2 weeks of immobilization and was significant if motion was delayed for longer than 6 weeks. Loss of fracture reduction was more common in the group treated with early motion and hospitalization was prolonged compared to the delayed group. After ORIF, a delay of up to 14 days in the initiation of motion is not detrimental to the final motion of the joint.

Late Reconstruction

Painful posttraumatic arthritis following tibial plateau fracture has been successfully treated by total knee arthroplasty in the age-appropriate patient. In one series addressing this problem, the authors noted that reconstruction was difficult and particular attention needed to be directed toward re-establishing plateau tilt and addressing proximal bone loss. Results more closely paralleled those of revision surgery than of primary arthroplasty.[50]

In the young active person, posttraumatic arthritis remains a difficult problem. Arthroplasty is generally unacceptable in this population due to the high incidence of loosening, and arthrodesis yields a less than ideal level of function. The use of fresh osteochondral allografts to replace the arthritic tibial condyle has received considerable attention. Long-term results of this technique have recently been reported by the Bone Bank Program at the University of Toronto. The approach of this group has been to use fresh (harvested less than 24 hours earlier) rigidly fixed thin segment osteochondral allografts. The recipient meniscus is preserved, if possible. If not, the donor meniscus is transplanted as well. Axial alignment was restored prior to placing the graft. Collapse due to creeping substitution of the graft was generally less than 3 mm and was not a significant problem in most knees. The patients with meniscal grafts did nearly as well as those with preserved menisci. The cartilage space was preserved in approximately 50% of patients 2 years after injury, with the remainder showing a variable loss of cartilage thickness.[51] Biopsy of the transplanted grafts showed 91% chondrocyte viability in the medial plateau of one patient at 41 months and 37% chondrocyte viability of the lateral plateau of another patient at 72 months.[52] By survivorship analysis, these authors report a 75% overall success rate at 5 years, 64% at 10 years, and 63% at 14 years. Contraindications include patellofemoral arthritis, persistent ligament instability, and 60 or more years of age. The mechanism of slow failure of these grafts, the importance of the immune response, and antigenic matching/mismatching are yet to be fully elucidated.

Conclusions and Controversies

Tibial plateau fractures encompass a broad spectrum of both osseous and soft-tissue injury. Imaging sufficient to fully understand the injury pattern and classify the fracture should be performed prior to determining the optimum treatment plan. Anatomic restoration and maintenance of both joint alignment and surface congruity has been shown to yield the best results. This goal may not always be realistic in situations of severe comminution, soft-tissue compromise, osteopenia, or severe associated injuries. The aggressiveness of treatment should be matched by the reduction and stabilization needs of the fracture pattern using the least invasive means possible to achieve the goals of a congruent and level joint surface with stability sufficient to allow early motion. The amount of residual joint incongruity or malalignment that is compatible with a good long-term result remains controversial. Several studies indicate that a lateral stepoff of 3 to 5 mm may be well tolerated, but this is largely due to the modifying effects of the intact meniscus on the cartilage contact stress level. The relative intolerance of the medial condyle to incongruity and malalignment (Outline 1) may be a reflection of the paucity of meniscal coverage of the medial condyle compared to the lateral side.[53]

The role of MRI in injury assessment appears promising, but the clinical significance of the soft-tissue changes requires further evaluation. The optimum role of arthroscopy, percutaneous techniques, and external fixation also require further refinement.

Annotated References

1. Kennedy JC, Bailey WH: Experimental tibial-plateau fractures: Studies of the mechanism and a classification. *J Bone Joint Surg* 1968;50A:1522–1534.

2. Honkonen SE: Indications for surgical treatment of tibial condyle fractures. *Clin Orthop* 1994;302:199–205.

3. Moore TM, Patzakis MJ, Harvey JP: Tibial plateau fractures: Definition, demographics, treatment rationale, and long-term results of closed traction management or operative reduction. *J Orthop Trauma* 1987;1:97–119.

    The authors reviewed 10 years' experience with 988 tibial plateau fractures, of which 44% were treated surgically and 56% were treated by traction and early motion. Anatomic reduction and early motion were thought to be major factors in a successful outcome. The complication rate of surgical cases was 19%, largely secondary to infection. Traction carried a complication rate of 8%.

4. Moore TM: Fracture-dislocation of the knee. *Clin Orthop* 1981;156:128–140.

5. Moore TM, Harvey JP Jr: Roentgenographic measurement of tibial-plateau depression due to fracture. *J Bone Joint Surg* 1974;56A:155–160.

6. Elstrom J, Pankovich AM, Sassoon H, et al: The use of tomography in the assessment of fractures of the tibial plateau. *J Bone Joint Surg* 1976;58A:551–555.

7. Rafii M, Lamont JG, Firooznia H: Tibial plateau fractures: CT evaluation and classification. *Crit Rev Diagn Imaging* 1987;27:91–112.

8. Dias JJ, Stirling AJ, Finlay DB, et al: Computerised axial tomography for tibial plateau fractures. *J Bone Joint Surg* 1987;69B:84–88.

9. Rafii M, Firooznia H, Golimbu C, et al: Computed tomography of tibial plateau fractures. *Am J Roentgenol* 1984;142:1181–1186.

10. Kode L, Lieberman JM, Motta AO, et al: Evaluation of tibial plateau fractures: Efficacy of MR imaging compared with CT. *Am J Roentgenol* 1994;163:141–147.

11. Schatzker J, McBroom R, Bruce D: The tibial plateau fracture: The Toronto experience 1968–1975. *Clin Orthop* 1979;138:94–104.

12. Honkonen SE, Jarvinen MJ: Classification of fractures of the tibial condyles. *J Bone Joint Surg* 1992;74B:840–847.

13. Müller ME, Nazarian S, Koch P, et al (eds): *The Comprehensive Classification of Fractures of Long Bones.* Berlin, Germany, Springer-Verlag, 1990.

14. Vangsness CT Jr, Ghaderi B, Hohl M, et al: Arthroscopy of meniscal injuries with tibial plateau fractures. *J Bone Joint Surg* 1994;76B:488–490.

15. Bennett WF, Browner B: Tibial plateau fractures: A study of associated soft tissue injuries. *J Orthop Trauma* 1994;8:183–188.

16. Delamarter RB, Hohl M, Hopp E Jr: Ligament injuries associated with tibial plateau fractures. *Clin Orthop* 1990;250:226–233.

    The authors evaluated 39 patients with tibial plateau fractures and ligament injuries 1 year after injury. Of the 19 patients in whom the collateral ligament was repaired, 12 had excellent or good results; four, fair; and three, poor. Of the 20 patients with unrepaired ligaments, 10 had excellent or good results; two, fair; and eight, poor. The poor results were thought to be secondary to residual instability of more than 10°. Cruciate repair did not improve the results over collateral repair alone.

17. DeCoster TA, Nepola JV, el-Khoury GY: Cast brace treatment of proximal tibia fractures: A ten-year follow-up study. *Clin Orthop* 1988;231:196–204.

    The authors report on 29 patients evaluated more than 10 years after cast bracing for a tibial plateau fracture. Clinically and radiographically, 61% had good results. Range of motion averaged 117° and Iowa knee score averaged 71. Moderate to severe radiographic posttraumatic arthritis developed in 32%, including 70% of displaced bicondylar fractures. The authors concluded that cast bracing of minimally displaced fractures gave satisfactory results. Results were variable in complex fractures.

18. Lansinger O, Bergman B, Korner L, et al: Tibial condylar fractures: A twenty-year follow-up. *J Bone Joint Surg* 1986;68A:13–19.

    This is the longest follow-up to date of 102 patients originally evaluated by Rasmussen at 7 years. The criterion for nonsurgical treatment was less than 10° varus/valgus instability in full extension irrespective of the radiographic appearance; 90% achieved a good or excellent result. Inferior results were seen in those patients with more than 10 mm of articular depression. The good results reported at the early follow-up were maintained.

19. Duwelius PJ, Connolly JF: Closed reduction of tibial plateau fractures: A comparison of functional and roentgenographic end results. *Clin Orthop* 1988;230:116–126.

    The authors evaluated 73 fractures treated by closed reduction and cast bracing, of which 89% had good or excellent results with a 12% complication rate at an average of 5.1 years. No correlation was found between the functional result and the radiographic appearance of the fracture.

20. Jensen DB, Rude C, Duus B, et al: Tibial plateau fractures: A comparison of conservative and surgical treatment. *J Bone Joint Surg* 1990;72B:49–52.

21. Lachiewicz PF, Funcik T: Factors influencing the results of open reduction and internal fixation of tibial plateau fractures. *Clin Orthop* 1990;259:210–215.

    The authors report on 43 displaced tibial plateau fractures treated by open reduction and internal fixation. Average follow-up was 2.7 years. Overall, the results were excellent in 35, good in five, and fair in three. There were no poor results. There were 10 postoperative complications and 14 patients required removal of implants. Radiographically, six knees had mild degenerative changes, two had moderate changes, and two had severe changes. The absence of bone grafting was associated with a less than excellent result.

22. Perry CR, Evans LG, Rice S, et al: A new surgical approach to fractures of the lateral tibial plateau. *J Bone Joint Surg* 1984;66A:1236–1240.

23. Georgiadis GM: Combined anterior and posterior approaches for complex tibial plateau fractures. *J Bone Joint Surg* 1994;76B:285–289.

24. Tscherne H, Lobenhoffer P: Tibial plateau fractures: Management and expected results: A review. *Clin Orthop* 1993;292:87–100.

25. Gossling HR, Peterson CA: A new surgical approach in the treatment of depressed lateral condylar fractures of the tibia. *Clin Orthop* 1979;140:96–102.

26. Fernandez DL: Anterior approach to the knee with osteotomy of the tibial tubercle for bicondylar tibial fractures. *J Bone Joint Surg* 1988;70A:208–219.

27. Delamarter R, Hohl M: The cast brace and tibial plateau fractures. *Clin Orthop* 1989;242:26–31.

28. Benirschke SK, Agnew SG, Mayo KA, et al: Immediate internal fixation of open, complex tibial plateau fractures: Treatment by a standard protocol. *J Orthop Trauma* 1992;6:78–86.

29. Fowble CD, Zimmer JW, Schepsis AA: The role of arthroscopy in the assessment and treatment of tibial plateau fractures. *Arthroscopy* 1993;9:584–590.

    The authors compared the results of standard open reduction and internal fixation to arthroscopic reduction and percutaneous fixation (ARPF) in 23 patients with split depression or depression fractures. The ARPF group had superior results because they had a higher percentage of anatomic reductions, fewer complications, shorter hospital stay, and shorter time to full weightbearing. In addition, concomitant knee pathology was addressed at the time of fixation.

30. Caspari RB, Hutton PM, Whipple TL, et al: The role of arthroscopy in the management of tibial plateau fractures. *Arthroscopy* 1985;1:76–82.

31. Jennings JE: Arthroscopic management of tibial plateau fractures. *Arthroscopy* 1985;1:160–168.

32. O'Dwyer KJ, Bobic VR: Arthroscopic management of tibial plateau fractures. *Injury* 1992;23:261–264.

33. Keogh P, Kelly C, Cashman WF, et al: Percutaneous screw fixation of tibial plateau fractures. *Injury* 1992;23:387–389.

34. Koval KJ, Sanders R, Borrelli J, et al: Indirect reduction and percutaneous screw fixation of displaced tibial plateau fractures. *J Orthop Trauma* 1992;6:340–346.

    Indirect reduction and percutaneous screw fixation were attempted in 20 displaced tibial plateau fractures. Closed indirect reduction was possible only in pure split fractures. Depressed fragments could not be reduced reliably with either ligamentotaxis or percutaneous elevation. The results were excellent in six (33%), good in 10 (56%) and fair in two (11%).

35. Guanche CA, Markman AW: Arthroscopic management of tibial plateau fractures. *Arthroscopy* 1993;9:467–471.

36. Mallik AR, Covall DJ, Whitelaw GP: Internal versus external fixation of bicondylar tibial plateau fractures. *Orthop Rev* 1992;21:1433–1436.

37. Murphy CP, D'Ambrosia R, Dabezies EJ: The small pin circular fixator for proximal tibial fractures with soft tissue compromise. *Orthopedics* 1991;14:273–280.

38. Bucholz RW, Carlton A, Holmes R: Interporous hydroxyapatite as a bone graft substitute in tibial plateau fractures. *Clin Orthop* 1989;240:53–62.

39. Itokazu M, Matsunaga T: Arthroscopic restoration of depressed tibial plateau fractures using bone and hydroxyapatite grafts. *Arthroscopy* 1993;9:103–108.

40. Blokker CP, Rorabeck CH, Bourne RB: Tibial plateau fractures: An analysis of the results of treatment in 60 patients. *Clin Orthop* 1984;182:193–199.

41. Stokel EA, Sadasivan KK: Tibial plateau fractures: Standardized evaluation of operative results. *Orthopedics* 1991;14:263–270.

42. Anglen JO, Healy WL: Tibial plateau fractures. *Orthopedics* 1988;11:1527–1534.

43. Savoie FH, Vander Griend RA, Ward EF, et al: Tibial plateau fractures: A review of operative treatment using AO technique. *Orthopedics* 1987;10:745–750.

44. Young MJ, Barrack RL: Complications of internal fixation of tibial plateau fractures. *Orthop Rev* 1994;23:149–154.

45. Andrews JR, Tedder JL, Godbout BP: Bicondylar tibial plateau fracture complicated by compartment syndrome. *Orthop Rev* 1992;21:317–319.

46. Keys GW, Walters J: Nonunion of intercondylar eminence fracture of the tibia. *J Trauma* 1988;28:870–871.

47. Schatzker J, Schulak DJ: Pseudarthrosis of a tibial plateau fracture: Report of a case. *Clin Orthop* 1979;145:146–149.

48. Kress KJ, Scuderi GR, Windsor RE, et al: Treatment of nonunions about the knee utilizing custom total knee arthroplasty with press-fit intramedullary stems. *J Arthroplasty* 1993;8:49–55.

49. Gausewitz S, Hohl M: The significance of early motion in the treatment of tibial plateau fractures. *Clin Orthop* 1986;202:135–138.

50. Roffi RP, Merritt PO: Total knee replacement after fractures about the knee. *Orthop Rev* 1990;19:614–620.

51. Locht RC, Gross AE, Langer F: Late osteochondral allograft resurfacing for tibial plateau fractures. *J Bone Joint Surg* 1984;66A:328–335.

52. Czitrom AA, Keating S, Gross AE: The viability of articular cartilage in fresh osteochondral allografts after clinical transplantation. *J Bone Joint Surg* 1990;72A:574–581.

17
Fractures of the Tibial Diaphysis

Introduction

Fractures of the tibial shaft are the most common of the long bone fractures. The National Center for Health Statistics has reported an occurrence rate of 492,000 fractures of tibia, fibula, and ankle per year in the United States.[1] Fractures of the tibia and fibula in the same time period resulted in 77,000 hospitalizations, accounting for 569,000 hospital days with an average length of stay of 7.4 days and 825,000 office visits to physicians. The frequency with which this fracture occurs belies the complexity of its treatment. Perhaps more than with any other long bone fracture, attempts to separate the treatment of the bony injury from its soft-tissue environment can lead to serious difficulties.

Fractures of the tibial diaphysis constitute a spectrum of injuries that result in a loss of unrestricted loadbearing of the extremity. This spectrum includes fatigue-type injuries (stress fractures), which are primarily osseous failures, stable nondisplaced fractures from low-energy trauma, and extreme energy-absorbing injuries that result in the loss of soft-tissue envelope continuity, neurologic dysfunction, vascular insufficiency, and loss of bone. With sufficient damage to the different tissue groups, viability of the limb may be sacrificed, resulting in amputation.

Anatomy

A thorough knowledge of both the topographic and structural anatomy of the leg is essential in planning surgical approaches to the extremity. The anteromedial surface of the tibia and anterior crest are easily palpated from the area of the tibial tuberosity and distally into its termination in the medial malleolus. The fibular shaft is palpable at the proximal portion of the fibular head and then is covered by the peroneal muscles until the distal third, where the lateral fibular shaft can be palpated to its termination in the lateral malleolus. These bony landmarks also serve as guides to closed reduction techniques and as points for preferential pin placement for external fixation. The four leg compartments (anterior, lateral, and superficial and deep posterior compartments) each confine specific neurovascular and musculotendinous units that must be assessed for determination of functional loss and reconstructive demands after tibial injury.

The medullary canal of the tibia is more triangular than circular in cross section. The lack of curvature of the tibial medullary canal as opposed to the femur makes it difficult to achieve a longitudinal interference fit using an intermedullary nail. At the metaphyseal-diaphyseal transitions proximally and distally, the cortex thins and the medullary canal expands. Clinically, this frequently presents difficulties when intramedullary or external fixation is required for fractures of the proximal and distal one fourth. In this region, external fixation half-pins engage less cortex and thus have less resistance to stress. Intramedullary nails do not fill the canal and thus offer little or no resistance to deforming forces without interlocking screw supplementation.

The anterior compartment of the leg contains the tibialis anterior, extensor digitorum longus, extensor hallucis longus, and peroneus tertius muscles. This compartment is primarily responsible for dorsiflexion of the foot and ankle. Loss of dorsiflexion may be due to neurologic damage, loss of functional integrity of the motor-tendon unit, or prolonged immobilization of the ankle. Because of the tough crural fascia and the prominent location of this compartment, compartment syndrome is a frequent complication in closed and open fractures.

The anterior crest of the tibia and the medial aspect of the tibia are preferred sites for percutaneous half-pin external fixation systems for two reasons. First, because of the unobstructed area, the fixator can be placed very close to the extremity, increasing its mechanical stability. Second, because no muscle-tendon units are transfixed by the pins, functional movement of the foot and ankle is not impaired.

The lateral compartment contains only two muscles, the peroneus brevis and peroneus longus, and the superficial peroneal nerve. This nerve is rarely injured with closed fractures of the fibular shaft, but is at risk with fractures of the fibular neck, traction injuries of the lower extremity (because of its relative fixed position proximally at the fibular neck), or fractures at the junction of the middle and distal thirds of the leg, where the subcutaneous superficial sensory branch lies between the peroneus brevis and extensor digitorum longus muscles.

The superficial posterior compartment contains the gastrocnemius, the soleus, the popliteus, and the plantaris muscles, the sural nerve, and the short and long saphenous veins and no arterial structures of significance. This compartment is important in plantarflexion of the foot. Compartment syndromes can occur in the superficial posterior compartment and, like the anterior compartment, the posterior compartment is easily palpable for clinical examination. This compartment also serves as a source for local muscle flaps for coverage of soft-tissue defects in the proximal and middle third of the tibia.

The deep posterior compartment contains the tibialis posterior, flexor digitorum longus, and flexor hallucis longus muscles. These structures are involved in plantarflexion of the foot and toes and inversion of the foot through the tibialis posterior muscle function. The posterior tibial nerve and the peroneal and posterior tibial arteries are present in this compartment. The posterior tibial artery, because of its protected nature, frequently is the major arterial supply after a significant open fracture and is a potential source for anastomosis with free flaps for soft-tissue reconstruction of the leg.

The blood supply of the tibial shaft from the nutrient artery and the periosteal vessels may undergo major changes after injury. The nutrient artery of the tibia arises from the posterior tibial artery and enters the posterolateral cortex of the bone at the origin of the soleus muscle just below the oblique line of the tibia posteriorly. This artery divides into three ascending branches and only one main descending branch, which gives off smaller branches to the endosteal surface. The periosteum has an abundant blood supply from branches of the anterior tibial artery as it courses down the interosseous membrane. The intramedullary vascular supply may be the most important in normal bone;[2] however, after an injury that disrupts the intramedullary vascular pattern, the periosteal blood vessels increase their contribution and become prominent in the formation of new bone. The periosteal vessels are especially important in distal third tibia fractures but there is no difference in intramedullary supply between proximal and distal regions.[3] The concern for the effect of reaming in intramedullary nailing of open tibial fractures has motivated much of the research into the use of modern nail design to allow interlocking nail techniques to be applied to open tibial fractures. The five major venous structures of the leg are the greater and lesser saphenous veins, the posterior and anterior tibial veins, and the peroneal vein. Study of these vessels has important implications in revascularization techniques and the occurrence of thromboembolic disease.

Cross-sectional anatomy of the leg is important in the application of conventional fixators and recently introduced circular fixators using transfixion wires. "Safezones" have been described for the insertion of transfixing pins[4] and a cross-sectional atlas should be consulted if these types of devices are to be used.

Mechanism of Injury

For the tibial shaft to fracture, a significant amount of energy must be applied in one of three modes. Torsional injuries are more common with low-energy trauma, in which the foot becomes fixed and the body rotates about this fixed point, ie, skiing injuries. These injuries radiographically are spiral in nature with varying degrees of comminution based on the energy applied and absorbed by the tibia at the time of failure. Three- and four-point bending forces produce short oblique and transverse fractures. As the points of bending are spread apart and the energy applied is increased, comminution increases and even segmental fractures develop. Direct force applications are crushing in nature with high concentrations of energy to a smaller area, causing more damage to the bone and soft tissues. These applications range from baseball bats[5] to industrial mechanized crush injuries.

In one study, tibial plating using an alphanumeric classification was used to evaluate the mechanical forces resulting in various fracture patterns (Fig. 1).[6] Their results documented that the incidence of complications rose as the complexity of the initial injury increased.

Classification of Injury

Classifications for diaphyseal tibial fractures that can be replicated from physician to physician are elusive. The more specific the grading system or classification becomes, the less agreement between physicians. This was most recently demonstrated at the 1992 Orthopaedic Trauma Association meeting.[7] Surgeons were asked to classify 12 open tibial fractures using the Gustilo and Anderson classification after presentation of the clinical history, radiographs, and intraoperative videotapes of the surgical debridement. Agreement on classification averaged only 60%.

Most classification systems include some type of bony injury grade, soft-tissue injury grade, and a locational description for the fracture. In 1958, displacement, comminution and wound severity in tibial fractures treated with nonsurgical methods were evaluated and a classification based on three grades (minor, moderate and major) was developed.[8] The significance of the grades was reflected in average time to union of 10, 15, and 23 weeks, respectively. The time to union has not significantly changed with any surgical modality. Henley[9] applied the classification system of Winquist and Hansen[10] for femur fractures to the tibia (Fig. 2). This classification relates the potential application of varying interlocking nail constructs to specific tibial fracture patterns. A classification that evaluated the mechanical forces resulting in various fracture pattern was adopted and modified by the AO/ASIF group to incorporate soft-tissue grading[11] along the lines of the classifications described by Tscherne[12] and Gustilo and Anderson[13] for soft tissue and open fractures. The OTA has published a classification of fractures that draws heavily from Tscherne's work in an attempt to standarize the literature for the future. However, until these systems have been validated in clinical settings with regard to reproducibility and interobserver agreement, the validity and comparability of the literature are open to speculation.

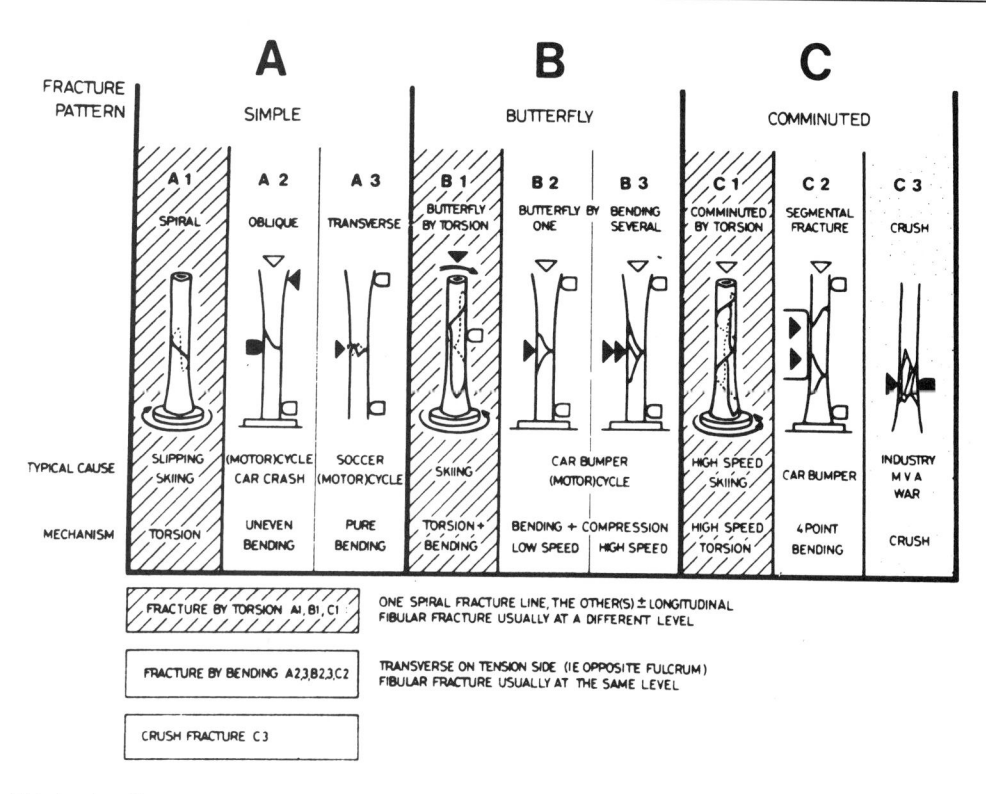

Fig. 1 Johner and Wruhs classification of fracture patterns of the tibia. (Reproduced with permission from Johner R, Wruhs O: Classification of tibial shaft fractures and correlation with results after rigid internal fixation. *Clin Orthop* 1983;178:7-25.)

Gustilo and Anderson's 1976 classification of types I, II, and III injuries[13] with Gustilo's 1984 modification in subgrouping type III injuries into IIIA, IIIB, and IIIC patterns[14] is still the most widely used system in North America (Outline 1).

Physical Examination and Diagnostic Evaluation

Because the tibia is subcutaneous for the majority of its length, deformity is usually readily apparent. The contralateral extremity serves as a useful control for examination. Stability of the fracture is one of the first assessments required during the physical examination. An obvious deformity or shortening confirms the diagnosis of mechanical instability of the tibial diaphysis. However, nondisplaced fractures may be tested by application of careful varus or valgus stress of the extremity. At the first indication of instability, the leg should be splinted and immobilized pending radiographic evaluation. The soft-tissue envelope of the tibia must be inspected throughout its circumference for ecchymosis and tissue turgidity. This is especially important because of the association of compartment syndromes with tibial fractures. Associated fractures of the fibula may give insight into the degree of initial displacement during the injury and also the potential for instability of the tibial fracture.

Assessment of the neurologic and vascular status of the foot is required because a tibial fracture may affect adjacent muscle-tendon units, nerves, and blood vessels. All wounds should be inspected to assess possible osseous communication and then dressed pending exploration under a controlled surgical environment, if required. It is suggested that true grading of the open fracture of the tibia is best made after formal surgical debridement and irrigation. Careful documentation of the degree of periosteal stripping, bone and soft-tissue loss, and size of the open wound may be more useful than characterization into a type I, II, or III.

The hallmark of tibial diaphyseal radiographic imaging is a standard anteroposterior and lateral full length view of the tibia from the knee to the ankle. More detailed and expensive procedures, such as computed tomography and magnetic resonance imaging, are rarely indicated for tibial diaphyseal fractures. The technetium bone scan is still the most cost-effective and useful indicator of occult injuries and stress fractures in the presence of continuing symptoms with negative plain radiographs. Arteriography and venography are applicable only in situations associated with vascular compromise and have little clinical

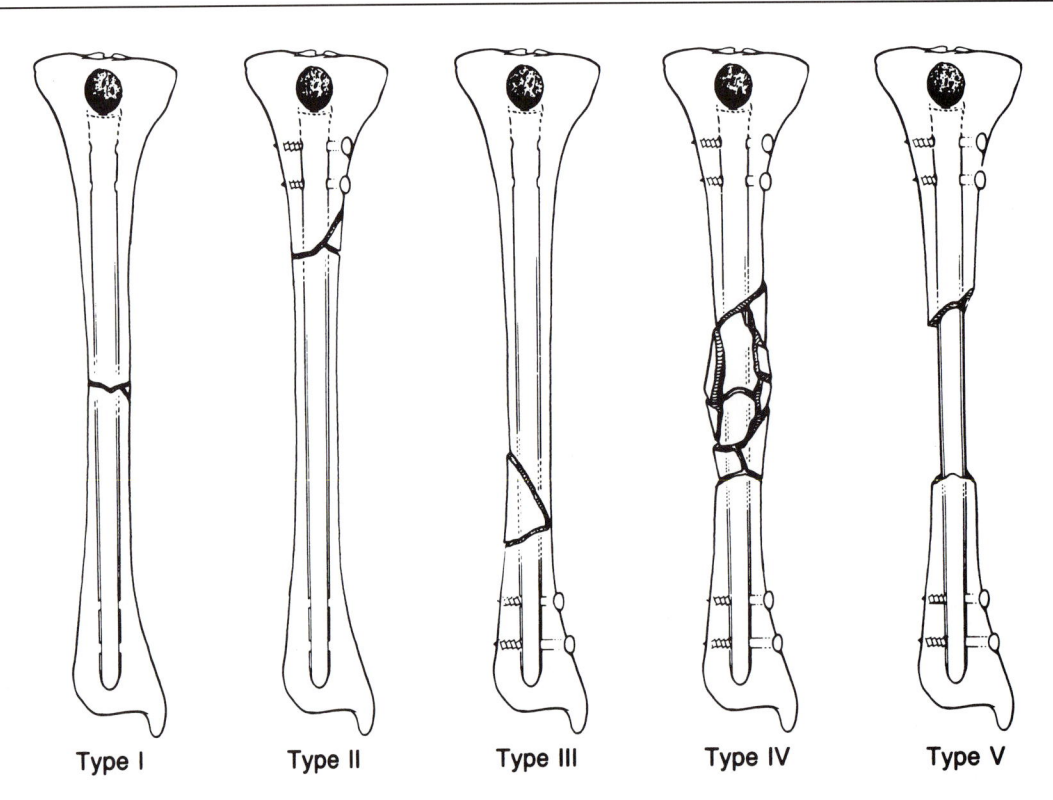

Fig. 2 Henley modification of Winquist-Hansen classification for diaphyseal tibial fractures. (Reproduced with permission from Henley MB: Intramedullary devices for tibial fracture stabilization. *Clin Orthop* 1989;240:87-96.)

Outline 1. Classification of open fractures (Gustilo)

Grade I	Skin opening of 1 cm or less, quite clean; most likely from inside to outside; minimal muscle contusion; simple transverse or short oblique fractures
Grade II	Laceration more than 1 cm long with extensive soft-tissue damage, flaps, or avulsion; minimal to moderate crushing component; simple transverse or short oblique fractures with minimal comminution
Grade III	Extensive soft-tissue damage, including muscles, skin, and neurovascular structures; often a high-energy injury with a severe crushing component
IIIA	Extensive soft-tissue laceration, adequate bone coverage; segmental fractures, gunshot injuries
IIIB	Extensive soft-tissue injury with periosteal stripping and bone exposure; usually associated with massive contamination
IIIC	Vascular injury requiring repair

usefulness in management decisions of the standard closed fracture.

Treatment Options and Results of Treatment

Much of the published literature over the past 50 years has focused on the mechanical orientation of treatment tibial fractures over the biologic aspects in the care of these injuries. Probably no other fracture has more treatment options available or more complications engendered by these treatment options. A shift is occurring in the outcome appreciation of the surgeon with regard to the patient's perception of the result with less tolerance for malunion and functional loss. Most texts and articles still reference acceptable guidelines of less than 1 cm of shortening, alignment within 5° to 10° varus and valgus with anterior-posterior tolerance of 5° to 10° and less than 20° of external rotation and 10° of internal rotation. Often with these strict criteria, results of nonsurgical treatment become less desirable.

Nonsurgical Treatment

Nonsurgical management of tibia fractures with long leg casts and braces has been in existence for hundreds of years. The results of an average community type experience of patients with tibial shaft fractures treated with closed weightbearing treatment program have been described.[15] Low-energy trauma accounted for the mechanism in 71% of the patients and high-energy trauma in 29%. The reported delayed union rate was 19%; nonunion rate 4%; anterior-posterior malunion rate 13%; varus valgus malunion rate, 21%; and significant length deformity rate, 5.3%. Rotational problems were not mentioned, but 43%

of the patients lost ankle range of motion. In an analysis of 780 tibial fractures treated with initial cast immobilization and conversion to prefabricated functional braces, initial treatment was with closed reduction and long leg casts.[16] Bracing was applied on an average of 3.8 weeks after closed fractures and 5.2 weeks after open fractures. Bracing was contraindicated in fractures with excessive initial shortening or in those that showed increasing angular deformity while in the cast. Patients who had significant neurologic and/or vascular damage, showed segmental bone loss, or required soft-tissue flaps were not candidates for bracing. Other complications of casting and bracing included skin irritation and maceration, occasionally requiring discontinuation of bracing. No comments were made with regard to range of motion after treatment. Most series report a 25% to 40% incidence of joint stiffness in the ankle and subtalar joint after prolonged casting and immobilization.

Surgical Treatment

Using the techniques described by the AO/ASIF of anatomic reduction and stable fixation with a dynamic compression plate, 93% good functional results were achieved in a closed group with a 6% failure rate.[17] In 101 open tibial fractures, there were 90% eventual good function results with a complication rate of 30%. In a study using the AO/ASIF techniques of plate and screw fixation, complications increased to 9.5% with simple fracture patterns and to 48% with comminuted fractures, with a respective increase in infection rates from 2.1% to 10%.[6] Nonunion was twice as common and infection five times as common when open fractures were plated compared to closed fractures. These complications and the inability of many surgeons to obtain the excellent results reported by Ruedi and associates[17] have dampened enthusiasm for open reduction and plate and screw fixation for tibial diaphyseal fractures in North America.

External fixation has been applied primarily to open fractures but it has been advocated for treatment of closed tibial fractures. It is useful in patients with tibial fractures in conjunction with compartment syndrome and in multitrauma patients with head injuries, burns, or impaired sensation. This technique was used to obtain a 95% rate in open and closed fractures, however, approximately 20% of cases obtained a significant malunion.[18]

A uniplanar fixator that has the capability of dynamization, allowing fracture impaction, has been used.[19] Research and clinical studies thus far have been inconclusive on the advantage of passive dynamization. Dynamization seems to aid primarily by closing gaps at fracture sites if activated within the first 6 weeks. A significant improvement in time to union has been shown with active dynamization,[20] but it has not yet reached clinical utility in North America. One study reported the results of a series of 219 patients with closed and open injuries in which the authors were able to use two different types of external fixators to actually measure the fracture stiffness using strain gauge measurement through the fixator.[21] The stiffness of 15 N·m/degree and the sagittal plane provided useful definition of union of the tibial fracture. With this protocol, refractures could be eliminated in the study group that achieved 15 N·m/degree of stiffness. These two aspects of external fixation, dynamization and telemetry through the frame exemplify the research that is being conducted with external fixation in closed and open fractures.

The use of intramedullary nails for tibial fracture stabilization effectively began with the era of Kuntscher and Lottes. However, in many cases, intramedullary nailing could not be used because of the frequent infraisthmal comminuted nature of most tibia fractures. Good results have been reported with the use of Ender nails with 95% or higher union rates and only 10% malunion rate.[22,23] The advantage of these Ender-type devices was that they were able to better control rotation in the tibial fracture with multiple pin fixation, however, they were not effective for axially unstable fractures. Subsequently, interlocking nails were introduced in North America. The addition of interlocking screws to aid in the prevention of axial and rotational deformities became widely accepted. In a study of 112 fractures of the tibia treated by reamed intramedullary nailing, 66 of the fractures were acute and were open.[24] Thirty-six of the fractures were treated for nonunions or malunions. A 99% union rate and a 6% infection rate were obtained. Twenty-eight of these patients were treated with Gross-Kemph nails, with 84 being treated with interlocked AO nails. They had a nonunion rate of less than 3% with 5% of the patients having shortening of 1 cm or more. A similar series of 93 fractures with similar results has been reported[25] and another similar reported series had an infection rate of 1.5%, a nonunion rate of 1.6%, a malunion rate of 2.4%, and an incidence of exhibiting some residual ankle or subtalar joint stiffness in 7.2% of the patients.[26] In later series, tibial fractures were usually treated within 78 hours after the injury. Immediate weightbearing was prescribed in 43% of the patients and 92% of the patients were weightbearing by 6 weeks. In another study, a non-reamed interlocking nail technique was used with quite different results; the average time to union was 32 weeks, with 11 of the patients (42%) requiring reoperations, including exchange nailing, dynamization, and bone grafting to obtain union.[27] These patients were in a delayed weightbearing program because of the concern for implant failure with smaller diameters of the interlocking nail design.

Difficulties have been encountered when surgeons have tried to extend tibial intramedullary nailing techniques to proximal and distal metaphyseal fractures.[28] Interlocking nails fail to provide sufficient stability in metaphyseal fractures alone. This can result in higher malunion and nonunion rates, particularly when the proximal and distal limits are pushed to the extreme. These problems are exacerbated when the surgeon dynamizes the interlocking nail construct, resulting in increased instability of the nail-bone construct and increased rate of fatigue failure and loss of reduction (Fig. 3).

In a comparative, prospective randomized study, traditional conservative management was compared with a

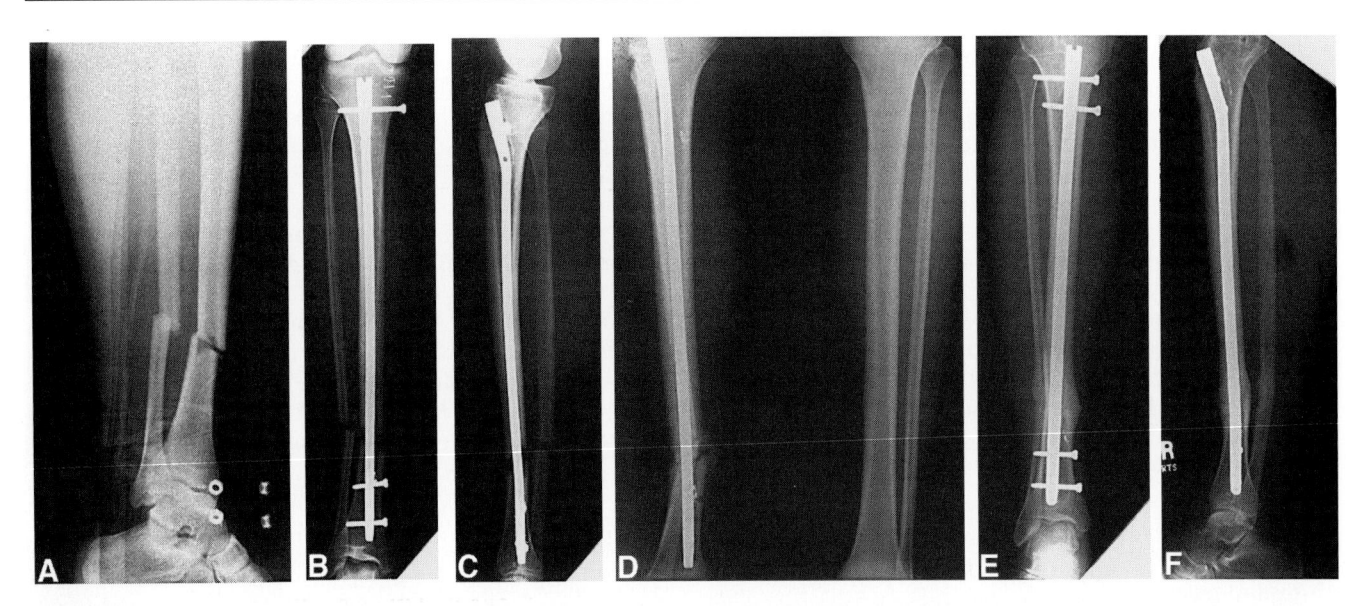

Fig. 3 **A,** Distal one third type 2 open tibia-fibula fracture. **B** and **C,** Tibia nailed in slight valgus and distraction (note fibula). **D,** Nail dynamized to close gap at 4 weeks postoperatively with loss of stability and valgus deformity. **E** and **F,** Nonunion treated with renailing with static reamed nail.

weightbearing program using reamed interlocking intramedullary nailing of the tibia.[29] The study groups included patients with isolated tibial fractures displaced 50% or more or angulated 10° or more, closed and grade I open fractures in skeletally mature patients with the fracture zone at least 5 cm from the knee and ankle. Nonsurgical treatments were indicated only in nondisplaced fractures. Significant importance was placed on the decreased time to union, rate of malunion, and the improved functional rehabilitation of the patients in the intramedullary nail treatment group.

For closed, isolated tibia-fibula fractures in the diaphyseal region within 5 cm of the joint proximally distally, the treatment with the highest recorded rate of success and functional improvement of the patients is the use of a reamed interlocking intramedullary nail with a closed technique.

Open Fractures

The treatment of open fractures of the tibia has undergone a major shift in philosophy over the past 10 years. As classification systems have become more focused in differentiating the severe tibia fracture, it has become apparent that soft-tissue damage, including periosteal stripping and tissue loss, is the primary determinant of infection and nonunion. Open tibial fractures with arterial interruption have also undergone increased scrutiny with regard to limb salvage versus acute amputation. As the reliability of soft-tissue microvascular tissue transfers has improved, attitudes toward debridement and irrigation of open tibias have also changed. It has been advocated that the surgeon treating a severe type III open tibial fracture will undertake this endeavor only if there is plastic surgical support. This is necessary because the surgeon must execute an aggressive debridement of bone and soft tissue, as necessary, with copious irrigation until the contaminated interface has been cleaned. The surgeon must have the capability of bony augmentation with either autologous leg grafting or bone transport techniques to repair the osseous loss. An increased success rate was noted with early application of a soft-tissue free flap coverage compared with delayed coverage, and infection rates and nonunion rates were lower in the former group.[30] This also has been related to earlier bone grafting that increased rates of union with decreased time to healing.

New techniques of bone regeneration as developed by Ilizarov[31] have facilitated the concept of more radical bony debridement and now allow reconstitution routinely of 5 to 7 cm with bone segment transport. Bone segment transport over an intramedullary nail can produce ample bone regeneration, giving support to the importance of periosteal blood supply of the tibia.[32]

Stabilization of the extremity benefits the treatment of the fracture and soft tissues. External fixation and interlocking intramedullary nails with a nonreamed technique have gained widespread acceptance over cast and plate and screw techniques in the open fracture. The general principles of external fixation of the tibia using half pin techniques have been outlined[33] and documented.[34] External fixation is used primarily in type III open fractures. External fixation is complicated with multiple problems partially due to the severe injuries in which they are used and partially due to the fixation technique. A loss of reduction and a higher malunion rate have been noted using external fixation initially and then transition to long leg casting.[35]

In a 1987 review of 62 type III open fractures (11 type IIIA, 42 type IIIB, and 9 type IIIC injuries), significant differences were shown between the subgroups.[36] These fractures were treated with debridement, irrigation, and external fixation. The type IIIA fractures had infections and a 28% nonunion rate. The 42 type IIIB fractures had a 35% nonunion rate, a 39% infection rate, and a 17% amputation rate. Initially in the IIIB subgroup that had early flap coverage, the nonunion rate, infection rate, and amputation rate were decreased up to 21% in the infection, and the amputation rate was decreased to 8%. In the type IIIC fractures, seven of nine (78%) resulted in amputation and the remaining 22% were considered poor results.

A uniaxial fixator with dynamization capability was used to treat 38 type II and 63 type III fractures (28 IIIA, 33 IIIB and six IIIC) using a protocol of irrigation and debridement, flap coverage, and bone grafting, as necessary, in 19 and 38 cases, respectively.[37] A 96% union rate was reported with treatment of the fracture to union in the fixator. Pin tract infections were frequent. Ninety-five percent of the cases had less than 10° of angulation. The infection rate in this selected group of patients was 6%.

Closed-section interlocking intramedullary nails have been designed with smaller diameters and modified section modulus characteristics to allow insertion with nonreamed techniques. In one report, 50 open tibial fractures were treated with this system (68% type III [A22, B12]).[38] The infection rate was 0% for grades I and II fractures, 5% for type IIIA fractures, and 25% for IIIB. The union rate was 96%. Thirty-six percent of the cases were dynamized and/or bone grafted. There were no malunions at follow-up.

In a prospective, randomized study presented in 1994 at the Orthopaedic Trauma Association's Annual Meeting, Henley and associates compared external fixation with intramedullary nails, and reported that the primary difference between external fixation and nonreamed interlocking intramedullary nails was a higher rate of malunion with external fixation (MB Henley and associates, unpublished data, 1994). In types II, IIIA, and IIIB open fractures, union rates for the nail group were 92% compared with 88% for external fixation, 0.6 secondary procedures were required for the nail group compared to 2.5 for the external fixation group. There were 24% malunions in the external fixation group with no malunions in the nail group. The loss of reduction during the course of treatment of the tibia in the external fixator system is believed to imply loss of stability of the fracture construct due to slippage of the connections with external fixation systems.

The type IIIA fractures can be treated either with non-reamed interlocking nail techniques or with external fixation; the results are equivalent with the exception that with current generation of external fixators, nonunion is higher in the external fixation group. It does appear that there may be a difference in the new generation of external fixators with regard to control of the fracture to avoid malunions. The type IIIB fracture in most series still has an infection rate of 5% to 50%, depending on soft-tissue viability; a malunion rate of 5% to 30%; and a nonunion rate of 10% to 20%. The type IIIC injury evokes the most controversy regarding limb salvage versus amputation.

Issues and controversy of limb salvage versus acute amputation exist for type IIIC severe open tibial fractures.[39] The surgeon is compromised by the lack of a sensitive and specific classification system to permit an early decision for amputation, by the emotional impact of amputation, and by the concern for litigation. Conversely, unsuccessful limb salvage may truly compromise a patient with regard to his or her ability to return as a functioning member of society.

Current reviews of prospective studies[40,41] have documented that severe open tibia fractures are frequently able to be salvaged. However, the literature is divided in its report on functional outcome. One series reports a high success rate with an aggressive salvage program and preservation of a weightbearing limb in a high percentage of cases.[40] In another study comparing function outcome, patients who underwent a long-limb salvage viewed themselves as more disabled than patients with below-the-knee amputation and documented a higher economic cost and a longer period of disability after limb salvage than patients with below-the-knee amputations.[41] When the American Medical Association guidelines for permanent physical impairment were used, the patient had a lower permanent physical impairment with limb salvage over amputation.[42] This may reflect less sensitivity in the rating system rather than improvement over the functional results of limb salvage over amputation.

Most authors currently recommend amputation in type IIIC open tibial fractures. The limb salvage scoring system advocated by Helfet and associates[43] compares amputation to limb salvage success based on time from injury, warm ischemia time, presence of shock, and severity of injury. McNamara and associates[44] modified the Mangled Extremity Severity Score (MESS) to include neural injury and separate soft-tissue and bone grading with a preliminary increased incidence of sensitivity. Although helpful in decision making, the classification has not been sufficiently validated by other studies to permit its endorsement by the general orthopaedic community for prospective amputations.

Complications

Complications of the tibia are somewhat dependent on treatment. Malunions and refracture are more likely to occur after closed treatment or external fixation but rarely seem to result in reconstructive surgery; whereas, intramedullary nails may result in implant failures, anterior knee pain, and malunion when applied to very proximal and distal metaphyseal fractures. There is no technique or treatment that completely prevents malunions. This problem is further complicated by a lack of functional outcomes studies documenting the long-term effect of malunions on adjacent joints. Nonunion, which occurs most frequently in unstable fractures with bone or soft-tissue loss, has been decreased by the use of aggressive early bone grafting in the treatment of tibial fractures.[45-47] Bone grafting has been shown to dramatically decrease the time to union in most series.

Nonunions

Reamed intramedullary nailing is an effective treatment for tibial nonunion with early weightbearing and return to functional activities with or without a fibular osteotomy to allow correction of deformity.[48-51] A useful technique for displaced fractures acutely and delayed using a femoral distractor on the tibia to correct deformity and to obtain length prior to nailing has been described.[52] The femoral distractor has been used for reduction and plate fixation with indirect reduction for displaced nonunion.[53] Excellent results have been reported with compression plating technique for nonunion of the tibia with deformity.[54,55] This technique offers significant advantages over intramedullary nailing if previous external fixation has been used to avoid osteomyelitis from old external fixation pin sites. In situations where there is impaired biologic response, as evidenced by poor callus formation or atrophic bone, autologous bone grafting should be added to the mechanical construct.

Infection

Detailed studies of all external fixation series using open tibial fractures demonstrate a fairly constant rate of pin tract infection, usually 50%. These complications usually respond to local conservative measures or exchange of pin or wire fixation. Pin tract infections are a source of concern because of the use of intramedullary nailing as a salvage procedure for nonunion.[56] Some surgeons now recommend plate fixation for nonunion following failed external fixation because of concern about intramedullary sepsis. Sepsis may be related more to previous pin tract infection and the time of external fixation application prior to nail treatment.[57] Intramedullary nailing is rarely recommended in the face of an acute infection. If there was preexisting pin tract deep sepsis, an exchange treatment from external fixation to nailing probably should be avoided. If, however, the surgeon is unable to obtain an adequate debridement initially and the patient is placed in external fixation, exchange to intramedullary nailing after soft-tissue closure within the first 2 weeks is an acceptable course of treatment.

The issue of infection with intramedullary nailing now seems to be more a factor of initial surgical debridement and soft-tissue coverage than of the nail technique. Infection rates of 1% to 5% are frequently reported in closed tibial nail studies. Infection after intramedullary nailing is more readily treatable than previously expected.[58] Current recommendations are to maintain the nail in place if it provides stability and to suppress the infection until fracture healing occurs and then remove the nail and debride the canal. If the implant is unstable, it should be removed with debridement, irrigation should be performed, and the extremity should be stabilized with external fixation along with appropriate antibiotics and soft-tissue treatment. Treatment of tibial infection after fracture should be based on the extent of the infection and the tissue planes involved. It is best handled in centers that specialize in these techniques.

Concern for implant failures of screws and nails when smaller diameter nails are used must be balanced by the potential benefits of decreased reaming with potential conservation of bone stock and less thermal damage from reaming. For closed fractures, reamed intramedullary nailing with appropriate interlocking is the most widely accepted treatment for diaphyseal fractures. Controversy exists over the indications for reamed versus unreamed techniques using interlocking tibial nailing in closed fractures. Implant failure rates are one focus in this controversy. Most manufacturers have modified their interlocking intramedullary nails with changes in design and manufacturing techniques to permit using smaller diameter nails with longer fatigue lives. An acceptably low implant failure rate of the nails has been found using 8 and 9 mm interlocking tibial nails of a closed section design.[59] Coldworking of the locking holes increases fatigue life. Screw failure occured in 11% of patients tested but affected outcome in only 1 of 106 fractures. All broken nails were in a dynamic mode, with a nail breakage rate of 2.8%. Changes have also been demonstrated by increasing the core diameter of the screws for interlocking nails to minimize screw breakage, which is the most common mode of implant failure. Dynamization of the tibial nail resulted in increased rate of nail failure and loss of reduction, especially in distal one fourth fractures. Exchanging nailing was recommended over dynamization in unstable tibial constructs.[59]

The surgeon must have a high index of suspicion and a low threshold for intervention for compartment syndrome even in open fractures.[60] Compartment pressure monitoring has become readily available and is especially helpful in patients who are comatose or unresponsive due to other injuries. A patient with symptoms and signs of compartment syndrome does not require compartment pressure measurements by the surgeon prior to proceeding with fasciotomy. The issue of compartment syndromes induced by intramedullary nailing has received a great deal of attention; however, the increase in compartment pressure was noted primarily at the time of reduction of the fracture both with closed and surgical treatment.[61] Compartment syndromes, if unrecognized, frequently result in contractures of the leg and foot, but contractures may also occur from trapping of muscle-tendon units in fracture fragments or fixation systems. Functional treatment of the extremity with early mobilization of the joints of the foot and ankle can help minimize this problem or alert the physician to its presence. Neurologic deficits occur with tibial fractures whether they are treated with closed or surgical modalities. Frequently these are neuropraxic injuries resulting in a peroneal nerve palsy and can be quite troublesome to the patient and a source of continued disability. Overdistraction of the tibia should especially be avoided. Nailing early rather than late may decrease the incidence of neurologic complications to minimize excessive traction to obtain reduction.[62]

Summary

As the limitations of closed treatment have been better defined and the technique of tibial interlocking intramedullary nailing has improved, nailing is assuming a larger role in the treatment of tibial shaft fractures. Difficulties relating to malunion occurring after fixator removal are still a frequent problem. New developments in external fixation may be effective in decreasing malunion rates. It is hoped that telemetry of the frames to ascertain sufficient fracture healing will decrease the complication of refracture. Controversy in the next decade will revolve around limb salvage versus acute amputation and refinement of these indications with regard to functional outcome and cost-benefit analysis from the prospective of the patient and society. The issue of reaming versus nonreaming will require that a large number of patients be studied to delineate the true advantages and disadvantages of these respective techniques. Continued improvements in internal and external fixation systems can be anticipated from a mechanical standpoint and will require clinical validation. However, the crux of the problem will always revolve around the biologic nature of the injury and its effects on the vascularity and the regeneration capability of the soft tissues. Refinements in the techniques of intramedullary nailing have led to improved results for closed unstable fractures. Improvements in surgical stabilization techniques and the philosophy of aggressive and repeated debridement coupled with early tissue augmentation (vascularized flaps and early bone grafts) have improved treatment results for open fractures. However, a higher expectation by the patient and society for improved functional outcome from treatment of the tibial fracture continues to challenge the treating physician.

Annotated References

1. Praemer A, Furner S, Rice DP (eds): *Musculoskeletal Conditions in the United States.* Park Ridge, IL, American Academy of Orthopaedic Surgeons, 1992.

2. Rhinelander FW: Tibial blood supply in relation to fracture healing. *Clin Orthop* 1974:105:34-81.

3. Macnab I, De Haas WG: The role of periosteal blood supply in the healing of fractures of the tibia. *Clin Orthop* 1974;105:27-33.

4. Green SA: *Complication of External Skeletal Fixation: Causes, Prevention, and Treatment.* Springfield, IL, Thomas, 1981.

5. Levy AS, Bromberg J, Jasper D, et al: Tibia fractures produced from the impact of a baseball bat. *J Orthop Trauma* 1994:8:154-158.

6. Johner R, Wruhs O: Classification of tibial shaft fractures and correlation with results after rigid internal fixation. *Clin Orthop* 1983;178:7-25.

7. Brumback RJ, Jones AL: Interobserver agreement in the classification of open fractures of the tibia: The results of a survey of two hundred forty-five orthopaedic surgeons. *J Bone Joint Surg* 1994;76A:1162-1166.

    The authors provide interesting results of an interactive video evaluation of open tibial fractures by audience participants during the Orthopaedic Trauma Association meeting in 1994. The results reveal poor sensitivity and reproducibility of Gustilo's 1984 grading system for open fractures among physicians.

8. Ellis H: The speed of healing after fracture of the tibial shaft. *J Bone Joint Surg* 1958;40B:42-46.

9. Henley MB: Intramedullary devices for tibial fracture stabilization. *Clin Orthop* 1989;240:87-96.

10. Winquist RA, Hansen ST Jr, Clawson DK: Closed intramedullary nailing of femoral fractures: A report of five hundred and twenty cases. *J Bone Joint Surg* 1984;66A:529-539.

11. Müller ME, Nazarian S, Koch P, et al (eds): *The Comprehensive Classification of Fractures of Long Bones.* Berlin, Germany, Springer-Verlag, 1990.

12. Tscherne H, Gotzen L (eds): *Fractures With Soft Tissue Injuries.* New York, NY, Springer-Verlag, 1984.

13. Gustilo RB, Anderson JT: Prevention of infection in the treatment of one thousand twenty-five open fractures of long bones: Retrospective and prospective analyses. *J Bone Joint Surg* 1976;58A:453-458.

14. Gustilo RB, Mendoza RM, Williams DN: Problems in the management of type III (severe) open fractures: A new classification of type III open fractures. *J Trauma* 1984;24:742-746.

15. Oni OO, Hui A, Gregg PJ: The healing of closed tibial shaft fractures: The natural history of union with closed treatment. *J Bone Joint Surg* 1988;70B:787-790.

16. Sarmiento A, Gersten LM, Sobol PA, et al: Tibial shaft fractures treated with functional braces: Experience with 780 fractures. *J Bone Joint Surg* 1989;71B:602-609.

    The authors reviewed their analysis of 7,809 tibial fractures treated initially with cast immobilization and conversion to prefabricated functional braces. Sixty-three percent of the study group was followed to union with 17% of the patients lost to follow-up. Six percent of the patients were converted early after failure of closed treatment methods because of loss of control. The nonunion rate was 2.5%. The average healing time for isolated tibial fractures was 17.4

weeks and average healing time for tibial and fibular fractures was 21.5 weeks. Sixty percent of the patients healed with shortening averaging 7.1 mm with a range of 1 to 31 mm. Twenty-five percent of the patients healed with more than 5° of varus with a higher incidence of residual malunion in proximal and distal third tibial fractures. Anterior and posterior angulation also occurred in approximately 20% to 30% of the cases. The authors do not comment on malrotation.

17. Ruedi T, Webb JK, Allgöwer M: Experience with the dynamic compression plate (DCP) in 418 recent fractures of the tibial shaft. *Injury* 1976;7:252-257.

18. Anderson LD, Hutchins WC, Wright PE, et al: Fractures of the tibia and fibula treated by casts and transfixing pins. *Clin Orthop* 1974;105:179-191.

19. De Bastinani G, Aldegheri R, Renzi-Brivio L: The treatment of fractures with a dynamic axial fixator. *J Bone Joint Surg* 1984;66B:538-545.

20. Kenwright J, Richardson JB, Cunningham JL, et al: Axial movement and tibial fractures: A randomised trial of treatment. *J Bone Joint Surg* 1991;73B:654-659.

21. Richardson JB, Cunningham JL, Goodship AE, et al: Measuring stiffness can define healing of tibial fractures. *J Bone Joint Surg* 1994;76B:389-394.

22. Mayer L, Werbie T, Schwab JP, et al: The use of Ender nails in fractures of the tibial shaft. *J Bone Joint Surg* 1985;67A:446-455.

23. Wiss DA, Segal D, Gumbs VL, et al: Flexible medullary nailing of tibial shaft fractures. *J Trauma* 1986;26:1106-1112.

24. Bone LB, Johnson KD: Treatment of tibial fractures by reaming and intramedullary nailing. *J Bone Joint Surg* 1986;68A:877-887.

25. Alho A, Ekeland A, Stromsoe K, et al: Locked intramedullary nailing for displaced tibial shaft fractures. *J Bone Joint Surg* 1990;72B:805-809.

26. Court-Brown CM, Christie J, McQueen MM: Closed intramedullary tibial nailing: Its use in closed and type I open fractures. *J Bone Joint Surg* 1990;72B:605-611.

27. Riemer BL, DiChristina DG, Cooper A, et al: Nonreamed nailing of tibial diaphyseal fractures in blunt polytrauma patients. *J Orthop Trauma* 1995;9:66-75.

28. Henley MB, Meier M, Tencer AF: Influences of some design parameters on the biomechanics of the unreamed tibial intramedullary nail. *J Orthop Trauma* 1993;7:311-319.

29. Hooper GJ, Keddell RG, Penny ID: Conservative management or closed nailing for tibial shaft fractures: A randomized prospective trial. *J Bone Joint Surg* 1991;73B:83-85.

30. Fischer MD, Gustilo RB, Varecka TF: The timing of flap coverage, bone-grafting, and intramedullary nailing in patients who have a fracture of the tibial shaft with extensive soft-tissue injury. *J Bone Joint Surg* 1991;73A:1316-1322.

31. Ilizarov GA: The tension-stress effect on the genesis and growth of tissues: Part II. The influence of the rate and frequency of distraction. *Clin Orthop* 1989;239:263-285.

32. Raschke MJ, Mann JW, Oedekoven G, et al: Segmental transport after unreamed intramedullary nailing: Preliminary report of a ''Monorail'' system. *Clin Orthop* 1992;282:233-240.

33. Behrens F, Searls K: External fixation of the tibia: Basic concepts and prospective evaluation. *J Bone Joint Surg* 1986;68B:246-254.

   The authors present an excellent review of external fixation design and basic construction using current terminology.

34. Behrens F, Comfort TH, Searls K, et al: Unilateral external fixation for severe open tibial fractures: Preliminary report of a prospective study. *Clin Orthop* 1983;178:111-120.

35. Court-Brown CM, Wheelwright EF, Christie J, et al: External fixation for type III open tibial fractures. *J Bone Joint Surg* 1990;72B:801-804.

36. Caudle RJ, Stern PJ: Severe open fractures of the tibia. *J Bone Joint Surg* 1987;69A:801-807.

   This classic article discusses the results of open Gustilo type IIIA, B, and C injuries and points to necessity of early soft-tissue control and need for objective criteria for early amputation in type IIIC open tibial fractures. The authors utilized external fixation and microvascular free flaps.

37. Marsh JL, Nepola JV, Wuest TK, et al: Unilateral external fixation until healing with the dynamic axial fixator for severe open tibial fractures. *J Orthop Trauma* 1991;5:341-348.

38. Whittle AP, Russell TA, Taylor JC, et al: Treatment of open fractures of the tibial shaft with the use of interlocking nailing without reaming. *J Bone Joint Surg* 1992;74A:1162-1171.

   The authors present a technique and rationale for small diameter interlocking nails engineered to maximize strength characteristics for nonreamed application. The clinical results document that the infection rate is not increased with intramedullary nailing and that there are clinical advantages to this procedure when compared to historical external fixation of improved malunion rates.

39. Hansen ST Jr: Editorial: Type III-C tibial fracture: Salvage or amputation. *J Bone Joint Surg* 1987;69A:799-800.

40. Trabulsy PP, Kerley SM, Hoffman WY: A prospective study of early soft tissue coverage of grade IIIB tibial fractures. *J Trauma* 1994;36:661-668.

41. Georgiadis GM, Behrens FF, Joyce MJ, et al: Open tibial fractures with severe soft-tissue loss: Limb salvage compared with below-the-knee amputation. *J Bone Joint Surg* 1993;75A:1431-1441.

42. Kemp AG, van Niekerk JL, van Meurs PA: Impairment scores of type III open tibial fractures. *Injury* 1993;24:161-162.

43. Helfet DL, Howey T, Sanders R, et al: Limb salvage versus amputation: Preliminary results of the mangled extremity severity score. *Clin Orthop* 1990;256:80-86.

44. McNamara MG, Heckman JD, Corley FG: Severe open fractures of the lower extremity: A retrospective evaluation of the mangled extremity severity score (MESS). *J Orthop Trauma* 1994;8:81-87.

45. Charnley J: Fractures of the shaft of the tibia, in *The Closed Treatment of Common Fractures*. Edinburgh, Scotland,

Churchill Livingstone, 1961, pp 204-249.

46. Edwards CC, Simmons SC, Browner BD, et al: Severe open tibial fractures: Results treating 202 injuries with external fixation. *Clin Orthop* 1988;230:98-115.

47. Burgess AR, Poka A, Brumback RJ, et al: Pedestrian tibial injuries. *J Trauma* 1987;27:596-601.

48. Clancey GJ, Winquist RA, Hansen ST Jr: Nonunion of the tibia treated with Kuntscher intramedullary nailing. *Clin Orthop* 1982;167:191-196.

49. Mayo KA, Benirschke SK: Treatment of tibial malunions and nonunions with reamed intramedullary nails. *Orthop Clin North Am* 1990;21:715-724.

50. Wiss DA, Stetson WB: Nonunion of the tibia treated with a reamed intramedullary nail. *J Orthop Trauma* 1994;8:189-194.

51. Johnson KD: Management of malunion and nonunion of the tibia. *Orthop Clin North Am* 1987;18:157-171.

52. Moed BR, Watson JT: Intramedullary nailing of the tibia without a fracture table: The transfixion pin distractor technique. *J Orthop Trauma* 1994;8:195-202.

53. Helfet DL, Jupiter JB, Gasser S: Indirect reduction and tension-band plating of tibial non-union with deformity. *J Bone Joint Surg* 1992;74A:1286-1297.

54. Wiss DA, Johnson DL, Miao M: Compression plating for non-union after failed external fixation of open tibial fractures. *J Bone Joint Surg* 1992;74A:1279-1285.

55. Johnson EE: Acute lengthening of shortened lower extremities after malunion or non-union of a fracture. *J Bone Joint Surg* 1994;76A:379-389.

56. McGraw JM, Lim EV: Treatment of open tibial-shaft fractures: External fixation and secondary intramedullary nailing. *J Bone Joint Surg* 1988;70A:900-911.

57. Maurer DJ, Merkow RL, Gustilo RB: Infection after intramedullary nailing of severe open tibial fractures initially treated with external fixation. *J Bone Joint Surg* 1989;71A:835-838.

58. Court-Brown CM, Keating JF, McQueen MM, et al: Infection after intramedullary nailing of the tibia: Incidence and protocol for management. *J Bone Joint Surg* 1992;74B:770-774.

59. Whittle AP, Wester W, Russell TA: Fatigue failure in small diameter interlocking tibial nails: Implications for postoperative care. *Clin Orthop* 1995, in press.

60. Blick SS, Brumback RJ, Poka A, et al: Compartment syndrome in open tibial fractures. *J Bone Joint Surg* 1986;68A:1348-1353.

The authors review their experiences with open fractures complicated by compartment syndromes at the Shock Trauma Center in Baltimore. The results dispel the false concept that compartment syndromes are rare in open fractures.

61. McQueen MM, Christie J, Court-Brown CM: Compartment pressures after intramedullary nailing of the tibia. *J Bone Joint Surg* 1990;72B:395-397.

62. Koval KJ, Clapper MF, Brumback RJ, et al: Complications of reamed intramedullary nailing of the tibia. *J Orthop Trauma* 1991;5:184-189.

Annotated Bibliography

Catagni M: Classification and treatment of nonunion, in *Operative Principles of Ilazarov*. Baltimore, MD, Williams & Wilkins, 1991, pp 191-198.

The authors present a logical classification of the types of nonunions with proposed Ilizarov approach to treatment.

Cattaneo RM, Catagni M, Johnson EE: The treatment of infected nonunions and segmental defects of the tibia by the methods of Ilizarov. *Clin Orthop* 1992;280:143-152.

The authors review a very difficult clinical problem with Ilizarov techniques.

Court-Brown CM: Fractures of the tibial diaphysis. *Int J Orthop Trauma* 1993;3:40-46.

This is an excellent review article from an experienced researcher who summarizes the results and questions regarding tibial shaft injuries.

Johnson EE, Urist MR, Finerman GA: Distal metaphyseal tibial nonunion: Deformity and bone loss treated by open reduction, internal fixation, and human bone morphogenetic protein (hBMP). *Clin Orthop* 1990;250:234-240.

This is a possible glimpse into the future of biologic intervention of difficult tibial problems.

Keating JF, Kuo RS, Court-Brown CM: Bifocal fractures of the tibia and fibula: Incidence, classification and treatment. *J Bone Joint Surg* 1994;76B:395-400.

The authors confirm the preferred treatment of segmental tibial fractures with intramedullary nail techniques.

Lonner JH, Jupiter JB, Healy WL: Ipsilateral tibia and ankle fractures. *J Orthop Trauma* 1993;7:130-137.

The authors suggest that although nonsurgical managment may be successful, this combination may best be treated with combined surgical fixation for mobilization of the extremity.

Templeman DC, Marder RA: Injuries of the knee associated with fractures of the tibial shaft: Detection by examination under anesthesia. A prospective study. *J Bone Joint Surg* 1989;71A:1392-1395.

The authors present a prospective study conducted in the knees of 50 patients who had sustained a fracture of the ipsilateral tibial shaft. The fractures were of varying severity. Patients were examined manually while the patient was under general anesthesia. Eleven patients (22%) sustained an injury to at least one ligament of the knee that resulted in increased laxity of 2+ or more. One knee had dislocated. Authors believe that after stabilization of a fracture of the tibial shaft, it is essential to examine the knee thoroughly to identify any associated ligamentous injuries.

Williams MO: Long-term cost comparison of major limb salvage using the Ilizarov method versus amputation. *Clin Orthop* 1994;301:156-158.

The author compared hospital costs and professional fees of Ilizarov limb reconstruction patients to hospital costs, professional fees, and prosthetic costs of lower-extremity amputation patients. Ten patients with tibial nonunions, osteomyelitis, infected nonunions, and/or bone defects underwent Ilizarov limb reconstruction while six patients with similar traumatic injuries underwent amputation (three acute and three delayed). Both the Ilizarov and the amputation groups required an average of four surgical procedures. The total average treatment time was 322 days for the Ilizarov group and 175 days for the amputation group. The total cost of the Ilizarov limb reconstruction averaged $59,213.71. The hospital costs and professional fees for the amputation group averaged $30,148.02 without prosthetic costs; with the projected lifetime prosthetic costs included, costs averaged $403,199.18. The author suggests that Ilizarov limb reconstruction is cost-effective when compared with amputation when prosthetic costs are also considered. This study may be indicative of the type of cost-benefit analysis that may help justify improved technologies.

Wu CC, Shih CH: Complicated open fractures of the distal tibia treated by secondary interlocking nailing. *J Trauma* 1993;34:792-796.

The authors demonstrate successful use of external fixation provisionally followed by early intramedullary nailing. This may demonstrate a time-dependent phenomenon of pin tract contamination versus infection.

18
Fractures of the Tibial Plafond

Introduction

Intra-articular fractures of the distal end of the tibia present a wide spectrum of articular and metaphyseal damage and are relatively infrequent injuries, representing approximately 1% of lower extremity fractures and 5% to 10% of all tibial fractures. These fractures have been referred to as pilon fractures, a description based on the talus acting like a hammer driving into the weightbearing surface of the distal tibia. These injuries are also called fractures of the tibial plafond, which is an anatomic analogy to the distal tibial articular surface acting like a roof over the talus.

Pilon injuries must be differentiated from the more common ankle fractures. The key to identifying pilon fractures is the disruption of the weightbearing articular surface of the tibia, most commonly from an axial loading mechanism of injury. This is distinct from rotational ankle injuries, in which the malleoli fail as medial and lateral bony restraints because of excessive talar rotation or translation. However, the distinction is not clearcut, because a percentage of ankle fractures have a component of axial compression of the tibial articular surface and some fractures of the tibial plafond can result from overwhelming rotational forces.

The direction of the force applied to the foot and the position of the foot at the time of impact help determine the fracture pattern involving the distal tibia.[1,2] If the foot is in plantarflexion during extreme axial compression of the limb, the posterior portion of the tibial articular surface is likely to be loaded, fracturing the posterior malleolus from the remainder of the distal tibia and impacting the central portion of the ankle joint. If forced dorsiflexion occurs instead, the anterior joint surface is compressed by the talus, leading to anterior ankle joint comminution. The pilon fracture may have the entire tibial articulation disrupted from the tibial shaft or it may cause only one portion of the joint to be separated from the otherwise intact distal tibia. Although the ipsilateral fibula is commonly fractured in tibial plafond injuries, it has been reported to remain intact, with or without injury to the syndesmosis, in up to 25% of pilon fractures.[2] Because some degree of rotational forces are common in these injuries, a wide spectrum of fracture patterns is created by the many variable mechanisms of injury.

Injuries from axial loading are thought to create more articular cartilage damage than the shear forces associated with rotational injuries and, thus, may have a greater propensity for poor clinical results.[3] The most common mechanisms of injury include falls and motor vehicle accidents. Because one mechanism of injury, such as skiing, may place more rotational forces on the distal tibia than another, ie, a fall from a height, some patient populations may be predisposed to better clinical outcomes than others. To explain the wide range of results reported with fractures of the tibial plafond, investigators have scrutinized the various published series on pilon fractures in terms of differences in the mechanism of injury and, hence, potential differences in the degree of articular damage.

Injury Evaluation

Clinically, pilon fractures have posed little difficulty in diagnosis. Marked pain and swelling, the inability to bear weight, and a mechanism of injury of axial loading should raise the suspicion for a fracture of the distal tibia. A careful neurovascular examination is mandatory. Plain radiographs, for the most part, disclose the degree of disruption of the articular surface. If comminution is mild, and the position of the osteocartilaginous fragments apparent, no further diagnostic tests are warranted. Comparison views of the contralateral uninjured ankle may also be helpful. With severe displacement or impaction of the weightbearing surface, however, tomograms or computed tomograms may provide the surgeon with a better understanding of the size and location of the articular fragments and assist in planning any surgical approach.

Because pilon fractures often result from high-energy trauma, the physician should have a high index of suspicion for other injuries that result from axial-load mechanisms, such as accompanying hindfoot fractures as well as lower extremity long bone fractures, vertical shear injuries of the pelvis, and compression or bursting fractures of the vertebral column. Certainly intracranial, intrathoracic, and intra-abdominal injuries must be considered in patients with pilon fractures from major accidents or falls.

Classification

Many classification schemes for fractures of the distal tibia have been published. Lauge-Hansen[4,5] classified this frac-

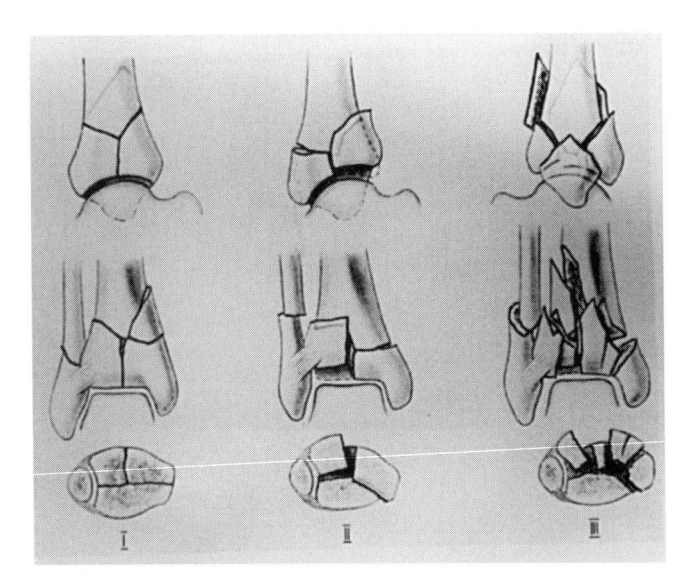

Fig. 1 The Ruedi and Allgöwer classification of fractures of the tibial plafond. (Reproduced with permission from Ruedi TP, Allgöwer M: Fractures of the lower end of the tibia into the ankle joint: Results 9 years after open reduction. *Injury* 1973;5:130.)

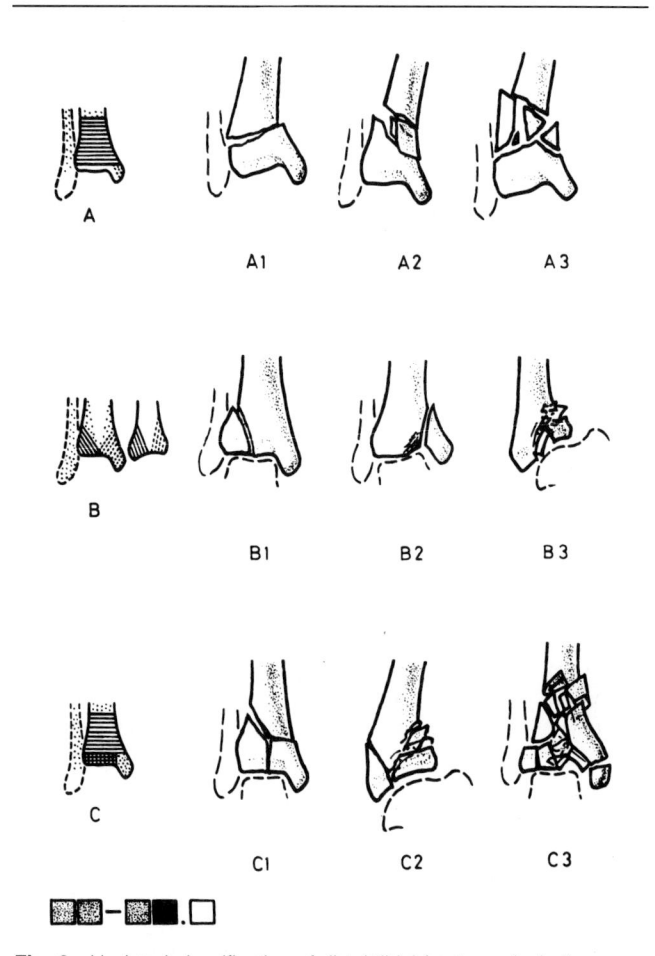

Fig. 2 Updated classification of distal tibial fractures, including nonarticular fractures as well as fractures of the tibial plafond. (Reproduced with permission from Müller ME, Nazarian S, Koch P, et al (eds): *The Comprehensive Classification of Fractures of Long Bones.* Berlin, Germany, Springer-Verlag, 1990, p 173.)

ture as a separate ankle fracture occurring from forced dorsiflexion, with a vertical fracture of the medial malleolus accompanied by impaction of the tibial plafond. Other authors have taken into account the varying degrees of rotational forces in some fractures of the distal tibia. Most notably, Kellam and Waddell[3] divided pilon fractures by mechanism of injury and fracture pattern into two types, rotational and axial loading. The importance of this distinction was that the fractures occurring from rotational injuries had a much greater chance of having a good clinical outcome. Rotational injuries tended to have large osteocartilaginous fragments, most notably a significant posterior malleolus fragment. Axial loading injuries more commonly presented with comminution and impaction of the articular surface.

The building block for more modern classifications is that of Ruedi and Allgöwer,[6] who subdivided pilon fractures into types I, II, and III according to increasing severity, based on the degree of joint surface comminution and displacement (Fig. 1). Variations on this classification have been published,[7-9] but none of these classifications has been widely accepted within the orthopaedic literature. The importance of the Ruedi and Allgöwer[6] classification is that it specifically addresses the difficult axial loading injuries of the tibial plafond and it has been shown by several studies to be predictive of clinical outcome.[8,10]

Unlike the classification of many other injuries, the classification of pilon fractures is still undergoing revision, leading to confusion over this issue. The early Ruedi and Allgöwer[6] classification used the accepted type I, II, and III grouping. Later, a new A, B, C system was proposed in which type A fractures are distal tibial metaphyseal injuries without joint involvement (supramalleolar) and types B and C represent the true pilon fractures (Fig. 2).[11] The older classification[6] is most representative of the current literature. However, with future investigations of pilon fractures, it is likely that one of the newer, but as yet untested, classification systems will be used.

Treatment Options

Nonsurgical treatment with casts or splints has not yielded a high percentage of acceptable results, except as management for nondisplaced fractures. Treatment with calcaneal traction, pins and plaster, transarticular pin fixation, and fibular fixation alone have likewise led to poor results, and these methods have been abandoned.[12,13] Before the era of open reduction and internal fixation, early ankle arthrodesis was the likely outcome for a moderate to severe fracture of the tibial plafond. Therefore, unless damage to the distal tibial surface is so extensive that reconstruction is not possible, displaced pilon fractures should be treated surgically.

The accepted principle of treatment is to restore anatomic alignment to the joint surface and obtain enough stability of the distal tibia to allow for early motion of the ankle joint. This can be provided with open reduction and plating or with lag screw fixation of the joint surface and external fixation.

Timing of Surgery

Most authors agree that surgical reconstruction of the distal tibia should be performed within 8 to 12 hours of injury or should be delayed for 7 to 10 days. Swelling, secondary to both the injury and surgery, may lead to difficulty with wound closure and/or skin slough. For cases that require delay, temporizing measures, eg, closed reduction with restoration of length to the leg, followed by the application of a well-padded splint and elevation of the limb to minimize further swelling, are recommended. If maintenance of limb length is difficult with splinting, calcaneal traction should be considered as a preoperative measure.

In critically ill patients undergoing lifesaving emergency surgery, it may be advisable to place an external fixator across the ankle joint to hold the limb at appropriate length. This maneuver permits a "ligamentotaxis" reduction of the distal tibial fragments. This select group of patients may not be medically cleared for surgery within a week or 10 days of injury, and the external fixator provides good stability and a partial reduction during the delay awaiting joint reconstruction. On the other hand, if the polytrauma patient's condition is stable, fixation of the tibial plafond is recommended on the day of injury.

Surgical Goals and Results

The Swiss, led by Ruedi and Allgöwer's classic work published in 1969,[2] addressed the surgical treatment of pilon fractures in a stepwise, logical manner. The first step was to repair the fibula. Usually, the fibula was not comminuted and restoration of anatomic alignment of the lateral column provided a guide to overall length of the comminuted distal tibia. The second step was to reconstruct the articular surface of the distal tibia, usually with lag screws. The third step was to insert cancellous bone graft into the distal tibial metaphysis to help support the articular surface, fill the dead space created by its impaction, and stimulate healing of the fracture. The fourth step was to plate the medial portion of the distal tibia. The goal was to create a stable distal tibia, permitting early range of motion of the ankle joint. These tenets of treatment remain the mainstay of surgical planning for the fixation of displaced fractures of the tibial plafond.

Before that 1969 series, most investigations of pilon fractures reported good results in fewer than 50% of the cases. Using exacting open reduction techniques, Ruedi and Allgöwer[2] obtained 74% good and excellent results at the 4-year follow-up. Five years later, long-term follow-up of the same patient population showed no attrition of these results over time.[14] Another confirmatory study, based primarily on skiing injuries, reported good to excellent results in 90% of patients with open reduction of pilon fractures[15] (Fig. 3).

One criticism of these investigations has been that the patient populations selected were young athletes involved in ski injuries, with a potential predisposition toward good results because of the low level of energy involved compared to that usually found in high-energy injuries from falls or motor vehicle accidents. Skiing, as a mechanism of injury, was believed to create a higher percentage of rotational fracture types without significant comminution or impaction of the articular surface. To answer this criticism, the authors published a study in which approximately 50% of the patients had fractures classified as type III, the more severe intra-articular injuries, all treated by open plating.[6] At follow-up, 80% of the patients judged their ankle fit for normal use and 52% had symmetric ankle motion with the uninjured side.

Many other investigators from both Europe and the United States began to report similar results with this difficult spectrum of injuries. No universal scoring system for functional outcome of pilon fractures has been employed by these various investigations, making a true comparison of results difficult. In one study, better results were reported with open reduction than with all other forms of treatment.[9] However, half of the comparison group was treated nonsurgically with closed reduction and casting, a method previously known to produce poor outcome. The authors concluded, as have many other investigators,[10,16] that the final functional result correlates well with the accuracy of the articular reduction. They reported an overall rate of 65% good or excellent results and an infection rate of 6%. One series reported, after an average 10-year follow-up, 95% good and fair results with open reduction techniques but also reported that an anatomic reduction with good early clinical results did not guarantee against the development of late arthrosis and pain.[16] These findings, in a low-energy injury population, differ from those of a previous report of long-term follow-up,[14] which noted no decline in results over time.

Although many studies reported low complication rates even with the inclusion of some high-energy trauma, other studies showed a directly proportional ratio between the incidence of high-energy trauma and the incidence of complications. In Swiss studies,[2,16] for example, high-energy trauma accounted for only 25% and 42% of the cases, respectively. In another study, 62% of the patients had high-energy injuries and still had excellent results.[9] However, Bourne and associates[17] reported an increase in complication rates as the incidence of high-energy trauma increased. The authors reported a high rate of complications, a 32% arthrodesis rate, and only 25% good results in type III fractures. These findings are in sharp contrast to the results previously quoted.

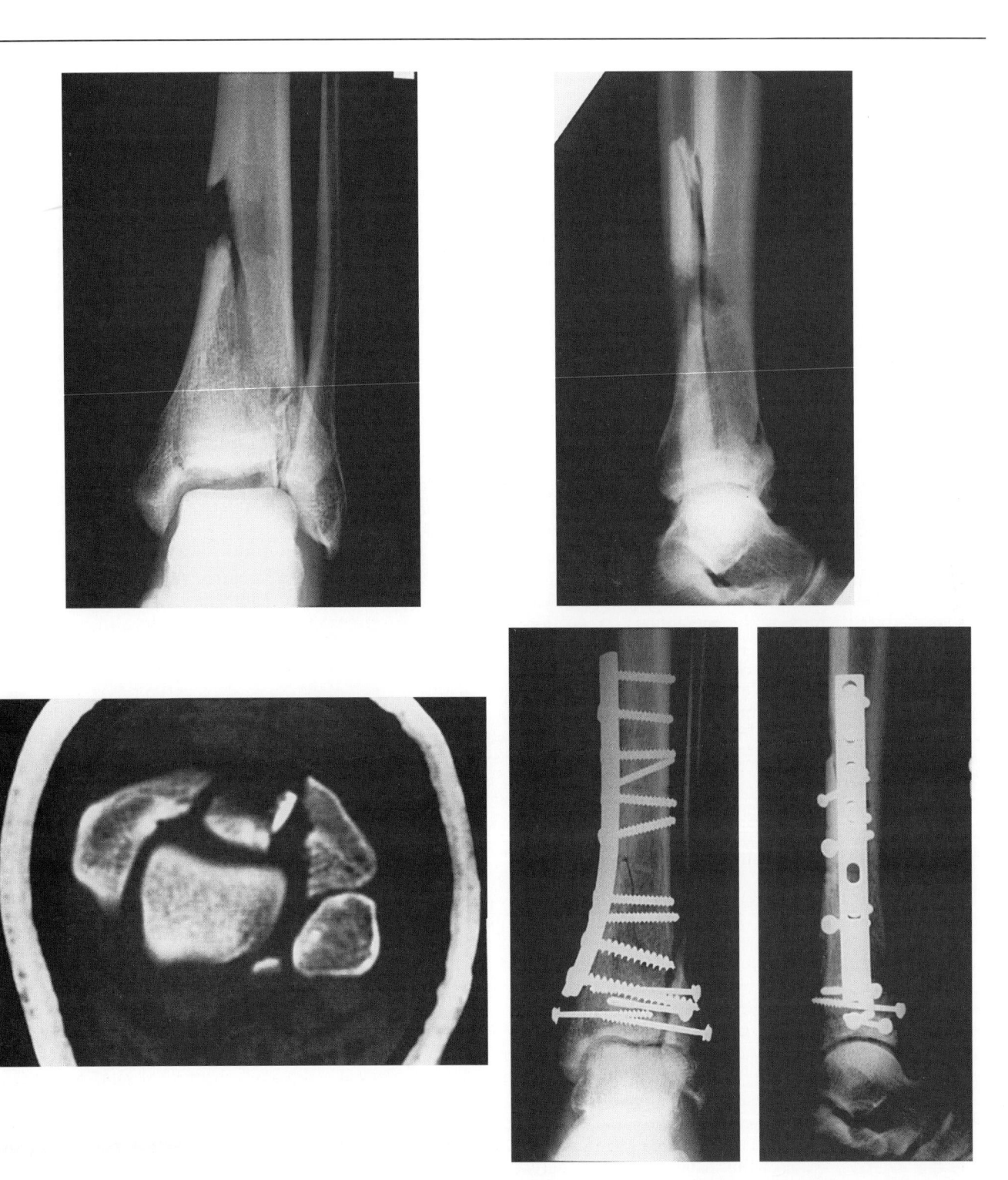

Fig. 3 An example of open reduction and internal fixation of a comminuted pilon fracture. **Top left** and **top right**, Anteroposterior (AP) and lateral radiographs demonstrate a comminuted distal tibial fracture; note the impaction of the articular surface on the lateral aspect of the tibial plafond as seen on the AP radiograph. **Bottom left**, Computed tomography scan at the level of the weightbearing surface of the talus and of the distal tibial metaphysis reveal a comminuted distal tibial articular surface. A large medial malleolar fragment and the anterolateral "Tillaux" fragment are easily identifiable. The talus has been driven superiorly and slightly posteriorly into the plafond of the distal tibia. **Bottom right**, AP and lateral radiographs after open reduction and plating. The joint surface has been anatomically restored and the distal tibia has been plated. Range of motion of the ankle at 1-year follow-up was 7° of dorsiflexion and 30° of plantarflexion. (Reproduced with permission from Brumback RJ, McGarvey WC: Fractures of the tibial plafond: The pilon fracture. Evolving treatment concepts. *Orthop Clin North Am* 1995;26:273-285.)

Other recent investigations support the caution expressed by Bourne and associates.[17] In a small series of 11 patients treated by surgeons whose experience in the management of severe pilon fractures was limited, disastrous results were reported, with a 55% incidence of osteomyelitis.[18] Only three of the 11 fractures united without complications after open reduction. In a larger retrospective review, 50% poor results were reported overall,[19] with 37% of the type III fractures complicated by infection. Infection occurred more often in patients with postoperative wound problems (dehiscence, failure of closure, drainage) and was not directly related to the presence of an open fracture. The rate of ankle arthrodesis for type I and II fractures was 10%. Arthrodesis was required in 26% of the type III injuries. In a recent report of 52 pilon fractures, in which 40% were type III injuries and 46 of 52 were treated with open reduction,[20] 40% of the fractures suffered some complication, including an infection rate of approximately 20%. These complications resulted in a total of 77 additional procedures for this patient population and, although more frequent in type III injuries, complications were not limited to this more severe fracture type.

Therefore, recent literature has demonstrated that the pilon fracture, although amenable to open reduction, carries a high risk of complications and the potential for repeat surgery. This has led orthopaedists to search for techniques to minimize bone and soft-tissue problems while achieving the surgical goals originally put forth by Ruedi and Allgöwer.[6] In the 1990s, more and more surgeons are using a combined internal fixation/external fixation technique to decrease the amount of iatrogenic damage and dissection in severe pilon fractures.[21,22] This technique is not new,[23] but several recent studies[24,25] verify a reduction in complications associated with this treatment of fractures of the tibial plafond.

The surgical technique, paralleling the principles of Ruedi, usually begins with open reduction and plating of the fibula. As the external fixator can be used to restore fibular length without the need for plating, some authors have elected to forego fibular plating in some instances.[21,26] After restoring appropriate length, the distal tibial articular surface is realigned. This may be attempted percutaneously, but more often requires open reduction of the fracture fragments. A 6- to 9-cm incision placed anteriorly over the major fracture line has been advocated.[21] Minimal periosteal stripping is performed and the anterior fractures serve as a "window" for reduction of the impacted articular fragments. The reduced articular surface is held in place with bone graft and cannulated lag screws. The metaphyseal portion is stabilized to the tibial diaphysis with external fixation, and bone graft is inserted into metaphyseal defects as necessary (Fig. 4). Some clinicians use small tension wire fixation of the distal tibia just proximal to the articular surface, permitting free ankle motion (Fig. 5).[21] Other investigators use external fixation to the calcaneus or talus (Fig. 4).[22] External fixation to the calcaneus has the theoretical disadvantage of restricting subtalar joint motion. The talus, due to its relatively small size and high percentage

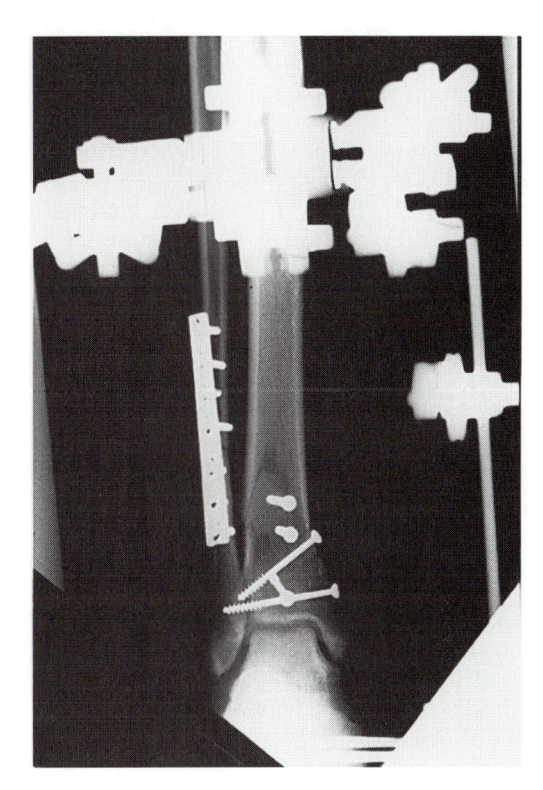

Fig. 4 An example of a healed intraarticular fracture of the distal tibia treated by lag screw fixation and fibular plating and supported by external fixation across the ankle joint. AP radiograph discloses an anatomic joint surface with acceptable alignment of the tibial metaphyseal portion of the fracture. (Reproduced with permission from Brumback RJ, McGarvey WC: Fractures of the tibial plafond: The pilon fracture. Evolving treatment concepts. *Orthop Clin North Am* 1995;26:273-285.)

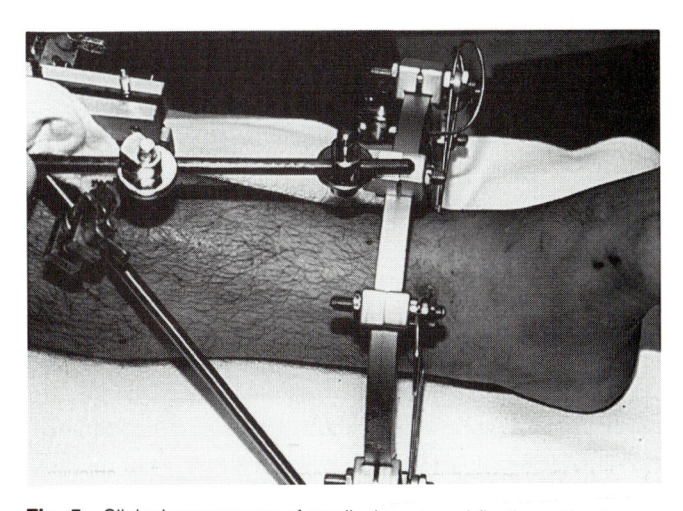

Fig. 5 Clinical appearance of small-wire external fixation with wires placed cephalad to the ankle joint, permitting ankle range of motion.

of articular cartilage surface, is not an ideal anchor for external fixation. Unilateral articulated fixators also have been used to permit ankle joint motion while maintaining external fixation across the ankle joint.[26] Early motion of the ankle joint after fixation with this technique has been investigated, but never in a well-controlled clinical environment.

The results of external fixation with minimal internal fixation have been promising. In one study of 17 pilon fractures, the authors obtained 69% good results in type III fractures with only one deep infection.[21] No wound sloughs were noted, but four patients had pin-tract infections. In another study, no infections were reported in 20 patients whose severe comminution or open pilon fractures were treated with external fixation and limited open reduction.[22] At follow-up, 75% had good to excellent range of motion of the ankle. Three delayed unions required repeat surgery. Two patients had pin-tract infections and two patients underwent eventual arthrodesis for posttraumatic arthritis. Several series have reported similar results with the unilateral external fixator. One recent presentation, however, demonstrated a high rate of pin-tract complications associated with articulated unilateral external fixation across the ankle.[27]

In the only study directly comparing surgical techniques, the authors analyzed the complications associated with open reduction with respect to those seen with external fixation and minimal internal fixation.[28] In a prospective, surgeon-randomized trial, unplanned surgery for complications was seen in 55% of those fractures treated by open reduction versus 18% of those treated by external fixation. The authors concluded that external fixation with minimal internal fixation is an excellent alternative to open reduction and plating.

Complications and Salvage Procedures

Certain pilon fractures are so comminuted that they preclude anatomic joint reduction. These injuries are best treated by early ankle arthrodesis. It is controversial whether the chance of a successful arthrodesis is improved by an attempt to reconstruct the bone stock of the distal tibia, even without anatomic restoration of the articular surface, or whether allowing the distal tibia to heal in its displaced position before attempting fusion is a more prudent course. The fragments in these injuries can be greatly displaced, making future arthrodesis difficult. Distraction via an external fixator device can provide gross alignment of the major fracture fragments and may negate any need to address surgically the distal tibial bone stock awaiting arthrodesis. Fortunately, these injuries are rare. These injuries have a marked soft-tissue injury component accompanying the joint destruction, and it is recommended that arthrodesis be delayed for a minimum of 6 to 12 weeks after injury.[29]

It is apparent that severely comminuted pilon fractures, or those with less than anatomic reconstructions, have a greater risk of posttraumatic arthritis. Ankle arthrodesis is an excellent salvage procedure when symptoms become disabling in these instances. The technique selected for ankle fusion must be individualized to the type and severity of the pilon fracture, the original method of surgical stabilization, and any previous history of infection. Despite the excellent functional results obtainable with ankle arthrodesis, many patients elect to live with restricted range of motion of the ankle and mild discomfort rather than give up what increased function their diminished ankle range provides.

No matter how carefully the reconstruction of the distal tibia is performed, surgery for pilon fractures occasionally results in wound problems. Coverage of the distal tibia by rotation of local tissue is not often successful, because these tissues are inherently involved with the injury. Wound problems are believed to be more common when the two incisions used for open reduction have a skin bridge less than 7 cm wide.[14,30] When possible, the distance between the fibular and tibial wounds should be maximized to prevent hypovascularity of the skin covering the anterior tibia. Several wound closure scenarios have been studied. Excessive tension at the time of wound closure is to be avoided. If both wounds cannot be closed after open reduction, closure of the medial tibia wound is performed with skin grafting of the lateral fibular wound.[31] This technique provides coverage of the exposed tibia fracture, the tendons and neurovascular structures anterior to the tibia, and the inserted hardware without resorting to tissue flaps.[32] The technique of "pie-crusting," with multiple small skin incisions, has been used to avoid the need for skin grafting while shifting the skin of the lower leg to cover medial defects.[31]

Wound dehiscence, failure of closure after open reduction, or closure of open fracture wounds can be performed with freely vascularized transfer of the latissimus dorsi or rectus abdominus. As these muscles may provide too much bulk around the ankle, some authors have suggested using the full-thickness radial forearm flap.[30] Although these are specialized procedures, full-thickness coverage about the ankle is desirable because of the paucity of soft tissue in this location and the high degree of bone necrosis associated with this comminuted intra-articular fracture. Full-thickness coverage also prevents adherence and desiccation of tendons and neurovascular structures, as well as providing a healthy soft-tissue bed for fracture healing.

Deep infection is the most feared complication in the treatment of pilon fractures. It can be adequately treated only by removal of all necrotic tissue and, most often, the stabilizing hardware. Although the infection can be temporarily allowed to drain while awaiting fracture healing in hopes of maintaining the ankle joint, comminuted pilon fractures often have many devitalized articular fragments. These necrotic osteocartilaginous fragments, which form the reconstructed weightbearing dome of the ankle joint, may be the nidus of the infection and their removal signals the demise of future ankle function. On the other hand, some pilon infections are centered in the crushed supramalleolar area and salvage of ankle joint function can be attempted.

Should infection lead to excision of all or part of the articular surface of the distal tibia, reconstruction of the leg with a bone transport and ankle fusion has been proposed. Although a specialized procedure, this salvage technique has prevented the need for a below-the-knee amputation in a patient with a normally sensate foot.[33]

Summary

Pilon fractures represent a most difficult challenge to the orthopaedist. Assessment of the degree of energy causing the fracture, as well as careful planning of the joint reconstruction, will lead to acceptable results in most cases. High-energy pilon fractures should be treated with great care and respect, because the risk of complications is high and the likelihood of a good functional ankle is less predictable. Treatment trends have moved away from formal open reduction and plating to limited surgical exposure for reduction of the articular surface with external fixation stabilization of the distal tibia and ankle. However, fear of complications should not deter the orthopaedist from attempting to gain anatomic restoration of joint alignment as this produces the best clinical results. Knowledge of the appropriate salvage procedures, should complications develop, is needed to treat the full spectrum of pilon injuries.

Annotated References

1. Bone LB: Fractures of the tibial plafond: The pilon fracture. *Orthop Clin North Am* 1987;18:95-104.

    This review article summarizes the classification schemes, the treatment options, and the results of pilon fractures treated with open reduction or external fixation.

2. Ruedi TP, Allgöwer M: Fractures of the lower end of the tibia into the ankle-joint. *Injury* 1969;1:92-99.

    This classic article describes the stepwise reconstruction of fractures of the distal tibia with open reduction. The authors obtained 74% good results with open plating techniques in a ski injury population.

3. Kellam JF, Waddell JP: Fractures of the distal tibial metaphysis with intra-articular extension: The distal tibial explosion fracture. *J Trauma* 1979;19:593-601.

    The authors investigated 26 distal tibial fractures classified into type A (rotational) and type B (compressive) fractures. Type A fractures had 84% acceptable results versus only 53% for type B injuries. Rotational pilon fractures were less common than compressive injuries (7 of 19) and had a better prognosis.

4. Lauge N: Fractures of the ankle: Analytic historic survey as the basis of new experimental, roentgenologic and clinical investigations. *Arch Surg* 1948;56:259-317.

5. Lauge-Hansen N: Fractures of the ankle: II. Combined experimental-surgical and experimental-roentgenologic investigations. *Arch Surg* 1950;60:957-985.

6. Ruedi TP, Allgöwer M: The operative treatment of intra-articular fractures of the lower end of the tibia. *Clin Orthop* 1979;138:105-110.

    This Swiss series presented 75 patients of whom 47% had sports-related injuries. In approximately 50%, fractures were classified as type III. The authors obtained 80% good functional results 6 years after open reduction and internal fixation. Only 5% of the series required ankle arthrodesis. There were no cases of osteomyelitis and only one nonunion. This article illustrates the Ruedi and Allgöwer classification and provides a good overview of previous Swiss publications.

7. Maale G, Seligson D: Fractures through the distal weight-bearing surface of the tibia. *Orthopedics* 1980;3:517-521.

    The authors propose a classification including (1) distal tibial compression fractures, (2) external rotation fractures with large posterior fragments, and (3) spiral fractures with extension surface. The authors emphasize the relationship between the mechanism of injury, the fracture into the distal tibial articular pattern, and the clinical prognosis, with rotational injuries having a better prognosis.

8. Mast JW, Spiegel PG, Pappas JN: Fractures of the tibial pilon. *Clin Orthop* 1988;230:68-82.

    This is a good review article that emphasizes open reduction with a detailed description of the surgical technique and the use of the femoral distractor for indirect reduction.

9. Ovadia DN, Beals RK: Fractures of the tibial plafond. *J Bone Joint Surg* 1986;68A:543-551.

    The authors present a retrospective review of 145 fractures of the distal tibia. Using traditional open reduction techniques, the authors achieved 65% good and excellent results. Arthrodesis was required in more than 30% of the severe injuries. These results parallel those reported by Reudi and associates.

10. Helfet DL, Koval K, Pappas J, et al: Intraarticular "pilon" fracture of the tibia. *Clin Orthop* 1994;298:221-228.

    The authors present a retrospective review of 34 high-energy pilon fractures, 28 treated by open reduction and six by external fixation and minimal internal fixation. Type II fractures had 65% good results; type III fractures had 50% good results. The final result was correlated to the accuracy of the articular reconstruction. This is a recent series that advocates open reduction and plating for most injuries.

11. Müller ME, Nazarian S, Koch P, et al (eds): *The Comprehensive Classification of Fractures of Long Bones.* Berlin, Germany, Springer-Verlag, 1990.

12. Ruwe PA, Randall RL, Baumgaertner MR: Pilon fractures of the distal tibia. *Orthop Rev* 1993;22:987-996.

13. Leach RE: A means of stabilizing comminuted distal tibial fractures. *J Trauma* 1964;4:722-725.

14. Ruedi T: Fractures of the lower end of the tibia into the ankle joint: Results 9 years after open reduction and internal fixation. *Injury* 1973;5:130-134.

15. Heim U, Naser M: Operative treatment of distal tibial fractures: Technique of osteosynthesis and results in 128 patients. *Arch Orthop Unfall-Chir* 1976;86:341-356.

16. Etter C, Ganz R: Long-term results of tibial plafond fractures treated with open reduction and internal fixation. *Arch Orthop Trauma Surg* 1991;110:277-283.

17. Bourne RB, Rorabeck CH, Macnab J: Intra-articular fractures of the distal tibia: The pilon fracture. *J Trauma* 1983;23:591-596.

18. Dillin L, Slabaugh P: Delayed wound healing, infection, and nonunion following open reduction and internal fixation of tibial plafond fractures. *J Trauma* 1986;26:1116-1119.

19. Teeny SM, Wiss DA: Open reduction and internal fixation of tibial plafond fractures: Variables contributing to poor results and complications. *Clin Orthop* 1993;292:108-117.

20. McFerran MA, Smith SW, Boulas HJ, et al: Complications encountered in the treatment of pilon fractures. *J Orthop Trauma* 1992;6:195-200.

21. Tornetta P III, Weiner L, Bergman M, et al: Pilon fractures: Treatment with combined internal and external fixation. *J Orthop Trauma* 1993;7:489-496.

    The authors present a good review of the surgical technique for external fixation and minimal internal fixation. Seventeen pilon fractures are presented with 69% good results in type III injuries. Only one deep infection occurred.

22. Bone L, Stegemann P, McNamara K, et al: External fixation of severely comminuted and open tibial pilon fractures. *Clin Orthop* 1993;292:101-107.

23. Scheck M: Treatment of comminuted distal tibial fractures by combined dual-pin fixation and limited open reduction. *J Bone Joint Surg* 1965;47A:1537-1553.

24. Saleh M, Shanahan MD, Fern ED: Intra-articular fractures of the distal tibia: Surgical management by limited internal fixation and articulated distraction. *Injury* 1993;24:37-40.

25. Murphy CP, D'Ambrosia R, Dabezies EJ: The small pin circular fixator for proximal tibial fractures with soft tissue compromise. *Orthopedics* 1991;14:273-280.

26. Bonar SK, Marsh JL: Unilateral external fixation for severe pilon fractures. *Foot Ankle* 1993;14:57-64.

    The authors present a retrospective review of 21 patients treated with unilateral external fixation and minimal internal fixation. Early ankle motion with an articulated unilateral external fixator is documented. There were no reported cases of osteomyelitis. Late ankle arthrodesis was necessary only for those injuries in which the articular surface was too comminuted to permit reconstruction.

27. DiChristina D, Riemer BL, Butterfield SL, et al: Pilon fractures treated with an articulated external fixator: A preliminary report of significant complications. *Orthop Trans* 1994;18:719-720.

28. Wyrsch B, McFerran MA, McAndrew MA, et al: A randomized, prospective study evaluating the surgical management of pilon fractures. *Orthop Trans* 1994;18:720.

    The authors present the only comparative study of open plating versus external fixation with minimal internal fixation currently available. Major complications occurred in 55% of the open reduction group versus 18% of the external fixation patients. The authors conclude that external fixation with minimal internal fixation of pilon fractures is safer with fewer soft-tissue complications than with traditional open reduction.

29. Brumback RJ, McGarvey WC: Fractures of the tibial plafond: The pilon fracture. Evolving treatment concepts. *Orthop Clin North Am* 1995;26:273-285.

    This review of the evolving changes in the treatment of pilon fractures includes discussion of the various classifications and a comparison of the results of open plating versus external fixation with minimal internal fixation.

30. Trumble TE, Benirschke SK, Vedder NB: Use of radial forearm flaps to treat complications of closed pilon fractures. *J Orthop Trauma* 1992;6:358-365.

31. DiStasio AJ II, Dugdale TW, Deafenbaugh MK: Multiple relaxing skin incisions in orthopaedic lower extremity trauma. *J Orthop Trauma* 1993;7:270-274.

32. Leone VJ, Ruland RT, Meinhard BP: The management of the soft tissues in pilon fractures. *Clin Orthop* 1993;292:315-320.

33. Stasikelis PJ, Calhoun JH, Ledbetter BR, et al: Treatment of infected pilon nonunions with small pin fixators. *Foot Ankle* 1993;14:373-379.

    The authors review the treatment of infected pilon fractures and present a technique used for limb salvage in six patients. Excision of infected, necrotic bone coupled with distraction osteogenesis and ankle arthrodesis is used to avoid amputation in this select group of complications after pilon fracture.

19
Ankle and Foot Injuries

Ankle Injuries

Lateral Ankle Ligament Injuries

Definition of Injury/Classification of Injury Injury to the lateral ligamentous complex of the ankle is a common clinical problem. Approximately 23,000 of these injuries occur daily in the United States, and they are the most common injury in sports. The lateral ligament complex consists of three ligaments: anterior talofibular, calcaneofibular, and posterior talofibular. The anterior talofibular ligament, which anatomically is a thickening in the anterior joint capsule, runs parallel to the axis of the foot in the neutral position. In plantar flexion this ligament runs parallel to the leg axis and functions as a collateral ligament. The calcaneofibular ligament is a discrete, extra-articular structure that courses perpendicular to the anterior talofibular ligament and is intimately associated with the overlying peroneal tendon sheath. The posterior talofibular ligament courses from the posterior aspect of the fibula to insert on the lateral tubercle of the posterior process of the talus.

Studies by Brostrom nearly 3 decades ago showed that approximately two thirds of sprains are isolated injuries to the anterior talofibular ligament. Combined rupture of the anterior talofibular ligament and calcaneofibular ligament occurred in 20% of patients. Isolated rupture of the calcaneofibular ligament was not observed in these studies, although it may occur rarely. These concepts continue to be accepted today. Extrapolating from concepts derived through study of the medial collateral ligament of the knee, injuries to the lateral ankle ligaments are most commonly classified as grade I, II, and III, according to the severity of histologic damage to the ligament in question. A grade I injury implies stretching only without macroscopic tearing, while a grade II injury involves partial macroscopic tearing. In a grade III injury the ligament is completely ruptured and loses all mechanical function. Some studies stage these injuries from a clinical perspective. In this scheme a stage I injury is a partial injury to the anterior talofibular ligament while the calcaneofibular ligament is completely intact. A stage II injury involves complete rupture of the anterior talofibular ligament and partial injury to the calcaneofibular ligament. Finally, a stage III injury implies complete rupture of the anterior talofibular and calcaneofibular ligaments.

Evaluation of Injury Physical examination is most important in the evaluation of a patient with an inversion injury of the ankle. Localization of swelling and point tenderness in the early hours after injury can implicate the specific ligaments involved. Although useful, stress examination (anterior drawer and talar tilt) is often too painful initially. Plain radiographs are useful to rule out fractures, and stress radiographs (anterior drawer and talar tilt) and arthrography can demonstrate complete ligamentous rupture. Stress radiographs are valuable in clinical trials to objectively stratify injuries, although they are rarely indicated with current treatment algorithms for isolated cases. Magnetic resonance imaging (MRI) can demonstrate the specific ligaments involved in an ankle sprain. These results show a qualitative correlation to the results of graded stress radiographs but do not correlate directly with the degree of clinical instability.[1]

Treatment Options Traditional protocols for the treatment of grade I and II injuries involve initial efforts to limit swelling (ice, compressive wrap, and elevation) followed by a period of protective wrapping or bracing. Finally, as pain subsides, range-of-motion exercises, progressive weightbearing, and proprioceptive training are increased. For grade I and II injuries the prognosis is almost universally excellent. Treatment of grade III injuries has been more controversial. Kannus and Renstrom performed a meta-analysis of all available randomized, prospective studies of surgical versus nonsurgical treatment of grade III ligamentous injuries of the ankle.[2] Twelve such studies are available in the English literature. Half compared primary surgical repair plus cast immobilization with cast immobilization alone. The other half compared these two treatment modalities with functional treatment as outlined above for grade I and II injuries. All patients in the 12 studies gave the typical history of an inversion injury, had typical clinical findings, and had complete ligamentous rupture demonstrated by at least one radiographic method. The total number of patients in this meta-analysis was approximately 1,500. The results throughout all series were, in general, excellent, regardless of the treatment method. No consistently significant difference could be found in the time required for return to work or physical activity, residual functional instability, mobility, reinjury, or objective mechanical stability. Surgical treatment had a significantly higher complication rate and was more expensive than other forms of treatment.

Based on this work, the recommendation for treatment of any ankle sprain is a functional program. Because all grades of ankle sprain are treated similarly, differentiation is helpful only in defining the prognosis and time to return to activity. For this reason, stress radiographs and arthrography are not routinely recommended. These recommendations hold true even for high-performance athletes.

Complications With nonsurgical treatment of ankle sprains, complications are rare. Functional and mechanical instability remains the most common problem. Mechanical instability can be demonstrated with stress radiographs (anterior drawer or talar tilt), but functional instability is more difficult to show objectively. Estimates of late instability range from 10% to 30% in various series. Treatments include nonsurgical methods directed at peroneal strengthening, improved proprioception, and bracing. Surgical treatments include delayed primary ligamentous repair and ligamentous reconstruction, but should be considered only if symptomatic instability persists after nonsurgical treatment. Because of its simplicity and efficacy, delayed primary repair is indicated in most situations.[3] Exceptions currently include patients with generalized ligamentous laxity and patients with instability of more than 10 years' duration. These patients as well as those few in whom delayed primary repair fails are candidates for reconstructive procedures. Of the many reconstructions described, the Chrisman-Snook technique seems to give the best clinical results.[4] The outcome of delayed reconstructive procedures has been shown to be similar to that of acute primary repair,[5] lending further support to the recommendation for early functional treatment.

Syndesmosis Sprains

Classification Acute injury to the syndesmotic ligaments of the ankle without fracture continues to be unusual and must be differentiated from the common ankle sprain. Four types of syndesmosis sprains have been described: lateral distal fibular subluxation, lateral subluxation with plastic deformation of the fibula, posterior dislocation of the distal fibula, and diastasis produced by superior talar dislocation. The diagnosis should be based primarily on the history and clinical examination findings. Pain occurs in the anterior ankle, not laterally. Patients generally have a positive response to the squeeze test.[6] In this test, compression of the tibia against the fibula at midcalf produces pain in the anterior ankle. Pain at the syndesmosis with external rotation stress of the ankle is also indicative of a syndesmosis injury. Stress radiographs can confirm the diagnosis if the patient can tolerate the discomfort. Scintigraphy has a sensitivity of 100% and a specificity of 71% when compared to stress radiography and therefore may be a useful test in certain patients. Arthrograms may confirm the diagnosis.

Treatment The importance of recognizing a syndesmotic ligament injury is related mainly to prognosis. Average time to full activity is 31 to 55 days, approximately double that for lateral ligament injuries. Functional treatment is generally preferred, resulting in 86% good and excellent results based on pain, stiffness, and persistent swelling.[6] Up to 50% to 90% of patients develop heterotopic ossification in the interosseous membrane, although this does not appear to influence outcome. Surgery should be reserved for those injuries in which obvious mortise widening is present on plain radiographs obtained without stressing.

Complications Patients recover good to excellent function in the affected ankle in most cases. Up to 23% of patients, however, will complain of mild to moderate pain on activity, and 36% will complain of mild to moderate stiffness.

Achilles Tendon Rupture

Definition of Injury Acute rupture of the Achilles tendon is an injury not infrequently misdiagnosed by the initial treating physician. The diagnosis is based on posterior calf or ankle pain, weakness of plantar flexion, a palpable gap in the tendon, and a positive result on the squeeze test (absence of ankle plantar flexion with compression of the proximal gastrocnemius-soleus muscle belly). The etiology in most instances is a combination of intratendon degeneration and mechanical stress.

Treatment Management consists of either primary repair or cast immobilization with the ankle held in equinus. Recent prospective, randomized studies have concluded that surgical repair is preferable but cast immobilization continues to be an acceptable alternative.[7] Surgically treated patients tend to have a higher rate of resuming their preinjury level of activity, fewer complaints, and fewer re-ruptures. Surgical treatment does have a higher complication rate than nonsurgical treatment.

Surgical treatment can be done in either an open or a percutaneous fashion.[7,8] Cadaveric studies have shown open repair to result in a significantly stronger repair, while a high incidence of sural nerve entrapment has been demonstrated when the percutaneous technique is used.[9] Clinical studies comparing open repair to percutaneous techniques have shown both methods to be effective. Re-rupture in percutaneous repairs ranges from 0 to 16%, while the rate of re-rupture is 0 to 6% after open repair. Wound complications are rare with percutaneous techniques but range from 0 to 13% with open repair. A transverse incision has been advocated to decrease wound problems, with a reported rate of 2% minor wound problems and 0% major wound complications.

Traumatic Subluxation/Dislocation of the Peroneal Tendons

Traumatic subluxation and dislocation of the peroneal tendons, although uncommon, is not rare. The most common mechanism is a sporting activity, especially snow skiing.

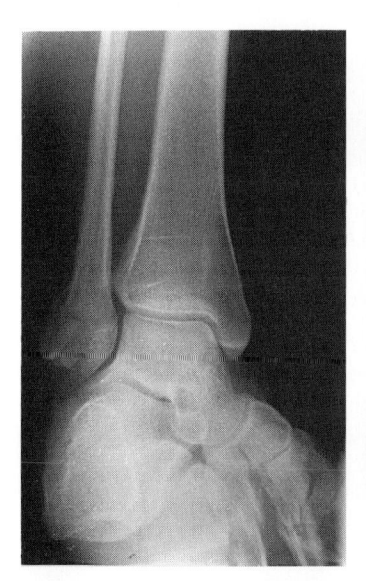

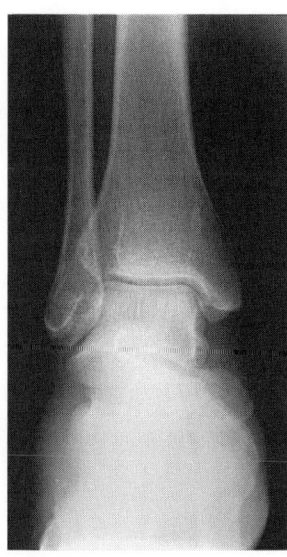

Fig. 1 Radiograph showing avulsion of a thin shell of lateral malleolar cortex associated with dislocation of the peroneal tendons.

Injury occurs as reflexic contracture of the peroneal musculature overcomes the restraining soft tissue. Anatomic variations of the posterolateral ankle may predispose to this injury. The pathoanatomy is variable but includes avulsion of a thin shell of lateral malleolar cortex (Fig. 1), tearing of the retinacular tissue, or detachment of the periosteum, creating a pouch on the undersurface of the distal end of the fibula similar to the Bankart lesion in the shoulder. The diagnosis is based on clinical examination, with intense pain on active eversion being a strong indicator of the injury. Treatment of the acute injury remains controversial, with advocates for both surgical and nonsurgical treatment. Surgical treatment in the acute case entails primary repair of the torn or fractured structures. Most chronic and recurrent cases require a more extensive procedure such as reconstruction of the peroneal retinaculum or deepening of the peroneal groove.[10]

Ankle Dislocation

Dislocation of the ankle without fracture is a rare injury. The mechanism of injury appears to be forced inversion of the foot, resulting in posteromedial dislocation. A majority of these injuries are open (63% to 93%), with injury to the anterolateral neurovascular structures occurring occasionally. In general, the recommendation for a closed dislocation is closed reduction with cast immobilization. Most authors recommend primary lateral ligament repair in open injuries at the time of debridement of the anterolateral wound. Long-term results are generally good with these methods of treatment. Instability is rare, although degenerative arthrosis may occur.[11]

Ankle Fractures

Classification of Injury Classification of unstable ankle fractures continues to be based on two systems: the Lauge-Hansen scheme and the Danis-Weber scheme. The Lauge-Hansen classification was derived from cadaver studies in which the pattern of injury was described by two parameters: the position of the foot at the time of the injury and the direction of the deforming force. Four types of ankle injuries were found: the supination-adduction injury, the supination-external rotation injury, the pronation-abduction injury, and the pronation-external rotation injury. Each type of injury is divided into stages, depending on the severity of the lesion (Fig. 2). The Danis-Weber scheme is based on the level of the fibula fracture; with type A being infrasyndesmotic, type B transyndesmotic, and type C suprasyndesmotic (Fig. 2). The recent literature has focused on comparing these two established classification systems. Both schemes have certain advantages and disadvantages. Three criteria have been proposed for an ideal ankle fracture classification. First, the scheme should be reproducibly usable among observers. Recent reports have shown an acceptable level of interobserver and intraobserver variability in both classification schemes, although neither was excellent. Observers have shown difficulty identifying the pronation-abduction injuries, which suggests a poor radiographic definition of this injury. Also, poor precision of staging in the Lauge-Hansen system must diminish its usefulness in daily practice. Second, the system should be simple, which seemingly would favor the Danis-Weber scheme. Third, the classification should provide relevant information that can be used to develop a treatment plan. Formerly, when closed manipulation and cast immobilization were standard treatment modalities, the Lauge-Hansen system influenced treatment significantly by implying the deforming forces that should be countered to be successful in a closed manipulation. Today surgical treatment predominates in the treatment of bimalleolar injuries, making thorough knowledge of such mechanisms relatively less important. Thus, by these criteria the Danis-Weber classification system seems preferable for current treatment algorithms. The Lauge-Hansen system, however, will not soon be forgotten. It describes the important pathoanatomic features of ankle fractures and should in some fundamental way be appreciated by all surgeons treating these injuries.

Evaluation of Injury The clinical evaluation of ankle fractures consists primarily of physical examination and plain radiography. Careful palpation for bony and ligamentous tenderness as well as observation of swelling is important. A systematic evaluation of both malleoli, fibular shaft, proximal fibula, deltoid ligament, and syndesmosis must be performed to identify the sites of injury and begin to formulate an assessment of ankle stability. Plain radiographic studies consist of the anteroposterior (AP), lateral, and mortise radiographs and must be done on all patients with significant tenderness over the malleoli. Any shift of the talus within the mortise creating asymmetry of the clear

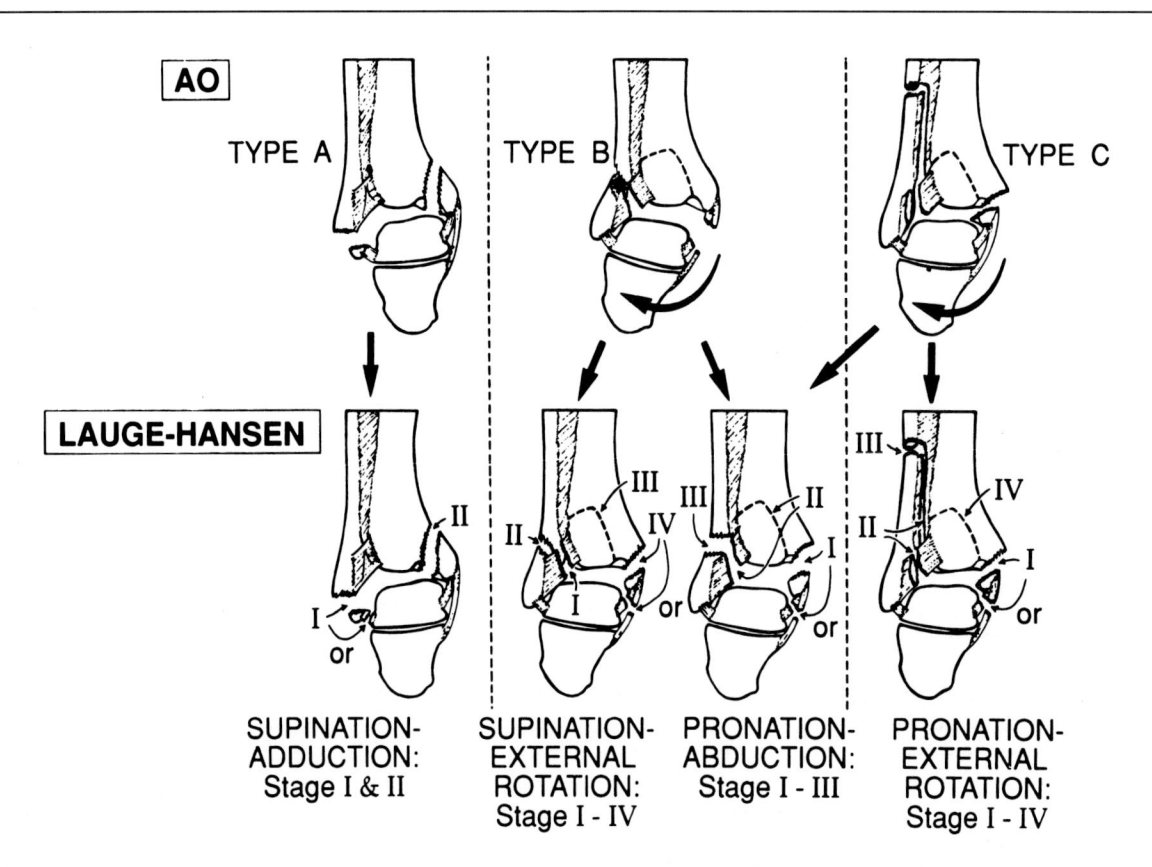

Fig. 2 Danis-Weber and Lauge-Hansen classification systems for ankle fractures. (Reproduced with permission from Sangeorzan BJ: Ankle and foot: Trauma, in Frymoyer JW (ed): *Orthopaedic Knowledge Update 4*. Rosemont IL, American Academy of Orthopaedic Surgeons, 1993, pp 635-644.)

space implies instability and must be recognized. Ankle fractures considered to be unstable should be considered for surgical reduction and fixation as the primary mode of treatment.

Criteria for evaluation of isolated lateral and medial malleolus fractures continue to be somewhat confusing. Minimally displaced lateral malleolus fractures are generally considered nonsurgical injuries, although the amount of displacement that is acceptable is not clearly defined. Recent work using CT evaluation has shown that plain radiographs consistently overestimate displacement of the lateral malleolus. CT has shown that the apparent external rotational deformity of the distal fibular fragment is relative only to the proximal fibular fragment and not to the tibia. Thus, the apparent external rotational deformity may not indicate derangement of the talofibular articulation itself. These findings may explain the good results reported in previous long-term studies of nonsurgical treatment of lateral malleolus fractures.

Recent work has helped clarify the anatomy and relative stability of the medial side of the ankle. Through both a radiographic review and cadaveric dissections, investigators have identified six types of injuries that can occur. This classification depends on an understanding of the anterior and posterior colliculi and the deltoid ligament. The anterior colliculus is narrower and serves as the primary proximal attachment for the superficial deltoid ligament. The posterior colliculus is somewhat broader and, along with the intercollicular groove, serves as the point of attachment of the deep deltoid ligament. The six injury types include rupture of the deep and superficial portions of the deltoid ligament, avulsion chip fractures (primarily of the anterior colliculus), anterior colliculus fractures, concurrent anterior colliculus fracture and deep deltoid ligament rupture, posterior colliculus fractures, and supracollicular fractures. Because of surrounding soft-tissue attachments, all but concurrent anterior colliculus fracture and deep deltoid rupture, and supracollicular injuries can be considered stable injuries. In addition to plain radiography, other studies may be indicated in selected cases. Stress radiography, for example, may be useful when stability cannot be determined by examination and standard radiography.

Treatment Options/Results of Treatment The treatment of ankle fractures depends on the stability of the ankle as judged clinically and radiographically. Isolated lateral malleolus fractures are generally treated nonsurgically. Even very minimal treatment of these injuries with an elastic wrap and immediate weightbearing as tolerated has been shown to result in satisfactory outcome. Bimalleolar injuries, on the other hand, often require surgical intervention. Clinical outcome appears to depend on the adequacy of achieving and maintaining appropriate reduction of the ankle mortise. Although adequate reduction may be achieved with closed treatment, early results appear to be more predictable with open reduction and internal fixation.[12] Studies with longer follow-up have shown little difference in the final outcome between surgical and nonsurgical treatment when reduction is achieved and maintained.[13]

When surgical treatment is required, internal fixation with plates and screws as advocated by the AO group is favored. These methods seem to give the most satisfactory maintenance of reduction until healing is complete. Significant experience, particularly in Scandinavia, has been gained with nonrigid fixation using cerclage wires and staples, but these methods appear less effective in retaining congruence of unstable bimalleolar and trimalleolar fractures. Fixation of medial malleolar fragments is commonly done with small cancellous screws, but tension band fixation has been shown to be effective even with large medial fragments. Repair of a deltoid ligament rupture in association with a lateral malleolus fracture is unnecessary provided reduction of the lateral malleolus and the medial joint space is accurate.

Classically, fixation of the lateral malleolus is done by placing a one-third tubular plate laterally on the distal fibula. Although generally effective, this method has several disadvantages, including wound healing problems and prominence beneath the skin, necessitating removal. Most Danis-Weber type B fractures can be fixed with a dorsally placed plate positioned as an antiglide plate. This technique is gaining popularity because of reports of good clinical results and better biomechanical properties than the traditional lateral positioning of the plate.

Many aspects of syndesmosis fixation continue to be controversial, including indications for fixation, the effect of fixation on ankle articulation, the duration of fixation required, and the necessity for removal. Fixation should be performed when clinical instability exists. This is generally determined by stressing the syndesmosis with lateral displacement of the distal fibula (Cotton test). Instability may not be predictable based purely on disruption of the distal tibiofibular joint as seen on radiographs. In vitro studies have shown that rigid fixation of the medial and lateral malleoli will impart clinical stability in most cases.[13] Cadaveric studies have also demonstrated that in bimalleolar injuries in which the medial injury cannot be rigidly stabilized (ie, deltoid ligament injuries), fibular fractures above a critical transition zone occurring 3.5 to 4.0 cm above the ankle joint require syndesmotic fixation.[14]

The need for internal fixation of posterior malleolar fractures is generally based on the size of the fragment. Recent work, however, has implied that even larger fragments (greater than 25% articular surface involvement)

may not require fixation. In a retrospective review, investigators noted no significant clinical difference with and without fixation.[15] They determined that as long as anatomic reduction and rigid fixation of the lateral and medial malleoli was achieved, posterior subluxation of the talus did not occur. Previous studies in which posterior subluxation was seen to be a problem had not used internal fixation of the medial and lateral sides of the ankle. Posterior malleolar fracture fragment size, however, has been shown to have prognostic significance. Investigators in two recent studies showed that even when perfectly reduced, large posterior fragments (greater than 25% to 33% of the articular surface) are associated with a worse prognosis than smaller fragments.

Much recent work has been done on the use of bioabsorbable implants in internal fixation of ankle fractures. The proposed advantages of these implants include avoidance of long-term irritation by the implant and avoidance of a second operation for implant removal. Although effective in maintaining reduction of the fragments, the polyglycolide screws have been associated with a high incidence of nonspecific foreign-body reaction (7% to 10%). This reaction generally results in a draining, sterile sinus over the implant but does not seem to interfere with bone healing. More recently, polylactide screws have been shown to be comparable to stainless steel in the fixation of medial malleolus fractures, and are not associated with the foreign-body reaction noted with polyglycolide implants.

Several investigators have addressed the treatment of open fractures of the ankle. In one recent comparative study, irrigation and debridement followed by immediate open reduction and internal fixation resulted in a shorter hospital stay and no increased incidence of infection when compared to cast immobilization.[16] In another series of open ankle fractures, 77% good and excellent results were reported, with no infection or nonunion. Controversy remains, however, with regard to the open grade IIIB ankle fracture. Despite eradication of infection and successful fusion of degenerated joints, patients often have significant ongoing functional and psychosocial disability.

Treatment of ankle fractures in the elderly, although common, has remained problematic. Despite the difficulty associated with internal fixation in osteoporotic bone, recent studies favor open reduction and internal fixation over cast immobilization. Surgical treatment resulted in a significantly better outcome, both radiographically and clinically, in two comparative studies of surgical fixation versus closed reduction and casting in this patient population. Because of concern about poor bone quality, alternatives to standard fibular plating have also been investigated in the elderly population.

One study concluded that fixation of unstable lateral malleoli in elderly patients with Rush rods gave a higher percentage of good and excellent results than the standard AO technique. Rush rod fixation also resulted in lower morbidity. Thus, for elderly patients, intramedullary rod fixation of the fibula may be a reasonable treatment alternative.

Laterally comminuted fracture-dislocations of the ankle constitute a specific entity that has not been well described until recently.[17] The injury consists of an avulsion-type fracture of the medial malleolus at the level of the plafond, lateral displacement of the talus, comminution of the fibula at or proximal to the syndesmosis, and often an impaction of the plafond in the lateral aspect. A majority of these injuries are open, with the soft-tissue wound occurring as a transverse tearing of the skin on the medial side of the ankle at the level of the plafond. These injuries are technically challenging because accurate assessment of fibular length is not possible. Success in treating these lesions has been gained by irrigation and debridement of the wound, followed by fixation of the medial fracture first. The lateral malleolus is then positioned anatomically into the lateral articular facet of the talus under direct vision and provisionally pinned to the talus with Kirschner wires. A fibular plate is then contoured appropriately and fixed definitively to the proximal and distal fibular fragments, bridging the region of comminution. When this method is used, anatomic restoration can be consistently achieved. Bone grafting of the fibula is often needed to gain union.

The Maisonneuve fracture of the fibula is a special ankle injury that in the past was considered unstable and an indication for internal fixation of the syndesmosis. This treatment recommendation was based on the belief that the injury constituted complete disruption of all syndesmotic ligaments (anterior tibiofibular, interosseous ligament, posterior tibiofibular ligament, and the transverse tibiofibular ligament) as well as the interosseous membrane up to the level of the fibula fracture. Recent clinical results with closed manipulation and casting of these injuries have led to a reevaluation of this belief. One investigator reported successful treatment of eight Maisonneuve injuries with nonsurgical methods. This success was attributed to the fact that these injuries are inherently stable except in external rotation. It seems likely that the injury often produces a rupture of only the anterior syndesmotic ligament. This allows external rotation of the fibular fragment below the fracture. With rupture of the deltoid ligament, widening of the medial clear space can occur. Because the posterior syndesmotic ligaments and the interosseous membrane remain intact, internal rotation reduces the mortise. Thus, nonsurgical treatment of these injuries may be effective if internal rotation is maintained with a long leg cast. Regardless of the mode of treatment (surgical or nonsurgical), reduction of the mortise must be achieved and maintained until ligamentous structures have completely healed.

The most effective postsurgical regimen following open reduction and internal fixation of ankle fractures has been the focus of several recent clinical studies. Concerns have centered on immobilization versus early motion, and on early versus delayed weightbearing. Regardless of whether patients were allowed early weightbearing with protection or were kept nonweightbearing, early range-of-motion exercise has not proved to have significant long-term benefits. Similarly, it has been difficult to demonstrate significant clinical differences in patients who are allowed early protected weightbearing with an ankle-foot orthosis and those who are kept nonweightbearing until healing is complete.

Firm conclusions are therefore difficult to make concerning either weightbearing or cast immobilization because all patients tested had similarly good results.

Complications

Complications of the treatment of ankle fractures vary with the treatment method. As the standard treatment has evolved from nonsurgical to surgical, so too has the spectrum of complications evolved from malunion and subsequent joint degeneration to complications related to surgery. Late arthrosis is rare in surgically treated fractures but may be as high as 28% in nonsurgically treated bimalleolar fractures. Fibular malunions are still encountered with some frequency and numerous recent reports have documented the benefit of osteotomy to correct this problem.[18] These studies have shown fibular osteotomy to be very effective even years after the original injury and in the presence of early degenerative changes.

Surgical complications are mainly those of infection and wound healing, as well as loss of reduction and fixation. Reported rates of postsurgical complications have varied significantly. In an early prospective study of 306 ankle fractures treated according to the AO method, investigators reported an infection rate of 1.8%, poor wound healing in 3.1%, and a reoperation rate of 5%. One recent study, however, that focused specifically on postoperative complications demonstrated these problems to be somewhat more frequent. In 121 patients treated surgically the major complication rate was found to be 12% while the minor complication rate was 18%. Findings in this series included a lower complication rate with early surgery than with late intervention: 5.3% of patients who underwent surgery in the first 24 hours had complications, whereas 44% of patients treated more than 24 hours after injury had problems. In addition, fracture-dislocations were associated with three times as many major complications as simple fractures, and fractures associated with blisters or abrasions had double the complication rate. Delay of fixation of more than 14 days has also been shown to significantly affect the ability to achieve an anatomic reduction, compared with surgical intervention in less than 24 hours.

Fracture blisters have recently been reported to affect patient care in up to 71% of the patients who develop them. Although blisters do seem to be associated with an increased complication rate, the exact correlation is unclear. They may actually only be a marker of an injury with more soft-tissue damage. Early surgical intervention decreases their occurrence, and thus early intervention would seem to be the best defense against blister-related problems. There is as yet no consensus as to the optimum method to manage this skin lesion or in what way it should influence surgical intervention.

Other surgical complications recently reported include prolonged venous dysfunction and adhesions of the distal tibiofibular joint. Although commonly seen by the active clinician, the magnitude and duration of swelling and ve-

Table 1. Staging system for classifying osteochondral lesions of the talus

Stage	Arthroscopic	MRI	Radiographs (Berndt & Harty)
Stage I	Irregularity and softening of articular cartilage, no definable fragment	Thickening of articular cartilage and low signal changes	Compression lesion, no visible fragment
Stage II	Articular cartilage breached, definable fragment, not displaceable	Articular cartilage breached, low signal rim behind fragment indicating fibrous attachment	Fragment attached
Stage III	Articular cartilage breached, definable fragment, displaceable, but attached by some overlying articular cartilage	Articular cartilage breached, high signal changes behind fragment indicating synovial fluid between fragment and underlying subchondral bone	Nondisplaced fragment without attachment
Stage IV	Loose body	Loose body	Displaced fragment

(Reproduced with permission from Dipaolo JD, Nelson DW, Colville MR: Characterizing osteochondral lesions by magnetic resonance imaging. *Arthroscopy* 1991;7:101-104.)

nous dysfunction have only recently been documented. This dysfunction was shown to require 18 months to return to baseline. Another newly reported complication is that of adhesions of the distal tibiofibular joint presenting as anterior ankle pain after fracture. Patients with this complication have normal radiographs and may benefit from arthroscopic resection of the adhesions.

Foot Injuries

Osteochondral Injuries of the Talus

Definition of Injury/Classification Osteochondral lesions of the talus remain a diagnostic and therapeutic challenge. Many lesions are initially misdiagnosed and treated as lateral ankle ligament injuries, only later to be recognized as osteochondral injuries. The terminology used in describing injuries that involve the chondral surface of the talar dome has varied significantly in the literature and includes the terms osteochondral fracture, transchondral fracture, osteochondral lesion, and osteochondritis dissecans. Probably all of these terms represent a portion of a larger spectrum of injury to the talar articular surface. Although the etiology of these lesions is thought to be primarily traumatic, an underlying ischemic problem resulting in pathologic fracture may contribute in varying degrees to these lesions. In 1959 a staging system was described by Berndt and Harty based on cadaveric observations and correlation with radiographs (Table 1). Using MRI, DiPaolo and associates have modified the standard classification to more accurately reflect the underlying pathology (Table 1).[19]

Clinical and Radiologic Evaluation The patient with an osteochondral lesion of the talus often has a history of an inversion injury to the ankle that was treated without recognition of the osteochondral injury. Chronic symptoms of pain, stiffness, swelling, locking, and occasionally a palpable loose body then result. Physical findings may include localized tenderness and decreased range of motion, although there are no signs that are pathognomonic for an osteochondral lesion of the talus. The diagnosis can be made in 70% to 100% of individuals with plain radiography. In patients with normal radiographs, a technetium bone scan is a very sensitive screening tool.[20] MRI, however, is the most useful method of noninvasive evaluation because of its ability to demonstrate the stability of the fragment as well as the condition of the overlying cartilage.[19,21]

Treatment and Results Treatment is based primarily on symptoms and the stage of the lesion as assessed with radiography and MRI. Asymptomatic stage 1, 2, and 3 lesions do not require treatment. Symptomatic stage 1 lesions can usually be treated with activity restriction, whereas symptomatic stage 2 lesions are best treated with immobilization for 6 weeks. This method has resulted in a 90% success rate in the treatment of these lesions. Stage 1 and 2 injuries involve stable fragments and thus require only protection to allow capillary ingrowth and healing. Treatment of symptomatic stage 3 lesions remains controversial. The medial stage 3 injury is thought to heal more readily than the lateral lesion, and a trial of nonsurgical care is recommended even though one third of these patients will eventually need surgery. The lateral stage 3 lesions do more poorly and immediate surgical intervention seems warranted. Surgery may be performed arthroscopically[22] or as an open procedure. The arthroscopic method results in less soft-tissue dissection and avoids the need for a malleolar osteotomy in some cases. The long-term results of these two methods, however, appear similar. Current recommendations for treatment of an osteochondral lesion are based on the condition of the overlying cartilage. If the cartilage is intact, drilling of the lesion through the cartilage is sufficient. If the overlying cartilage is frayed, debridement followed by drilling of the subchondral bone in the defect is necessary. Acute stage 4 injuries should be treated with open reduction and internal fixation (utilizing bone pegs, Herbert screws, or countersunk cancellous screws) when the fragment is large enough. Fibrin sealant (containing human fibrinogen, bovine aprotinin, calcium chloride, and bovine thrombin) has also been used successfully to fix these fragments. If the fragment is too small to be fixed, it should be excised and the base drilled to stimulate ingrowth of fibrocartilage.

Surgical treatment of stage 3 and 4 lesions may have good early results in 63% to 88% of patients. For a significant number of these patients, however, the results deterio-

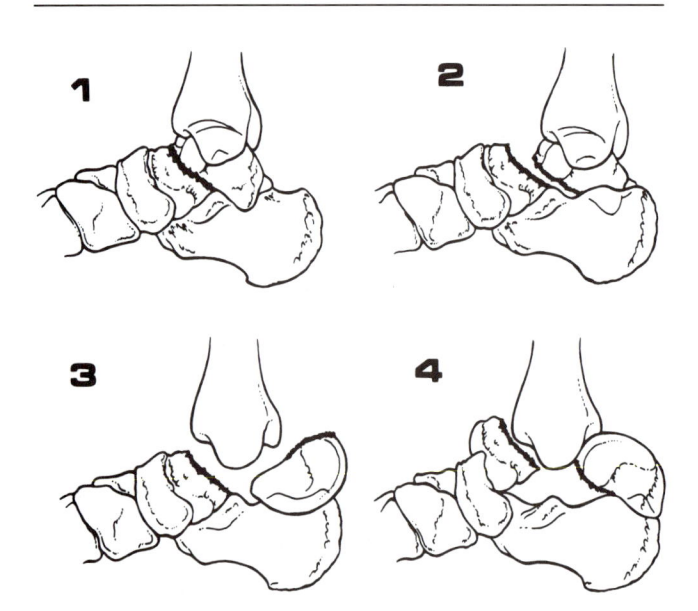

Fig. 3 Hawkins classification of talar neck fractures. (Reproduced with permission from Sangeorzan BJ: Ankle and foot: Trauma, in Frymoyer JW (ed): *Orthopaedic Knowledge Update 4*. Rosemont IL, American Academy of Orthopaedic Surgeons, 1993, pp 635-644.)

rate with time, and up to 75% develop some evidence of degenerative joint disease. One important prognostic factor seems to be the condition of the overlying articular cartilage. An inherent problem with the standard radiographic classification of these lesions, on which most long-term results are based, is failure to account for the condition of the cartilage. More accurate prognostic information may be gained in the future through the use of MRI or arthroscopic staging, both of which can be used to accurately evaluate the condition of the cartilage.[22]

Talus Fractures

Definition of Injury/Classification Fractures of the talus include the relatively common talar neck fracture as well as the less common fractures of the talar head, body, and lateral and posterior processes. With the exception of the talar neck fracture, the literature on talus fractures is sparse. The classification of talar neck fractures as originally outlined by Hawkins in 1970 continues to be widely applied (Fig. 3). In this classification three types of fractures are recognized. Type 1 fractures are nondisplaced vertical fractures, type 2 fractures are displaced fractures with subluxation or dislocation of the subtalar joint, and type 3 fractures are displaced with subluxation or dislocation of the talar body from both the subtalar and ankle joints. A rare variant of the type 3 injury in which the head of the talus is also dislocated from the talonavicular joint has been described and referred to as a type 4 injury.

Radiologic and Clinical Evaluation Standard AP and lateral radiographs are usually sufficient to assess and classify talus fractures. Complex fractures of the talus, as well as those associated with the multiply injured foot, may benefit from examination with CT, but the need to surgically reduce and stabilize these fractures in a timely manner may preclude performing further diagnostic studies.

Treatment The preferred method of treatment of talar neck fractures continues to be based on achieving an anatomic reduction and maintaining it until healing occurs. With nondisplaced, type 1 fractures, closed treatment in a nonweightbearing short leg cast is usually sufficient, and the risk of osteonecrosis is low. Recent reports have advocated meticulous attention to achieving an anatomic reduction in displaced fractures because malunion of the talar neck is poorly tolerated. This generally implies an open reduction in type 2 and 3 fractures. Several different methods of internal fixation using screws have been advocated. These include anterior-to-posterior screws placed through an anteromedial incision alone, anterior-to-posterior screws placed through both an anteromedial and an anterolateral incision (Fig. 4), and posterior-to-anterior screws placed through a posterior incision. Use of screws made of titanium allows better MRI when concerns about osteonecrosis arise.[23]

The postoperative treatment of patients with talar neck fractures remains poorly defined. Initially patients are kept nonweightbearing and assessed both for union and for osteonecrosis. Absence of osteonecrosis is usually inferred from the presence of Hawkins' sign (subchondral lucency in the talar dome, thought to be secondary to hypervascularity). If osteonecrosis is suspected, prolonged protection, either by nonweightbearing or by a patellar tendon-bearing orthosis, is recommended. MRI will most likely play a larger role in determining postoperative management in the future.

Results of treating talar neck fractures appear to depend on the severity of the initial injury and on the method of treatment employed. Series of talus fractures reported in the 1970s included patients who had been treated with closed reduction and cast immobilization and patients who had been treated with open reduction and internal fixation.[24] In this combined group of patients, a satisfactory outcome was achieved in 93% to 100% of patients with type I injuries, in 44% to 57% of patients with type II injuries, but in only 15% to 48% of patients with type III injuries. Osteonecrosis was found to correlate with the severity of the injury, occurring in 13% of type I fractures, 42% to 50% of type II injuries, and 84% to 91% of type III injuries. Interestingly, two thirds of the patients with radiographic evidence of osteonecrosis did well enough clinically to never require additional surgical intervention after an average follow-up of 15 years. Thus, although weightbearing should be delayed in the setting of osteonecrosis, the eventual outcome may still be satisfactory.

In a recent multicenter investigation of talus fractures, Szyszkowitz and associates described the benefits of internal fixation.[25] Seventy-one fractures of the neck and body of the talus were treated surgically; 66 with open reduction and internal fixation and five with primary fusion or talec-

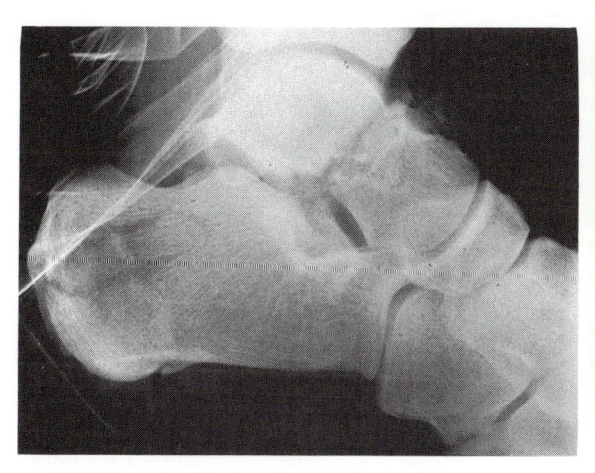

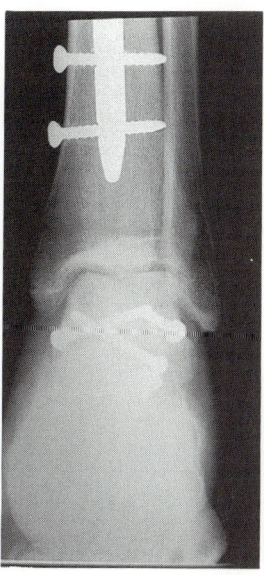

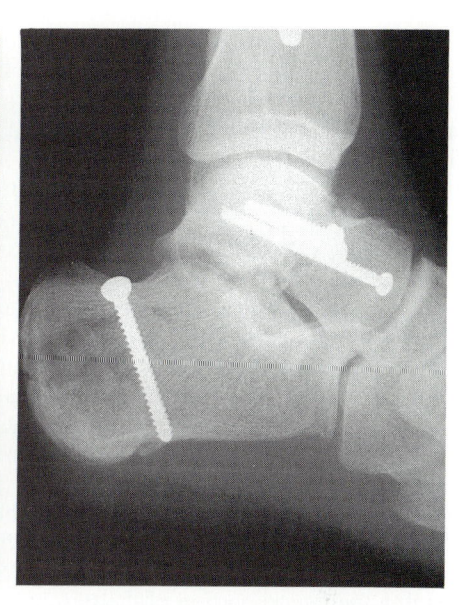

Fig. 4 Radiograph showing a Hawkins type 2 talar neck fracture (**left**) treated with open reduction and internal fixation using crossing lag screws placed through two incisions (**center** and **right**).

tomy. The final outcome in this group was good or very good for 82% of patients. In the most severe group of fractures, referred to as dislocation fractures and comparable to Hawkins type III injuries, the outcome was good or very good in 73%. Osteonecrosis was not specifically addressed, but the authors did demonstrate that the severity of arthrosis worsened as the injury worsened. In the dislocation fracture group (comparable to Hawkins type 3), 47% of patients had ankle arthrosis and 67% had subtalar arthrosis by radiographic criteria. The clinical effect of this was not specifically addressed.

Complications Osteonecrosis is a result of disruption of the blood supply to the talus. As such, the probability of osteonecrosis occurring is related to the Hawkins class of the fracture, with osteonecrosis occurring in 0 to 13% of type 1 injuries, 42% to 50% of type 2 injuries, and 84% to 91% of type 3 injuries. Although these rates are significant, especially in the more severe injuries, it is important to realize that osteonecrosis is a radiologic diagnosis and that the resulting symptoms may vary from mild to severe. Early osteonecrosis is suspected if there is no subchondral lucency in the talar dome (Hawkins' sign) by 6 weeks after injury. As time passes, the talus will show progressive sclerosis as the surrounding skeleton becomes more radiolucent secondary to disuse osteoporosis. MRI can demonstrate the presence and extent of the process as early as 3 weeks after injury. Ideally the patient would remain nonweightbearing until complete revascularization has occurred, to protect against collapse of the talus. Complete revascularization, however, may take months to years,

making patient compliance poor. Protection with a patellar tendon-bearing orthosis may help prevent collapse. This will allow the patient to be fully ambulatory once the fracture is healed, which can occur even when the talar body is avascular.

Posttraumatic arthrosis of the ankle or subtalar joints has been identified in patients who have sustained fractures of the talus. This complication is related either to osteonecrosis or chondral surface damage at the time of injury. When symptomatic, this problem can initially be managed by either an ankle-foot orthosis, a University of California Biomechanics Laboratory orthosis, or an orthosis that combines the two. If conservative management fails, a Blair fusion, a tibiocalcaneal fusion, or a pantalar fusion will be needed. Although these procedures generally relieve the arthritic pain, hindfoot function is usually significantly impaired.

Malunion of talar neck fractures is well recognized, and strict attention to detail is required to prevent this complication. Hawkins has stressed the importance of classifying only nondisplaced fractures as type 1. Residual dorsal angulation can limit ankle dorsiflexion, while the more common varus malunion can result in excessive weight being borne on the lateral border of the foot, causing a painful gait. Cadaveric studies of talar neck malalignment, however, have failed to show a significant change in overall joint contact area, although increased localization of stresses with as little as 2 mm of displacement has been observed. Although delayed union is fairly common, nonunion of talar neck fractures is rare.

Calcaneal Fractures

Definition of Injury/Classification Fractures of the calcaneus are divided into those that involve the subtalar joint (intra-articular) and those that do not (extra-articular). Extra-articular fractures make up approximately 25% of all calcaneal fractures and include anterior process fractures, posterosuperior tuberosity fractures, extra-articular fractures of the body, and fractures of the medial and lateral processes. Many of these are minimally displaced or represent avulsion-type fractures. These can be effectively treated nonsurgically. Intra-articular fractures, however, present a much more confusing picture. Much of the problem in understanding and classifying intra-articular fractures revolves around both the complex bony anatomy and the variety of fracture lines present. Vertical loading of the calcaneus through the talus initially results in the production of a primary fracture line that progresses from posteromedial to anterolateral, dividing the posterior facet. If sufficient energy is present, an additional, secondary fracture line appears and produces a third fragment containing the lateral portion of the posterior facet, known as the superolateral fragment. Some studies have proposed the existence of a fourth important and consistent fragment, the anterolateral fragment. This fragment results from an additional fracture line that progresses anteriorly, away from the primary fracture line, often entering the calcaneocuboid joint. If this fragment is not reduced properly, limitation of eversion of the hindfoot and calcaneocuboid articular degeneration may occur.

Classification systems for intra-articular fractures of the calcaneus have been limited in the past by difficulties inherent in imaging the calcaneus with standard radiography. CT is increasingly recognized as essential in understanding the nature of a calcaneal fracture. As such, classification systems based on CT analysis of these fractures have been proposed and shown to reflect accurately the prognosis of these injuries. Crosby and Fitzgibbons proposed a simple three-level CT classification based on the posterior facet.[26] In this system, type 1 injuries are those in which the posterior facet fragments are nondisplaced. Type 2 injuries are those in which the facet fragments are displaced but not comminuted, and type 3 injuries are those in which the posterior facet is comminuted. With nonsurgical treatment, Crosby and Fitzgibbons showed that type 1 injuries did uniformly well, type 2 injuries had mixed results, and type 3 injuries generally did poorly. Sanders and associates, using both coronal and transverse CT scans, identified four types of intra-articular fractures based on the number of displaced fragments of the posterior facet (Fig. 5).[27] Each type of fracture is subdivided according to the medial-to-lateral position of the intra-articular fracture line seen on the CT scan. In this system a type I fracture is a nondisplaced or extra-articular fracture, a type II fracture has one displaced fracture line resulting in two main fragments of the posterior facet, a type III fracture has two main fracture lines resulting in three fragments, and a type IV fracture has at least three fracture lines and four fragments in the posterior facet. This scheme is relatively simple if appropriate CT scans are obtained, and it has been shown to be prognostic for surgical treatment of these fractures.

Clinical and Radiographic Assessment The diagnosis of a calcaneal fracture is generally made from a standard lateral radiograph of the foot. Additional information can be gained from AP and axial radiographs. Broden's views, which are obtained by internally rotating the foot 45° with the heel resting on the radiographic plate and directing the beam cephalad in angles varying from 10° to 40°, can still be useful, particularly in the intraoperative setting, to assess posterior facet reduction. Recently, however, increasing emphasis has been placed on the use of CT to assess these fractures, and several reports have demonstrated the value of CT when compared to plain radiography. Maximum information can be obtained by imaging the calcaneus in two planes oriented 90° to one another, one parallel and one perpendicular to the posterior facet. Images perpendicular to the posterior facet are best obtained with the knee flexed. The ability to produce three-dimensional images of the calcaneus with CT analysis has been demonstrated. Although this technique can highlight the position of the major fragments, its usefulness in routine treatment of calcaneal fractures has not been clearly shown. CT can also be helpful in assessing peroneal tendon subluxation and dislocation, and this injury complex should be carefully sought in each case.

MRI of acute fractures of the os calcis has also been investigated. Changes in the marrow signal due to contusion, hemorrhage, and edema obscure visualization of the bony anatomy, making this study minimally helpful. Evaluation of the calcaneal fat pad with MRI has uncovered no significant difference between patients with calcaneal fractures and healthy volunteers, thus bringing into question the contribution of fat pad injury to chronic pain.

Treatment Controversy continues to surround nearly every aspect of calcaneal fracture management. With improved methods of assessing and classifying fractures, surgical treatment has become more popular. Nonetheless, a variety of closed treatment methods continue to be used and supported by many surgeons. Closed treatment can be carried out with or without manipulation and with or without immobilization. Much of what is known about these methods was published in the literature over the past 50 years. The results are quite varied and difficult to interpret, in large part because of inconsistent classifications and lack of CT analysis. Many of the goals of closed manipulation, such as narrowing the heel and reestablishing the height of the calcaneus, remain constant regardless of whether treatment is administered as a closed or open procedure. Authors who favor closed treatment without manipulation believe that the deformity that is accepted will be less bothersome than the stiffness that results from immobilization. The remaining problem with closed treatment, however, is inability to accurately restore the articu-

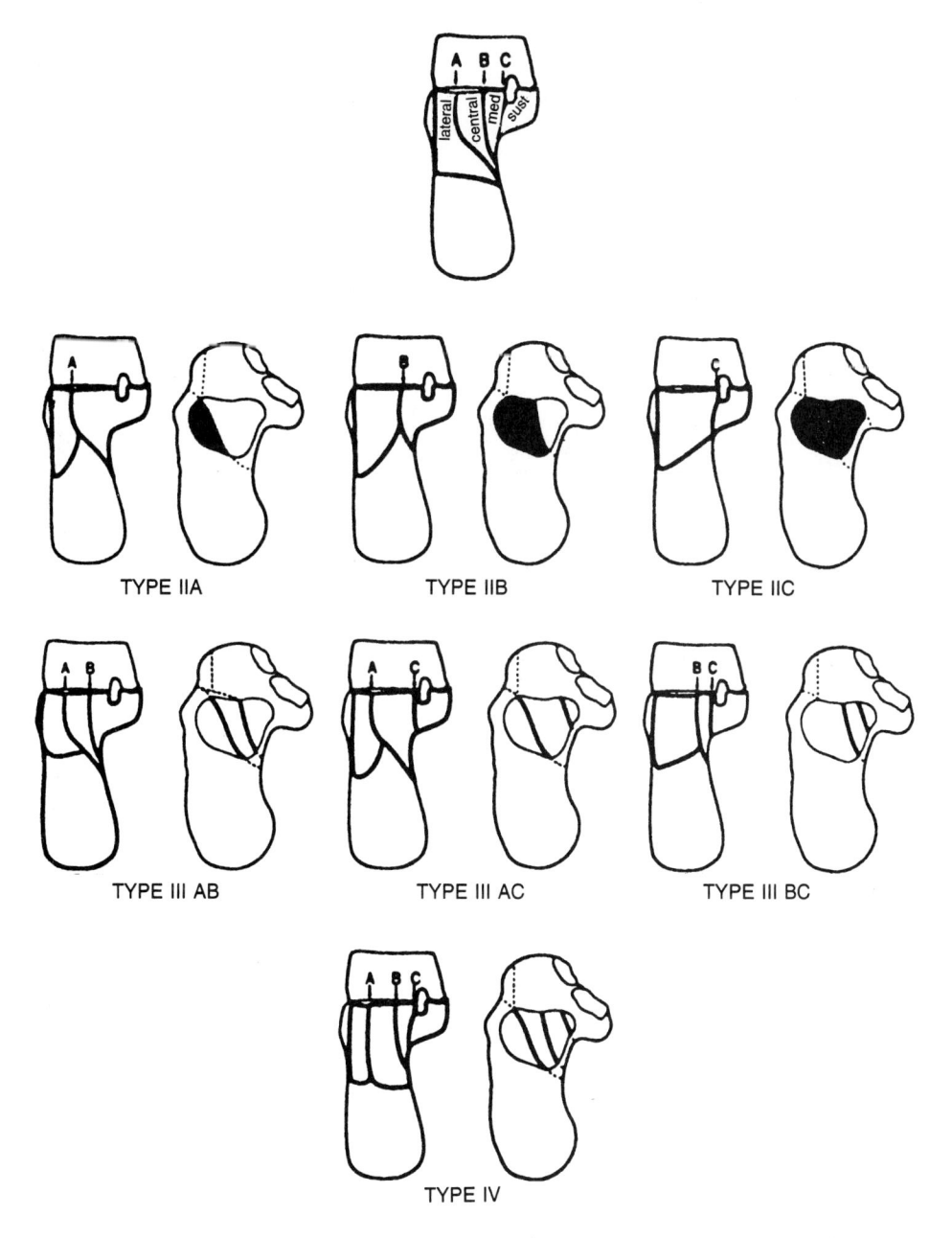

Fig. 5 Sanders classification of intra-articular calcaneal fractures. Each pair of schematics represents a coronal CT image (**left**) and a transverse CT image (**right**) of the posterior facet. (Reproduced with permission from Sanders RW: Intraarticular fractures of the calcaneus: Present state of the art. *J Orthop Trauma* 1992;6:252-265.)

lar surface of the posterior facet. This fact is well supported in recent work in which CT was used to analyze calcaneal fractures. When intra-articular calcaneal fractures treated with closed methods were assessed with CT, the severity of intra-articular disruption correlated well with clinical outcome. Nondisplaced fractures had a good outcome whereas displaced and comminuted fractures did not.[26]

The surgical treatment of calcaneal fractures has received increasing attention over the past decade.[27,28] All authors recognize the same surgical treatment goals: anatomic restoration of calcaneal shape, correction of hindfoot varus, and restoration of the posterior facet joint surface (Fig. 6). The surgical techniques to achieve these results, however, are numerous, with a large number of reports

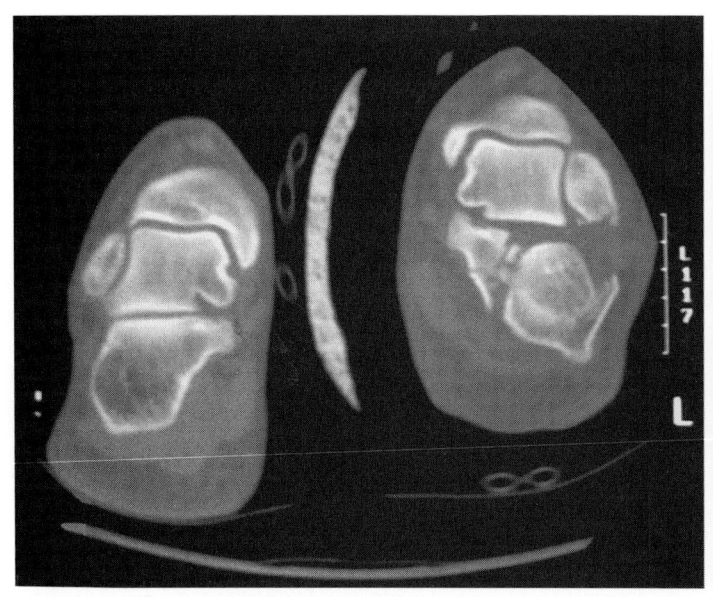

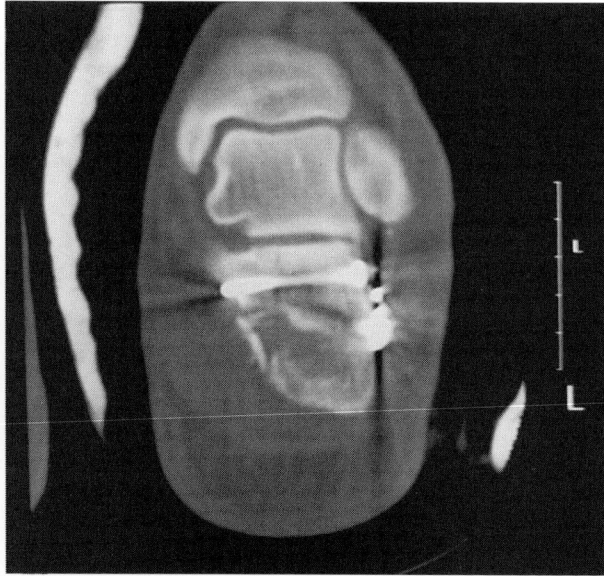

Fig. 6 Preoperative (**left**) and postoperative (**right**) coronal CT scans of a Sanders type II intra-articular calcaneal fracture.

advocating a variety of different methods of approaching, reducing, and internally fixing these fractures.

The use of small tensioned wires and ring fixators has been reported to be successful in treating fractures of the os calcis. Through distraction techniques, heel height and hindfoot varus can be restored. Articular reduction requires a lateral incision for reduction under direct vision. The advantages of this technique are reported to be early weightbearing and avoidance of an extensile exposure.

Formal surgical treatment may be classified into medial, lateral, and combined approaches. Authors who advocate a formal medial approach state that this approach permits direct reduction of the constant sustentacular fragment to the tuberosity. Advocates of this approach admit, however, that accurate reduction of the posterior facet requires a lateral incision. Authors who have reported results achieved with an extensile, lateral approach believe that reduction of the posterior facet is the most important aspect of this procedure and that this is best accomplished by direct lateral exposure of the subtalar joint. Restoration of calcaneal shape and articular congruity and correction of hindfoot varus can also be directly performed with this approach. Finally, some authors advocate the routine use of both a lateral and a medial incision, either sequentially or simultaneously. The reported advantages of this technique are improved accuracy of reduction and a decrease in the size of the implant required laterally if secure fixation is achieved on the medial side. The results achieved with the extensile lateral incision alone, however, probably make routine use of the medial incision superfluous. Although bone grafting has been advocated by some authors to maintain the height of the posterior facet, the fact that equal results have been seen with or without it makes the use of a supplementary bone graft questionable.

Using these varied methods, different groups state that 70% to 85% of patients have had good or excellent results on follow-up.[27,28] Long-term studies (5 years) of outcome, however, are still needed to adequately assess the efficacy of any of these techniques. Further, despite the many recent reports of success with surgical intervention, clear documentation (with long-term follow-up) of the superiority of open reduction and internal fixation over closed treatment is lacking. Two small series that compared surgical versus closed treatment favored surgical treatment, although the length of follow-up was short and assignment of patients to each treatment limb was not random. In addition, clinical parameters that have been associated with a poor outcome have not been consistently employed in these studies. These parameters include age older than 50, increased body weight, work involving strenuous labor, and more time missed from work because of the injury. Radiographic parameters correlating with poor outcome include subtalar incongruity, arthrosis of the talonavicular and ankle joint, increased heel width, decreased fibulocalcaneal space, and a decreased Bohler's angle.[29] Heel height, fat pad height, talocalcaneal angle, and length of the Achilles tendon fulcrum did not relate to outcome. Correlation of the CT evaluation postoperatively with functional evaluation has been mixed. Some authors have found that CT changes indicative of degeneration and incongruity of the posterior facet correlate with a poor functional outcome. Others have been unable to find a good correlation between CT parameters and functional evaluation.

Complications Complications related to calcaneal fractures consist of those that occur as part of the injury itself and those that are secondary to the treatment instituted. Compartment syndrome occurs in up to 10% of calcaneal fractures, with clawing of the lesser toes or other foot deformities developing in one half. The plantar aponeurosis is the structure responsible for most compartment syndromes that occur with calcaneal fractures. Significantly increased compartment pressures in the plantar muscle compartment should be relieved by a longitudinal incision of the plantar aponeurosis. Injury to the peroneal tendon structures is another long-term complication of calcaneal fractures and one that previously was difficult to diagnose radiographically.[30] CT has been shown to be effective in demonstrating lateral displacement, impingement by bony fragments, subluxation, and dislocation. Subluxation and dislocation have been identified in as many as 39% of acute cases when assessed with CT. Routine radiographs have been only about half as sensitive in demonstrating these problems. Complications of the nonsurgical treatment of calcaneal fractures include subtalar arthrosis, peroneal tendon impingement, hindfoot varus, and widening. Some authors have recommended osteotomy of the calcaneus through the primary fracture line to correct the deformity, followed by subtalar fusion. Others have recommended subtalar fusion with a distraction bone block technique to restore the height of the hindfoot. Complications that arise with the lateral approach relate mainly to the soft tissues. Superficial wound necrosis occurs in approximately 5% of patients, but can lead to deep infection with disastrous results. For fractures treated with open reduction and internal fixation in which wound breakdown occurs, early aggressive treatment with local or free flap coverage is recommended to prevent progression to osteomyelitis. If calcaneal osteomyelitis does occur, bony and soft-tissue debridement followed by flap coverage and antibiotics is recommended. Finally, sural nerve injury can also occur, but it is less common when an extensile approach is used in place of a limited lateral exposure.

Subtalar Dislocation

Subtalar or peritalar dislocation is defined as simultaneous dislocation of the talocalcaneal and the talonavicular joints, with the calcaneocuboid joint left undisturbed. These are unusual injuries, so that large series with long follow-up are difficult to compile. Recent reports, however, have provided additional information. These injuries continue to be classified as to the direction of displacement of the distal segment (foot) relative to the proximal. These are mainly medially displaced injuries (74% to 80%). Some authors have also found examples of anterior and posterior dislocations but these are very rare. Subtalar dislocations are associated with an open wound in 25% to 44% of cases and with fractures in well over 50% of cases. The diagnosis is made primarily from standard radiographic views of the foot. Associated fractures that must be sought on these radiographs include fractures of the medial malleolus, navicular, talus, and calcaneus. CT evaluation is rarely helpful except in some cases to evaluate associated fractures.

Treatment of these injuries includes an initial attempt at closed reduction with the patient heavily sedated or under general anesthesia. The success rate of closed reduction in closed dislocations has been reported to be 91% to 100%. Irreducible dislocations must be reduced with a formal open technique. Trapped tendons or large fracture fragments are usually found preventing the reduction. After closed or open reduction and fixation if needed, the foot is immobilized with a short leg cast for 6 weeks. Associated fractures may require additional surgical procedures or prolonged immobilization time. Authors give varying opinions regarding patients' weightbearing status while casted. Follow-up results at an average of 5 years have been somewhat disappointing. Using a combined scoring system that included subjective and objective parameters, one series found that 54% of patients had poor results and only 11% had good results.[30] Many of the poor results were associated with reflex sympathetic dystrophy, which occurred in 25% of patients. Other series have shown somewhat better outcomes, with 62% of patients reporting no pain and 88% reporting no activity restriction. Moderate subjective instability, however, was reported in 50% of this group. Investigators recommend a minimum of 6 weeks of immobilization post injury in younger patients, stating that some loss of subtalar motion is acceptable in an effort to prevent chronic subtalar instability. The need for triple arthrodesis following this injury has been unusual.

Navicular Fractures

Fractures of the tarsal navicular are divided into three types: stress fractures, acute fractures, and avulsion fractures. Displaced, intra-articular fractures of the navicular have been classified recently by Sangeorzan and associates[4] into three types. Type 1 injuries involve a fracture in the coronal plane without angulation in the forefoot. Type 2 injuries are those with a dorsolateral to plantar-medial fracture line with medial displacement of the main fragment and adduction of the forefoot. Type 3 injuries are those with a comminuted sagittal fracture line and lateral angulation of the forefoot. Treatment requires meticulous attention to detail with the goal of restoration of the anatomic configuration of the navicular and surrounding bones while maintaining mobility of the talonavicular joint. Type 1 fractures can often be treated with dorsal-to-plantar lag screws without violating surrounding joints. Type 2 and 3 injuries, however, may require fixation of fragments of the navicular to the surrounding cuneiforms to maintain reduction. If talonavicular instability persists, smooth K-wires may be used to temporarily fix this joint. More definitive fixation of this joint should be avoided because of the importance of motion in this joint to normal foot mechanics. The type of fracture correlates directly with the ability to achieve an anatomic reduction, as well as with the clinical outcome. At final evaluation with an average follow-up of 44 months in one series, 67% of patients had a good result, 19% a fair result, and 14% a poor result.

Cuboid Fractures

Cuboid fractures may be of the avulsion or compression type. In the compression fracture the body of the cuboid is often comminuted, resulting in shortening of the lateral column of the foot. These injuries are often associated with other midfoot injuries. Recent treatment recommendations for cuboid fractures include restoration of cuboid anatomy with open reduction followed by bone grafting, when necessary, and internal fixation. This approach allows articular reconstruction and maintenance of the lateral column of the foot. Early results in a limited series of patients have been superior to nonsurgical treatment or a late midtarsal fusion.

Cuneiform Fractures and Fracture-Dislocations

Isolated case reports of fractures and fracture-dislocations involving the cuneiforms continue to appear. These reports vary from cases of isolated fractures of various types to cases of multiple fractures and dislocations involving more than one cuneiform. Unfortunately, no large series of these injuries has yet appeared to allow development of a meaningful system of classification or treatment.

Lisfranc Joint Injuries

Injuries to the tarsometatarsal joint complex are complex and difficult to treat. The appearance of these injuries on superficial inspection is usually complex because of the variety of fractures that often accompany the joint dislocations. These features have also made it difficult to establish an adequate classification system. Quenu and Kuss in the early 1900s divided these injuries into three types. Type 1 injuries are homolateral dislocations, with all five metatarsals being displaced in the coronal plane. Type 2 injuries are isolated dislocations, with one or two metatarsals being displaced in the coronal plane. Type 3 injuries are divergent dislocations, with separation between the first and second metatarsals and displacement in both the coronal and sagittal planes. Hardcastle modified this classification, recognizing that displacement rarely occurs solely in the coronal plane. He divided these injuries into total, partial, and divergent (Fig. 7). In all of these, displacement could potentially occur in the coronal, sagittal, or a combined plane. In total tarsometatarsal dislocation there is incongruity of the entire joint complex. The partial injury may be medial or lateral but results in disruption of only part of the tarsometatarsal joint complex. In the divergent injury type, the first metatarsal is displaced medially and some portion of the lateral four metatarsals is displaced laterally. Incongruence may be partial or total in the divergent injury.

Recent work has confirmed the high rate of association between Lisfranc joint injuries and fractures involving the metatarsal and tarsal bones. As many as 95% of patients with Lisfranc joint dislocations have been found to have associated metatarsal fractures. In addition, it has been noted that fractures of the metatarsals occur in different locations when associated with a Lisfranc joint injury. When associated with this type of dislocation, metatarsal fractures occur more commonly in the proximal second metatarsal and less commonly in the fifth metatarsal. Further, fractures of the midtarsal bones (cuneiforms, cuboid, and navicular) have been seen in up to 39% of patients. Often the full extent of the midfoot dislocation is not appreciated initially and attention is focused instead on the more obvious fractures.

The diagnosis of tarsometatarsal dislocations is still generally made with standard radiographic evaluation, which must include AP, oblique, and lateral views. These films should be assessed for both the relationship of the bases of the metatarsals to the tarsal bones and for fractures that have a known association with Lisfranc dislocations, including avulsion fractures of the bases of the first or second metatarsals, avulsion fractures of the medial pole of the navicular, crush injuries of the cuboid, and anterior process fractures of the calcaneus. Recently a weight-bearing lateral radiograph has been shown to be beneficial in diagnosing subtle Lisfranc joint injuries by showing flattening of the longitudinal arch.[32] This can be detected by measuring the distance between the base of the fifth metatarsal and the base of the medial cuneiform on this film. Stress radiographs can also be helpful in identifying

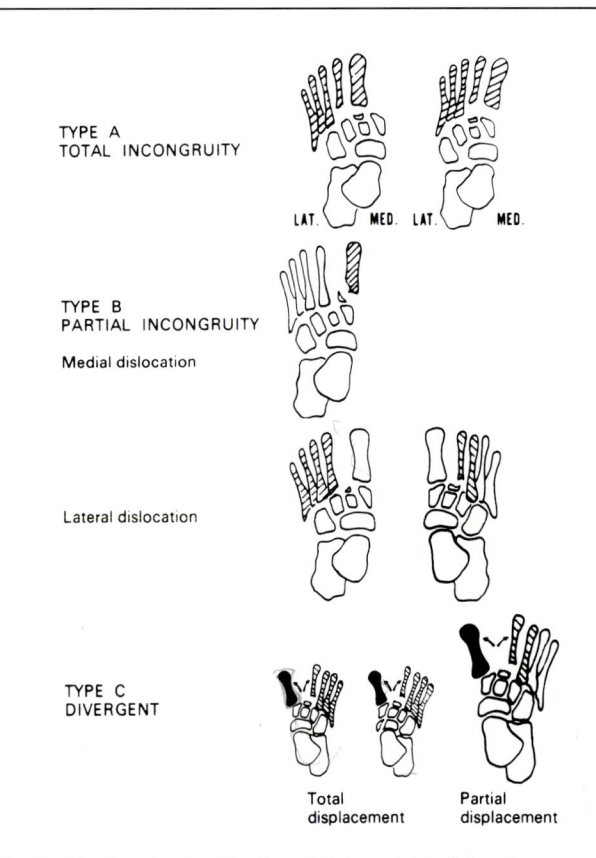

Fig. 7 Hardcastle classification of Lisfranc joint dislocations. (Reproduced with permission from Hardcastle PH, Reschauer R, Kutscha-Lissberg E, et al: Injuries to the tarsometatarsal joint. *J Bone Joint Surg* 1982;64B:349-356.)

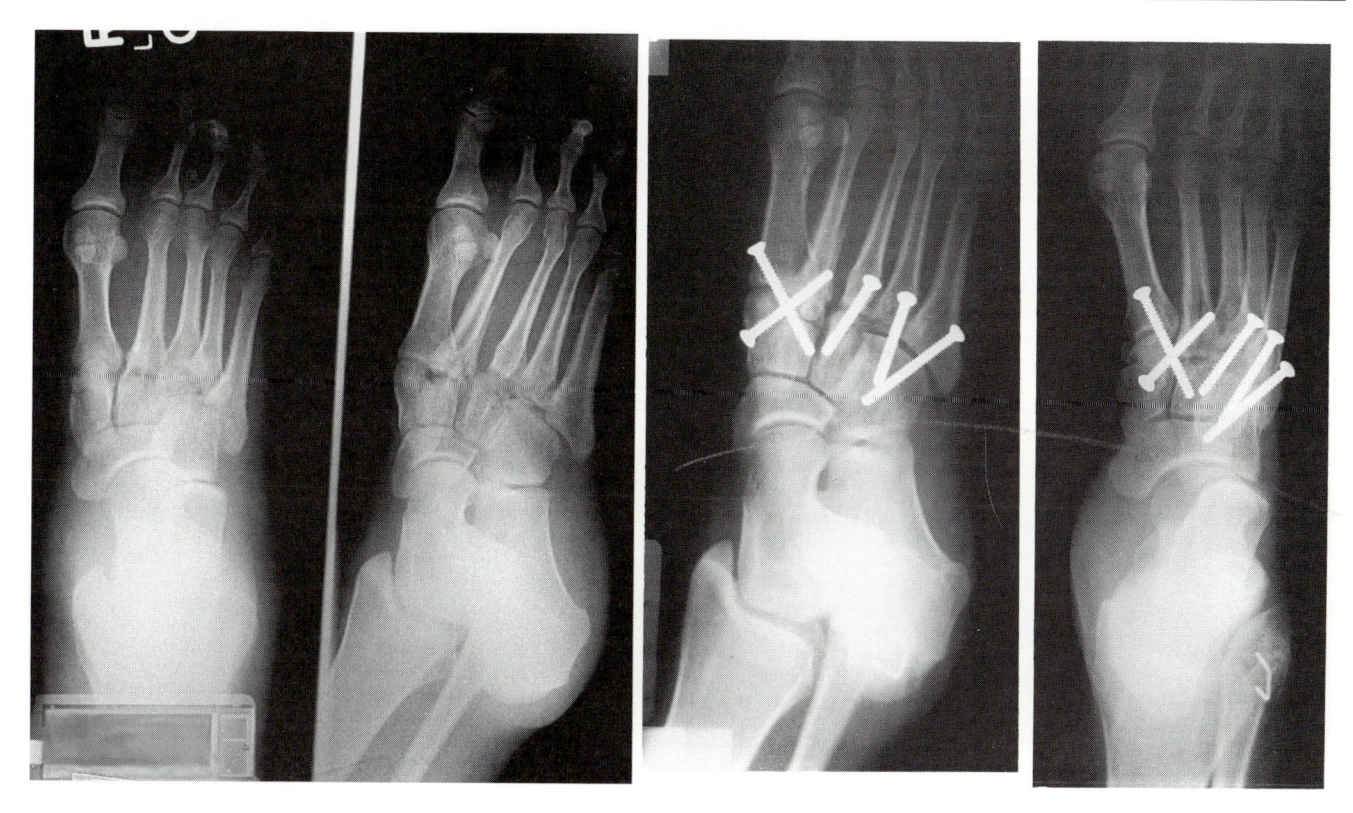

Fig. 8 **Left** and **center left,** Radiographs of a partial, lateral Lisfranc dislocation with lateral displacement of the lateral three rays. **Right** and **center right,** Open reduction was performed, followed by internal fixation with temporary lag screws.

subtle injuries. Although rarely indicated in initial assessment, CT studies of patients with Lisfranc joint injuries support the accuracy of this modality in demonstrating the amount of displacement in the sagittal plane.

The cornerstone of success in the treatment of tarsometatarsal joint injuries is achieving and maintaining anatomic reduction of the joints while the ligaments heal. Although closed reduction and percutaneous pinning may be effective in selected cases, few recent authors have recommended this approach. If closed reduction is attempted, the surgeon must be critical in assessing the postreduction radiographs, since this will directly affect outcome. Difficulty in achieving and assessing the closed reduction has led most authors to recommend proceeding directly to open reduction. Open reduction is generally performed through two or three longitudinal incisions. Once reduced, the tarsometatarsal joints should be stabilized with 3.5-mm screws (Fig. 8). This technique has been quite successful in maintaining the reduction without the problems associated with smooth pins, such as pin migration, pin-tract infection, and loss of reduction.[33] Further, studies advocating screw fixation have found that these implants contribute little to the development of arthrosis of the joints they fix. Typically, patients begin to ambulate with the screws still in place by 3 months, with the implants being removed by 6 months.

Results

Results of the treatment of Lisfranc joint injuries improved with recognition of the importance of anatomic reduction of all joints. Even with anatomic reduction, however, the prognosis is somewhat guarded.[34] Treatment with closed or open reduction followed by K-wire fixation has resulted in a 49% to 71% rate of good or excellent results. Arntz and associates[33] reported on 34 patients in whom AO screws were used for temporary internal fixation. They found good or excellent results in 28 of 30 patients in whom anatomic reduction was achieved. Six of 34 patients had fair or poor results, but 67% did not have an anatomic reduction and 83% had associated grade II or grade III open injuries. The authors concluded that posttraumatic arthrosis was directly related to damage to the articular surface or to inadequate reduction, or both. In another study, gait analysis of 11 patients with previously displaced Lisfranc fractures revealed that none had a normal gait. Limp was found to be due to a prolonged hindfoot period and a shortened period of weight transfer through the midfoot to the forefoot as a result of pain inhibition. The most normal gait pattern in this group of patients was seen in those who had undergone anatomic reduction of their dislocation. Patients with persistent deformity or pain despite conservative or surgical treatment after a Lisfranc dislocation or fracture-dislocation may benefit from arthrodesis of the affected joints. Arthrodesis by open reduction and internal fixation yielded good to excellent results in 69% of a small series of patients.[35]

Fractures of the Proximal Fifth Metatarsal

Proximal fifth metatarsal fractures are divided into tuberosity avulsion fractures and proximal diaphyseal fractures, often referred to as the Jones fracture. Fractures occurring in the proximal diaphysis may be acute or fatigue fractures, and chronic nonunion is well recognized in this region as well. Recognition of the category into which each individual fracture fits will influence treatment and prognosis.[36,37]

The appropriate treatment of a proximal diaphyseal fracture is controversial. Treatment must be individualized and depends on careful evaluation of the history and radiographs to distinguish acute, chronic, and stress fractures. Most authors agree that nonsurgical treatment with nonweightbearing using either a short leg cast or an elastic bandage is indicated initially for acute fractures.[36,37] They would recommend this approach even for athletes, in whom expeditious return to sports participation is paramount. Others, however, have reported excellent results when treating athletes with acute fractures with percutaneous screw fixation performed in an outpatient setting. Average time to return to full activity with this protocol has been about 8.5 weeks. Late surgery, which generally results in full return of function, is required in about 12% of patients with acute fractures that were initially treated nonsurgically. Although chronic fractures or stress fractures may heal without surgical intervention, as many as 50% may eventually require surgical intervention. Intramedullary sclerosis about the fracture is viewed as a poor prognostic sign for the healing of chronic fractures. The recommended treatment for chronic fractures is placement of an intramedullary compression screw. Use of a bone graft is still advocated as an effective surgical alternative by some authors.

Recent investigations have attempted to clarify the underlying cause of the propensity for poor healing in the proximal diaphyseal fracture. Using India ink or barium sulfate injections, it was found that the blood supply to the proximal metaphysis was from multiple vessels that penetrated the nonarticular portion of the metaphysis in a random, radiate pattern. The vascular supply to the proximal diaphysis, on the other hand, was primarily from the nutrient artery, which gave rise to multiple intramedullary branches. A watershed region was identified just distal to the tuberosity that corresponds to the region of poor prognosis for healing. This relative paucity of blood flow may contribute to delayed and nonunions in this region.

Metatarsophalangeal Joint Injuries

Injury to the first metatarsophalangeal joint may vary from a mild sprain to severe tearing of the capsuloligamentous structures and even fracture-dislocation of the joint. This has become a fairly common sporting injury, particularly in football, as more flexible shoeware and artificial playing surfaces have been introduced. This condition is commonly referred to as "turf toe." In a group of 80 professional football players who sustained this injury, the mechanism was found to be hyperextension in 85%. Eighty-three percent of these players had sustained their initial injury on artificial turf. The injury resulted in significant loss of motion of the toe. Treatment recommendations include a standard regimen of ice, taping, and anti-inflammatory medications, with a gradual return to sports as symptoms decrease. Possible modes of prevention include forefoot stiffening in shoeware and use of an orthotic device.[38]

Compartment Syndrome of the Foot

Description of Injury Recognition of the compartment syndrome in the foot came slightly more than a decade ago. This condition tends to occur in association with crushing and high-energy injuries. Although the foot classically is thought to contain four compartments (medial, central, interosseous, and central), recent anatomic studies have identified nine distinct compartments.[39] This description is similar to the classic description in terms of the medial and lateral compartments but has significant variation in the remaining compartments. The central compartment has a superficial and deep component, with the latter known as the calcaneal compartment. The interossei are contained within four separate compartments, and the adductor muscle is within yet another deep forefoot compartment.

Diagnosis The diagnosis of foot compartment syndrome is best made by maintaining a high index of suspicion. This condition is associated with multiple metatarsal fractures, Lisfranc dislocation, calcaneal fractures, and other injuries associated with high-energy or crushing mechanisms. Although clinical findings may be inconsistent, tense swelling of the foot and intense pain are common. Interstitial compartment pressures should be measured if any clinical suspicion exists. With the availability of the previously mentioned anatomic description, authors have begun to recommend multiple sites of catheterization prior to ruling out the condition. Based on results of studies on the forearm and leg, most authors recommend release of the compartments if pressures exceed 30 mm Hg or 10 to 30 mm Hg below diastolic blood pressure.

Treatment Experimental studies on fresh cadaver feet have shown that both the single medial incision and the double dorsal incision technique can result in adequate decompression of fascial compartments. The investigators did note that intracompartmental pressures equalized faster after the medial incision release, although the clinical relevance of this observation was unclear. Thus, no consensus opinion exists favoring one technique over the other. With recognition of nine distinct compartments, concern has been raised about whether dorsal incisions alone are sufficient for decompression of the deep central compartment (the calcaneal compartment). Use of the dorsal incisions to release the forefoot compartments and a small medial incision to decompress the medial and calcaneal compartments may be the most predictable way to decompress the foot.

Complication When recognized and treated promptly with fascial release, compartment syndrome rarely results in significant complications. With insufficient or delayed release, clawing of the toes is the most common problem. Fasciotomy wounds can occasionally be closed in a delayed primary fashion but more often require split-thickness skin grafting. With the two-dorsal-incision technique, loss of the skin bridge has been reported in 11% of cases.

Partial Foot Amputations
With severe injury to the foot, amputation of all or part of the foot may be required. Often toe or ray amputation is sufficient and will give a very good functional result. If transmetatarsal amputation is necessary, function will still be quite good. Most of these patients can wear off-the-shelf shoes with a toe filler in the area of the missing foot.

Controversy surrounds the topic of partial foot amputation proximal to the transmetatarsal level. Chopart amputation—disarticulation through the calcaneocuboid and talonavicular joints—has fallen into some disfavor in recent years because of the equinus deformity that results from unopposed pull of the triceps surae. This problem can be lessened by lengthening or releasing the Achilles tendon at the time of the amputation. The advantages of this procedure over a Syme's amputation (disarticulation through the ankle joint), are the ease of the operation and the ability of the patient to wear a regular shoe when fitted with an ankle-foot orthosis.

In a recent retrospective review of 260 partial foot amputees, 113 patients were evaluated at a mean 16 year follow-up. The end results were found to be good in 43%, fair in 38%, and poor in 19%. Of the original group, 19% required revision to a Syme's or below-knee amputation. Patients with amputations through Lisfranc's joint or Chopart's joint did well, and in fact often had a better result than patients with digital or transmetatarsal amputations.

Annotated References

1. Rijke AM, Goitz HT, McCue FC III, et al: Magnetic resonance imaging of injury to the lateral ankle ligaments. *Am J Sports Med* 1993;21:528-534.

2. Kannus P, Renstrom P: Treatment for acute tears of the lateral ligaments of the ankle: Operation, cast, or early controlled mobilization. *J Bone Joint Surg* 1991;73A:305-312.

    The authors performed a meta-analysis of randomized prospective studies of the treatment of grade III lateral ankle sprains. All 12 studies available in the English language were evaluated. The meta-analysis included a total of 1,500 patients. The authors concluded that functional treatment with early range of motion and progressive weightbearing is as effective as casting or acute primary surgical repair and avoids the cost and complications of these more invasive methods.

3. Karlsson J, Bergsten T, Lansinger O, et al: Reconstruction of the lateral ligaments of the ankle for chronic lateral instability. *J Bone Joint Surg* 1988;70A:581-588.

    One hundred seventy-six patients with chronic lateral instability of the ankle were treated with transection and imbrication of the anterior talofibular ligament. Sixty-eight also underwent reconstruction of the calcaneofibular ligament. One hundred fifty-two ankles were evaluated 2 to 12 years postoperatively. An excellent or good result was achieved in 132. Most patients with an unsatisfactory result had generalized joint hypermobility, long-standing ligamentous insufficiency or had undergone a previous operation. Reconstruction of both ligaments gave a better result than did reconstruction of the anterior talofibular ligament alone.

4. Sangeorzan BJ, Veith RG, Hansen ST Jr: Salvage of Lisfranc's tarsometatarsal joint by arthrodesis. *Foot Ankle* 1990;10:193-200.

    Sixteen patients with fracture-dislocations of the tarsometatarsal (Lisfranc) joint and in whom initial treatment failed underwent arthrodesis. Presurgical symptoms included pain and progressive deformity. A method of rigid internal fixation was used to achieve fusion. A total of 49 joints were fused, and symptomatic nonunion occurred in four sites in three patients. Good or excellent results were achieved in 11 patients and fair or poor results in five patients. All but one patient improved subjectively.

5. Cass JR, Morrey BF, Katoh Y, et al: Ankle instability: Comparison of primary repair and delayed reconstruction after long-term follow-up study. *Clin Orthop* 1985;198:110-117.

6. Hopkinson WJ, St.Pierre P, Ryan JB, et al: Syndesmosis sprains of the ankle. *Foot Ankle* 1990;10:325-330.

7. Cetti R, Christensen SE, Ejsted R, et al: Operative versus nonsurgical treatment of Achilles tendon rupture: A prospective randomized study and review of the literature. *Am J Sports Med* 1993;21:791-799.

8. FitzGibbons RE, Hefferon J, Hill J: Percutaneous Achilles tendon repair. *Am J Sports Med* 1993;21:724-727.

9. Hockenbury RT, Johns JC: A biomechanical in vitro comparison of open versus percutaneous repair of tendon Achilles. *Foot Ankle* 1990;11:67-72.

10. Arrowsmith SR, Fleming LL, Allman FL: Traumatic dislocations of the peroneal tendons. *Am J Sports Med* 1983;11:142-146.

   Traumatic dislocation of the peroneal tendons is reviewed. This is a diagnosis often missed initially. Intense retromalleolar pain on active eversion is a specific and highly suggestive finding. Fracture of a thin shell of the lateral malleolar cortex is diagnostic. Surgical repair is controversial in the acute case, but nonsurgical treatment is unpredictable. If surgical treatment is undertaken for the acute case, simple repair of the torn or fractured structures is generally successful. Chronic cases require surgery that often involves reconstruction of the peroneal retinaculum or deepening of the peroneal groove.

11. Moehring HD, Tan RT, Marder RA, et al: Ankle dislocation. *J Orthop Trauma* 1994;8:167-172.

   Fourteen patients with pure dislocation (without associated fracture) of the ankle were identified. Twelve of 14 were followed up from 15 months to more than 10 years after injury. All dislocations were posteromedial, and most were open on the anterolateral side. Simple repair of the lateral ligaments was routinely done in the open injuries. Eighty-three percent of patients had good or excellent results. No patient had evidence of instability.

12. Phillips WA, Schwartz HS, Keller CS, et al: A prospective randomized study of the management of severe ankle fractures. *J Bone Joint Surg* 1985;67A:67-78.

13. Bauer M, Bergstrom B, Hemborg A, et al: Malleolar fractures: Nonsurgical versus surgical treatment. A controlled study. *Clin Orthop* 1985;199:17-27.

14. Boden SD, Labropoulos PA, McCowin P, et al: Mechanical considerations for the syndesmosis screw: A cadaver study. *J Bone Joint Surg* 1989;71A:1548-1555.

   The need for a syndesmosis screw was tested on cadavers in which the syndesmotic ligaments had been divided and the interosseous membrane sectioned to various levels. Models simulating both a deltoid ligament rupture and a medial malleolar fracture were tested. When rigid fixation of both the medial and lateral injuries could be achieved, minimal widening of the syndesmosis occurred, even with division of the membrane 15 cm proximal to the ankle. When the medial injury could not be rigidly fixed, as with a deltoid ligament injury, the syndesmosis showed significant instability once the interosseous membrane had been divided higher than 4.5 cm above the ankle.

15. Harper MC, Hardin G: Posterior malleolar fractures of the ankle associated with external rotation-abduction injuries: Results with and without internal fixation. *J Bone Joint Surg* 1988;70A:1348-1356.

   Thirty-eight patients in whom a fracture of the posterior malleolus was shown to comprise 25% or more of the articular surface on the lateral radiograph were followed up for an average of 44 months. Open reduction with internal fixation was done on all fractures of the medial and lateral malleoli. No significant difference was noted between the 15 patients who had internal fixation of the posterior malleolus and the 23 patients who did not. Satisfactory reduction of the posterior malleolus was usually achieved when the fibula was reduced and was maintained without the aid of internal fixation. No posterior subluxation of the talus occurred in either group.

16. Bray TJ, Endicott M, Capra SE: Treatment of open ankle fractures: Immediate internal fixation versus closed immobilization and delayed fixation. *Clin Orthop* 1989;240:47-52.

17. Limbird RS, Aaron RK: Laterally comminuted fracture-dislocation of the ankle. *J Bone Joint Surg* 1987;69A:881-885.

   Eight patients with a previously undescribed laterally comminuted fracture-dislocation of the ankle were described. This is a rare injury that is usually associated with an avulsion fracture of the medial malleolus lateral displacement of the talus comminution of the fibula at or proximal to the syndesmosis and an impaction fracture of the lateral plafond. Discontinuity of the fibula makes accurate restoration of fibular length and rotation difficult. The authors recommend accurately reducing and fixing the medial malleolus first. The fibula is then reduced anatomically to the lateral articular facet of the talus and temporarily pinned in this position. Plate fixation of the fibula is then used to maintain this position. Bone grafting is often necessary to achieve complete healing of the fibula. Clinical and radiographic results were highly satisfactory when these methods were used.

18. Marti RK, Raaymakers EL, Nolte PA: Malunited ankle fractures: The late results of reconstruction. *J Bone Joint Surg* 1990;72B:709-713.

19. Dipaolo JD, Nelson DW, Colville MR: Characterizing osteochondral lesions by magnetic resonance imaging. *Arthroscopy* 1991;7:101-104.

20. Anderson IF, Crichton KJ, Grattan-Smith T, et al: Osteochondral fractures of the dome of the talus. *J Bone Joint Surg* 1989;71A:1143-1152.

21. De Smet AA, Fisher DR, Burnstein MI, et al: Value of MR imaging in staging osteochondral lesions of the talus (osteochondritis dissecans): Results in 14 patients. *AJR Am J Roentgenol* 1990;154:555-558.

   The value of MRI of patients with osteochondral lesions of the talus was studied. Fourteen patients underwent both MRI and surgical evaluation of an osteochondral lesion of the talus (usually arthroscopic). Investigators were able to correctly predict the surgical findings by MRI in 13 patients. The 14th patient had an incorrect diagnosis of a chondral fragment. Partially attached fragments had an irregular high-intensity signal zone at the fragment-talar interface. Unattached fragments had a complete ring of fluid surrounding the lesion.

22. Pritsch M, Horoshovski H, Farine I: Arthroscopic treatment of osteochondral lesions of the talus. *J Bone Joint Surg* 1986;68A:862-865.

   Twenty-four patients with symptomatic osteochondral lesions of the talus were graded and treated based on arthroscopic findings. Patients were evaluated after an average of 30 months. Lesions in which the cartilage is intact are best treated by restriction of activity. Those in which the overlying cartilage is soft can be treated with drilling of the lesion and those in which the cartilage is frayed can be treated with curettage. These methods of treatment give good results with minimum morbidity.

23. Ebraheim NA, Coombs RE, Jackson WT, et al: The effect of metallic implants on magnetic resonance imaging: A brief note. *J Bone Joint Surg* 1991;73A:1397-1398.

24. Canale ST, Kelly FB Jr: Fractures of the neck of the talus: Long-term evaluation of seventy-one cases. *J Bone Joint Surg* 1978;60A:143-156.

   Seventy-one fractures of the neck of the talus were reviewed after an average of 12.7 years. Accurate anatomic reduction is recommended if necessary by open reduction and internal fixation. Osteonecrosis was seen in 52% of patients, but many of these patients had satisfactory clinical results. Other complications, including malunion and subtalar arthrosis, are discussed.

25. Szyszkowitz R, Reschauer R, Seggl W: Eighty-five talus fractures treated by ORIF with five to eight years of follow-up study of 69 patients. *Clin Orthop* 1985;199:97-107.

   The results of surgical treatment of 69 displaced talus fractures are discussed. Radiographically, a significant number of patients had arthrosis in the ankle or the subtalar joints. Clinically, however, 82% of patients with talar neck or body fractures had good or very good results. The authors conclude that open reduction with internal fixation offers significantly better results for displaced fractures than closed treatment.

26. Crosby LA, Fitzgibbons T: Computerized tomography scanning of acute intra articular fractures of the calcaneus: A new classification system. *J Bone Joint Surg* 1990;72A:852-859.

27. Sanders R, Fortin P, Dipasquale T, et al: Operative treatment in 120 displaced intraarticular calcaneal fractures: Results using a prognostic computed tomography scan classification. *Clin Orthop* 1993;290:87-95.

   One hundred twenty intra-articular fractures of the calcaneus were treated surgically. To evaluate results a classification scheme based on CT findings was developed. In this system the number of intra-articular fragments of the posterior facet of the calcaneus is identified. Both the ability to achieve an anatomic reduction and the clinical result decline as the number of intra-articular fragments increases. Type IV fractures, in which the posterior facet is broken into four or more fragments, resulted in predictably poor results. Consideration should be given in these cases to primary subtalar arthrodesis. A significant learning curve was identified for the surgeons involved in the study.

28. Zwipp H, Tscherne H, Thermann H, et al: Osteosynthesis of displaced intraarticular fractures of the calcaneus: Results in 123 cases. *Clin Orthop* 1993;290:76-86.

29. Paley D, Hall H: Intra-articular fractures of the calcaneus: A critical analysis of results and prognostic factors. *J Bone Joint Surg* 1993;75A:342-354.

30. Ebraheim NA, Zeiss J, Skie MC, et al: Radiological evaluation of peroneal tendon pathology associated with calcaneal fractures. *J Orthop Trauma* 1991;5:365-369.

   Eight cases of peroneal tendon subluxation or dislocation associated with intra-articular calcaneal fractures are reported. Routine radiographs failed to show the soft tissue lesion in five of the eight. CT and MRI both demonstrated well the relationship between the tendons retinaculum and the fibular groove.

31. Merchan EC: Subtalar dislocations: Long-term follow-up of 39 cases. *Injury* 1992;23:97-100.

   Thirty-nine subtalar dislocations were reviewed after an average follow-up of 5.5 years. Seventy-four percent were medial dislocations and 41% were open. Open reduction was used only if closed reduction was unsuccessful. Results were good in 11 cases, fair in seven, and poor in 21. Associated fractures were common and correlated with poor results. Good results were associated with accurate reduction. Open reduction with K-wire fixation is recommended if minor displacement persists.

32. Faciszewski T, Burks RT, Manaster BJ: Subtle injuries of the Lisfranc joint. *J Bone Joint Surg* 1990;72A:1519-1522.

33. Arntz CT, Veith RG, Hansen ST Jr: Fractures and fracture-dislocations of the tarsometatarsal joint. *J Bone Joint Surg* 1988;70A:173-181.

   Forty-one fracture-dislocations of the tarsometatarsal joints were treated with open reduction and temporary internal fixation with AO screws. Thirty-four patients returned for follow-up evaluation at an average of 3.4 years. An anatomic or near anatomic reduction was achieved in 30 patients, and 28 of these had a good or excellent result. Of the six patients who had a fair or poor result, five had a grade II or III open injury and four had nonanatomic reduction. Screws were removed at an average of 16 weeks.

34. Brunet JA, Wiley JJ: The late results of tarsometatarsal joint injuries. *J Bone Joint Surg* 1987;69B:437-440.

35. Sangeorzan BJ, Benirschke SK, Mosca V, et al: Displaced intra-articular fractures of the tarsal navicular. *J Bone Joint Surg* 1989;71A:1504-1510.

   Twenty-one patients with displaced fractures of the body of the tarsal navicular were treated with open reduction and internal fixation. Results were reviewed after an average follow-up of 44 months. Three fracture types were identified: coronal, oblique in the dorsolateral to plantar-medial plane, and comminuted. A good result was achieved in 14 patients, a fair result in four, and a poor result in three. The fracture type correlated with the clinical outcome.

36. Josefsson PO, Karlsson M, Redlund-Johnell I, et al: Jones fracture: Surgical versus nonsurgical treatment. *Clin Orthop* 1994;299:252-255.

37. Torg JS, Balduini FC, Zelko RR, et al: Fractures of the base of the fifth metatarsal distal to the tuberosity: Classification and guidelines for non-surgical and surgical management. *J Bone Joint Surg* 1984;66A:209-214.

   Forty-six fractures of the base of the fifth metatarsal distal to the tuberosity were treated and then evaluated at a mean follow-up of 40 months. Three types of fractures were identified by radiographic criteria: acute fractures with a narrow fracture line and no intramedullary sclerosis, delayed union with widening of the fracture line and evidence of intramedullary sclerosis, and those with nonunion and complete obliteration of the medullary canal by sclerotic bone. Success was achieved for acute fractures with nonweightbearing cast immobilization. Delayed unions may be successfully treated with non-surgical methods but may require extended periods of treatment. Active individuals with delayed unions and those with symptomatic nonunion can be treated effectively with medullary curretage and bone grafting.

38. Clanton TO, Butler JE, Eggert A: Injuries to the metatarsophalangeal joints in athletes. *Foot Ankle* 1986;7:162-176.

39. Manoli A II, Weber TG: Fasciotomy of the foot: An anatomical study with special reference to release of the calcaneal compartment. *Foot Ankle* 1990;10:267-275.

   An investigation of the anatomic compartments of the foot was performed. The various compartments of the feet of fresh cadaver specimens were injected with dyed gelatin. The feet were then frozen and sectioned either transversely or sagittally. Nine compartments were identified—the medial, superficial, lateral, adductor, four interossei, and calcaneal compartments. The calcaneal compartment is a previously undescribed compartment that lies deep to the superficial compartment of the hindfoot and contains the quadratus plantae muscle. Compartment syndrome of this compartment may be the cause of claw toe deformity following a fracture of the os calcis.

III
Pelvis and Acetabulum

James F. Kellam, MD, FRCS(C), FACS
Section Editor

Fractures of the Pelvis and Acetabulum: An Overview

In fractures of the pelvis and acetabulum there is a unique relationship between the soft-tissue injury and the fracture. The pelvic fracture is the key to recognizing the associated injuries in the initial phase of management of the polytrauma patient. Therefore, the orthopaedic surgeon must be involved in the management of polytrauma patients to recognize those injuries that will lead to significant hemorrhagic problems either from the pelvic fracture or from the associated injuries secondary to the trauma that caused the fracture. The acetabular fracture does not have the same implication with regard to life-threatening problems but has a significant relationship to long-term disability. The fracture is through a major weightbearing joint, and anatomic repositioning of the joint is imperative for maximal functional result. This is complicated by the soft tissues about the fracture, thus making surgical approaches and treatment difficult. It is very important to understand the relationship between the fracture and the associated soft-tissue components before these individual fractures are definitely treated.

In the acute management of pelvic injury, including acetabular fractures, it is imperative that the orthopaedic surgeon understand what will cause mortality. If there has been any major accomplishment in the management of pelvic ring injuries it has been in recognizing that diagnosis and treatment can be predicted based on force vector and fracture pattern. The common lateral compression injury to the pelvis is usually associated with head injuries and intra-abdominal injuries that are more severe and more life-threatening than the pelvic ring injury itself. However, injuries that are caused by shear or by avulsions where the hemipelvis is torn from the axial skeleton, such as motorcycle or pedestrian injuries, have more of a direct relationship to pelvic hemorrhage than to the other injuries not associated with the pelvis. In cooperation with the trauma surgeon, the orthopaedic surgeon can have an integral role in the acute life-saving management of the patient and, hence, transfer to an appropriate facility, which can then provide long-term management of the major pelvic or acetabular disruption appropriately. It is imperative to recognize that the orthopaedic surgeon's role in the acute referral center is the use of simple orthopaedic techniques, such as skeletal traction, limb positioning, the use of an antishock garment, or appropriate external methods of pelvic stabilization to prevent ongoing hemorrhage. Even the use of external fixation devices or emergency pelvic percutaneous clamps by the orthopaedic surgeon may prove very useful in this management.

Most important is the need for any orthopaedic surgeon who is involved in the treatment of pelvic injuries to be well versed in the Advanced Trauma Life Support® (ATLS) protocol for trauma assessment. Recognizing and managing airway and breathing injuries as well as circulatory problems will improve the patient's chances for survival.

The second role of the orthopaedic surgeon is the appropriate assessment and the definite decision-making in pelvic and acetabular fractures. It is well recognized that these injuries usually are associated with a polytrauma patient. The injury and the associated problems take priority in the first 5 to 7 days of management. However, the orthopaedic surgeon's role is to assess the pelvic and acetabular injury and to make a rapid decision as to what is going to be the appropriate treatment for this injury. This requires an indepth understanding of the available assessment techniques. For the pelvis, anteroposterior, inlet, and outlet radiographs are necessary; for the acetabulum, anteroposterior and Judet radiographs are necessary. These views will provide the orthopaedic surgeon with most of the information needed to make an appropriate treatment decision. More sophisticated investigations using computed tomography and its associated manipulations of axial and three-dimensional scans are usually necessary for detailed preoperative planning and occasionally for surgical decision-making. Ultimately, the surgeon must decide whether the patient requires surgical intervention by reduction and traction or nonsurgical management by traction and/or bed rest alone (Outlines 1 and 2).

If the orthopaedic surgeon is unable to appropriately assess the patient and the injury and make a decision regarding treatment within the first 24 to 48 hours, the patient or the radiographs must be referred to an orthopaedic traumatologist. It is unacceptable for patients with displaced pelvic and acetabular fractures not to have these appropriate decisions made early.

Outline 1. Transfer criteria for pelvic fractures

Posterior instability/displacement with hemodynamic instability after resuscitation and external stabilization have been started

Bladder/urethral injuries and pelvic fractures

Open pelvic fractures

Laterally directed force causing fractures through iliac wing, sacral ala, or foramina, which are displaced internally

Anteroposterior compression injury with anterior displacement of greater than 2.5 mm

Complete translational instability: sacroiliac joint dislocation, complete displacement of sacral fracture

Acetabular fractures associated with pelvic ring injuries

Outline 2. Transfer criteria for acetabular fractures

Incongruent reduction out of traction seen on any radiograph
    Articular step greater than 2 mm
    Lack of parallelism between femoral head and acetabular roof
    Medial subluxation femoral head

Instability out of traction after closed reduction
    Subluxation/dislocation (anterior, posterior, medial)
    Persistent displacement of wall and/or column following closed reduction of fracture

Numerous techniques have been developed for internal fixation of pelvic ring injuries. Because of the importance of the soft-tissue injury, and the damage that occurs to the muscles and nerve tissue around the pelvic ring, indirect reduction and percutaneous or limited open reduction are now used to minimize the surgical trauma to these tissues. These techniques as well as the open techniques require significant expertise and a long learning period. Simpler techniques such as plating of the symphysis or application of external fixator may be needed for stabilization of a pelvic ring at the time of life-saving surgery.

Most of the other techniques used for pelvic fracture fixation are associated with significant complications. They should be undertaken only by orthopaedic traumatologists trained in the surgical management of pelvic and acetabular fractures. Anatomic reduction and precise placement of the fixation are mandatory.

The biomechanical evaluation of these fixation techniques shows that there is a very small margin of safety. Consequently, any variation or any inability to obtain an acceptable reduction and appropriate fixation may lead to a failure, even in the hands of skilled orthopaedic traumatologists.

To date, the results of surgical intervention in the treatment of pelvic fractures has at least decreased the malunion and nonunion rates. However, the ability to achieve a pain-free, fully functional result through open reduction and internal fixation of the pelvic ring injury has not occurred. It is well known that reduction and stabilization of the sacroiliac joint will lead to the best results with this injury. However, even these patients will continue to have pain in the posterior pelvis. If neurologic injury to the lumbar sacral trunk has occurred, causalgic-type pain and decreased neurologic function will be evident. Extra-articular injuries through the sacrum, particularly those that involve the sacral foramina, and nerve root injury are also particularly disabling with regard to function and pain. Injuries through the iliac wing probably give the best results.

What is most important is to recognize the cause of the pelvic instability and then what needs to be stabilized. It certainly is much easier to maintain a reduction by internal fixation than to attempt to treat a functionally significant malunion or nonunion at 1 year after injury. Again, assessment and diagnosis of those cases that have potential instability which is either rotational or translational are extremely important.

Acetabular fractures require a precise understanding in order to make the appropriate surgical decisions with regard to reduction and the approach that should be used. The common dislocation of the hip associated with the posterior wall is one fracture pattern that should be well recognized by all orthopaedic surgeons. This requires prompt reduction and stabilization of the fracture to obtain a stable hip. Hence, the surgeon must be thoroughly familiar with how to evaluate and assess the patient and the patient's radiographs. The more complex acetabular fractures require complex decision-making with regard to the type of approach that will be used to stabilize the fracture. The nonextensile approaches are used to avoid iatrogenic surgical injury to the already injured soft tissues. Because of this, the definitive management of acetabular fractures is best carried out by orthopaedic traumatologists trained in surgery for acetabular fractures. A knowledge of all approaches to the acetabulum is required because no one approach is better than another and each must be considered when deciding how to maximize this exposure and facilitate reduction and fixation.

The pelvic classification system has been developed by Pennal, Tile, Burgess, and Young based on mechanism and force vector analysis as well as the radiographic appearance of the injury.

Pelvic stability, or the ability of the pelvis to resist displacement by physiologic forces, is dependent on the bony ring and, most importantly, on the ligamentous structures that maintain the posterior sacroiliac joint complex and the symphysis as well as the muscular and fibrous structures of the pelvic floor.

Disruption either of the pelvic floor or of the posterior structures, but not both, usually will lead to an incomplete or partial instability, which is evidenced through a rotational displacement of hemipelvis. This can cause internal rotation with or without superior rotation if the force has been directed from the outer aspect of the pelvis over the lateral iliac wing. The more posteriorly associated lateral force tends to cause a direct compression through the sacrum, leading to a very stable fracture pattern because the cancellous bone of the sacrum is impacted, and the pelvic floor is intact. The pelvis is rotated internally and stable in this position. If the force is directed to the more anterior aspect of the iliac wing and in a superior direction, however, the hemipelvis pivots about the anterior aspect of the sacrum and either will fracture through the iliac wing or through the sacral ala or foramina. In this situation, the major posterior ligamentous structures of the pelvis are bypassed by the fracture pattern but the pelvic floor remains intact; hence, the pelvis will displace internally. These fractures are particularly prone to displacement and deformity unless they are stabilized.

If the force is applied either directly posterior over the sacrum or anteriorly over the symphysis, or if the leg is externally rotated, the pelvis will tend to open through the symphysis and continue through the pelvic floor into the anterior sacroiliac joint ligaments. This produces the open book injury, anteroposterior compression injury, or external rotation deformities. These injuries are rotationally unstable externally and rarely will have global instability or posterior disruption of the major ligaments.

Any of these injuries either through a lateral compression or anteroposterior compression force may completely disrupt the pelvic floor and the posterior structures. If this occurs, the hemipelvis is completely unstable and will assume any position at any time, depending on the forces applied to it. This is a completely unstable pelvic fracture, which has been referred to as a vertical shear fracture, a Malgaigne fracture, or a type III anteroposterior compression injury.

The basis of the classification is an appreciation of the soft-tissue disruption and its associated fracture patterns. With this understanding one can appreciate which injuries will be stable and remain so throughout treatment, which are potentially unstable (such as the rotational injuries), and which are completely unstable. It is not imperative so much to give these injuries names and numbers as to understand how the injuries occur.

Acetabular fractures have been adequately classified by Letournel. This classification is based on fractures of the columns that support the acetabulum. Elementary fractures comprise part or all of one supporting acetabular column and these include the fractures of the posterior wall, posterior column, anterior wall, anterior column, and transverse fractures.

The associated fractures of the second group include at least two of the elementary forms above and include T-shaped fractures, fractures involving both components of the columns, and the associated both column fracture. This diagnosis is particularly useful because it helps determine the surgical approach, which is an important aspect of acetabular fracture decision-making. Posterior injuries will be approached posteriorly and anterior injuries approached anteriorly. Associated fractures that are more complex require more extensile approaches or an understanding of how to use a single approach to its maximum benefit. Specific publications provide more-detailed analyses of the classifications.

Bibliography

American College of Surgeons: *Advanced Trauma Life Support: Programs for Physicians*. Chicago, IL, American College of Surgeons, 1993.

Letournel E, Judet R (eds): *Fractures of the Acetabulum*, ed 2. Berlin, Germany, Springer-Verlag, 1993.

Müller ME, Allgöwer M, Schneider R, et al (eds): *Manual of Internal Fixation*: Techniques Recommended by the AO-ASIF Group, ed 3. Berlin, Germany, Springer-Verlag, 1991, pp 485–500.

Tile M (ed): *Fractures of Pelvis and Acetabulum*. Baltimore, MD, Williams & Wilkins, 1995.

Young JWR, Burgess AR (eds): *Radiologic Management of Pelvic Ring Fractures: Systematic Radiographic Diagnosis*. Baltimore, MD, Urban & Schwarzenberg, 1987.

21

The Acute Management of Pelvic Ring Injuries

Injury to the Pelvic Ring

Injuries to the pelvic ring are not uncommon in the patient with blunt trauma. The significant forces required to disrupt the pelvic ring produce a spectrum of injuries related to the direction and magnitude of the injury force. The treatment requirements for each patient are related to the degree of osseous ligamentous injury, displacement, and the presence of associated pelvic, abdominal, thoracic, and head injury. Approximately 12% to 20% of the patients with *high-energy pelvic injuries* will have urogenital injuries, 8% will have injuries to the lumbosacral plexus, and approximately 20% will have hemodynamic instability directly related to blood loss from the pelvic injury (hemorrhage remains the leading cause of death in pelvic fractures, with an overall mortality rate of greater than 15%).

The force vector that causes the injury to the pelvis is usually associated with a major crush or deceleration event and extra-pelvic injuries that are often more significant and more immediately life-threatening than the pelvic trauma.[1-3] In one series, only 32 (9%) of 348 patients with pelvic fractures had isolated injury to the pelvic ring.[1] Closed head injuries, abdominal trauma and pulmonary injury are highly correlated with the presence of the pelvic fracture. Pelvic fracture survivors sustain an average of 1.89 injuries in addition to their pelvic fractures and nonsurvivors, 2.95 injuries.[2] Sixty percent to 85% of patients with pelvic fractures will have fractures in other extremities.[3]

Treatment Priorities

The patient's clinical presentation and the significant physical findings of the initial examination define the magnitude of the pelvic injury. Pelvic ring injuries can be divided into two major groups according to the presence or absence of related pelvic hemorrhage and/or the presence of an open fracture pattern. Pelvic fracture blood loss contributing to hemodynamic instability or open pelvic fractures have a significant risk of death (more than 15%). Numerous series have demonstrated that recognition of these comorbid conditions in the acute treatment phase and initiation of treatment to address these problems can positively affect the clinical outcome.

The decision to definitely stabilize the pelvis is a far less critical decision pathway at this time. Prioritizing and timing the care of nonlethal pelvic trauma is dependent on the condition of the patient, the experience of the surgeon, and the capabilities of the hospital. The reduction of a dislocated hip requires semi-emergent attention. Surgical stabilization of an unstable acetabular fracture or of a rotationally or vertically unstable pelvic ring injury is usually nonemergent, but early temporary stabilization to mobilize the patient probably has beneficial effects.

Evaluation of the Patient

The alert and oriented trauma patient will direct the examining team to pelvic injuries. History obtained from the paramedics will assist the surgeon in determining the degree of injury and the force vectors. A lateral compression pelvic fracture in a pedestrian struck by a car will have a different injury constellation than a lateral compression pelvic fracture resulting from a motor vehicle collision. Crash scene data, including vehicle sizes and direction of impact, has been correlated to injury pattern. The patient's position in the vehicle and the direction of the impact (lateral, frontal, or oblique) will assist the examiner with the understanding of the patient's clinical presentation. More pelvic fractures occur from lateral (25%) than from frontal (8%) impact motor vehicle collisions.[4,5] The patient's location in the car correlates with the severity of injury. Occupants on the side of impact have been shown to have greater injury (mean injury severity score, or ISS, is 24) than occupants on the contralateral side (mean ISS, 11).[6]

Physical examination signs that usually herald significant pelvic trauma are listed in Outline 1. Hypotension in the patient suspected of having a pelvic fracture is a critical

Outline 1. Pelvic fracture: Physical findings

Scrotal or labial swelling and ecchymosis

Abnormal position of the lower extremity with excessive internal rotation, external rotation, flexion, adduction, or abduction

Abnormal motion of the pelvis on provocative examination

Painful response to provocative examination

Outline 2. Etiology: Hypovolemic shock

Intrathoracic bleeding
Intraperitoneal bleeding
Retroperitoneal bleeding
Blood loss from open wounds
Bleeding at closed extremity fracture sites

finding. A prolonged low-flow state can aggravate a pulmonary contusion, head and visceral injuries, as well as increase the chances of developing sepsis, adult respiratory distress syndrome (ARDS), and multiple organ failure.[7] A rapid and logical search for the source of the hypotension must be initiated. Decision pathways will be determined based on the ability of the evaluators to associate the hypotension with a pelvic injury. The usual causes of hypovolemia in the trauma patient are listed in Outline 2. The severity of the blood loss can be determined on the initial evaluation by assessing the pulse, blood pressure, and capillary refill (Table 1). A patient can be hypotensive from blood loss associated with one or a combination of many bleeding sites.

Physical examination, chest radiographs, and tube thoracostomy will detect the presence and the severity of intrathoracic blood loss. Physical examination of the abdomen might be remarkable for signs of injury, or absolutely benign in the unresponsive patient. In the hemodynamically unstable patient, the intra-abdominal space must be excluded as a possible bleeding source. Emergent evaluation is provided by a peritoneal aspirate. In hemodynamically normal patients, computed tomography (CT) can be used to assess the peritoneal cavity. If the peritoneal aspiration or lavage is performed in a patient suspected of having a pelvic fracture, the *entry point must be placed supraumbilical to avoid inadvertent puncture of a large hematoma.*

A complete examination of the perineal region must be performed. The examiner is searching for signs of open wounds in the perineum or communication with the vagina or rectum. Evaluation of the bladder and urethra is required because of the high incidence of injury in pelvic fracture patterns. Blood from the urethral meatus suggests an injury. The male rectal examination determines the position and morphology of the prostate. Passage of the coronary catheter should be considered to be part of the physical examination. Inability to freely pass the catheter into the bladder signifies the need for urethrography to establish the continuity of the bladder neck and the urethra.

Lastly, in the alert patient, a neurologic examination of the lumbosacral plexus should be performed to determine the presence of a plexus injury. There is a 50% incidence of plexus injuries in the patients with unstable pelvic fractures or fractures that involve the sacral ala or foramina.[8]

Radiographic Evaluation: Force Vector Analysis

The anteroposterior (AP) radiograph is required in all patients with blunt trauma, unless they are awake, alert, and without pain on examination.[9] The radiograph rapidly identifies the major pelvic injury. In one study, the authors were able to correctly classify the pelvic fracture and identify the dominant force vector based on the portable AP film in 90% of the patients.[10] The classification of the fracture and recognition of the injury "force vector" as AP compression (APC), lateral compression (LC), vertical shear (VS), or combined mechanism injury (CMI) is useful in directing the resuscitation of the trauma patient. A modification of the Pennal classification system is presented in Figure 1 and Table 2.

There is a correlation between the "force vector" and the pattern of organ injury, resuscitative requirements, and mortality.[11] Early recognition of the "force vector" can direct patient care intervention protocols and reduce the mortality associated with the pelvic fracture.[3] In one study, 49% of the patients had LC injuries, 21% had APC injuries, 6% had VS injuries, and 14% had a combined fracture pattern (Table 2).[10] Pelvic classification based on the initial AP radiograph was found to be predictive of the patient population at high risk for massive hemorrhage.[7] Fifty percent to 69% of the patients with unstable pelvic fractures

Table 1. Estimated fluid and blood losses* based on patient's initial presentation†

Parameters	Class I	Class II	Class III	Class IV
Blood loss (ml)	Up to 750	750 to 1,500	1,500 to 2,000	> 2,000
Blood loss (% BV)	Up to 15%	15% to 30%	30% to 40%	> 40%
Pulse rate	< 100	> 100	> 120	> 140
Blood pressure	Normal	Normal	Decreased	Decreased
Pulse Pressure (mm HG)	Normal or increased	Decreased	Decreased	Decreased
Respiratory rate	14 to 20	20 to 30	30 to 40	> 35
Urine output (ml/hr)	> 30	20 to 30	5 to 15	Negligible
CNS/mental status	Slightly anxious	Mildly anxious	Anxious and confused	Confused and lethargic
Fluid replacement (3:1 rule)	Crystalloid	Crystalloid	Crystalloid and blood	Crystalloid and blood

*For a 70–kg male
†The guidelines in Table 1 are based on the "three-for-one" rule. This rule derives from the empiric observation that most patients in hemorrhagic shock require as much as 300 ml of electrolyte solution for each 100 ml of blood loss. Applied blindly, these guidelines can result in excessive or inadequate fluid administration. For example, a patient with a crush injury to the extremity may have hypotension out of proportion to his blood loss and require fluids in excess of the 3:1 guideline. In contrast, a patient whose ongoing blood loss is being replaced requires less than 3:1. The use of bolus therapy with careful monitoring of the patient's response can moderate these extremes.

will require four units or more of blood and 30% to 40% will require 10 units or more.[7]

Inlet and outlet radiographs are often required to supplement the AP film and better define the position and degree of pelvic instability and the severity of the force vector injury. The inlet view provides information on the status of the sacral ala, the displacement of the hemipelvis in the AP plane, and the fracture pattern of the pubic ramus. The outlet view provides the best view of the sacrum and the sacral foramina. This view also detects the presence of superior migration of the injured hemipelvis. Lumbosacral spine films usually should be added to radiographic evaluation in patients with documented pelvic fractures because of the high incidence of associated fractures of the lower lumbar spine. These radiographs are delayed until the patient is satisfactorily resuscitated. In resuscitated patients with acetabular fractures detected on an initial AP pelvic radiograph, Judet views are used to further assess the anterior and posterior columns of the acetabulum and classify the injury pattern.

CT is extremely valuable in the definite evaluation of pelvic ring trauma to define posterior ring instability. In the polytrauma patient, diagnostic services must be efficient in terms of both time and expense. In patients who are stable, scanning of the pelvis should be completed in concert with the required CT of the head, spine, or abdomen. If possible, isolated cuts through the level of the sacroiliac joint should be obtained in unstable patients who are undergoing CT for evaluation of head or abdominal trauma. The limited information from this study can often help direct the early management of the patient, particularly if it can help define the magnitude of the posterior ring injury. A more formal CT of the pelvis can be completed when the patient is stable enough to tolerate the procedure. CT of pelvic injuries in stable patients is nonemergent.

As directed by the patient's hemodynamic stability and the findings of the clinical examination, other radiographic examinations might be required on an emergent or semiemergent basis. The indications for angiography will be discussed later. A retrograde ureterogram is performed in patients with meatal blood or if the passage of a catheter is not possible. A cystogram is performed on patients suspected of urinary tract trauma by history and physical examination or hematuria to determine the presence of intra- or extraperitoneal bladder rupture.

In addition to providing information about pelvic ring stability, the screening AP radiograph also demonstrates dislocation of the hip joint and fractures of the femoral neck or intertrochanteric region.

Patients with pelvic fractures require assessment of the clinical and radiographic findings to determine the "stability" of the pelvic ring, or the tendency to resist displacement of the posterior sacroiliac complex. A significant correlation has been identified between posterior pelvic disruption and patient mortality.[12]

Common radiographic signs of pelvic instability include: (1) displacement of the posterior sacroiliac complex more than 5 mm in any plane; (2) presence of a posterior fracture gap, rather than an impaction; and (3) presence of an avulsion fracture of the transverse process of the fifth lumbar vertebra or the sacral ischial end of the sacrospinous ligaments.

Force Vector Recognition: Clinical Utilization

The ability to recognize the dominant injury force can assist the resuscitation team in anticipating blood/fluid requirements and angiographic intervention and can help direct assessment and treatment[3] (Tables 3 and 4). Patients with complete posterior instability can be anticipated to present with a severe hemorrhage.

A type 3 AP compression fracture in a hemodynamically abnormal patient has a high incidence of circulatory shock (67%), adult respiratory distress syndrome (18.5%), sepsis (59%), and death (37%).[11] In a study of LC injuries, type 1 and type 2 rotational instability injuries had a significant associated brain injury component (50%) as well as an increased incidence of lung, liver, spleen, and bladder injury. The LC 1 and LC 2 patterns had a low incidence of pelvic vascular injury. The LC 3 subgroup had a distinctly different pattern of associated organ injury. Because the mechanism of injury to create the LC 3 fracture pattern is usually a direct crush/rollover of the pelvis, no incidence of brain, lung, liver, or spleen injury was noted. The LC 3 patients, however, had a 20% incidence of bowel injury, a 40% incidence of lower extremity fractures, and a 60% incidence of retroperitoneal hematoma. The vertical shear injuries had a high incidence of brain injury (56.2%), lung injury (23%), splenic injury (25%), and shock (62.5%), and a 25% mortality rate.

There is a significantly higher risk of transsection of the thoracic aorta (8:1) in blunt trauma patients with pelvic fracture compared to blunt trauma patients without pelvic fracture. The majority of the aortic injuries were related to an APC injury vector.[13] It is the pattern of organ injury, especially traumatic brain injury, that is associated with a more severe type of pelvic disruption. The combination of injuries determines the patient's risk of mortality and pattern of complications.[11]

Burgess and associates[3] reviewed the outcomes of 210 pelvic fracture patients. The overall mortality was 8.6%. They noted that 20% of the APC patients and 6.6% of the LC patients died. Of the 14 deaths from the series, the pelvic fracture was thought to be the primary cause of death in only two patients, contributing to the death in ten patients, and related to the death in two patients. The major cause of death in the LC fracture was the closed head injury. The LC nonsurvivors had an average ISS of 54, an average Glasgow Coma Score (GCS) of 4.7, and an average first day blood utilization of 5.8 units. The major cause of death in APC patients was combined pelvic and visceral injury. APC nonsurvivors had an average ISS of 39, a GCS of 10.2, and an average first day blood replacement of 28.4 units.

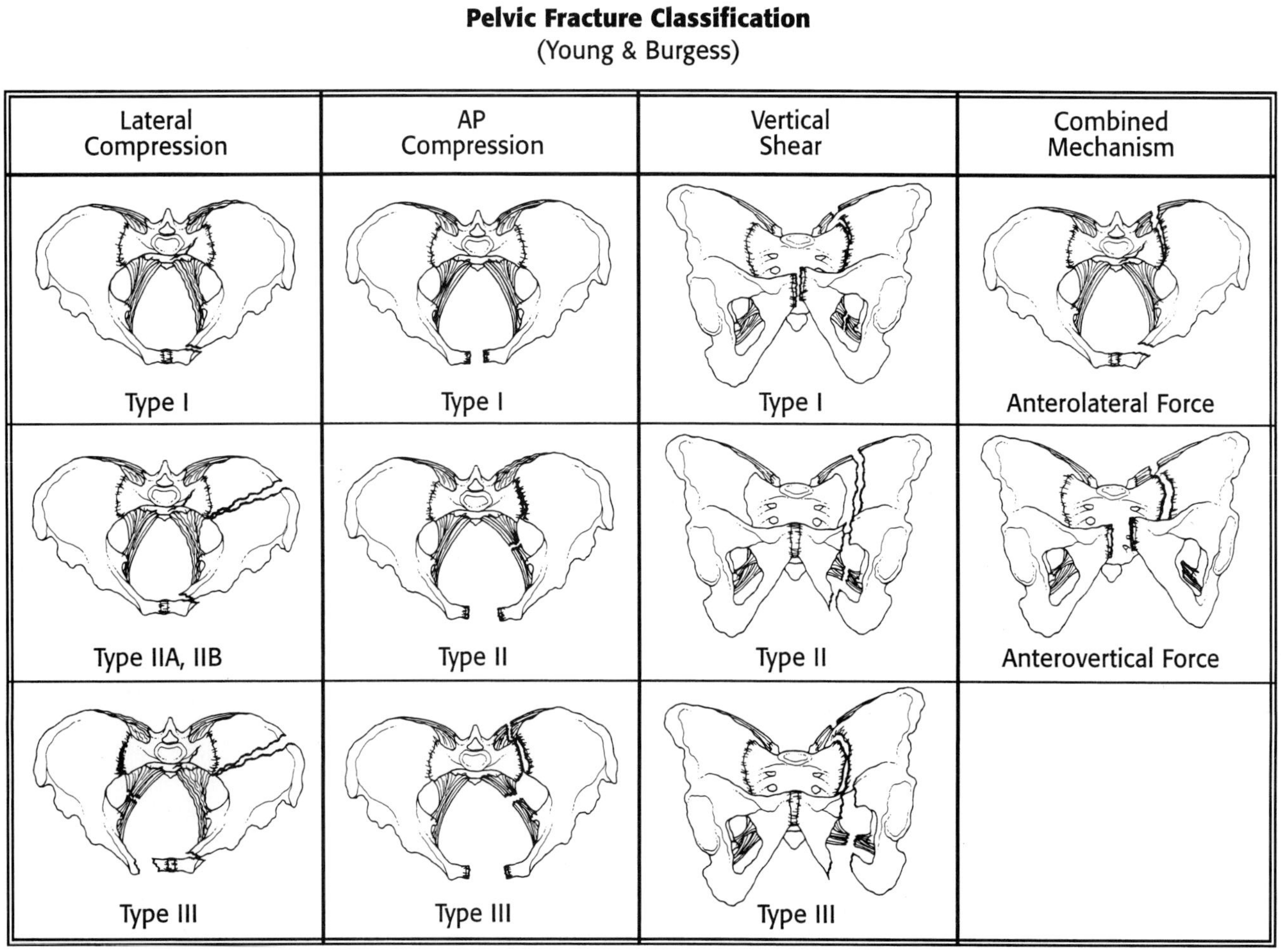

Pelvic Fracture Classification
(Young & Burgess)

Lateral Compression	AP Compression	Vertical Shear	Combined Mechanism
Type I	Type I	Type I	Anterolateral Force
Type IIA, IIB	Type II	Type II	Anterovertical Force
Type III	Type III	Type III	

Fig. 1 Modified Pennal classification system (see Table 2).

Acute Management

The immediate care of the polytrauma patient with a pelvic fracture must address associated retroperitoneal hemorrhage, pelvic ring instability, injuries to the genitourinary system and rectum, as well as fractures open to the perineum. Cessation of blood loss, minimization of septic sequelae, and stabilization of the fracture allowing early, safe patient mobilization are the immediate goals of the treatment team. Hemorrhage is the leading cause of death in the patient with a pelvic fracture, attributing to 60% of the mortality. Most of the blood loss is from the fracture site or injured retroperitoneal veins, only 20% of the deaths are associated with major arterial injury.[14] An average blood replacement of 5.9 units (LC = 3.6, AP = 14.8, VS = 9.2, and CMI = 8.5) has been reported.[3]

The Hemodynamically Abnormal Patient

The patient's admission vital signs (Table 1) indicate the severity of the hemorrhagic state. A 3% mortality was noted in pelvic fracture patients admitted hemodynamically normal compared to a 38% mortality rate for patients admitted hypotensive.[15] Aggressive resuscitation is initiated to obtain an adequate tissue perfusion. The search for the hemorrhagic site evaluates the thoracic cavity, the intraperitoneal cavity, and the retroperitoneal space. *Before assuming that hypotension in a pelvic fracture patient is secondary to the fracture, other bleeding sources must be ruled out.* Knowledge of intraperitoneal pathology is critical in deciding the best management of the unstable patient. As soon as possible after admission, ultrasound or a supraumbilical peritoneal lavage should be performed. Aspiration of 10 to 20 cc of blood confirms significant intraperitoneal injury and emergency exploratory laparotomy should be performed. If the peritoneal aspiration is negative, the trauma team should assume that the cause of the patient's hemodynamic instability *is not from* an intra-abdominal source and bleeding into the retroperitoneal space must be a primary concern. Efforts to identify the retroperitoneal bleeding site and control the blood loss are initiated.

Table 2. Injury classification keys

Category*	Common Characteristic	Differentiating Characteristic
LC 1	Anterior transverse fracture (pubic rami)	Sacral compression on side of impact
LC 2	Anterior transverse fracture (pubic rami)	Crescent (iliac wing) fracture
LC 3	Anterior transverse fracture (pubic rami)	Contralateral open-book (APC) injury
APC 1	Symphyseal diastasis	Slight widening of pubic symphysis and/or SI joint; stretched but intact anterior and posterior ligaments
APC 2	Symphyseal diastasis or anterior vertical fracture	Widened SI joint, disrupted anterior ligaments; intact posterior ligaments
APC 3	Symphyseal diastasis or anterior vertical fracture	Complete hemipelvis separation, but no vertical displacement; complete sacroiliac joint disruption; complete anterior and posterior ligament disruption
VS	Symphyseal diastasis or anterior vertical fracture	Vertical displacement anteriorly and posteriorly, usually through SI joint, occasionally through iliac wing and/or sacrum
CM	Anterior and/or posterior, vertical and/or transverse components	Combination of other injury patterns; LC/VS or LC/APC

* LC, lateral compression; APC, anteroposterior compression; VS, vertical shear; CM, combined mechanism
(Reproduced with permission from Burgess AR, Eastridge BJ, Young JW, et al: Pelvic ring disruptions: Effective classification system and treatment protocols. J Trauma 1990;83:848–856.)

Bleeding due to the pelvic fracture is from three sources: cancellous bone at the fracture sites, retroperitoneal lumbar plexus venous injury, and pelvic arterial injury. The bleeding sources can be considered as low-pressure and high-pressure systems.

In most cases, blood loss from pelvic injury is from a low-pressure source. Major arterial injury has been associated with only 20% of pelvic hemorrhage related deaths.[14] Arterial injury was noted (in order of decreasing frequency) from the superior gluteal, the internal pudendal, the obturator, and the lateral sacral artery. Active bleeding was most commonly found at the internal pudendal artery.[16]

Because of complexity and the acuity of the decision making process in the polytrauma patient, an institutional protocol that outlines the suggested *management guidelines* is useful to direct the treatment team to the evaluation and intervention sequences (Fig. 2).

A hemodynamically abnormal patient with a pelvic fracture and a *positive peritoneal* aspirate or ultrasound is emergently explored to identify and control the intraperitoneal bleeding site. The orthopaedic surgeon *must be present* at the laparotomy to assess the abdominal injury and the size and stability of the retroperitoneal hematoma. Provisional control of an unstable pelvic injury can be obtained prior to laparotomy by application of an external fixator,[3,17] a pelvic clamp,[18] MAST trousers, or a bean bag in the trauma admitting area. The provisional pelvic fixation can be modified or definitive fixation applied at the conclusion of the laparotomy, depending on the patient's response to resuscitation and laparotomy and the dynamics of the retroperitoneal hematoma.

If after addressing the abdominal injury the patient and the retroperitoneal hematoma stabilize, extension of the midline laparotomy incision will allow for plating of a pubic symphysis diastasis, if required. After closure of the abdomen, percutaneous iliosacral screw fixation of a *reduced* posterior pelvic injury can be considered. If the patient's condition prohibits additional operating room time or wound extension, control of the anterior pelvis is obtained with a external fixation frame. Supplemental, ipsilateral femoral traction is added, if necessary, to control cephalad migration in fractures with complete instability.

If the patient has a large or rapidly expanding or pulsatile retroperitoneal hematoma at the initiation of the abdominal exploration, angiographic evaluation is imperative. The intraventional radiologist is emergently called and an angi-

Table 3. Injuries associated with pelvic fractures

Pelvic Fracture Pattern*	Frequency	Average Blood Loss	Shock	Sepsis	Death	ARDS†	Brain Injury	Chest	SPL-LIV†	Bowel	GU†	Retroperitoneal Hematoma
LC												
Type 1	1.5		30	30	13.9	6.3	44	26	7	5	8	5.2
Type 2	6.4		31.8	54.6	13.6	18.2	50	40	8	5	10	13.6
Type 3	33.5 (41.4)	3.6	40	0	0	0	0	0	0	20	0	60
PC												
Type 1	90		30	29	16.1	8	67.7	26	13	5	8	25.8
Type 2	8.7		30	33.3	25	10	33.3	43.4	20/20	10	10	30
Type 3	7.9 (25.7)	14.8	67	59.2	37	18.5	59.3	18.5	20/20	12	0	519.
VS	4.7	9.2	62	41	25	10	56	25	25/10	5	16	47
CM	9.9	8.5	43	31	20	12	50	25	17/5	5	10	20
Acetabular fracture with ring disruptions	18.4		25	20	1.6	8	26.9	26	0	0	0	4.8

* LC, lateral compression; APC, anteroposterior compression; VS, vertical shear; CM, combined mechanism.
† ARDS, Adult respiratory distress syndrome; SPL-LIV, spleen-liver; GU, genitourinary

Table 4. Vascular injuries associated with pelvic fractures

Pelvic Fracture Pattern*	Retroperitoneal Hematoma	Pelvic Vascular Injury
APC		
Type 1	25.8%	6.5%
Type 2	30.0%	10.0%
Type 3	51.9%	22.2%
LC		
Type 1	5.2%	0.0%
Type 2	13.6%	8.0%
Type 3	60.0%	23.0%
VS	48.0%	10.0%
CM	20.0%	10.0%
Acetabular fractures	4.8%	0.0%

* LC, lateral compression; APC, anteroposterior compression; VS, vertical shear; CM, combined mechanism

ography suite is placed on immediate stand-by. At the conclusion of the laparotomy, an external fixator or pelvic resuscitation clamp is applied to the pelvis (if the fracture pattern requires and the frame has not been previously applied in the emergency room) and the patient is transported to the angiography suite. Resuscitation with appropriate blood product continues.

In some cases, laparotomy *decompresses* the abdominal content and allows for rapid expansion of the pelvic hematoma. The pressure rapidly falls and massive fluid volumes are required. Closure of the abdomen is sometimes impossible. If the patient is "in extremis" and cannot be stabilized for transport to the angiography suite, temporary cross clamping of the abdominal aorta must be considered to allow for transport and initiation of the angiography procedure or for immediate exploration and packing of the retroperitoneal space.

Although the practice of exploration of the hematoma and ligation of bleeding sites and packing of the retroperitoneal space has been largely abandoned in the United States, reports indicate that a growing series of hemorrhagic patients have been successfully controlled with this technique.[10,19] The injury is approached in a manner similar to the management of a massive liver injury. The retroperitoneal space is opened and the hematoma is evacuated. Accessible bleeding sites are ligated. The space is packed and closed and packings are changed every 2 to 3 days.

After the patient's pelvic bleeding is controlled and the hemipelvis is stabilized, intensive care monitoring, pulmonary and vascular support, and normalization of coagulation parameters are the major elements needed for patient survival.

Control of Retroperitoneal Bleeding: Modality Overview

The control of retroperitoneal hemorrhage has focused on three interventions: (1) decreasing blood loss from the fracture sites and lacerated soft tissue by stabilizing the fracture and the forming hematoma, (2) limiting of low-pressure bleeding by normalization of the pelvic volume and evoking a retroperitoneal tamponade effect, and (3) localizing and controlling arterial bleeding sites via therapeutic angiography or surgical exploration.

External Fixation

Although it has not been validated by prospective randomized trials, many clinical series have advocated the use of immediate external fixation to stabilize the pelvis, reduce the pelvic volume, and initiate a retroperitoneal tamponade effect.[20,21] One author reported that the external fixator was more successful in controlling hemorrhage than the MAST trousers (95% vs 71%) and noted that blood replacement was reduced from 7.4 to 3.7 units with application of the fixator.[22] Another author noted a decrease in the mortality rate (from 41% to 21%) in patients with pelvic fracture who were admitted with a systolic blood pressure < 100 mm Hg after initiation of an early external fixation protocol.[17] In one study at the Maryland Shock Trauma Center, the author reported a 28% incidence in the use of external fixation.[3] The recent development of "resuscitation clamps" allows for potentially rapid and effective stabilization of the pelvic fracture in the emergency room.[18,23]

Noninvasive external fixation is used in the emergency room in some centers. Deflatable, deforming bean bags are placed under the patient and conformed around the pelvis as it is manually reduced. The bags are deflated and the provisional cast mold helps maintain reduction and limit pelvic motion. The pneumatic antishock garment (PASG) has application in the treatment of pelvic injuries. It can be utilized as a field stabilization and transport device as a method of "tamponade" for patients with persistent hypotension, pending the availability of an operating suite or angiography.

Therapeutic Angiography

Continued, unexplained blood loss, despite fracture stabilization and aggressive resuscitation, mandates angiographic exploration. In one study, 8% of the 162 patients reviewed by the authors required angiography. Embolization was needed in 20% of APC and VS injuries and CMIs, but in only 1.7% of LC injuries.[3] In a series of 63 patients referred for angiography, the authors reported 123 arterial injuries in 49 patients.[16] Angiography successfully stopped arterial bleeding in 86% of patients in another study.[24] One author advocates "preemptive embolization," stressing that if an artery is found at angiography to be transected, it should be embolized to avoid the risk of delayed hemorrhage than can occur with clot lysis.[25]

Unstable Pelvic Fractures: Hemodynamically Normal

For reasons that are still unclear, early fixation and mobilization of polytrauma patients with major injuries positively

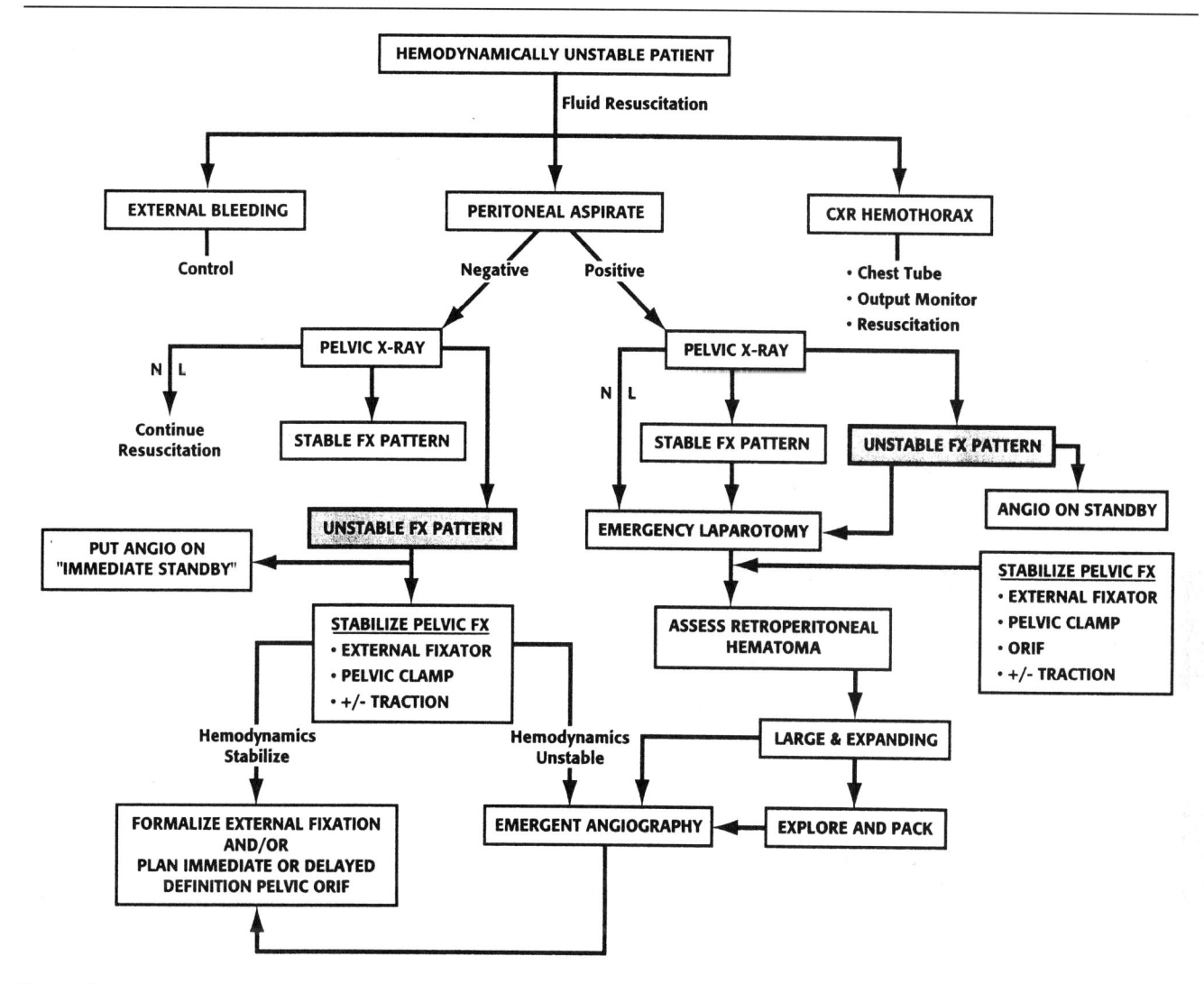

Fig. 2 Suggested management guidelines in the hemodynamically unstable patient.

affects the outcome of the patient. Improved outcomes in patients with unstable pelvic fractures treated by early stabilization have been reported.[17,26] Utilizing early external fixation of the pelvis, one author reported a significant decrease in the mortality rate (from 26% to 6%) among patients with pelvic fracture with initiation of an early fixation and mobilization protocol. The mortality rate for patients with pelvic fracture and closed head injuries fell from 43% to 7% with the use of early external fixation.[17]

A large number of patients, however, will have unstable pelvic fracture patterns and no associated injuries. They do not require monitoring in the intensive care unit. In this patient group, bed rest and traction on the ipsilateral femur (if required by the fracture pattern) can be utilized until the patient is available for an elective reduction and stabilization of the pelvis.

Open Pelvic Fractures

Isolated iliac wing fracture and a soft-tissue wound are managed like open fractures in other regions of the body. Major pelvic injuries that communicate with the rectum, colon, vagina, perineum, or gluteal regions present a more complex treatment challenge. The surgeon must recognize the significance of the open fractures and individualize management of the pelvis to address the problems of fracture stability, bleeding, and wound sepsis.

Early diverting colostomy is recommended for pelvic fractures that communicate with the colon, rectum, or perineum. Aggressive wound exploration and debridement, local packing to control hemorrhage, use of angiography, and external fixation have significantly decreased the morbidity and mortality for this injury complex. Richardson reports a 94.5% survival rate in 37 patients.[27]

Early detection and repair of vaginal laceration can minimize subsequent formation of a pelvic abscess. Four of 110 females with pelvic fracture had associated vaginal lacerations. A 72-hour delay in diagnosis occurred in one patient who developed an extensive associated pelvic abscess. Detection, irrigation, debridement, and surgical repair of the injury are recommended.[28]

Prophylaxis for Deep Vein Thrombosis

Patients with major pelvic injuries are at high risk for deep vein thrombosis. Pulmonary embolism rate in pelvic fracture patients has been reported to be 2%, compared to a 0.2% rate in polytrauma patients without pelvic fractures.[29] A graded prophylaxis protocol for deep vein thrombosis should be established for patients with these injuries. Vena caval filters should be considered in patients who cannot receive coagulation altering medications.

Interinstitutional Transfers

Successful management of patients with major pelvic and acetabular injuries often requires that the initial resuscitation team recognize the unique requirements of the patient and rapidly transfer the patient to a level 1 trauma facility capable of addressing the specific needs. A skilled interventional radiology team is required to treat hemodynamically abnormal pelvic fracture patients. The patient should be en route to a capable center *as soon as* the magnitude of the pelvic injury is recognized. Likewise, if a patient requires an emergent procedure for an acetabular fracture, a transfer of the patient to a facility staffed with a pelvic reconstruction team should be considered if expertise is not available at the initial admitting facility.

Annotated References

1. Poole GV, Ward EF: Causes of mortality in patients with pelvic fractures. *Orthopedics* 1994;17:691–696.

2. Fox MA, Mangiante EC, Fabian TC, et al: Pelvic fractures: An analysis of factors affecting pre-hospital triage and patient outcome. *South Med J* 1990;83:785–788.

3. Burgess AR, Eastridge BJ, Young JW, et al: Pelvic ring disruptions: Effective classification system and treatment protocols. *J Trauma* 1990;30:848–856.

    In a review of 210 consecutive pelvic fractures admitted to the Baltimore Shock Trauma Center over a 3-year period, the authors noted that 68% were related to motor vehicle or motorcycle accidents. Fifteen percent of the patients were admitted in shock. The Injury Severity Score (ISS) averaged 25.8 and the Glasgow Coma Score (GCS) averaged 13.2. Sixty-six percent of the patients had closed head injuries, 25% had major chest injuries, and 20% had injuries to the spleen, liver, or bowel. The argument is presented that pelvic fractures result from predictable force vectors. These forces affect other systems and the recognition of the injury force vector can direct resuscitation and care of the trauma patient. LC injuries averaged 3.6 units of PRBCs; APCs, 14.8 units; VSI, 9.2 units; and combined mechanism, 8.5 units. The overall mortality rate was 8.6%; injuries were as follows, LC = 7%, APC = 20%, VS = 0%, CM = 18%.

4. Gokcen EC, Burgess AR, Siegel JH, et al: Pelvic fracture mechanism of injury in vehicular trauma patients. *J Trauma* 1994;36:789–796.

5. Pattimore D, Thomas P, Dave SH: Torso injury patterns and mechanisms in car crashes: An additional diagnostic tool. *Injury* 1992;23:123–126.

6. McCoy GF, Johnstone RA, Kenwright J: Biomechanical aspects of pelvic and hip injuries in road traffic accidents. *J Orthop Trauma* 1989;3:118–123.

7. Cryer HM, Miller FB, Evers BM, et al: Pelvic fracture classification: Correlation with hemorrhage. *J Trauma* 1988;28:973–980.

8. Helfet DL, Koval KJ, Hissa EA, et al: Intraoperative somatosensory evoked potential monitoring during acute pelvic fracture surgery. *J Orthop Trauma* 1995;9:28–34.

9. Civil ID, Ross SE, Botehlo G, et al: Routine pelvic radiography in severe blunt trauma: Is it necessary? *Ann Emerg Med* 1988;17:488–490.

10. Young JWR, Burgess AR (eds): *Radiologic Management of Pelvic Ring Fractures: Systematic Radiographic Diagnosis.* Baltimore, MD, Urban & Schwarzenberg, 1987.

11. Dalal SA, Burgess AR, Siegel JH, et al: Pelvic fracture in multiple trauma: Classification by mechanism is key to pattern of organ injury, resuscitative requirements, and outcome. *J Trauma* 1989;29:981–1002.

    The 343 patients reported had a high incidence of multiple organ injuries and extremity injuries, and a 44.9% incidence of brain injury. Of the patients in the study, 39.1% were classified as having severe pelvic fractures (APC 2 and 3, LC 2 and 3, VS, and CMI). The overall incidence of shock was 35% and there was a 30% sepsis rate. Adult respiratory distress syndrome occurred in 8.2% of the cases. The overall mortality rate was low (15.5%) and was distributed to AP injuries (26.1%), LC injuries (13.4%), VS injuries (25%) and combined mechanism injuries (CMI) (17.7%). Anteroposterior injury deaths were related to blood loss from pelvic vascular and visceral injuries. LC injury deaths were related to brain injury. A detailed analysis of the associated injury patterns and resuscitation requirements of polytrauma patients with pelvic fractures is provided. The fractures are classified by the vector pattern (LC, APC, VS, and CM). LC mortalities were associated with brain injury and shock, while APC injury mortalities were associated with shocks, sepsis, and ARDS.

12. McMurtry R, Walton D, Dickinson D, et al: Pelvic disruption in the polytraumatized patient: A management protocol. *Clin Orthop* 1980;151:22–30.
13. Ochsner MG Jr, Hoffman AP, DiPasquale D, et al: Associated aortic rupture-pelvic fracture: An alert for orthopedic and general surgeons. *J Trauma* 1992;33:429–434.
14. Brown JJ, Greene FL, McMillin RD: Vascular injuries associated with pelvic fractures. *Am Surg* 1984;50:150–154.
15. Naam NH, Brown WH, Hurd R, et al: Major pelvic fractures. *Arch Surg* 1983;118:610–616.
16. Kam J, Jackson H, Ben-Menachem Y: Vascular injuries in blunt pelvic trauma. *Radiol Clin North Am* 1981;19:171–186.
17. Riemer BL, Butterfield SL, Diamond DL, et al: Acute mortality associated with injuries to the pelvic ring: The role of early patient mobilization and external fixation. *J Trauma* 1993;35:671–677.

   The effect on mortality is reviewed after initiation of an external fixation/early mobilization protocol for pelvic fracture patients. Mortality rates were decreased from 26% to 6% overall. The mortality rate for hypotensive patients dropped from 41% to 21% and the rate for patients with associated closed head injuries fell from 43% to 7%.

18. Ganz R, Krushell RJ, Jakob RP, et al: The antishock pelvic clamp. *Clin Orthop* 1991;267:71–78.
19. Pohlemann T, Gänsslen A, Bosch U, et al: The technique of packing for control of hemorrhage in complex pelvic fractures. *Tech Orthop* 1994;9:267–270.

   The rationale and techniques for direct (ligation) or indirect (packing) surgical control of retroperitoneal hemorrhage is presented in detail.

20. Edwards CC, Meier PJ, Browner BD, et al: Results treating 50 unstable pelvic injuries using primary external fixation. *Orthop Trans* 1985;9:434.
21. Gylling SF, Ward RE, Holcroft JW, et al: Immediate external fixation of unstable pelvic fractures. *Am J Surg* 1985;150:721–724.
22. Moreno C, Moore EE, Rosenberger A, et al: Hemorrhage associated with major pelvic fracture: A multispecialty challenge. *J Trauma* 1986;26:987–994.
23. Buckle R, Browner BD, Morandi M: Emergency reduction for pelvic ring disruptions and control of associated hemorrhage using the pelvic stabilizer. *Tech Orthop* 1994;9:258-266.
24. Mucha P Jr, Farnell MB: Analysis of pelvic fracture management. *J Trauma* 1984; 24:379–386.
25. Ben-Menachem Y, Coldwell DM, Young JW, et al: Hemorrhage associated with pelvic fractures: Causes, diagnosis and emergent management. *Am J Rad* 1991;157:1005–1014.

    The diagnosis and angiographic management techniques for the control of hemorrhage associated with pelvic fractures is presented in detail. The authors emphasize preemptive embolization of occluded pelvic vessels to prevent delayed hemorrhage associated with lysis of the clot.

26. Latenser BA, Gentilello LM, Tarver AA, et al: Improved outcome with early fixation of skeletally unstable pelvic fractures. *J Trauma* 1991;31:28–31.
27. Richardson JD, Harty J, Amin M, et al: Open pelvic fractures. *J Trauma* 1982;22:533-538.
28. Niemi TA, Norton LW: Vaginal injuries in patients with pelvic fractures. *J Trauma* 1985;25:547–551.
29. Buerger PM, Peoples JB, Lemmon GW, et al: Risk of pulmonary emboli in patients with pelvic fractures. *Am Surg* 1993;59:505–508.

22
Acute Care and Evaluation of Acetabular Fractures

Acute Management

Clinical Evaluation

Most acetabular fractures are the result of high-energy blunt trauma. Significant life-threatening injury may accompany acetabular fractures. Initial resuscitation of the patient with pelvic and acetabular fractures may involve fluid resuscitation, angiography, massive transfusion protocols, and various forms of internal fixation or skeletal/roller-type traction. External fixation has no role in the management of acetabular fractures. Emergent injuries must be stabilized prior to acetabular fracture surgery. In the hemodynamically unstable patient, laparotomy or angiography may be needed to control bleeding. Angiography is particularly useful in stopping bleeding from lacerations of the superior gluteal artery from fractures that extend into the sciatic notch. Open pelvic and acetabular fractures are associated with a high mortality and need prompt evaluation and stabilization.[1] The most frequently associated musculoskeletal injury is fracture of a long bone.[2,3] Once the patient has been fully resuscitated, the acetabular fracture can be further assessed.

The screening anteroposterior (AP) pelvic radiograph usually defines the magnitude of the acetabular injury. Judet views and computed tomographic (CT) scans assist with the final classification of the fracture, with the decision supporting surgical or conservative management, and with the preferred surgical exposure should internal fixation be required. The fractures described in this chapter demand a particularly thorough physical examination and radiographic evaluation to optimize results, to more accurately assess the outcome for an individual fracture, and to avoid the preventable complications that can occur with these fracture types.

Damage to the sciatic nerve can occur by direct compression with posterior wall fractures and associated posterior hip dislocations, and by entrapment of the nerve in the fracture site with posterior column and transverse fractures that occur near the greater sciatic notch.[4] Patients with preoperative nerve injuries are more likely to have measurable intraoperative changes on somatosensory-evoked potential nerve monitoring than patients with no nerve damage.[5] More important, severe involvement of the peroneal component of the sciatic nerve correlates closely with poor functional recovery. A thorough preoperative assessment will help avoid confusion in cases in which a nerve palsy is noted postoperatively.

If the femoral head is dislocated, reduction should be attempted as soon as possible. Anesthesia is required in some cases. After successful reduction, the ipsilateral femur is placed in traction, if the reduction is unstable, and surgical reconstruction of the acetabulum, if required, is sequenced into the care of associated conditions.

Except for patients with open injuries or irreducible hip dislocations, surgical treatment of the acetabular fracture is nonemergent. Acetabular fracture-dislocations are orthopaedic emergencies as the rate of osteonecrosis increases significantly if reduction is not accomplished within 6 to 12 hours after injury. Open fractures require debridement and, if possible, open reduction and internal fixation (ORIF) on the initial visit to the operating room. Irreducible hip dislocations require surgical relocation and ORIF of unstable acetabular components to maintain the reduction. The presence of intra-articular loose bodies is an indication for elective as opposed to emergency management of irreducible hip dislocations.

Local soft-tissue injuries need to be evaluated carefully. These include lacerations, abrasions, and degloving injuries (Morel-Lavale lesions), which may increase infection rates and may lead to a change in the surgical approach. In the absence of other associated injuries and with minimal local soft-tissue injury, the incidence of infection is between 3% and 6% in most large series. However, most patients with acetabular fractures do have other associated injuries or local soft-tissue injury. The risk of infection is increased by associated urologic and gastrointestinal injuries, and the presence of suprapubic catheters and colostomies may necessitate changing the planned surgical approach.[2] Similarly, open wounds, obesity, and open fractures of the ipsilateral extremity may increase the incidence of wound infection. Use of a prior incision such as the entry site for femoral rodding jeopardizes the posterior approach to the hip. Perioperative intravenous antibiotics, adequate debridement of nonviable tissue at the time of surgery, and

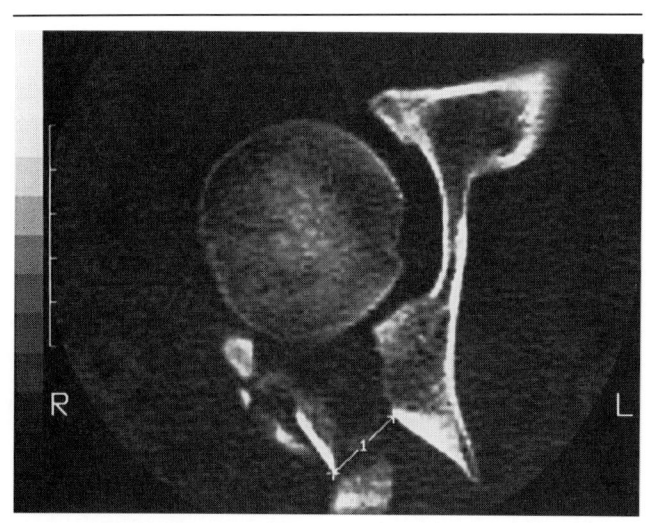

Fig. 1 Marginal impaction of the posterior wall.

careful surgical techniques should be employed to help decrease the incidence of infection. If deep infection does occur, early surgical debridement is required. Management of these difficult injuries requires a standardized institutional protocol that is constantly modified to provide optimal care for the patient.[2]

Heterotopic ossification is a common complication associated with posterior or extended acetabular approaches. Indomethacin has been effective in reducing the incidence of this complication. Low-dose irradiation has also been effective in preventing heterotopic ossification.[6–9]

Patients who are at high risk for deep vein thrombosis should be placed on some type of prophylaxis. This can include pneumatic compression stockings, aspirin, or other anticoagulants. A Greenfield filter may be indicated if bleeding is a concern.[10]

Radiographic Evaluation

Acetabular fractures are best assessed by studying the AP and the 45° oblique Judet views. These standard AP and 45° iliac and obturator oblique views recommended by

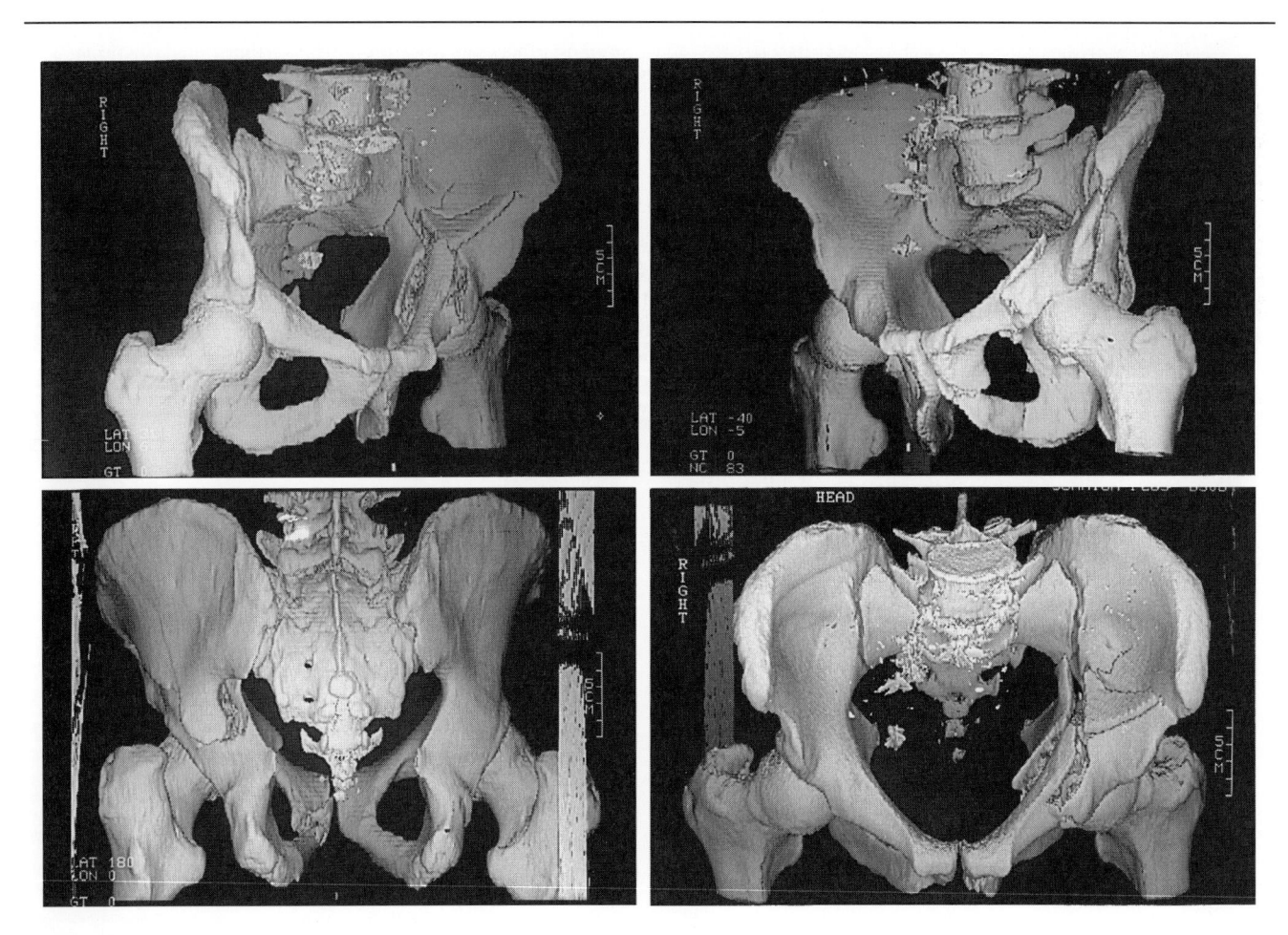

Fig. 2 Three-dimensional reconstruction of a both-column acetabular fracture.

Letournel and Judet remain the essential radiographic evaluation, even with the availability of newer imaging techniques. Careful preoperative evaluation of these three views is essential to avoid mistakes in the diagnosis and surgical approach. The two-dimensional CT scan allows definition of fracture lines, evaluation of intra-articular loose bodies, concentric reduction, definition of marginal impaction, evaluation of medial displacement, identification of femoral head impaction or fracture, and estimation of the size of the posterior wall fragment. The CT scan is excellent for evaluation of sacral fractures, sacroiliac joint dislocations, and difficult acetabular-pelvic fracture patterns (Fig. 1). Newer three-dimensional CT scans are useful in the evaluation of late reconstructions that require osteotomy for surgical correction of acetabular nonunion or malunion (Fig. 2). The fracture can be rotated and visualized on the screen for preoperative planning. Newer software techniques allow subtraction of the femoral head.

Judet and Letournel[11,12] developed a two-column concept of the acetabulum based on an inverted Y. The ilioischial component represents the posterior column and the iliopectineal component represents the anterior column (Fig. 3). Letournel's radiographic analysis provides identification of anterior column, posterior column, and composite landmarks. Evaluation of these landmarks on the AP and 45° iliac and obturator oblique views best determines the extent of bony injury.

The AP view demonstrates best the six fundamental radiographic landmarks (Fig. 4). The AP view should be examined for disruption of the standard radiographic lines of the pelvis and acetabulum. Successful preoperative planning involves drawing the lines of the pelvis on tracing paper placed over x-ray film. Examination of the AP view with sufficient clinical experience should lead to the proper fracture classification in the majority of cases. Disruption of the posterior rim indicates a posterior wall fracture. Disruption of the ilioischial line and posterior rim indicates a posterior column or associated posterior column/wall combination fracture. Disruption of the iliopectineal line and anterior rim indicates an anterior column or anterior wall fracture. If the iliopectineal line, ilioischial line, and anterior and posterior rims are disrupted together, a portion of the roof remains attached to the ilium, and if the obturator foramen is intact, the diagnosis is a transverse fracture or an associated transverse plus posterior wall fracture. The presence of a fracture through the obturator foramen distinguishes the transverse T fracture. Involvement of all of the radiographic landmarks of the acetabulum, as well as a fracture that separates the roof from the iliac wing or sacroiliac joint as well as a fracture of the obturator foramen, describes a both-column fracture.

The iliac oblique view best shows the posterior column and anterior wall. This view shows the anterior border of the iliac wing and crest, the iliac wing, the quadrilateral surface of the ischium, and the posterior border of the innominate bone (Fig. 5). The obturator oblique view best shows the anterior column and posterior wall. This view projects a radiographic image above the center of the cotyloid fossae and shows the opening of the obturator foramen maximally. Several features are identified: the true pelvic brim or the iliopectineal line, the anterior aspect of the obturator ring, the posterior border of the acetabulum, and the obturator foramen (Fig. 6).

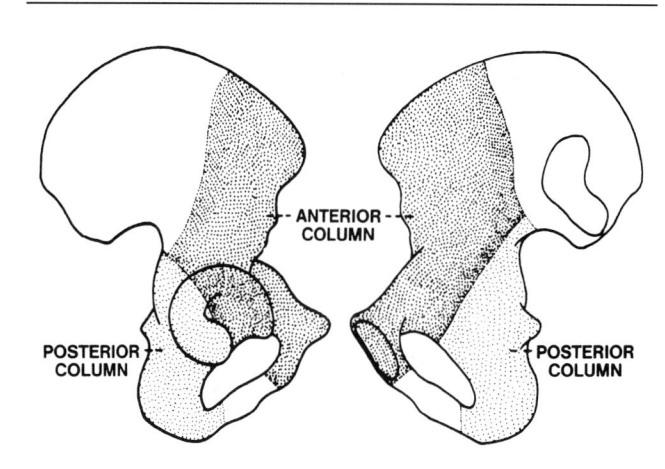

Fig. 3 Letournel's column concept for acetabular fracture classification. (Reproduced with permission from Mayo KA: Fractures of the acetabulum. *Orthop Clin North Am* 1987;18:43–57.)

Acetabular Fracture Classification

The Judet-Letournel classification was the first to integrate pelvic anatomy and fracture biomechanics into useful clinical material that allows the surgeon to correctly approach these difficult fractures. Acetabular surgery requires a comprehensive understanding of the three-dimensional anatomy of the hemipelvis and the radiographic landmarks of the normal and fractured hemipelvis to accurately classify fractures of the acetabulum. Judet and Letournel identified two major fracture categories: simple and complex fractures. The five simple fracture types encompass single fractures of the respective walls and columns and an additional solitary transverse pattern. All or part of one column is involved, as in a posterior wall, posterior column, anterior wall, anterior column, or transverse fracture. Transverse fractures, although involving both columns, have a portion of the superior weightbearing dome attached to the iliac wing and therefore have a better prognosis than the more complex both-column fracture, in which the entire weightbearing dome is separated from the iliac wing or sacroiliac joint (Fig. 7).

The five complex or associated types of fracture combine at least two of the simple forms. These have been divided into five principal fracture types: T-type fracture, fractures of the posterior column and wall, transverse and posterior wall fractures, fractures of the anterior column and wall associated with hemitransverse fractures posteriorly, and complete both-column fractures (Fig. 8). These fractures

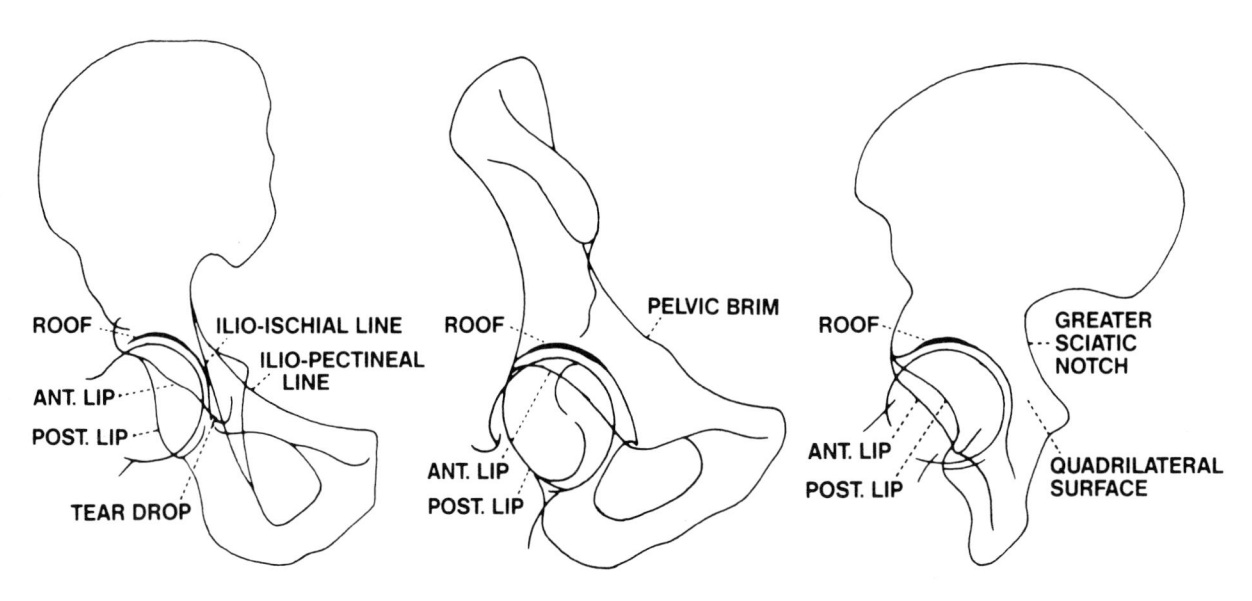

Fig. 4 **Left,** Anteroposterior radiographic landmarks. **Center,** Obturator oblique radiographic landmarks. **Right,** Iliac oblique radiographic landmarks. (Reproduced with permission from Mayo KA: Fractures of the acetabulum. *Orthop Clin North Am* 1987;18:43–57.)

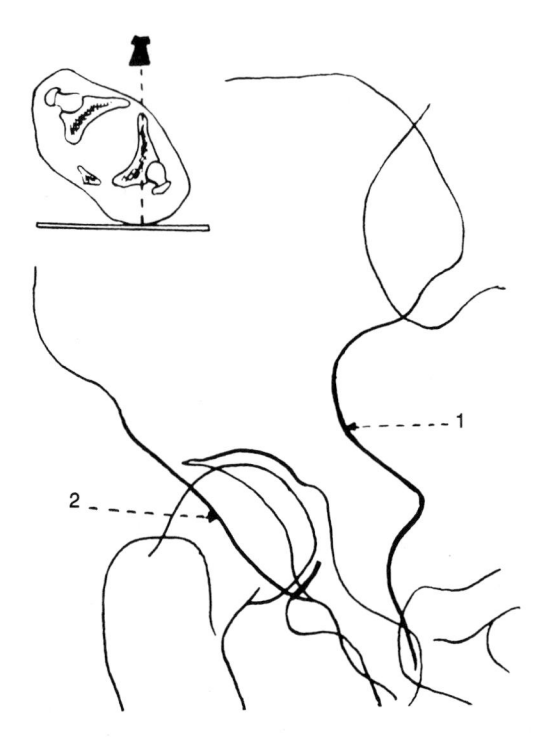

Fig. 5 Iliac oblique view: best visualized landmarks. **1,** Posterior column. **2,** Anterior wall. (Reproduced with permission from Judet R, Judet J, Letournel E: Fractures of the acetabulum: Classification and surgical approaches for open reduction. Preliminary report. *J Bone Joint Surg* 1964;46A:1615–1646.)

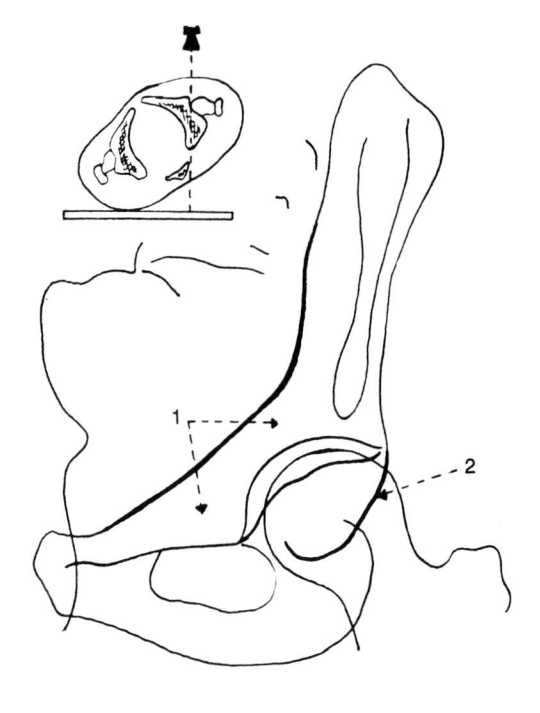

Fig. 6 Obturator oblique view: best visualized landmarks. **1,** Anterior wall. **2,** Posterior column. (Reproduced with permission from Judet R, Judet J, Letournel E: Fractures of the acetabulum: Classification and surgical approaches for open reduction. Preliminary report. *J Bone Joint Surg* 1964;46A:1615–1646.)

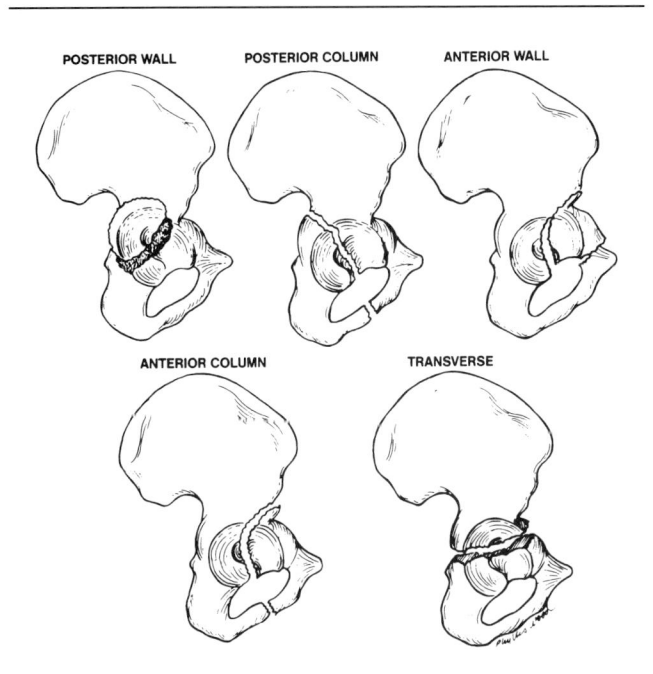

Fig. 7 Simple acetabular fracture types. (Reproduced with permission from Mayo KA: Fractures of the acetabulum. *Orthop Clin North Am* 1987;18:43–57.)

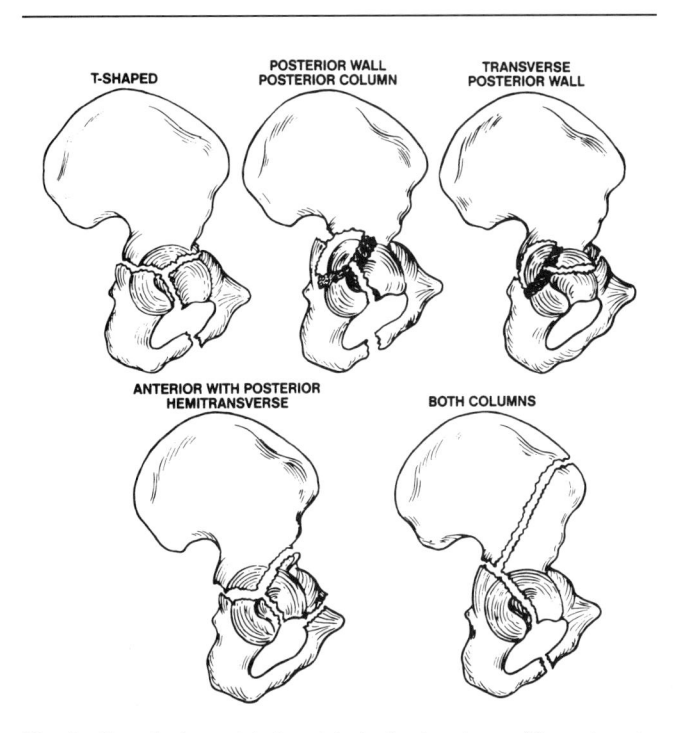

Fig. 8 Complex/associated acetabular fracture types. (Reproduced with permission from Mayo KA: Fractures of the acetabulum. *Orthop Clin North Am* 1987;18:43–57.)

are more complex and have a poorer prognosis because of the difficulty in restoring both columns separately.

Simple Acetabular Fractures

Posterior Wall Fractures Posterior wall fractures can occur at any level of the posterior column. Posterior wall fractures are perceived as being a rather straightforward fracture pattern that is easy to treat. Significant problems can be associated with these fracture patterns, however. Biomechanical studies have addressed many of these problems.[13] Major problems include marginal impaction, abrasions of the femoral head, and inability to reduce the femoral head in a fracture-dislocation in an appropriate time period.

Five of six fundamental radiographic landmarks remain intact in the radiographic evaluation of the posterior wall fracture: the roof, pelvic rim, ilioischial line, teardrop, and anterior border of the acetabulum. Only the posterior border, seen best on the obturator oblique view, is disrupted. The CT scan is helpful for evaluation of marginal impaction of the posterior wall fragments, evaluation of joint concentricity, and estimation of the size of the posterior wall fragment.

Posterior Column Fractures The posterior column fracture is characterized by complete detachment of the posterior column. The fracture pattern usually originates superiorly at the greater sciatic notch, extends inferiorly through the roof or weightbearing dome, and exits through the obturator ring.

The radiographic characteristic in the AP view is medial displacement of the femoral head, driving the quadrilateral surface and the sciatic buttress into the true pelvis. The ilioischial line is clearly disrupted, and the roof of the acetabulum usually maintains its normal position. The iliac oblique view shows the internal and superior boundaries of the displaced fragment and the normal anterior border of the acetabulum. The obturator oblique view shows the intact iliopectineal line and the anterior column structures.

Anterior Wall Fractures The anterior wall fracture crosses the articular surface, detaching the anterior wall at the anteroinferior spine, passing inferiorly through the cotyloid fossa, and usually exiting at the junction of the articular dome and the superior ramus interface. The roof segment is usually minimally involved.

Radiographs show a fracture through the iliopectineal line that is best seen in the obturator oblique view. This view also demonstrates the degree of involvement of the superior weightbearing dome. The iliac oblique view is normal.

Anterior Column Fractures The anterior column fracture is characterized by a large anterior segment separated by a fracture line extending from the middle of the pubic ramus inferiorly to any point above the anterior segment of the iliac crest.

The AP radiograph shows the principal landmarks of the posterior column, with the ilioischial line completely intact. The iliopectineal line, the principal anterior column landmark, which is best seen in the obturator oblique view, is always disrupted. The iliac oblique view reveals the intact posterior elements. The CT scan shows displacement of the anterior column and is useful in preoperative evaluation in determining the involvement of the roof segment.

Transverse Fractures The pure transverse fracture must be separated from the more complex both-column fracture. Both fractures involve the anterior and posterior columns. In a transverse fracture the fracture line extends transversely from the anterior to posterior column. The entire roof arc or weightbearing dome portion remains attached to the ilium or sacroiliac joint, as opposed to a both-column fracture.

The transverse fracture is further subdivided according to the levels at which these fractures occur. Transtectal fractures pass through the weightbearing dome or roof segment and are the most superior fracture pattern. Juxtatectal fractures divide the anterior and posterior columns just superior to the cotyloid fossa, leaving a large portion of the roof segment intact. Infratectal fracture patterns transect the anterior and posterior columns well below the weightbearing dome.

The radiographic characteristics reveal disruption of all vertical lines. The obturator ring, best seen in the obturator oblique view, is intact, which distinguishes this simple pattern from the more complex T-type fracture pattern. The iliac oblique view best shows the transverse fracture fragment and level through the posterior column. There is incongruity of the femoral head in relation to the intact roof segment. In all views, a section of the roof remains intact with the iliac wing, which distinguishes this simple pattern from the complex both-column acetabular fracture pattern. The CT scan is valuable in distinguishing between transverse and T-type fractures and can aid in determining the type of surgical approach.

Complex Acetabular Fractures

T-Type Acetabular Fracture The T-type acetabular fracture is a transverse fracture with a vertical fracture component splitting the cotyloid fossa, thereby rendering the posterior column a free fragment. All landmarks are disrupted, as seen in the transverse fracture. The radiographic key to identifying this fracture pattern is the vertical stem component. The vertical fracture component must be sought on the Judet views. The iliac oblique view shows fracture components that would reveal associated both-column injury.

Associated Posterior Column and Posterior Wall Fracture The fracture line of the posterior column extends from the sciatic notch through the cotyloid fossa, and the fracture extends into the obturator ring. The AP view shows the intact iliopectineal line, with disruption of the ilioischial line and central displacement of the femoral head. The obturator oblique view shows a fracture in the ischium or obturator ring and projects the displaced posterior wall fragment into the soft tissues. The iliac oblique view shows the integrity of the anterior column with the fracture line extending along the quadrilateral surface. Often the posterior column fracture is nondisplaced and the posterior wall fracture is the major fracture component.

Associated Transverse Plus Posterior Wall Fracture The transverse component of this associated injury resembles that previously described, yet the posterior wall fragment rarely reduces when the head is repositioned under the acetabular roof. The associated posterior wall fracture can be juxtatectal or infratectal, depending on the direction of the deforming force. There can be great variation in the extent of the posterior wall fragment. Variants exist that may make differentiation from transverse T types difficult.

The radiographic characteristics of this pattern are essentially a combination of the two distinct patterns previously described. On the AP view, there is typically a posterior fracture-dislocation of the hip, with all vertical landmarks disrupted. The iliopectineal line and ilioischial line are transversely separated. The iliac oblique view shows an intact iliac wing and a well-defined fracture of the quadrilateral surface. The obturator oblique view shows the posterior wall deficiency, posterior displacement, and level of the transverse fracture segment.

Associated transverse plus posterior wall fractures include the rotational component seen with the transverse fracture pattern. The obturator foraminal segment can rotate around a vertical axis passing through the symphysis pubis in addition to the horizontal axis forces. The inferior segments of this pattern may protrude inward by the force of the femoral head. The CT scan is of little value in classification or treatment of this fracture pattern.

Associated Anterior Wall or Column Fracture plus Posterior Hemitransverse Fracture This unusual pattern has the same characteristics as the anterior wall or column pattern in the isolated injury. The fracture line routinely detaches from the anterior wall at the anteroinferior spine and passes inferiorly through the cotyloid fossa, usually exiting at the junction of the superior ramus. The posterior hemitransverse component is a pure transverse fracture of the posterior column only. Generally, this is a nondisplaced fracture that is located in the lower half of the posterior column. The size of the anterior component varies with the mechanism of injury. Unlike the associated both-column fracture there is always an intact articulated fragment that remains attached to the iliac wing. The posterior column usually remains intact to the obturator ring.

Radiographically, the AP view demonstrates a nondisplaced fracture of the posterior column. The iliopectineal line is always displaced with this fracture pattern. The iliac oblique view demonstrates a fracture through the quadrilateral surface. The obturator oblique view depicts the size of the anterior wall or column. The CT scan is of little value in this fracture pattern but may help to distinguish it from a transverse T or associated both-column pattern.

Associated Both-Column Fractures The associated both-column acetabular fracture pattern involves both the anterior and posterior columns which actually separate from one another. This complex fracture pattern is distinguished from all other classification types in that no articular surface remains intact from the remainder of the iliac wing or sacroiliac joint. The principal posterior column fragment has a fracture line that characteristically begins at the greater sciatic notch and exits inferiorly. Secondary fracture lines may be transmitted anywhere in the retroacetabular surface. Anterior column involvement includes the iliac wing and anterior wall comminution. The obturator ring frequently is disrupted in several places.

Central dislocation of the femoral head is usually seen on the AP view, with the acetabular roof or dome segment demonstrating severe comminution. Malrotation frequently obliterates the ilioischial line, but obvious iliac wing fractures exist on the iliac oblique view with severe comminution of the anterior wall or column. The iliac oblique view also demonstrates the loss of all articular relationships of the acetabulum to the iliac wing. The classic radiographic hallmark of an associated both-column fracture is the spur sign. This characteristic obturator oblique view finding distinguishes this pattern from the transverse or T-type fracture pattern. Associated both-column fractures always have a break in the obturator foramen.

CT demonstrates severe fracture comminution and size of the fracture fragments. Three-dimensional CT scanning may be useful in determining accessibility for fracture stabilization through the single anterior approach versus an extensile or dual approach.

Treatment Principles

Nondisplaced or minimally displaced acetabular fractures require mobilization with crutches or walker touchdown weightbearing as permitted. Displaced acetabular fractures require exact restoration of the articular surface of the acetabulum with respect to the femoral head and rigid internal fixation, thereby avoiding prolonged postoperative traction or splinting while allowing early postoperative ambulation. Skeletal traction or roller traction is indicated when the patient's condition precludes surgery, such as when systemic illness, infection, or wound problems are present.

The indications for surgical management are based on the realization that anatomic restoration of the joint surface leads to excellent long-term results in the hands of experienced surgeons.[2,3,11,14–22] Many attempts have been made to define the limits of acetabular disruption that can be tolerated without surgical intervention before significant arthritis develops.[11,12,23] Secondary congruence seen with some both-column acetabular fractures can be treated by closed reduction techniques. However, fairly reliable indications for surgical reduction of acetabular fractures exist. The indications for ORIF include a 2- to 3-mm step-off, a nonconcentric hip reduction, and intra-articular debris.[11,12]

Irreducible anterior or posterior hip dislocations are considered true orthopaedic emergencies. These dislocations must be reduced immediately to decrease the incidence of osteonecrosis. Reduction should be done under a paralytic anesthetic to minimize trauma to the femoral head. All other acetabular fractures can be reduced on a more elective basis once the patient is stabilized and the surgical team that deals with these injuries is available. Fractures become more difficult to reduce after about 10 days. After 3 weeks the fracture has consolidated with callous, and an osteotomy via an extensile approach is required.

Acetabular results have been good in the older patient population.[11] Restoring the socket anatomy provides a foundation for a more successful subsequent total hip replacement should one be indicated. The goal in acetabular fracture surgery is to restore the joint surface. The primary goal should not be primary total hip replacement.[24] The results of total hip replacement after acetabular fracture are not nearly as good as for primary arthritis. Best results are usually obtained by addressing the displaced acetabular fracture with ORIF.[18]

References

1. Faringer PD, Mullins RJ, Feliciano PD, et al: Selective fecal diversion in complex open pelvic fractures from blunt trauma. *Arch Surg* 1994;129:958–964.
2. Matta JM, Letournel E, Browner BD: Surgical management of acetabular fractures, in Anderson LD (ed): American Academy of Orthopaedic Surgeons *Instructional Course Lectures XXXV*. St. Louis, MO, CV Mosby, 1986, pp 382–397.
3. Mayo KA: Fractures of the acetabulum. *Orthop Clin North Am* 1987;18:43–57.
4. Fassler PR, Swiontkowski MF, Kilroy AW, et al: Injury of the sciatic nerve associated with acetabular fracture. *J Bone Joint Surg* 1993;75A:1157–1166.
5. Vrahas M, Gordon RG, Mears DC, et al: Intraoperative somatosensory evoked potential monitoring of pelvic and acetabular fractures. *J Orthop Trauma* 1992;6:50–58.
6. Moed BR, Maxey JW: The effect of indomethacin on heterotopic ossification following acetabular fracture surgery. *J Orthop Trauma* 1993;7:33–38.

7. Kaempffe FA, Bone LB, Border JR: Open reduction and internal fixation of acetabular fractures: Heterotopic ossification and other complications of treatment. *J Orthop Trauma* 1991;5:439–445.

8. McLaren AC: Prophylaxis with indomethacin for heterotopic bone: After open reduction of fractures of the acetabulum. *J Bone Joint Surg* 1990;72A:245–247.

9. Bosse MJ, Poka A, Reinert CM, et al: Heterotopic ossification as a complication of acetabular fracture: Prophylaxis with low-dose irradiation. *J Bone Joint Surg* 1988;70A:1231–1237.

10. Webb LX, Rush PT, Fuller SB, et al: Greenfield filter prophylaxis of pulmonary embolism in patients undergoing surgery for acetabular fracture. *J Orthop Trauma* 1992;6:139–145.

11. Letournel E, Judet R (eds): *Fractures of the Acetabulum*, ed 2. Berlin, Germany, Springer-Verlag, 1993.

12. Judet R, Judet J, Letournel E: Fractures of the acetabulum: Classification and surgical approaches for open reduction. Preliminary report. *J Bone Joint Surg* 1964;46A:1615–1646.

13. Goulet JA, Rouleau JP, Mason DJ, et al: Comminuted fractures of the posterior wall of the acetabulum: A biomechanical evaluation of fixation methods. *J Bone Joint Surg* 1994;76A:1457–1463.

14. Bray TJ, Esser M, Fulkerson L: Osteotomy of the trochanter in open reduction and internal fixation of acetabular fractures. *J Bone Joint Surg* 1987;69A:711–717.

15. Matta JM, Mehne DK, Roffi R: Fractures of the acetabulum: Early results of a prospective study. *Clin Orthop* 1986;205:241–250.

16. Webb LX, Bosse MJ, Mayo KA, et al: Results in patients with craniocerebral trauma and an operatively managed acetabular fracture. *J Orthop Trauma* 1990;4:376–382.

17. Routt ML Jr, Swiontkowski MF: Operative treatment of complex acetabular fractures: Combined anterior and posterior exposures during the same procedure. *J Bone Joint Surg* 1990;72A:897–904.

18. Helfet DL, Borrelli J Jr, DiPasquale T, et al: Stabilization of acetabular fractures in elderly patients. *J Bone Joint Surg* 1992;74A:753–765.

19. Goulet JA, Bray TJ: Complex acetabular fractures. *Clin Orthop* 1989;240:9–20.

20. Matta JM, Anderson LM, Epstein HC, et al: Fractures of the acetabulum: A retrospective analysis. *Clin Orthop* 1986;205:230–240.

21. Matta JM, Merritt PO: Displaced acetabular fractures. *Clin Orthop* 1988;230:83–97.

22. Reinert CM, Bosse MJ, Poka A, et al: A modified extensile exposure for the treatment of complex or malunited acetabular fractures. *J Bone Joint Surg* 1988;70A:329–337.

23. Rowe CR, Lowell JD: Prognosis of fractures of the acetabulum. *J Bone Joint Surg* 1961;43A:30–59.

24. Romness DW, Lewallen DG: Total hip arthroplasty after fracture of the acetabulum: Long-term results. *J Bone Joint Surg* 1990;72B:761–764.

23
Biomechanics of Injuries of the Acetabulum and Pelvic Ring, and Fracture Fixation

Acetabular Biomechanics

An understanding of basic acetabular biomechanics provides a framework for evaluating and managing acetabular fractures. The mechanics of injury predict fracture patterns likely to occur. The mechanics of articular incongruities help predict which patients are at risk for posttraumatic arthritis. The mechanics of force transmission help guide surgical fixation and postoperative management. This section reviews basic acetabular biomechanics with a view toward clinical applicability.

In general, the acetabulum is disrupted when the femoral head is forcefully driven into the acetabulum. The energy to do this most often results from a blow to the foot, knee, or greater trochanter. The direction of the disrupting force can be determined by drawing a straight line from the point where the energy is applied through the center of the femoral head.[1] This direction determines the position of the fracture. For example, with a dashboard injury, the hip and knee are flexed 90°. If at the time of injury the victim's hip is in neutral abduction or adduction, then the force will be directed posteriorly, resulting in a posterior wall fracture. Conversely, if the victim's hip is abducted, the force will be directed more medially, resulting in a posterior column fracture. The injuries resulting from forces due to blows to the foot and to the greater trochanter can be similarly analyzed. Unfortunately, it is impossible to predict the specific details of each fracture. Such details depend not only on the direction of the injuring force but also on the force's specific characteristics and the quality of the patient's bone. Nevertheless, it is useful to keep the direction of the injuring force in mind when analyzing fracture patterns.

Although the exact pathogenesis of posttraumatic arthritis is not known, biomechanical factors are thought to be important. The most widely accepted theory suggests that articular incongruities decrease the available weightbearing area and thereby increase contact stresses (stress = force/area).[2] Over time, elevated stresses damage cartilage hemostasis and lead to arthritis. A second theory suggests that incongruities cause either major or minor hip instabilities.[3] These instabilities result in sheer stresses that, again, damage cartilage and lead to arthritis. Assuming that one or both of these theories is correct, it follows that preventing posttraumatic arthritis requires preventing elevated contact stresses and hip instabilities. Therefore, the management of nondisplaced fractures should be aimed at preventing secondary displacements. Fractures not affecting normal contact characteristics or hip stability can be considered insignificant, while fractures altering these factors must be reduced anatomically.

Unfortunately, we know very little about how acetabular fractures affect contact stresses. Normal hip contact stresses for level walking range from 0.5 to 5.5 MPa, depending on the hip's position and the stage of gait. Peak stresses range from 4.93 to 9.57 Mpa.[4] However, stresses as high as 18 MPa have been reported for subjects rising from a chair.[5] The stress magnitudes over the contact area are not equal. Higher stresses are noted in the center of the weightbearing area and lower stresses are observed toward the periphery.[6] During normal activities, forces are generally directed superiorly, medially, and posteriorly. However, the normal acetabular contact area is not well defined. Displaced fractures crossing the superior acetabulum are more likely to affect contact stresses than fractures located more inferiorly, but the exact fracture resulting in elevated contact stresses is not known. Presently, the best evidence for determining which fractures affect the weightbearing area comes from clinical reviews.[7]

Similar difficulties occur when one tries to identify significant fractures based on joint stability. Although reasonable data exist that delineate hip stability with posterior wall fractures, no studies have examined stability with other fracture patterns. The depth of the acetabulum can be described as the distance from the lateral edge of the posterior wall to the quadrilateral plate. If a posterior wall fragment involves no more than 20% of this depth, the hip will remain stable. If the fragment involves more than 40%, the hip will be unstable. A gray zone exists for fragments comprising 20% to 40% of the posterior wall.[8] With fragments of this size, some hips will remain stable while others will be unstable. It is important to remember that these guidelines are based on a cadaveric model in which a limited number of specimens were loaded under specific conditions. Although this study provides reasonable guidelines, the exact determinants of hip stability in vivo are not known. For fractures involving the acetabular dome, the direction of instability would be medial rather than posterior. The exact portion of the dome that ensures normal joint stability is not known.

Forces generated during the normal activities of daily living are better delineated for the hip than for any other joint. Peak forces during level walking range from 2.4 to 4.8 times body weight, depending on the subject and the technique used to estimate the force.[9] Fast walking and jogging increase the force to as high as 5.5 times body weight. These peak forces generally occur just after heel strike and decrease somewhat during the remainder of stance phase. During swing phase, forces drop to approximately 0.1 to 0.8 times body weight. Similar forces would be expected for a nonweightbearing patient on crutches. Even simple activities can generate substantial loads. Straight leg raising generates a force of 1.0 to 1.8 times body weight; getting out of bed, 0.8 to 1.4 times body weight; and getting into bed, 0.8 to 1.5 times body weight. The highest forces measured to date have resulted from experimental subjects stumbling (7.2 to 8.2 times body weight). These normal loads not only provide a framework for prescribing postoperative therapy but also give some idea of the forces that operative fixation must withstand.

In light of these high normal forces, it makes sense to choose the most stable fixation possible. Studies on cadaveric models have provided some limited information in this regard. Several methods of fixation were tested on a cadaveric transverse fracture model.[10] The anterior column was stabilized using a 6.5-mm lag screw, a 3.5-mm dynamic compression plate, a 3.5-mm reconstruction plate, or a Letournel plate. The posterior column was stabilized using a dynamic compression plate, a reconstruction plate, or a Letournel plate. No combination of fixation devices was found to be significantly more stable than the others. More important, none of the fixations failed, even at loads of up to 200% of body weight. However, all of the fixation methods allowed substantial fracture gapping. Gaps from 2 mm to 4 mm were noted under full load, but the fractures returned to their reduced positions once the load was removed. Slightly different results were noted when an isolated posterior column fracture model was used.[11] Posterior column fractures were stabilized by one 3.5-mm reconstruction plate, two 3.5-mm reconstruction plates, or a reconstruction plate plus a 3.5-mm lag screw. The lag screw–plate combination allowed significantly less motion than did the other fixation methods. Again, none of the fixations failed, but the specimens were loaded to only 75% of body weight.

These studies point out several limitations in using cadaveric models to study fracture fixation methods. Technical limitations and specimen availability make it possible to study only a limited number of very specific loading conditions, and the conditions chosen may greatly affect the results. In the posterior column fracture model, the specimens were loaded with the hip in two different positions. No differences in the fixation methods were noted with the hip at 30° of flexion. However, at 60° of flexion, the lag screw–plate combination proved significantly more stable. Similarly, the transverse fracture model evaluated fixation methods on a juxtatectal fracture. Had a high transtectal fracture been tested instead, all of the fixations might have failed. An even greater limitation may be our ignorance of the best conditions for fracture healing. Clearly, we do not want the fractures to displace. Within this limit, however, is absolute stability or is a small amount of motion best for fracture healing? Moreover, in the case of acetabular fracture fixation, the best biomechanical data come from clinical series. Letournel has applied standard techniques for stabilizing acetabular fractures in a large number of cases.[12] His results provide the best evidence available to date that these techniques are biomechanically sound.

Pelvic Biomechanics

An understanding of pelvic biomechanics can be useful in evaluating and treating pelvic injuries. Biomechanical considerations not only help to define the injury, they also help to determine whether or not surgery is indicated and what types of fixation are best. This section reviews pelvic biomechanics in relation to the clinical management of pelvic injuries.

To understand pelvic biomechanics, it is essential to understand the concept of stability. Biomechanical stability is defined as the ability of the pelvis to withstand normal physiologic loads without displacing. The stable pelvis can withstand normal physiologic loads; the unstable pelvis cannot. Although this definition seems straightforward, in reality it is somewhat arbitrary. Physiologic loads crossing the pelvis differ in magnitude and direction, depending on activity. Thus, a particular pelvic fracture may be stable with the patient in bed but may displace when the patient ambulates. Similarly, pelvic displacements can occur in any direction. However, certain displacements mean little clinically, while others have critical significance. To organize our clinical thinking, it is useful to make certain generalizations. When vertical displacement at the sacroiliac joint is possible at minimal physiologic loads (eg, during bed rest), the pelvis is described as vertically unstable. Similarly, when the pelvis is free to open like a book or to close so that the rami overlap, the pelvis is said to be rotationally unstable. These categories of instability are frequently referred to in both the clinical and biomechanical literature.[13] Nevertheless, they remain somewhat ambiguous generalizations. When evaluating this literature, one should keep in mind the basic questions of stability: How much load can the pelvis withstand, and in what direction are displacements likely to occur?

The bony pelvis has no inherent stability, but rather, its integrity is maintained by several strong ligaments. In front are the pubic symphysial ligaments. In back are the anterior sacroiliac ligaments, the interosseous ligaments, and the posterior sacroiliac ligaments. Inferiorly, the sacrotuberous and sacrospinous ligaments cross from the ilia to the sacrum and are continuous with the pelvic floor. Overall, the composite structure is extremely stable. Several in vivo and in vitro studies have demonstrated that translations at the sacroiliac joint and pubic symphysis are no greater than 6 mm and that rotations are no greater than 6°. Indeed, most studies note motions on the order of only a few millimeters.[14] In addition, biomechanical tests of pelvic strength have demonstrated that the normal pelvis can withstand vertical loads from 3,630 N (816 lb) to 5,837 N (1,312 lb) without failing.[15] In one study of isolated sacroiliac joints, some specimens withstood loads of 1,440 N (324 lb) without failing.[16]

To better understand the basic mechanics of pelvic stability, it is useful to draw certain analogies. One analogy is to think of the pelvis as a suspension bridge. The iliac wings act as the bridge's pillars, while the interosseous and posterior sacroiliac ligaments act as the bridge's suspension wires to prevent inferior sacral displacements.[17] To some extent, the pelvis also behaves as an arch, with the sacrum as the keystone.[15] The sacroiliac articulations are angled slightly from superolateral to inferomedial, so that they provide some resistance to inferior sacral displacements.[14] These analogies hold true, however, only when the pelvis is loaded through both acetabula (double leg stance). It has been demonstrated that when a person is in double leg stance, the pubic symphysis is in tension and the sacroiliac joints are in compression.[18] The opposite is true for a person standing on one leg or sitting. In both of the latter situations the pubic symphysis is in compression and the sacroiliac joints are in tension. Thus, the mechanisms by which the ligaments function to maintain pelvic stability depend greatly on how the pelvis is loaded.

Based on work by Pennal, a number of consequences of cutting the major pelvic ligaments can be described.[17] Disrupting the pubic symphysis allows the iliac wings to rotate outward slightly. The symphysis can spread 2.5 cm, but the sacroiliac ligaments and the other remaining pelvic ligaments prevent further rotational displacements. Because the sacroiliac ligaments remain intact, no vertical displacement is possible. If the anterior sacroiliac ligaments are then cut, the iliac wings can rotate laterally and open the pelvis like a book until the posterior spines lie against the sacrum. However, the intact interosseous and posterior sacroiliac ligaments continue to maintain vertical stability at the sacroiliac joint. Once these ligaments are disrupted, all stability is lost, and the pelvic bones are free to translate and rotate in any direction. The role of the sacrotuberous and sacrospinous ligaments is not clear. However, compared to the contributions of the other major ligaments, the contributions of these ligaments are most likely relatively small.[19]

Although these biomechanical analyses do improve our understanding, several difficulties arise when one tries to apply biomechanical data generated in the laboratory to the clinical situation. To date, biomechanical studies have concentrated on the effects of completely disrupting only major ligamentous structures. In the clinical situation, various combinations of complete and incomplete ligamentous lesions of major as well as minor supporting structures are possible. More important, it is very difficult to reproduce the clinical situation in a biomechanical model. Thus, it is impossible to rely solely on biomechanical data to determine pelvic stability. The ultimate test of stability in the living patient is whether the pelvis can withstand physiologic loads without displacing.[20]

To evaluate pelvic biomechanics appropriately, it is important to have a general idea of the loads crossing the pelvis. To date, no one has measured these loads directly. Nachemsom[21] has measured loads at the third lumbar disk, and it is reasonable to assume that sacral loads would be at least as high if not higher. For a 70-kg (154-lb) man sitting upright in a chair, Nachemson measured loads of 1,421 N (319 lb) at the L3-4 intervertebral disk.[21] At the pelvis, this load would be distributed equally across both sacroiliac joints. Thus, for a patient sitting in a chair, the load crossing each sacroiliac joint would be approximately 710 N (160 lb). For a subject lying supine, spinal loads measured 196 N (44 lb). When the subject rolled to the lateral decubitus position, loads rose to 686 N (154 lb). When the subject stood, loads rose to 980 N (220 lb). These measurements suggest that sacroiliac loads are substantial. It is important to keep this in mind when evaluating the strength of the various fixations.

It is generally accepted that anterior fixation alone will not adequately stabilize the posterior pelvis in a vertically unstable injury (posterior sacroiliac complex disrupted). In one study in which several external fixator designs were tested,[22] a frame constructed on double pin clusters (Pittsburgh Triangular Frame) was found to provide the greatest stability. However, even this frame failed at loads of only 300 N. Similarly, in a comparison of the Pittsburgh Triangular Frame with the Orthofix frame, both frames were found to fail at loads of less than 250 N.[23] In a study of several frame designs (a double cluster frame, a rectangular frame, a trapezoidal frame) all frames tested failed at loads of less than 200 N.[17] Internal fixation with either one plate anteriorly or two plates anteriorly was also tested.[17] Fixation failed at loads of less than 200 N. Because of the large forces that cross the sacroiliac joints, most surgeons believe that stabilizing the vertically unstable pelvis requires both anterior and posterior fixation. This does not mean that anterior fixation alone is not biomechanically sound in some situations. In a pelvis that is rotationally unstable but vertically stable (eg, the anterior pelvis is disrupted but the posterior ligaments are intact), anterior fixation can provide excellent stability.[13]

Clinical situations also exist in which anterior fixation alone may provide adequate stability, at least in the short term. External fixators are frequently used to control pelvic bleeding.[24] In these situations the fixator's role is not to provide vertical stability but rather to stabilize the pelvis against radial expansion. Theoretically, this controls pelvic volume and thereby provides tamponade.

Some patients are too sick to undergo the surgery necessary to provide stable internal fixation, making external fixation the only feasible option in the short term. Biomechanical studies have indicated some factors that can optimize the fixation in these situations. Three pins are stronger than two pins, and 5-mm pins are stronger than 4-mm pins.[25] Augmenting an anterior fixator with two anterior plates can substantially increase the stability. An anterior rectangular frame augmented by two anterior plates fails at 300 N, whereas a rectangular frame alone fails at approximately 20 N.[17]

Internal fixation of the posterior sacroiliac complex combined with either internal or external fixation of the anterior pelvis returns the greatest stability to the vertically unstable pelvis. Vertically unstable cadaveric pelves stabilized with sacral bars plus one anterior plate, sacral bars plus two anterior plates, or sacral bars plus an anterior frame all failed at loads of greater than 1,000 N.[26] In similar tests, it was reported that while the Slatis frame alone failed at loads of less than 50 N, the same frame augmented with either a cobra plate across the posterior pelvis or a three-holed dynamic compression plate across the anterior sacroiliac joint remained stable at loads of greater than 700 N.[22] Whether or not posterior pelvic fixation alone can provide adequate stability has not been tested biomechanically. It seems likely that posterior fixation alone would be adequate in situations where the anterior soft tissues remain intact and only the posterior soft tissues have been disrupted. However, in the vertically unstable pelvis, it is most likely important to fix both the anterior and posterior pelvis to provide adequate stability.[27]

Annotated References

1. Judet R, Judet J, Letournel E: Fractures of the acetabulum: Classification and surgical approaches for open reduction. Preliminary report. *J Bone Joint Surg* 1994;96A:1615–1636.

2. Hadley NA, Brown TD, Weinstein SL: The effects of contact pressure elevations and aseptic necrosis on the long-term outcome of congenital hip dislocations. *J Orthop Res* 1990;8:504–513.

   A radiographic technique was used to estimate hip contact stresses in patients with successfully treated congenital dislocated hips. Contact stresses estimated at the time of skeletal maturity were correlated with long-term clinical results. The cumulative overpressure index (Pc) was defined as the time-pressure product. Ninety percent of patients with Pc > 10 Mpa-years had a poor clinical outcome. The outcome was satisfactory in 80.9% of patients with Pc > 10 Mpa-years.

3. Vrahas MS, Fu F, Veenis B: Intraarticular contact stresses with simulated ankle malunions. *J Orthop Trauma* 1994;8:159–166.

4. Adams D, Swanson SAV: Direct measurement of local pressures in the cadaveric human hip joint during simulated level walking. *Ann Rheum Dis* 1985;44:658–666.

   Piezoelectric pressure transducers were placed in the acetabula of nine cadaveric hip joints. The joints were loaded to simulate normal gait, and acetabular contact pressures were recorded. Peak pressures ranged from 4.94 to 9.57 Mpa. Pressures were highest when the acetabula were maximally loaded.

5. Hodge WA, Carlson SM, Fijan RS, et al: Contact pressures from an instrumented hip endoprosthesis. *J Bone Joint Surg* 1989;71A:1378–1386.

6. Brown TD, Shaw DT: In vitro contact stress distributions in the natural human hip. *J Biomech* 1983;16:373–384.

7. Heeg MD, Oostrogrogel JHM, Klasen JH: Conservative treatment of acetabular fractures: The role of the weight-bearing dome and anatomic reduction in the ultimate results. *J Trauma* 1987;27:555–559.

8. Keith JE, Brashear HR, Gilford B: Stability of posterior fracture dislocations of the hip. *J Bone Joint Surg* 1988;70A:711–714.

   Hip stability with simulated posterior wall fractures was evaluated in nine cadavers. The depth of the acetabulum was determined by measuring the distance from the lateral lip of the acetabulum to the quadrilateral plate. Progressively larger posterior wall fragments were removed, and hip stability was tested. With fragments comprising 20% of the total depth, all hips remained stable. With 40% fragments, all hips were unstable. With 20% to 40% fragments, some hips were stable and some were unstable.

9. Bergman G, Graichen F, Rohlmann A: Hip joint loading during walking and running. *J Biomech* 1993;26:969–990.

   Instrumented total hip prostheses were implanted in two patients. In vivo hip joint forces were measured for various activities, including sitting, walking slowly, walking fast, jogging, and stumbling. Forces recorded while the patients were sitting and lying were very small. Forces for slow walking ranged from 2.8 × body weight to 4.8 × body weight. Fast walking and jogging raised forces to approximately 5.5 × body weight. The highest forces were recorded when the patients stumbled (7.2 × to 8.7 × body weight).

10. Sawaguchi T, Brown TD, Rubash HE, et al: Stability of acetabular fractures after internal fixation: A cadaveric study. *Acta Orthop Scand* 1984;55:601–605.

11. Schopfer A, DiAngelo D, Hearn T, et al: Biomechanical comparison of methods of fixation of isolated osteotomies of the posterior acetabular column. *Int Orthop* 1994;18:96–101.

12. Letournel E: *Fractures of the Pelvis and Acetabulum,* ed 2. New York, NY, Springer-Verlag, 1993.

13. Tile M: Pelvic ring fractures: Should they be fixed? *J Bone Joint Surg* 1988;70B:1–12.

14. Vukicevic S, Marusic A, Stavljenic A, et al: Holographic analysis of the human pelvis. *Spine* 1991;16:209–214.

15. Gunterberg B, Romanus B, Stener B: Pelvic strength after major amputation of the sacrum: An experimental study. *Acta Orthop Scand* 1976;47:635–642.

    The sacrums of five cadaveric pelves were loaded to failure with the pelves configured to simulate upright stance. Mean failure loads were 4,856 N. The pelves failed through the sacrum, first on one side, then on the other.

16. Miller JA, Schultz AB, Andersson GBJ: Load-displacement behavior of sacroiliac joints. *J Orthop Res* 1987;5:92–101.

17. Tile M: *Fractures of the Pelvis and Acetabulum.* Baltimore, MD, Williams & Wilkins, 1984.

18. Pawels F: *Biomechanics of the Locomotor Apparatus.* Berlin, Germany, Springer-Verlag, 1980.

19. Scholten PJM, Schultz AB, Luchies CW, et al: Motions and loads within the human pelvis: A biomechanical model study. *J Orthop Res* 1988;6:840–850.

20. Edeiken-Monroe BS, Browner BD, Jackson H: The role of standard roentgenograms in the evaluation of instability of the pelvic ring disruption. *Clin Orthop* 1989;240:63–76.

21. Nachemson A: Electromyographic studies on the vertebral portion of the PSOAS muscle. *Acta Orthop Scand* 1966;37:177–190.

    Forces crossing the lumbar spine during various activities were determined from intradiskal pressure measures. Loads with the patient supine were 196 N. Lying in the lateral decubitus position generated loads of 196 N. Standing upright generated loads of 980 N. Sitting generated loads of 1,421 N, and bending generated loads of 1,470 N.

22. Rubash HE, Brown TD, Nelson DD, et al: Comparative mechanical performances of some new devices for fixation of unstable pelvic ring fractures. *Med Biol Eng Comput* 1983;21:657–663.

23. Bell A, Smith R, Brown T, et al: Comparative studies of the Orthofix and Pittsburgh frame for external fixation of unstable pelvic ring fractures. *J Orthop Trauma* 1988;2:130–138.

24. Dalal S, Burgess AR, Siegel JH, et al: Pelvic fracture in multiple trauma: Classification by mechanism is the key to pattern of organ injury, resuscitative requirements and outcome. *J Trauma* 1989;29:981–1000.

25. Dathers LE, Jacobs RR, Jayaraman G, et al: A study of skeletal systems for unstable pelvic fractures. *J Trauma* 1984;24:876–881.

26. Stocks G, Gabel G, Noble PC, et al: Anterior and posterior internal fixation of vertical sheer fractures of the pelvis. *J Orthop Res* 1991;9:237–245.

27. Shaw JA, Mino D, Werner FW, et al: Posterior stabilization of pelvic fractures by use of threaded compression rods. *Clin Orthop* 1985;192:240–254.

24
Fixation of Pelvic Ring Disruptions

Introduction

Pelvic ring fractures and dislocations may be difficult to treat sucessfully. Low-energy pelvic fractures due to minor traumatic events, such as a fall from standing, rarely require surgical intervention. Conversely, complex pelvic ring disruptions result from severe injuries. High mortality rates in these polytrauma patients are usually due to rapid torrential hemorrhage, head trauma, and other primary system injuries[1,2] (Fig. 1). The complex bone and soft-tissue anatomy of the pelvis is unfamiliar to many orthopaedic surgeons and complicates surgical treatment. Classification schemes for pelvic fractures and dislocations are based on zones of injury, instability patterns, and load applications.[2,3] These classifications are difficult to remember and may not guide treatment, especially in the polytrauma patient.

Early pelvic stability diminishes bleeding and provides patient comfort, allowing mobilization from the recumbent position.[4] Many techniques can stabilize the disrupted pelvis.[4-8] These techniques include, but are not limited to, various and creative traction devices, body casting, and external fixation. Internal fixation of the unstable pelvic ring has received more attention recently for many reasons. Early field resuscitation and rapid transport techniques deliver patients with previously devastating pelvic injuries to regional trauma centers for treatment. Aggressive surgical management of the other primary system injuries often mandates a similar approach to the disrupted pelvic ring. Improved radiologic imaging modalities, especially intraoperative fluoroscopy, have improved the safety of performing pelvic internal fixation. Early internal fixation of the disrupted pelvis following a coordinated team approach is optimal according to recent studies.[9-12] More importantly, pelvic internal fixation is mechanically superior to even the most complicated external fixation constructs.[13,14]

Specific Injuries

Symphysis Pubis Disruption

Disruptions of the symphysis pubis are variable. Complete dislocations may result from compression, distraction, or other combined forces. The symphyseal ligaments, the pubic meniscus, and the arcuate ligament may be disrupted. Lateral compression loads can disrupt the symphysis pubis.

Fractures of the adjacent pubic superior and inferior rami may be present in association with symphyseal dislocations. Resultant deformities of the anterior pelvis due to the disrupted symphysis pubis include external/internal rotation, flexion/extension, and cephalad/caudad translation (Fig. 2).

For isolated disruptions of the symphysis pubis, most authors advocate closed, nonsurgical management, especially when the symphysis diastasis is less than 2.5 cm.[2,8,15] In cases where the diastasis exceeds this limit, stabilization should be pursued. A Pfannenstiehl exposure allows symphyseal access for reduction and plate fixation. Alternatively, in patients undergoing exploratory laparotomy, the caudal portion of the wound can be used to reduce and stabilize the symphysis pubis. Bladder and urethral repairs are performed by the urologist prior to symphyseal reduction and fixation, except in cases of ongoing hemorrhage. The symphysis is reduced using a variety of techniques. Manual compression of each iliac crest, a temporary anterior pelvic external fixation frame, or a reduction clamp approximates the two pubic areas while the bladder and urethra are protected with a malleable retractor.

Plate fixation of the symphysis pubis is accomplished using a variety of plating techniques. A two-holed 4.5-mm narrow dynamic compression plate secured to the cephalad surface of the symphysis pubis using 6.5-mm fully threaded cancellous screws has been advocated[8,15] in order to resist distraction forces while allowing physiologic rotational movements. This two-holed implant may be too flexible, especially in patients with severe posterior pelvic ring disruptions/instabilities.[16] A more rigid, multiplane symphyseal fixation approach using two plates oriented at right angles to one another has been advocated, especially in patients with posterior pelvic instability.[2] Application of the second (anterior/caudal) plate requires more extensive dissection of the anterior pelvic soft tissues, including the rectus abdominus insertions bilaterally. An alternative technique of locking a recessed caudal plate with a cephalad plate in a box configuration was more rigid than other symphyseal fixation techniques in a recent biomechanical study.[17] This "box plate" method has not been evaluated clinically. Another biomechanical study demonstrated that posterior pelvic ring fixation significantly improved the stability of simple uniplanar symphyseal plating (Fig. 3).[16]

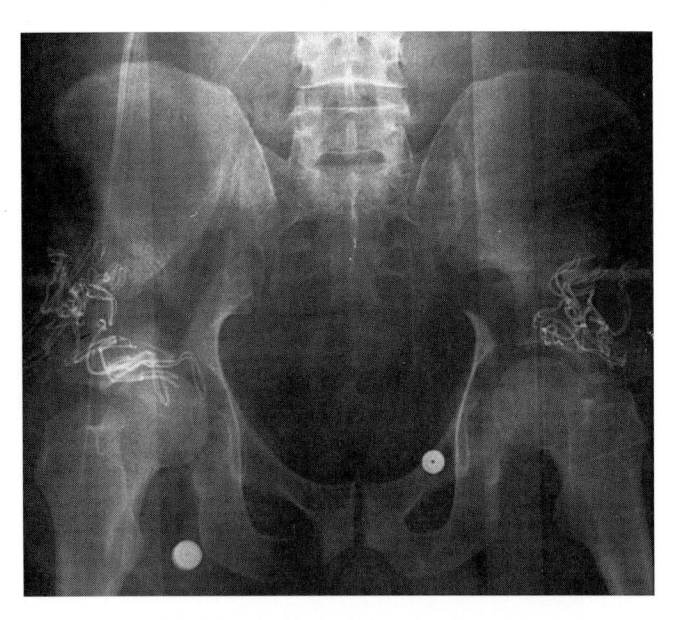

Fig. 1 This patient was crushed by a heavy trailer at the level of his waist. He had bilateral open acetabular fractures with eviscerations, a transverse sacral fracture, and bilateral complete neurovascular disruptions distal to the level of his injury. He died of torrential hemorrhage.

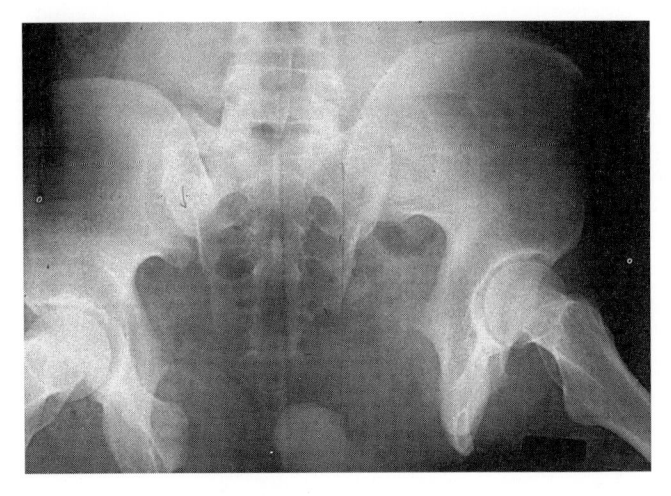

Fig. 2 Wide disruption of the symphysis pubis is seen in this patient after a motorcycle crash. Both sacroiliac articulations were injured.

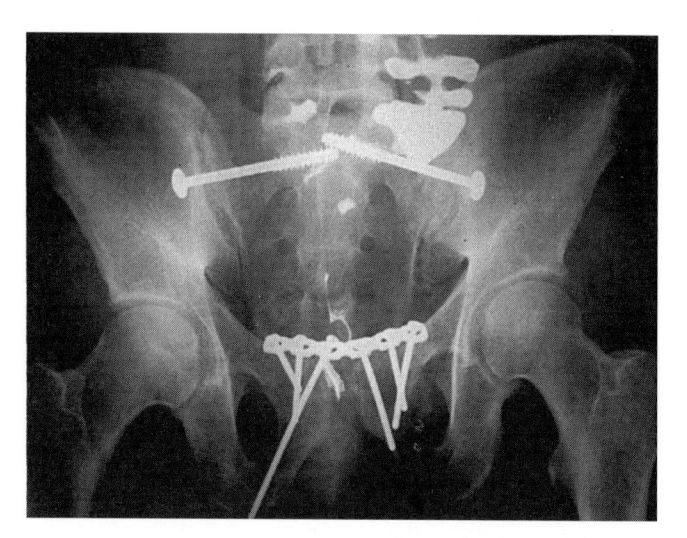

Fig. 3 This patient had plate fixation of the symphysis pubis using a Pfannenstiel surgical exposure. A six-hole, 3.5-mm reconstruction plate was used to stabilize the symphysis pubis. Bilateral iliosacral lag screws were used to stabilize the sacroiliac joint disruptions.

Pubic Ramus Fractures

Fractures occur at different locations along the pubic ramus. In most patients, these injuries do not require surgical intervention. Some form of ramus fixation does, however, support the posterior implants in patients with severe instabilities while also protecting the local anterior pelvic soft tissues.[16,18] Internal fixation of superior pubic ramus fractures is accomplished with either plate/screw constructs or medullary screw techniques. Parasymphyseal (medial) pubic fractures are often noted in association with symphyseal dislocations. These ramus fractures are reduced and fixed using a Pfannenstiehl exposure. Plate fixation is performed using a 3.5-mm reconstruction plate in most cases. More laterally located ramus (pubic root) fractures usually require an ilioinguinal exposure to reduce and stabilize.[7] Retrograde medullary superior pubic ramus screws may be used alternatively. Medullary superior pubic ramus screws have been shown to provide equivalent biomechanical stability when compared to more standard plate fixations.[18] These screws are difficult to insert accurately, even under direct visualization of the fracture. Experience and quality fluoroscopic imaging are mandatory for this fixation technique to be safe and effective (Fig. 4).[19]

Pubic ramus fractures in association with symphysis pubis dislocation are more difficult to treat. In some cases after the symphysis is reduced and stabilized, the ramus fracture is indirectly controlled by the local soft tissues, including the inguinal ligament, and requires no fixation. Other more unstable situations may mandate ramus reduction/fixation in order to reduce the symphysis pubis accurately. In these patients, the two injuries are treated either using a plate to stabilize both or inserting a medullary screw initially to control the ramus fracture, followed by reduction and plate fixation of the symphysis.[19]

Iliac Wing Fractures

Iliac fractures occur in a variety of patterns, yet all follow the structurally frail "fault lines" of the ilium. These fractures may result from direct high-energy loads applied to the subcutaneous iliac crest. Severe local contusions and open wounds may complicate these fractures. In such pa-

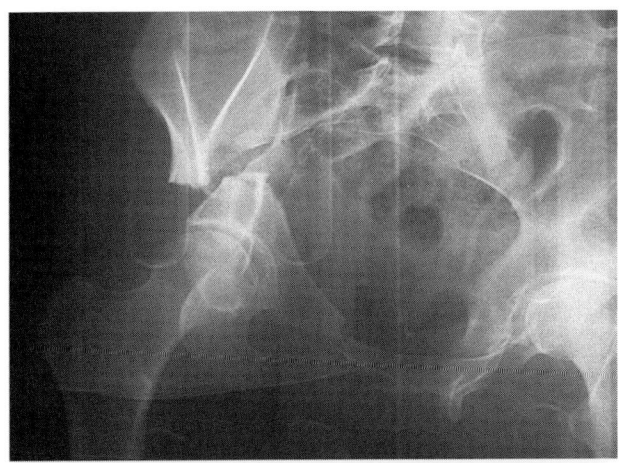

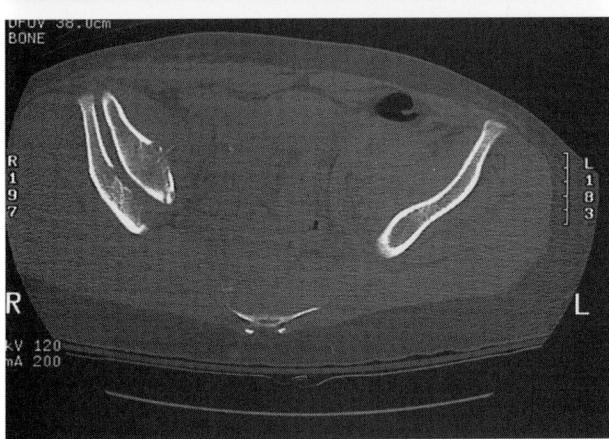

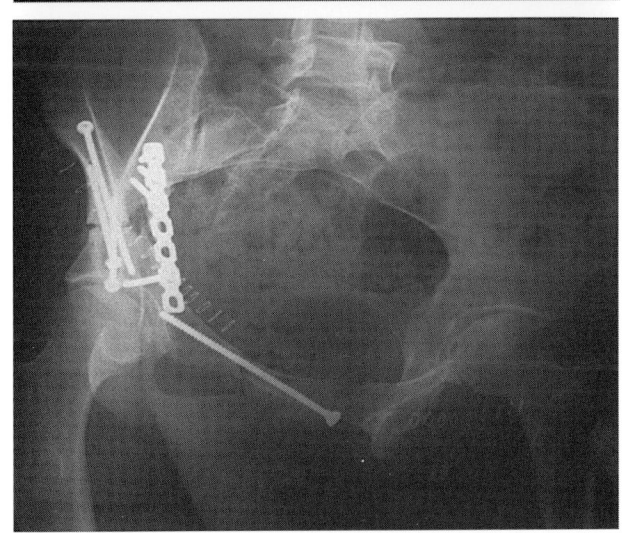

Fig. 4 Top, This patient has an unstable right hemipelvis after an automobile accident. **Center,** The CT scan demonstrates the degree of iliac fracture displacement. **Bottom,** The iliac fracture was reduced using an internal iliac exposure, and stabilized with a reconstruction plate and lag screws. The unstable mid-portion pubic ramus fracture was reduced using a Pfannenstiel exposure, and stabilized with a retrograde superior pubic ramus medullary lag screw.

tients, the buttock and flank may be ecchymotic and swollen. Careful evaluation for intra-abdominal pathology should be performed. Iliac fractures with displacement through or involvement of the greater sciatic notch area may injure the gluteal vascular structures. Angiographic evaluation is recommended prior to open treatment in such patients.[9,11,20] Open reduction of an iliac fracture is performed using either an internal or external iliac exposure. The internal iliac approach is the lateral window of the ilioinguinal extensile exposure.[21] Reconstruction of the iliac fracture is facilitated by using clamps or small pins as "joysticks" to manipulate the fragments. An assistant may be needed to pull distal traction through the femur, especially in delayed reconstructions. Lag screws between the iliac tables may be used to secure the reductions, and are supported using plates (Fig. 5).[7]

Sacroiliac Joint Dislocations

The sacroiliac joint is a complex articulation with an array of anatomic variations. The undulating articular surfaces occupy the anterior and cephalad areas, while dense interosseus ligaments tether the posterior ilium to the lateral sacrum. The inclination or slope of the cephalad portions of the joint usually parallel the sacral ala. Abnormal sacral alar morphology affects the sacroiliac articulation. Disruptions of the sacroiliac joint may present as complete dislocations due to severe trauma, or in varying degrees of anterior joint injury with incomplete interosseus ligament disruptions.

Internal fixation after anatomic reduction is recommended for an unstable or displaced sacroiliac joint disruption. The techniques and options for sacroiliac joint reduction and fixation are numerous. The choices of surgical exposure and fixation constructs should be individualized for each patient. The surgeon must consider the radiographic findings as well as the patient's body habitus, local soft-tissue injuries, and overall medical condition.

Stabilization of the sacroiliac joint from a posterior approach has been evaluated clinically.[2,7,22,23] The patient is positioned prone. Prone positioning and posterior fixation has been advocated in patients previously treated with anterior pelvic external fixation. Two operating tables were positioned end to end with a space left between the tables. This space allowed the anterior external fixation frame to be suspended between the opposing tables. A posterior surgical exposure visualizes the posterior portions of the sacroiliac joint. Deep dissection accesses the greater sciatic notch, allowing digital assessment of the anterior portions of the joint. Clamps are used to control the manipulative reduction. Use of plates, sacral bars, and iliosacral lag screws have been described with this posterior approach.[2,7,23] High complication rates, including skin breakdown, have been reported for these posterior incisions.[1,24]

Anterior exposure of the sacroiliac joint is accomplished using an internal iliac exposure. The fifth lumbar nerve root is located within a periosteal gutter along the sacral ala and limits medial retraction. Visualization of the joint surfaces is improved with headlamp illumination. Using

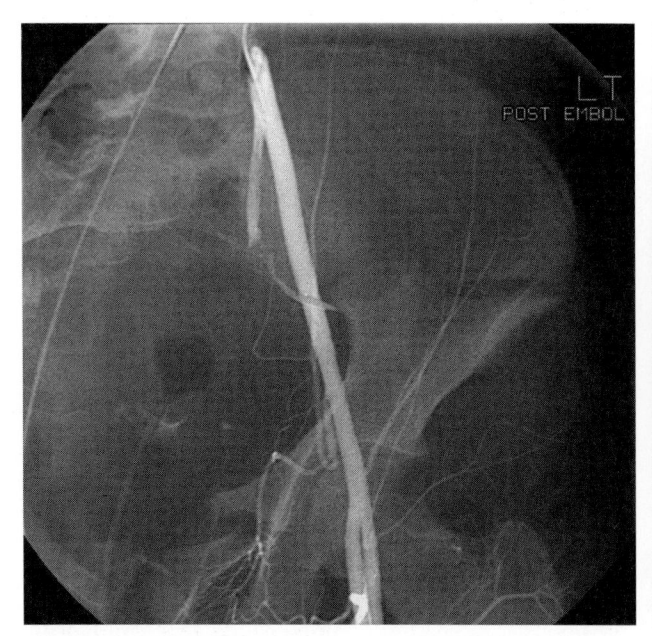

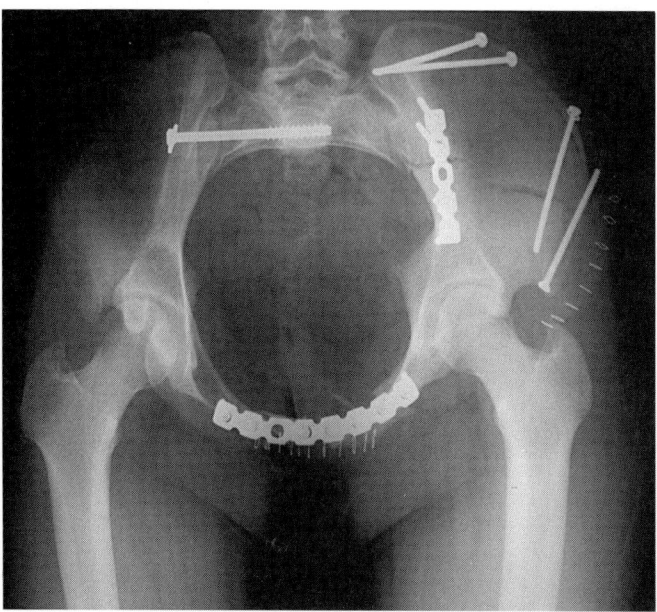

Fig. 5 Left, This patient had a displaced iliac fracture in association with a superior gluteal arterial disruption. Angiographic embolization was used prior to surgical fixation. **Right,** Plate fixation was used for the rami fractures, and lag screws stabilized the iliac fractures.

this exposure, external rotation of the ilium is accomplished using a clamp and osteochondral fragments are debrided from the sacroiliac joint. Reduction of the sacroiliac joint is somewhat difficult using the anterior exposure, especially in the obese patient. Overcompression of the visible anterior articular sacroiliac joint surfaces may cause distraction of the posterior/caudal aspects of the joint. Reduction clamps can obstruct plate applications, further complicating the procedure. In one series of patients, sacroiliac joint disruptions were treated successfully by anterior plating of the joint.[21] The biomechanical properties of sacroiliac joint plates have been described.[25]

Iliosacral lag screws stabilize disruptions of the sacroiliac joint. Bony landmarks have been identified along the posterior ilium to facilitate iliosacral lag screw insertion via the posterior exposure.[7] A thorough understanding of the bony, vascular, and neurologic anatomy of the posterior pelvis and the spatial relationships of the various elements is necessary.[7] Iliosacral screw insertion using biplanar fluoroscopy to guide implant placement also has been described.[7] Computed tomography (CT) has been used for safe percutaneous insertion of iliosacral screws.[26,27] Because the patients were positioned prone in the CT scanner and the screws were inserted percutaneously, reductions of the sacroiliac joints were not possible.

Iliosacral screws can also be inserted with the patient positioned supine.[28] The patient is elevated slightly from the operating table on a soft lumbosacral support. Supine positioning is advantageous for several reasons. The anterior pelvic ring injury (as well as abdominal, genitourinary, and lower extremity injuries) can be surgically treated using the same skin preparation and draping. Valuable surgical time is saved. When indicated, open reduction of the sacroiliac joint is accomplished via the internal iliac exposure. Reduction clamps do not obstruct the percutaneous insertion of the iliosacral lag screw. Successful closed reduction and percutaneous iliosacral lag screw stabilization of the sacroiliac joint is limited to incomplete sacroiliac joint disruptions treated early. Anatomic reduction of the anterior pelvic disruption "indirectly" reduces the sacroiliac joint. Final reduction and compression is possible when the iliosacral lag screw is oriented perpendicularly to the sacroiliac articulation. Triplanar (inlet, outlet, and lateral sacral) pelvic fluoroscopic imaging guides iliosacral lag screw insertion into the safest upper sacral vertebral body according to the preoperative plan. Alar screws are biomechanically inferior in pull-out testing to those situated within the sacral vertebral body.[29] Morphologic variations of the upper sacrum are not uncommon and must be identified preoperatively if iliosacral screw insertion is to be performed safely (Fig. 6). Blood loss is minimal when closed reduction and percutaneous screw insertion techniques are used. An increased rate of fixation failures and screw complications are seen: (1) if the patient is obese, (2) when the posterior pelvic anatomy is poorly understood, (3) if pelvic fluoroscopic imaging is of poor quality, (4) when sacroiliac joint malreductions are accepted, (5) when anterior external fixation frames are used to treat definitively the anterior pelvic injuries, and (6) in those patients with craniocerebral trauma.

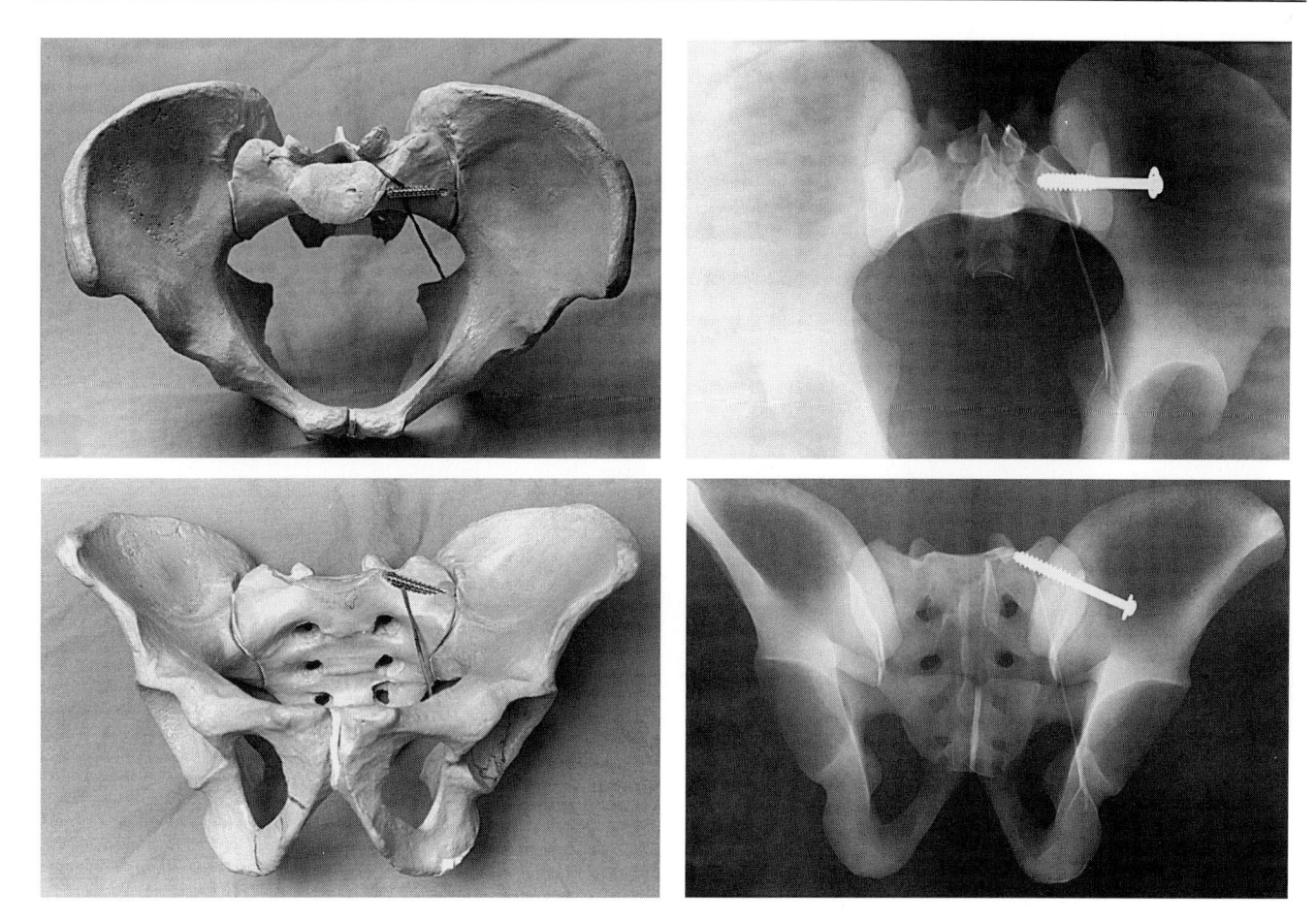

Fig. 6 This pelvic model (**top left** and **bottom left**) and its inlet (**top right**) and outlet (**bottom right**) pelvic radiographs demonstrate the problem of bi-planar imaging for iliosacral screw insertions. Because of the sacral alar slope, the iliosacral screw may appear to be interosseus, even when it is not. The fifth lumbar nerve root is represented on the models. The lateral sacral fluoroscopic view guides safe insertion of iliosacral screws, except in cases of upper sacral morphological abnormalities.

Crescent Fractures

Fracture-dislocation of the sacroiliac joint ("crescent fractures") are combination disruptions of the posterior pelvic ring. In these patients, the anterior sacroiliac joint capsular and ligamentous structures are injured, producing distraction or compression through the articular surfaces, depending on the application of load. As the disruptive force encounters the dense interosseus ligaments, either the iliac or the sacral bone fractures. When these traumatic events are caused by laterally applied loads, the iliac fracture is oblique and the anterior sacral ala sustains an associated impaction fracture.

Open reduction of crescent fractures is performed using either an anterior or posterior exposure. Each has its advantages. The anterior internal iliac approach provides direct visualization of the sacroiliac joint articular surfaces, which facilitates debridement and joint reduction. Reduction clamps for this injury may be difficult to use effectively through this exposure. Implant choice is dependent on the size of the intact posterior iliac crescent fracture fragment. Lag screws are placed from the internal iliac fossa into the crescent fragment. Iliosacral lag screws are used when possible. The external iliac exposure requires subperiosteal elevation of the hip abductors from the lateral ilium. The sacroiliac joint is accessed for debridement through the fracture. The fracture is accurately reduced along the crescent fragment and secured with clamps. Stability is achieved using lag screws and plates through this exposure.

Sacral Fractures

Sacral fractures occur in a variety of patterns. Certain alar fractures may involve the sacroiliac joint. Transforaminal sacral fractures risk lumbosacral nerve root injuries. These nerve root lesions may be caused by stretch, by compression from comminuted foraminal debris, or by laceration.[2,20,30] Transverse sacral fractures are difficult to diagnose because of their orientation. True lateral sacral radiographs are recommended for accurate evaluation or exclusion of these potential fractures.

Many of the principles of sacroiliac joint disruptions apply to management of sacral fractures. Stabilization of the sacrum from a posterior approach has been evaluated clinically. The biomechanical and clinical stability of threaded compressive transiliac rods have been demonstrated in the unstable posterior ring.[2,14] Small plates applied to the posterior sacrum locally were comparable to more standard forms of internal fixation according to another biomechanical study.[31] Open reduction of sacral fractures is indicated in displaced patterns and when foraminal bone debris correlates with specific nerve root symptoms and signs. The patient is positioned prone. Ipsilateral lower extremity (femoral or tibial) traction and nerve monitoring may be used.[32] A vertical paramedian skin incision is centered over the posterior iliac spine. The gluteal origin is divided, leaving a tendinous cuff for later repair, and is retracted laterally. The hematoma is evacuated, visible nerve roots are protected, and the fracture margins debrided. Foraminal comminuted bone fragments are removed with care. Reduction maneuvers are performed slowly and cautiously, avoiding overcompression. Internal fixation is used to secure the open reduction and protect the local nerve roots from further potential damage. Posterior tension plates, sacral bars, and other techniques have been recommended. "Local osteosynthesis" has been used to treat sacral fractures.[31] All forms of compression fixation are used cautiously to avoid iatrogenic nerve root damage, especially in the transforaminal fracture patterns.

Closed manipulative reductions of sacral fractures can be performed acutely. Anatomic restoration of the anterior pelvic ring disruption combined with distal skeletal traction often will reduce accurately the unstable sacral fracture. In these patients, the sacral fracture is stabilized with a percutaneously inserted iliosacral screw. The iliosacral screw direction is different for a sacral fracture than for a sacroiliac joint dislocation. Because the sacral injury is more medial than the sacroiliac joint, a longer screw is needed to obtain balanced fixation. The transforaminal fractures are usually oriented more vertically than the sacroiliac joint and therefore the screw is targeted to be perpendicular to the fracture. This horizontal screw orientation actually facilitates additional screw length within the safe zone, and consequently improves medial fixation. A fully threaded screw can be used to avoid compression of the sacral neural foramina (Fig. 7).[28] Because the screw(s) are placed percutaneously, the potential problems of wound infection and bleeding are greatly diminished.

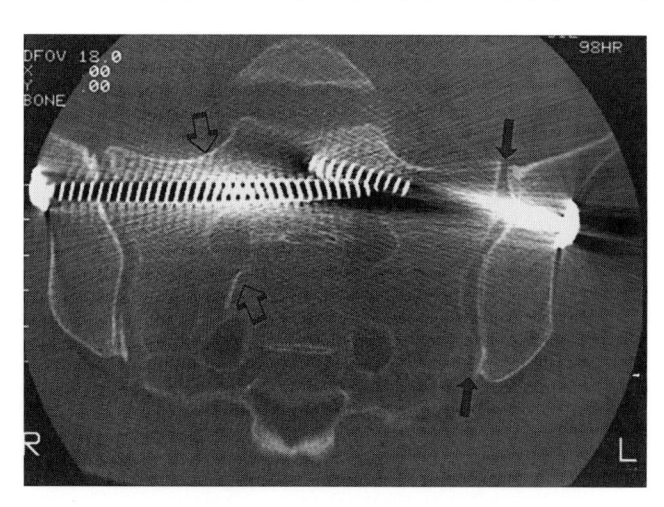

Fig. 7 A postoperative CT scan demonstrates a right-sided transforaminal sacral fracture (open arrows) and a left-sided sacroiliac joint disruption (solid arrows). The right-sided "sacral" screw is oriented more horizontally in order to achieve additional medial fixation. The "sacral" screw is fully threaded in order to avoid overcompression of the nerve roots. The left-sided "sacroiliac" screw is a lag screw directed perpendicular to the sacroiliac joint producing compression. Since the sacroiliac joint disruption is more lateral than the transforaminal sacral fracture, a shorter screw length may be used to achieve balanced fixation. In situations of bilateral injuries, such as this, the screws may be locked upon one another by cross threading as is shown.

Conclusion

The polytrauma patient with an unstable pelvic ring injury remains a treatment challenge. Rapid pelvic ring stability should diminish pelvic hemorrhage, provide comfort, and allow chair mobility. Improved functional outcomes are expected. In order to optimize the potential of pelvic internal fixation, the treating orthopaedic surgeon must possess a thorough knowledge of (1) pelvic and local soft-tissue anatomy, (2) pelvic surgical exposures, (3) modern techniques of fluoroscopic pelvic imaging, and (4) reduction and implant strategies. An aggressive team approach to these complex patients with pelvic trauma, especially including general surgical and urologic support staffs, provides a favorable environment for pelvic internal fixation.

Annotated References

1. Goldstein A, Phillips T, Sclafani SJ, et al: Early open reduction and internal fixation of the disrupted pelvic ring. *J Trauma* 1986;26:325–333.

2. Tile M: Pelvic ring fractures: Should they be fixed? *J Bone Joint Surg* 1988;70B:1–12.

3. Burgess AR, Eastridge BJ, Young JW, et al: Pelvic ring disruptions: Effective classification system and treatment protocols. *J Trauma* 1990;30:848–856.

4. Mears DC, Fu F: External fixation in pelvic fractures. *Orthop Clin North Am* 1980;11:465–479.

5. Kellam JF: The role of external fixation in pelvic disruptions. *Clin Orthop* 1989;241:66-82.

6. Mattox KL, Bickell W, Pepe PE, et al: Prospective MAST study in 911 patients. *J Trauma* 1989;29:1104–1112.

7. Matta JM, Saucedo T: Internal fixation of pelvic ring fractures. *Clin Orthop* 1989;242:83–97.

8. Lange RH, Hansen ST Jr: Pelvic ring disruptions with symphysis pubis diastasis: Indications, technique, and limitations of anterior internal fixation. *Clin Orthop* 1985;201:130–137.

9. Gruen GS, Leit ME, Gruen RJ, et al: The acute management of hemodynamically unstable multiple trauma patients with pelvic ring fractures. *J Trauma* 1994;36:706–713.

    Aggressive resuscitation of these patients included early internal pelvic fixation. Uncontrolled hemorrhage from the pelvic injury and/or surgery was not encountered. Anterior and posterior internal fixation of the pelvis after anatomic reduction provided stability while avoiding the complications of external fixation.

10. Latenser BA, Gentilello LM, Tarver AA, et al: Improved outcome with early fixation of skeletally unstable pelvic fractures. *J Trauma* 1991;31:28–31.

    Early fixation of pelvic fractures is advocated in this clinical series. Mortality and complication rates were low.

11. Poole GV, Ward EF, Muakkassa FF, et al: Pelvic fracture from major blunt trauma: Outcome is determined by associated injuries. *Ann Surg* 1991;213:532–539.

12. Zingg EJ, Casanova GA, Isler B, et al: Pelvic fractures and traumatic lesions of the posterior urethra. *Eur Urol* 1990;18:27–32.

13. Shaw JA, Mino DE, Werner FW, et al: Posterior stabilization of pelvic fractures by use of threaded compression rods: Case reports and mechanical testing. *Clin Orthop* 1985;192:240–254.

14. Stocks GW, Gabel GT, Nobel PC, et al: Anterior and posterior internal fixation of vertical shear fractures of the pelvis. *J Orthop Res* 1991;9:237–245.

    This biomechanical study evaluates different methods of internal and external pelvic fixation. An unstable pelvic fracture-dislocation model was used to simulate Malgaigne injuries. External fixation alone provided poor control of pelvic mobility. In interforaminal sacral fractures, sacral bars provided adequate rigidity, especially when anterior plate fixation or external fixation was used. Sacroiliac joint dislocations were less adequately treated with similar fixation constructs.

15. Webb LX, Gristina AG, Wilson JR, et al: Two-hole plate fixation for traumatic symphysis pubis diastasis. *J Trauma* 1988;28:813–817.

16. Simonian PT, Routt ML Jr, Harrington RM, et al: Biomechanical simulation of the anteroposterior compression injury of the pelvis: An understanding of instability and fixation. *Clin Orthop* 1994;309:245–256.

    Internal fixation constructs of pelvic ring disruptions were evaluated in this biomechanical study. The most rigid overall pelvic fixation was achieved when both the symphyseal and sacroiliac disruptions were stabilized internally. Sacroiliac joint fixation using either an iliosacral lag screw or two anterior sacroiliac joint plates was comparable.

17. Simonian PT, Routt MLC Jr, Harrington RM, et al: Box plate fixation of the symphysis pubis: Biomechanical evaluation of a new technique. *J Orthop Trauma* 1994;8:483–489.

    The authors of this biomechanical study evaluate a new technique of symphyseal fixation. The box plate construct was more rigid than other routine forms of symphyseal fixation.

18. Simonian PT, Routt MLC Jr, Harrington RM, et al: Internal fixation of the unstable anterior pelvic ring: A biomechanical comparison of standard plating techniques and the retrograde medullary superior pubic ramus screw. *J Orthop Trauma* 1994;8:476–482.

    This biomechanical study compared the retrograde medullary superior pubic ramus screw to standard plate fixation for pubic ramus fractures. Both techniques provided equivalent stability.

19. Routt MLC, Simonian PT, Grujic L: Preliminary report: The retrograde medullary superior ramus screw for the treatment of anterior pelvic ring disruptions. *J Orthop Trauma* 1995;9:35–44.

20. Slatis P, Huittinen VM: Double vertical fractures of the pelvis: A report on 163 patients. *Acta Chir Scand* 1972;138:799–807.

21. Simpson LA, Waddell JP, Leighton RK, et al: Anterior approach and stabilization of the disrupted sacroiliac joint. *J Trauma* 1987;27:1332–1339.

22. Browner BD, Cole JD, Graham JM, et al: Delayed posterior internal fixation of unstable pelvic fractures. *J Trauma* 1987;27:998–1006.

23. Mears DC, Capito CP, Deleeuw H: Posterior pelvic disruptions managed by the use of the double cobra plate, in Bassett FH III (ed): *Instructional Course Lectures XXXVII.* Park Ridge, IL, American Academy of Orthopaedic Surgeons, 1988, pp 143–150.

24. Kellam JF, McMurtry RY, Paley D, et al: The unstable pelvic fracture: Operative treatment. *Orthop Clin North Am* 1987;18:25–41.

25. Leighton RK, Waddell JP, Bray TJ, et al: Biomechanical testing of new and old fixation devices for vertical shear fractures of the pelvis. *J Orthop Trauma* 1991;5:313–317.

26. Ebraheim NA, Rusin JJ, Coombs RJ, et al: Percutaneous computed-tomography-stabilization of pelvic fractures: Preliminary report. *J Orthop Trauma* 1987;1:197–204.

27. Nelson DW, Duwelius PJ: CT-guided fixation of sacral fractures and sacroiliac joint disruptions. *Radiology* 1991;180:527–532.
28. Routt MLC Jr, Meier MC, Kregor PJ, et al: Percutaneous iliosacral screws with the patient supine technique. *Operative Tech Orthop* 1993;3:35–45.
29. Kraemer W, Hearn T, Tile M, et al: The effect of thread length and location on extraction strengths of iliosacral lag screws. *Injury* 1994;25:5–9.
30. Goodell CL: Neurological deficits associated with pelvic fractures. *J Neurosurg* 1966;24:837–842.
31. Pohlemann T, Angst M, Schneider E, et al: Fixation of transforaminal sacrum fractures: A biomechanical study. *J Orthop Trauma* 1993;7:107–117.

    A new technique of plate fixation of unstable sacral fractures is shown to be comparable to standard fixation techniques.
32. Helfet DL, Koval KJ, Hissa EA, et al: Intraoperative somatosensory evoked potential monitoring during acute pelvic fracture surgery. *J Orthop Trauma* 1995;9:28–34.

Annotated Bibliography

Pohlemann T, Bosch U, Gansslen, A, et al: The Hannover experience in management of pelvic fractures. *Clin Orthop* 1994;305:9–80.

The authors advocate accurate reduction and stable fixation of unstable pelvic ring injuries. An aggressive management protocol is outlined according to a strict timetable.

Bone LB, McNamara K, Shine B, et al: Mortality in multiple trauma patients with fractures. *J Trauma* 1994;37:262–265.

Early fracture fixation, including pelvic ring injuries, reduces mortality rates, as demonstrated in this multicentered study of polytrauma patients.

Ganz R, Krushell RJ, Jakob RP, et al: The antishock pelvic clamp. *Clin Orthop* 1991;267:71–78.

The pelvic antishock clamp is introduced. The technique of application is illustrated.

Albert MJ, Miller ME, MacNaughton M, et al: Posterior pelvic fixation using a transiliac 4.5-mm reconstruction plate: A clinical and biomechanical study. *J Orthop Trauma* 1993;7:226–232.

The authors of this combined study advocate posterior transiliac tension band plate fixation. The surgical exposures are outlined. Both infection and complication rates were low. Mechanical evaluations demonstrate comparable stability with sacral bars.

Duwelius PJ, Van Allen M, Bray TJ, et al: Computed tomography-guided fixation of unstable posterior pelvic ring disruptions. *J Orthop Trauma* 1992;6:420–426.

In this clinical series, iliosacral and transiliac screws are inserted using CT guidance in order to stabilize posterior pelvic disruptions. The screws were inserted with the patients in either the lateral or prone position. Reductions were obtained prior to screw insertion using skeletal traction and/or anterior external fixation. This iliosacral screw insertion technique may be indicated for nondisplaced posterior pelvic ring disruptions.

Koury HI, Peschiera JL, Welling RE: Selective use of pelvic roentgenograms in blunt trauma patients. *J Trauma* 1993;34:236–237.

The authors of this series conclude that alert, oriented and reliable patients involved in blunt trauma do not need routine pelvic radiographs if the physical findings are negative.

25
Functional Outcomes of Pelvic Ring Injuries

Following resuscitation, three alternatives exist for the definitive orthopaedic management of pelvic ring injuries: open reduction and internal fixation, nonsurgical treatment, and the intermittent use of external fixation. Each alternative is associated with a significant incidence of long-term disability. Surgical intervention, further, carries a risk of surgical complications. In the absence of a randomized prospective study, the results are not sufficiently disparate that a clear advantage to any one form of treatment emerges.

It seems intuitive that anatomic restoration of any displacement fracture should optimize functional recovery, whereas the scars from surgery to reduce displaced anatomy may add to the stiffness of "fracture disease." Complications, particularly infection, add to residual functional deficits.

The definition of a satisfactory reduction is arbitrary. Long bone deformities are considered acceptable based on a perceived potential for degeneration of surrounding joints. Articular reductions are often considered acceptable at 2 mm, the technical limit of surgical correction. Some other injuries—acromioclavicular joint separations, for example—have superior results if left unreduced because the complications may outweigh the functional benefits of an anatomic restoration.

Despite successful surgical reduction and stabilization of the displaced pelvis, surgical and functional deficits may occur. Surgical results in aggregate are a statistical picture, often arbitrary, of standards for analysis of results. The relative weight of each complication is not measured.[1,2] A satisfactory surgical result is a subjective, physician-generated analysis of the results of perhaps only one injury (out of several possible). Acceptable results can be defined by comparison with a preconceived notion of "the best that can be done." Pelvic fractures in young patients, however, infrequently occur as isolated injuries. Physician-generated analyses of the results in those cases tend to focus on only the pelvic fracture, ignoring other potential sources of disability, whether systemic or orthopaedic.

Acceptable surgical results differ from functional outcomes.[1,2] Functional outcome studies focus on the patients' perception of their ability to function in society, without regard to the source of injury, disease, or disability. Comparisons are made with a statistical analysis of societal norms.[3] Long-term functional outcomes after pelvic ring fractures have not been adequately reported. If a pelvic fracture occurs in a multiply traumatized patient, an excellent "surgical" result might be obviated by not altering the ability of the patient to function in society. Functional outcome studies thereby indirectly weigh the effects of complications and associated injuries. Determining the likelihood of altering long-term societal function is an alternative means of assessing the risk-benefit ratio of pelvic fixation.[1-3]

The natural history of unstable pelvic ring injuries has been described. All studies show residual disabilities. As early as 1948, in Holdsworth's[4] study of Malgaigne fractures, 17 (40%) of 42 patients were noted to have had pain after a minimum follow-up of 2 years (average, 5 years). Half of the patients returned to their previous occupation as heavy laborers. In addition to a standard medical questionnaire, Holdsworth graded functional outcomes by return to previous occupation. Tile,[5] in a more recent retrospective review, studied 218 patients with pelvic fractures. One hundred eighty were treated at community hospitals with no fixation and an additional 100 patients were treated at Tile's institution with intermittent external fixation. Sixty percent of patients with vertically unstable fractures continued to have pain. Patients with stable injuries had fewer complaints of pain, without a statistical analysis. Only 4% had leg length inequality of greater than 2.5 cm, and 3.5% had nonunions. The degree of functional impairment in these patients was not analyzed.

The authors of two studies have reported that patients with residual displacement of more than 1 cm have a higher incidence of late back pain.[6,7] However, in one study, the authors could not demonstrate an increase in the prevalence of back pain over that in the general population.[6]

An increase in severity of complaints of back difficulties as the severity of the initial trauma increased has been reported. None of these patients were treated with posterior internal fixation. Fractures were classified according to Tile's classification.[5] Class A fractures were undisplaced. Patients with class B fractures had sustained "rotational" forces that led to lateral compression fractures (overlap of anterior ring and, often, compression of the anterior sacrum) or "open book" fractures (rupture of the symphysis and anterior sacroiliac ligament). Tile class C fractures were vertically displaced. Only 16% of Tile class A patients—those with undisplaced fractures—complained of back pain, whereas 30% of Tile class B patients and 48% of Tile class C patients complained of residual back pain. The translation of these complaints into functional deficits was not clear, however, as roughly 30% of patients in each category altered their employment and approximately 30% of patients in each group reported altering their sexual practices as a result of pelvic pain.

A lack of correlation has been reported between residual displacement and late symptoms. A retrospective review of 50 pelvic fractures did not show any correlation between reduction and late disability and further noted that patients with more displacement seemed to have less pain. One theory for this is that the "close" reduction allowed irregular joint surfaces to rub, causing pain. The completely displaced, noncontiguous sacroiliac joint might be more comfortable in the long run. In a similar study of long-term results, Majeed[3] found that no correlation existed between final reduction and long-term functional outcome and that symptoms improved for 18 months after trauma. The author stressed the need for prolonged conservative treatment. Other studies have stated that patients with more than 1 cm of residual displacement may have more symptoms of late pain than patients with anatomic reductions.

Although most authors believe that residual displacement may correlate with late pain, the corollary has not been established. Completing a reduction may not alter long-term results. Fractures that are incompletely reduced by excellent and experienced surgeons are likely the worst injuries, accounting for the less than ideal results. The worst functional and anatomic results might reflect the magnitude of the original trauma. It is also possible that a higher incidence of associated injuries could be present, leading to more complaints of pain.

External fixation should not be equated with the natural history of pelvic ring disruptions. The anterior pelvic ring can often be partially reduced and held.[8-10] The posterior pelvic ring can generally be reduced in the immediate posttrauma period, but the ability of an anterior frame to hold posterior instability is inconsistent.[11-14] Some vertically unstable fractures will be held well, but most will slip at least partially. It is this partial reduction and stabilization that separates treatment by external fixation from the natural history of pelvic ring injuries. The authors of one study noted that patients treated by external fixation had less back pain than those treated nonsurgically.[10]

The indications for external fixation include radiographic instability, severe pain, and inability to mobilize in the immediate posttrauma period, proximal femoral or pelvic wounds, and hemodynamic or systemic instability. In a long-term study, external fixators were used on 58% of the study patients. In rotationally (Tile class B) and vertically (Tile class C) unstable fractures, one third of the patients with displaced fractures had residual pain and more than two thirds returned to employment.

Patients who undergo reduction and posterior internal fixation of the pelvic ring are also left with significant residual disabilities.[8,13] Approximately 50% of patients have late pain, the degree of which varies according to the technique of anterior fixation used. Two thirds of patients return to their previous occupation and less than 20% change jobs due to pelvic pain. Less than 20% of patients have residual causalgia, one quarter have residual neurologic injuries, and more than two thirds have pain. More than two thirds of patients have impaired gait, either from the pelvic injury, from neurologic deficits, or from associated injuries. A 4-mm incongruity of the posterior pelvis was accepted, not based on any observed functional results but on an inability to reduce fractures beyond this point.

Complication rates with open techniques have been high; an infection rate of 27% with open posterior techniques[8,11] and infection rates between 18% and 27%, depending on the timing of surgery,[13] have been reported. The L5 nerve root is at risk with anterior fixation.[14] With newer techniques, complication rates have diminished. A 2% infection rate and 5% reduction loss rate have been reported with open techniques. Neurologic injuries and infections are rare with percutaneous screws.

Some patients with displaced fractures (Tile classes B and C) that are left unreduced may function well. It is likewise clear that some patients with Tile class A fractures will have residual difficulties. Theoretically, the best a Tile class C fracture can be made is conversion to an undisplaced, stable Tile class A fracture.

Reports have focused on vertically unstable (Tile class C) and some rotationally unstable (Tile class B) fractures. Little attention has been paid to undisplaced (Tile class A) fractures, because it has been assumed that these patients would do well. Even simple fractures, however, require substantial forces and frequently occur in polytrauma patients. Michael Miranda and Barry L. Riemer, MD undertook a long-term functional outcome study, comparing patients with Tile classes A, B, and C fractures. Although complaints of pain were progressively more frequent from class A to class C, at an average 7.5-year follow-up, Tile class A patients functioned surprisingly poorly. On a physician-generated questionnaire, approximately 30% reported changes in occupation and sexual function due to pelvic pain—a rate similar to that in Tile class B and C patients. On SF-36 Functional Outcome testing, there were no statistical differences between Tile classes A, B, and C, with no notable trend, other than a slight tendency for Tile class C patients to complain of greater pain. There are numerous methodologic flaws in this study, primarily the attrition rate of the population base. These results should be taken only as a pilot study, calling into question whether the initial trauma creates a significant disability that cannot be improved by reduction and stabilization.

External fixation controls the interior pelvic ring but may allow posterior vertical displacement, possibly creating a length discrepancy. Pinning a vertically reduced symphysis pubis and progressively displacing a sacroiliac joint has not been found to affect limb lengths. The hip joint moves anteriorly and laterally, not vertically. Limb length is thought to be more sensitive to anterior fixation, either internal or external, than to posterior pelvic fixation.

Whether patients are treated nonsurgically, by external fixation, or by open reduction and internal fixation, significant residual disabilities will exist. Two thirds of patients return to previous work after open reduction and internal fixation and more than two thirds of patients with vertically unstable fractures treated by external fixation alone return to work, similar to the percentage of those with stable pelvic fractures. A 50% rate of return to heavy labor after nonsurgical treatment for unstable pelvic ring injuries has been reported.[4] These numbers are surprisingly similar. One must question the use of open reduction and internal fixation of even vertically unstable pelvic ring injuries until a valid statistical analysis of these three categories of patients has been performed.

A distinction must be made between science and treatment protocols. The differences between the natural history of pelvic ring injuries and the results of external fixation or open reduction and internal fixation are not sufficiently great that a retrospective historical comparison between series can be reliably performed. The only way to determine the risk-benefit ratio of pelvic fixation is through a randomized prospective study with standardized indications for surgery and outcome vehicles. Both surgical and functional outcome studies are needed.

Annotated References

1. MacKenzie EJ, Cushing BM, Jurkovich GJ, et al: Physical impairment and functional outcomes six months after severe lower extremity fractures. *J Trauma* 1993;34:528-539.

   In a 6-month review of 376 patients with unilateral lower extremity fractures, disability (SIP score) correlated well with extremity impairment (range of motion, muscle strength, and pain). Ability to function, however, correlated poorly.

2. Ware JE (ed): *SF-36 Health Survey: Manual and Interpretation Guide*. Boston, MA, The Health Institute New England Medical Center, 1993.

3. Majeed SA: Grading the outcome of pelvic fractures. *J Bone Joint Surg* 1989;71B:304-306.

4. Holdsworth FW: Dislocation and fracture-dislocation of the pelvis. *J Bone Joint Surg* 1948;30B:461-466.

   In a patient population of heavy laborers, unstable pelvic ring (Malgaigne) fractures were treated by a combination of bed rest, traction, and pelvic slings. In a minimum 2-year follow-up (average follow-up, 5 years), 50% of patients returned to their previous occupations as heavy laborers. Results were better in patients with sacral or iliac fractures than in patients with sacroiliac disruptions. The article is a classic review of the natural history of pelvic ring injuries.

5. Tile M: Pelvic ring fractures: Should they be fixed? *J Bone Joint Surg* 1988;70B:1-12.

   The potential natural history of pelvic ring injuries is presented in this retrospective review of 218 patients treated without the option of internal fixation. Sixty percent complained of pain. Tile's A, B, and C classification is presented, with biomechanical studies and management protocols for each class. In the author's series of 494 pelvic fractures, 19% required stabilization, with internal fixation used in only 5%. Although a protocol for treating each class of injury is presented, functional outcomes are not documented.

6. Henderson RC: The long-term results of nonoperatively treated major pelvic disruptions. *J Orthop Trauma* 1989;3:41-47.

   Twenty-six patients were reevaluated an average of 8 years after trauma. All fractures had been treated nonsurgically. Fifty percent had low back pain, 46% had neurologic complaints, 32% had gait abnormalities, and 38% had altered their employment. A correlation was seen between residual deformity and outcomes.

7. Semba RT, Yasukawa K, Gustilo RB: Critical analysis of results of 53 Malgaigne fractures of the pelvis. *J Trauma* 1983;23:535-537.

8. Kellam JF: The role of external fixation in pelvic disruptions. *Clin Orthop* 1989;241:66-82.

9. Riemer BL, Butterfield SL, Diamond DL, et al: Acute mortality associated with injuries to the pelvic ring: The role of early patient mobilization and external fixation. *J Trauma* 1993;35:671-677.

10. Slatis P, Karaharju EO: External fixation of unstable pelvic fractures: Experiences in 22 patients treated with a trapezoid compression frame. *Clin Orthop* 1980;151:73-80.

    In an early article on the results of external fixation, 15 patients had excellent reductions (0 to 5 mm), five had fair reductions (5 to 10 mm), and two had poor reductions (greater than 10 mm). Ten percent had gait abnormalities and 5% had pain. Fifty-four percent returned to work. These results were superior to those previously reported with nonoperative treatment.

11. Kellam JF, McMurtry RY, Paley D, et al: The unstable pelvic fracture: Operative treatment. *Orthop Clin North Am* 1987;18:25-41.

    The authors present indications and techniques for fixation of several types of pelvic fractures. Of 22 patients with unstable pelvic fractures that had been treated by open reduction and external fixation, 60% had a "satisfactory" outcome, being able to return to work. A 25% infection rate was noted, as well as a "significant problem" with failure of reduction and loss of fixation with the posterior approach to the sacroiliac joint.

12. Matta JM, Saucedo T: Internal fixation of pelvic ring fractures. *Clin Orthop* 1989;242:83-97.

13. Goldstein A, Phillips T, Sclafani SJ, et al: Early open reduction and internal fixation of the disrupted pelvic ring. *J Trauma* 1986;26:325-333.

14. Simpson LA, Waddell JP, Leighton RK, et al: Anterior approach and stabilization of the disrupted sacroiliac joint. *J Trauma* 1987;27:1332-1339.

26

Posterior Wall, Posterior Column, and Transverse Acetabular Fractures: Surgical Indications and Techniques

Introduction

Posterior wall, posterior column, and transverse acetabular fractures are among the elementary fracture types defined by Letournel. Fractures of the posterior wall of the acetabulum involve separation of a segment of the posterior articular surface, without injury to most of the posterior column (Fig. 1, *left*). A posterior dislocation usually accompanies the fracture. Fractures of the posterior wall occur more frequently than any other acetabular fracture. They account for 15% to 28% of all acetabular fractures, with smaller percentages of posterior wall fractures represented in the practices of highly specialized pelvic surgeons.[1-8]

Posterior column acetabular fractures involve detachment of the entire posterior column in one fragment (Fig. 1, *center*). The posterior column is driven medially and posteriorly and is most often accompanied by the femoral head, which is centrally dislocated. Posterior column fractures make up less than 5% of acetabular fractures in most large series.[2-8]

Transverse fractures of the acetabulum are created by a single fracture line that divides the innominate bone into two segments (Fig. 1, *right*). Transverse fractures transversely divide both the anterior and posterior column into two parts. The upper and lower sections of the divided columns remain intact with respect to each other, however. The fracture line transects a single plane, which may be oriented either horizontally or obliquely. In contrast to both column acetabular fractures, all types of transverse fractures contain an unfractured segment of roof that remains attached to the iliac wing fragment. Transverse fractures make up 5% to 19% of the acetabular fractures in most large series.[2-9]

Progress in the management of these groups of fractures has been marked by a better understanding of the specific requirements for preoperative imaging and better definition of the role of intraoperative nerve monitoring, especially with posterior approaches to the acetabulum. More stable forms of fixation have been proposed and tested, particularly for posterior wall fractures. Better recognition of the problems associated with posterior approaches to the acetabulum have led to an expanding role for anterior approaches to the acetabulum, especially for high transverse acetabular fractures. Finally, compromised results with delayed or revision surgery for each of these fracture types have been documented, further emphasizing the importance of early, accurate surgical management of even the most straightforward acetabular fractures. These developments are the focus of this chapter.

Evaluation of Injury

The general evaluation of patients with pelvic and acetabular fractures is described in Chapter 23. In addition to those general considerations, the fractures described in this chapter demand a particularly thorough physical examination to evaluate the preoperative status of the sciatic nerve. The sciatic nerve can be damaged by direct compression with posterior wall fractures and associated posterior hip dislocations, and by entrapment of the nerve in the fracture site with posterior column and transverse fractures that occur near the greater sciatic notch. Patients with preoperative nerve injuries are more likely to have measurable intraoperative changes on somatosensory-evoked potential (SSEP) nerve monitoring than patients with no nerve damage. More important, severe involvement of the peroneal component of the sciatic nerve correlates closely with poor functional recovery. A thorough preoperative assessment will help to avoid confusion in cases where a nerve palsy is noted postoperatively.

In one study of patients with delayed diagnoses of posteriorly dislocated hips, the delay may be avoidable by careful reading of even a single anteroposterior radiograph of the pelvis which shows superior displacement of the femoral head on the intact acetabular roof.[10] The diagnosis is more obvious, however, with oblique views and computed tomography (CT). Prompt diagnosis and treatment of poste-

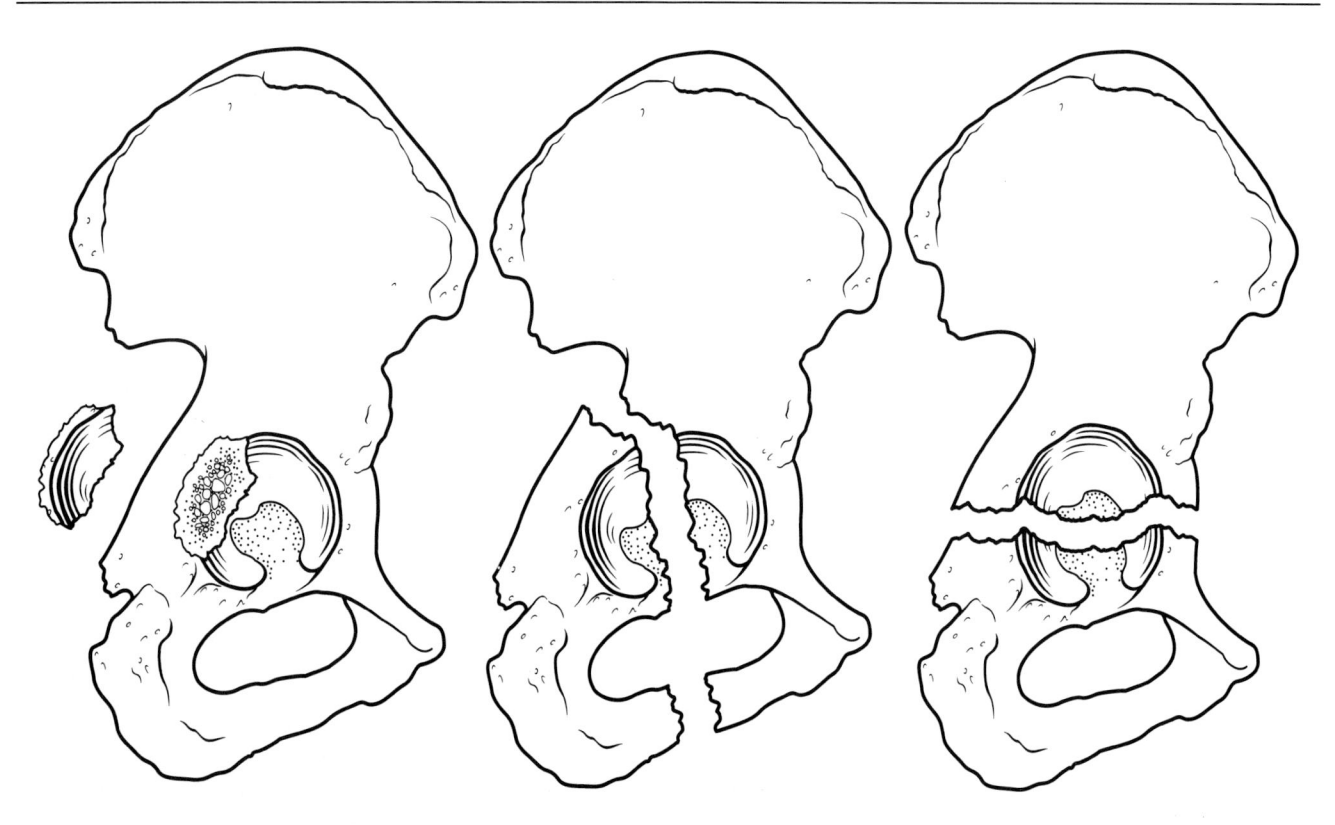

Fig. 1 **Left,** Posterior wall acetabular fracture. **Center,** Posterior column acetabular fracture. **Right,** Transverse acetabular fracture.

rior hip dislocations will lead to a decreased incidence of osteonecrosis of the femoral head, nerve palsy, and femoral head articular cartilage damage in these patients.[10]

Treatment and Results

Posterior Wall Fractures

Unlike most types of acetabular fractures, posterior wall acetabular fractures are commonly treated by surgeons who operate on acetabular fractures only occasionally. Although treatment of these fractures is frequently straightforward, reduction and fixation can be demanding. Failure to recognize the more complex presentations of these fractures and technical errors made at surgery can lead to poor outcomes and failure of treatment.

Preoperative evaluation of posterior wall fractures should include CT, which allows an assessment of the size and degree of comminution of posterior wall fractures and clearly demonstrates the presence of intra-articular osteochondral fragments. Laboratory studies of cadaver specimens have demonstrated that posterior wall fractures involving more than 50% of the posterior wall result in instability, whereas posterior wall fractures involving less than 25% of the acetabulum seldom affect joint stability in the absence of marginal impaction.[11] CT studies in patients with posterior wall acetabular fractures have demonstrated similar parameters of stability.[12] Nonsurgical management, generally consisting of 3 months of nonweightbearing or toe-touch weightbearing ambulation, may be appropriate for these stable fractures with no marginal impaction component and no intra-articular fracture fragments.

CT is especially valuable in the recognition of marginal impression fractures accompanying posterior wall fractures. The marginal impaction fracture is defined as rotated, impacted, osteocartilaginous fragments of the posteromedial acetabulum that occur in association with a posterior fracture dislocation of the hip (Fig. 2). Marginal impaction fractures occur in approximately 20% to 25% of all posterior wall acetabular fractures. Displacement of these fracture fragments create incongruity of the posterior acetabular articular surface and the potential for hip joint instability. Only by freeing these fragments and restoring them to proper alignment can the complete articular surface be reconstituted.[13]

Posterior wall fractures requiring surgical repair are exposed using a Kocher-Langenbeck approach. Patients are most commonly placed in the lateral position on a standard operating table. Because iatrogenic nerve injury is most frequently associated with fractures requiring a posterior approach, some surgeons advocate the routine use of SSEP monitoring with surgical repair of these

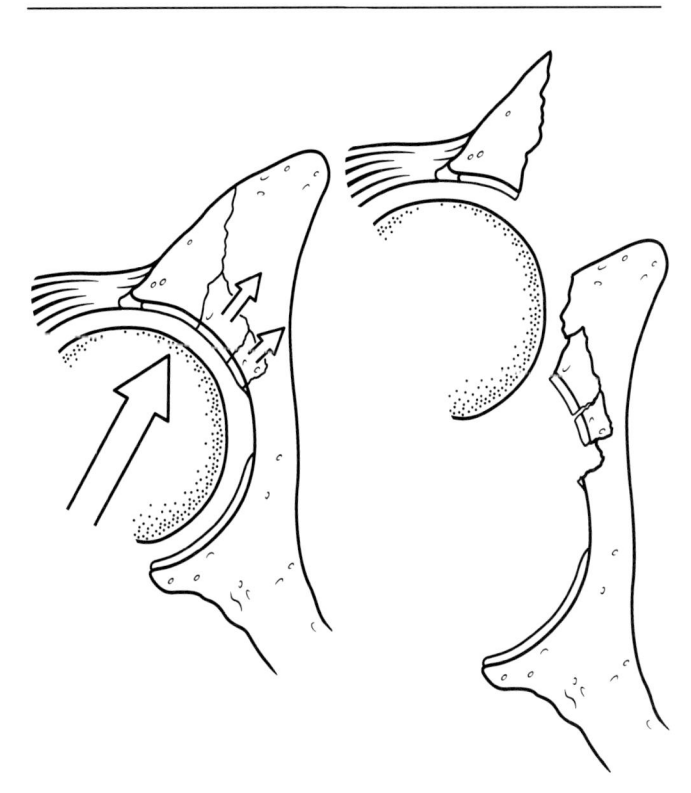

Fig. 2 Marginal impaction fracture. **Left,** The femoral head is directed posteriorly, creating a comminuted posterior wall fracture. The small arrows indicate the path of the osteochondral fragments, which will be crushed and remain attached to the acetabulum. **Right,** The femoral head has dislocated posteriorly. Part of the posterior wall remains attached to the hip capsule and has been displaced posteriorly and superiorly. The osteochondral fragments have been crushed and the congruity of the remaining acetabulum has been lost.

fractures. Removal of intra-articular fragments and excision of the torn ligamentum teres are facilitated by dislocating the femoral head posteriorly. Alternatively, a distraction instrument may be applied between the supra-acetabular area and the femur to enhance the exposure. The femoral head is then reduced, and distraction is released. If present, impacted segments of the articular surface should next be elevated using a small elevator, leaving as much cancellous bone as possible beneath the subchondral bone of the impacted fragment. Autogenous cancellous bone graft is placed in the resulting bone defect, with the greater trochanter as the customary source of bone graft for this application.[13]

Care should be taken to preserve the vascular supply to posterior wall fragments. Stripping of 2 to 3 mm at the fracture margins is all that is required to achieve an anatomic reduction while avoiding devascularization of the fragments. Preservation of soft-tissue attachments in comminuted fractures not only seems to prevent osteonecrosis of the posterior wall fragments, but frequently facilitates reduction of these fragments. Fracture fragments should be reduced in their anatomic position, with the femoral head used as a template to accurately reduce all retroacetabular fragments.

Posterior wall fractures are stabilized with a buttress plate spanning from the inferior iliac wing to the superior pole of the ischium. The plate is curved to parallel the rim of the acetabulum. Fixation with one or more lag screws through posterior wall fragments can supplement the buttress plate and may help maintain reduction of the fracture if the screws are placed prior to plate application. Care should be taken to direct the screws away from the joint. Auscultation with a sterile stethoscope has been used to ensure that screws are not placed into the joint when these fractures are repaired.[14] Intraoperative image intensification can also be used to prevent screw violation of the joint.

Comminution of posterior wall fractures may be associated with an increased rate of fixation failure. For transversely comminuted fractures, screws alone have been shown in laboratory testing to provide significantly less stability than a screw–buttress plate combination. Because they provide a minimal safety margin, interfragmentary screws should only be used for supplementary stabilization of comminuted posterior wall fractures when a buttress plate is also used. If the fracture comminution is concentric with the rim of the acetabulum, screw fixation cannot safely augment plate fixation without penetration of the articular surface. In these cases, spring plates can augment buttress plate fixation, forming a retaining wall behind the comminuted fracture fragments. Spring plates can be fashioned from thin one-third tubular plates, secured to the posterior ilium with a single screw, and buttressed into position using a pelvic reconstruction plate (Fig. 3). The application of spring plates has been shown in laboratory testing to significantly increase the stability achieved with buttress plate fixation alone.[15]

As with all acetabular fracture types, stable and accurate reduction of posterior wall fractures is the most important prerequisite for a good result. Unstable posterior wall fractures treated nonsurgically have been shown to proceed rapidly to poor results in approximately 80% of cases. Late surgical management results in a much lower percentage of good results than early, prompt surgical management, underscoring the need for early intervention and surgical management of unstable or displaced fractures.

Of the fractures discussed in this chapter, surgical treatment of posterior wall fractures has resulted in the highest percentage of perfect reduction. Letournel and Judet[4] reported 94% perfectly reduced posterior wall fractures and 98% nearly perfectly reduced posterior wall fractures. Other experienced acetabular fracture surgeons have reported variable results, ranging from 50% to 98% perfect reductions, but most series report anatomic reductions in more than 90% of surgically treated fractures.[1–3,5,7,8] As isolated fractures, posterior wall fractures seem to offer a slightly better chance for a satisfactory outcome than most fracture types if surgical treatment is instituted in timely fashion. In contrast to the high percentage of good results following early surgical management of these fractures, the authors of one study reported that only 18 of 35 posterior wall fractures treated

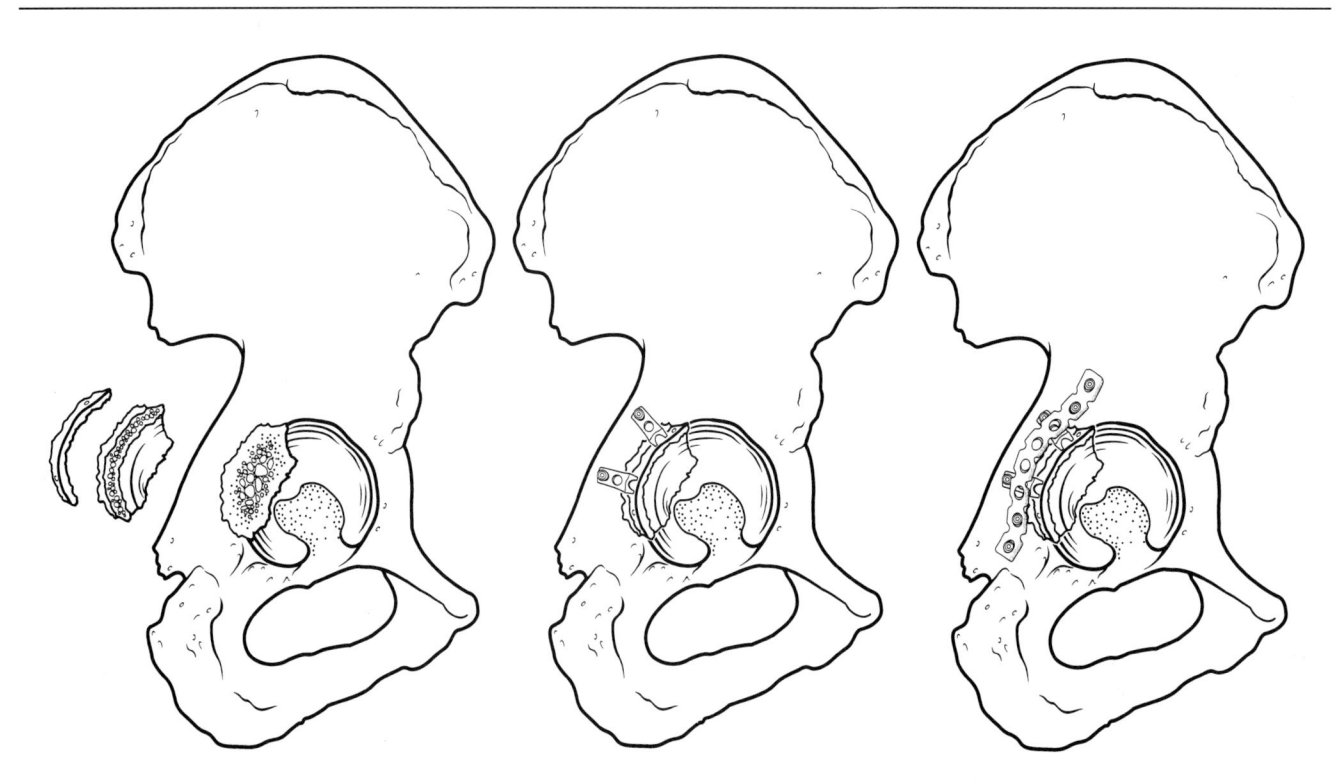

Fig. 3 Fixation of a comminuted posterior wall fracture with spring plates. **Left,** Concentrically comminuted posterior wall fracture. This fracture cannot be fixed with interfragmentary screw fixation without intra-articular penetration. **Center,** The fracture has been reduced and partially stabilized with spring plates. A thin tubular plate is flattened and a notch is cut through one of the end holes, creating prongs that may be bent over into the comminuted fragment. Care should be taken to avoid penetration of the joint through the labrum. Each spring plate is held in place with a single screw situated posterior to the anticipated buttress plate placement. **Right,** A buttress plate has been contoured and placed over the spring plates, forming a retaining wall behind the fracture fragments.

more than 3 weeks after fracture occurrence had good or excellent results.[16] Repeated surgery for malreduced posterior wall fractures results in an even lower percentage of good or excellent results. Of 22 patients with posterior wall acetabular fractures that were malreduced, only 45% had good or excellent results after revision surgery.[17] Although late surgical repair and repeated surgery to achieve acceptable stable reductions can result in successful salvage in many cases, delayed treatment and initial malreduction of these fractures lead to an appreciably lower percentage of good results, compared to results achieved with early intervention with stable fixation.

Posterior Column Fractures

Posterior column fractures with significant displacement are treated surgically. Posterior column fractures are exposed using the Kocher-Langenbeck approach. Patients may be placed in the lateral position. The prone position has been advocated by most surgeons, however, to improve visualization of the fracture and to overcome the effect of gravity redisplacing the fracture. After fracture lines are identified, bone fragments and debris are removed from the fracture site. Fracture displacement is rotational, along the longitudinal axis of the posterior column. An initial reduction of the fracture is achieved with a lever, frequently a 5- to 6-mm threaded pin, placed into the ischial tuberosity. This lever is used to derotate the ischial tuberosity into a more nearly anatomic position. After an approximate reduction has been achieved, a standard pelvic reduction forceps may be used with a two-screw technique to achieve final fracture reduction. The standard pelvic reduction forceps offers the advantage of providing better rotational and translational control than other reduction forceps. Farabeuf forceps may work better if adequate space for plate placement cannot be achieved in the presence of more bulky instruments. The adequacy of reduction is assessed by direct visualization of the joint as distraction is applied, and by palpation of the quadrilateral surface. Direct visualization of part of the quadrilateral surface can also be used to assess the adequacy of reduction when a prone position is utilized. Fixation is usually achieved with a lag screw and is augmented with placement of a curved plate on the retroacetabular surface.

As with posterior wall acetabular fractures, stable and accurate reduction of posterior column fractures is the most important prerequisite for a good result. Displaced posterior column fractures treated nonoperatively proceed rapidly to poor results in approximately 80% of patients. Late surgical management is expected to result in a lower percentage of good results than early, prompt surgical management, underscoring the need for early intervention and surgical management of unstable or displaced fractures. On the other hand, one group of experienced acetabular fracture surgeons reported good or excellent results in eight of nine patients with posterior column fractures who were treated with delayed surgery, demonstrating the utility of skilled surgical treatment even when surgery is delayed.[16]

In a series by Letournel and Judet,[4] perfect reductions were achieved in 77% of posterior column fractures and nearly perfect reductions in 90%. Other experienced acetabular fracture surgeons have reported similar results, with lower percentages of acceptable reductions associated with less surgical experience. Satisfactory clinical results can be anticipated in 75% to 80% of all patients with displaced posterior column acetabular fractures treated surgically.[2,3,7,8]

Transverse Fractures

The approach to transverse fractures varies according to the level and obliquity of the transverse fracture line. Most transverse fractures are exposed with a Kocher-Langenbeck approach. The lateral position on a standard operating table can be used for these fractures. The prone position on a standard operating table or on a Judet table has been advocated by many surgeons, however, to improve visualization of the fracture and to minimize the effect of gravity redisplacing the fracture.[4,7] Reduction of the transverse fracture is achieved in a manner similar to posterior column fracture reduction, with a lever placed into the ischial tuberosity to derotate the ischiopubic segment into a more nearly anatomic position. Provisional fixation of the fracture may be achieved using a two-screw technique with a standard pelvic reduction forceps or with Farabeuf forceps, as described above for posterior column fractures. In some cases, provisional reduction may be achieved with one end of an offset pointed reduction forceps placed through the greater sciatic notch onto the intrapelvic surface of the ischiopubic segment and the other end of forceps placed on the retroacetabular surface superior to the fracture line. The adequacy of reduction of the anterior column is assessed by digital palpation of the pelvic brim and quadrilateral surface.

Fixation of the anterior column component of transverse fractures is achieved with a lag screw directed from the retroacetabular surface toward the anterior column. In placing this screw, care must be taken to avoid joint penetration while maintaining the inferomedial tip of the screw within the pubis. Johnson and associates[18] have recommended that the entry point for this screw be within a narrow (2-cm) zone located 3 cm above the superior edge of the acetabulum (Fig. 4). Intraoperative radiographic confirmation of appropriate screw placement may help to avoid malposition of this screw. A plate placed along the retroacetabular surface completes the fixation.

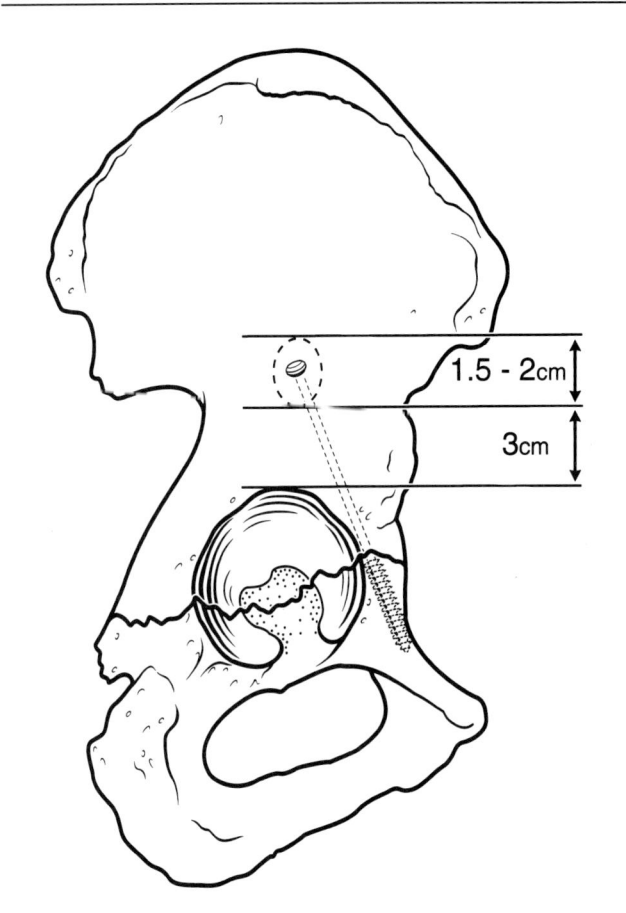

Fig. 4 An anterior to posterior lag screw for fixation of transverse fractures. A narrow zone of entry allows proper screw placement.

More proximal transverse fractures (transtectal fractures) may require a different approach. Precise reduction of the anterior column component of these fractures through the Kocher-Langenbeck approach is more difficult than reduction of more distal (juxtatectal or infratectal) fractures. If the fracture line is high on the anterior column and low on the posterior column, the fracture may be treated with the patient in a supine position through an ilioinguinal approach. Reduction can be achieved with pointed reduction forceps, or with a two-screw technique and Farabeuf forceps (Fig. 5). Alternately, high transverse fractures are well visualized and reduced through an extensile approach, using either an extended iliofemoral or triradiate approach. Although better visualization of the fracture reduction is possible through extensile approaches, problems associated with ectopic bone formation and prolonged rehabilitation reduce the appeal of these approaches when other alternatives are available. Some surgeons have also advocated a dual approach using simultaneous anterior and posterior surgical incisions for treatment of transtectal transverse fractures.[19] All of the patients with transverse fractures included in one recently published series required anterior as well as posterior approaches to achieve anatomic

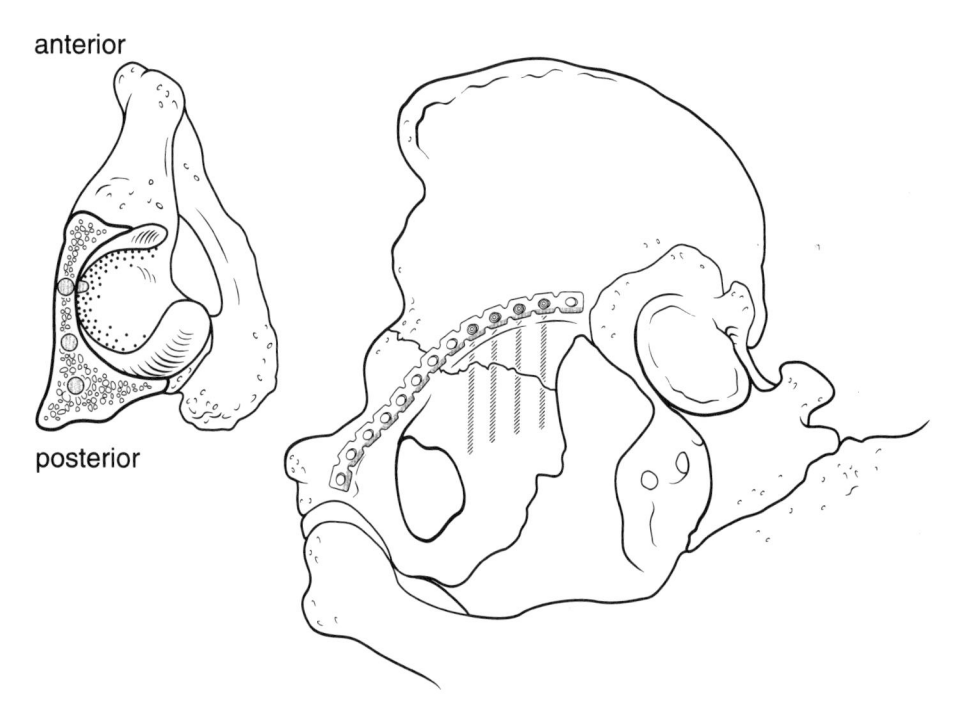

Fig. 5 Placement of anterior to posterior screws through a plate for fixation of a transverse fracture exposed through an ilioinguinal approach. Screws placed closer to the ischial spine are less likely to result in inadvertent intra-articular placement (see inset). The margin for error in placement of screws in the quadrilateral surface medial to the acetabulum is small.

reductions.[2] The dual approach appears to be most useful when an acceptable reduction of both columns of the transverse fracture is anticipated but cannot be achieved through a single posterior approach. When simultaneous anterior and posterior approaches to transverse acetabular fractures are used, care must be taken during the first part of the procedure to avoid placement of screws that may malreduce or block precise reduction of the second unreduced column of the fracture.

Stable and accurate reduction of transverse fractures is the most important prerequisite for a good result. Nonsurgical management of transverse fractures with displacement of more than 5 mm has been associated with a high rate of osteoarthritis appearing within months to years of fracture occurrence.

Letournel and Judet[4] reported a 77% rate of perfectly reduced transverse fractures, with nearly perfect reductions achieved overall in 90% of patients with transverse acetabular fractures. Other centers with experienced acetabular fracture surgeons that have published outcomes specific to fracture pattern have reported similar results.[5,7,9] Among the small number of cases of transverse fractures treated by highly experienced acetabular surgeons with open reduction and internal fixation using an ilioinguinal approach only, acceptable reductions have been reported in 83%.[9,20]

Late surgical management of transverse acetabular fractures results in a much lower percentage of good results than early prompt surgical management. Johnson and associates[16] reported that only nine (69%) of 13 transverse fractures treated late had good or excellent results. The decrease in good to excellent results resulted from several factors, including cartilage damage, femoral head erosion, and necrosis. The utility of reoperation by an experienced acetabular fracture surgeon in salvaging an acceptable result is clear, even if these results are less favorable than those achieved with earlier intervention. This finding underscores the need for early intervention and surgical management of unstable or displaced fractures.

Abductor muscle weakness is a common impediment to good early function following fractures exposed by posterior or extensile approaches. Abductor weakness following the Kocher-Langenbeck approach has been shown to be more profound in patients treated for transverse fractures than in patients treated for posterior wall fractures. Retention of abductor strength is highly correlated with hip outcome scores.[21]

Complications

Surgical wound infections, iatrogenic nerve palsy, ectopic bone formation, thromboembolism, osteonecrosis, and posttraumatic arthritis are the most common serious complications associated with all acetabular fractures, including the fractures described in this chapter. These complications are reviewed in general in Chapter 29. The current discussion focuses on problems that seem to be aggravated by the posterior hip dislocations associated with posterior wall fractures and by the posterolateral or extensile surgical approaches most commonly used to repair posterior wall, posterior column, and transverse acetabular fractures.

Significant ectopic bone formation results from a combination of initial trauma to the gluteal muscle mass and surgical exposure of the lateral surface of the pelvis. Extensile (extended iliofemoral or triradiate) approaches are associated with the highest incidence of ectopic bone formation, whereas the ilioinguinal approach is rarely associated with this complication. Many of the fractures described in this chapter require a posterolateral or extensile approach in order to achieve acceptable fracture reduction. When these approaches must be used, local measures may be helpful in reducing the incidence of heterotopic ossification. Debridement of devitalized muscle, particularly the gluteus minimus, has been shown to limit the extent of ectopic bone formation.

Some recent series have demonstrated that good reductions of high (transtectal) transverse fractures can be achieved by experienced surgeons through an ilioinguinal approach.[6,7,9,20] Choosing an ilioinguinal approach, when possible, reduces the incidence of ectopic bone formation. Regardless of the type of surgical approach, indomethacin and irradiation may be used to reduce the incidence of ectopic ossification associated with the surgical management of acetabular fractures. Low-dose irradiation (10 to 20 Gy) has been shown in small series of patients to be an effective method of decreasing the incidence of ectopic ossification after surgical treatment with an extensile approach, without complications attributed to the radiation treatment. The long-term effects of this radiation, even with low dosages and the use of selective portals, are unknown. For this reason, many centers limit the use of radiation treatment to older patients with a previous history of ectopic ossification. Indomethacin has also been demonstrated to be effective in preventing the development of heterotopic ossification in association with the surgical treatment of acetabular fractures.[22,23] Reported dosages have varied from 25 mg to 75 mg of indomethacin three times per day. The use of indomethacin to decrease the incidence of heterotopic ossification appears to be well supported and may have less potential for iatrogenic complications than prophylactic radiation therapy.

Sciatic nerve palsy, a potentially devastating complication of acetabular fracture surgery, occurs as an iatrogenic problem most frequently in posterior column, posterior wall, and transverse acetabular fractures. The sciatic nerve is most susceptible to compression or to entrapment in the fracture site with these fracture patterns. Dense impairment of the peroneal component of the sciatic nerve correlates closely with poor functional recovery. A permanent sciatic nerve palsy is severely limiting, but even transient sciatic nerve palsies are troublesome and can cause considerable and lengthy disability.[24] Any means of preventing or limiting damage to the sciatic nerve is therefore highly desirable.

Several centers have reported a decrease in the frequency of sciatic nerve palsy in patients who are monitored with intraoperative SSEP. When SSEP changes of decreased amplitude or increased latency are recorded, decreasing traction on the limb and relaxing all retraction in the vicinity of the nerve until the amplitude and latency return to normal baseline values has been reported to significantly reduce the incidence of iatrogenic sciatic and peroneal neurapraxia.[25,26] If the technique is available, therefore, the use of SSEP recording as an adjunctive monitoring tool would seem to be useful in patients with posterior fracture patterns and in patients with preoperative nerve involvement.

Osteonecrosis of the femoral head most frequently occurs as a late complication of acetabular fractures when the fracture is associated with a posterior hip dislocation, commonly found with any of the three fracture types discussed in this chapter. In one series, 30% of patients with posterior wall fractures developed this complication, all in association with delayed closed hip reductions.[1] Prompt reduction of the dislocated hip prior to surgical management of the posterior wall fracture is essential to limiting the incidence of this complication.[1,10]

Although uncommon, vascular injury is a dramatic complication that can arise from internal fixation of acetabular fractures. Injuries to the superior gluteal vessels have been reported to occur with posterior surgical approaches, and to the internal iliac and superficial femoral vessels with the ilioinguinal approach. Malposition of a posterior to anterior lag screw has also been reported to result in penetration of the superior pubic ramus at a point adjacent to the superficial femoral artery, with extrinsic compression of this vessel. Adherence to the guidelines described earlier and intraoperative radiographic confirmation of correct screw placement should prevent this complication.[18]

Conclusion

Progress in the management of fractures of the acetabulum with posterior wall, posterior column, and transverse patterns has been marked by a better understanding of the specific requirements for preoperative imaging and by better definition of the role of intraoperative nerve monitoring, especially with posterior approaches to the acetabulum. More stable forms of fixation have been proposed and tested, particularly for posterior wall fractures. Better recognition of the problems associated with posterior approaches to the acetabulum have led to an expanding role for anterior approaches to the acetabulum, especially for high transverse acetabular fractures. Documentation of compromised results with delayed or revision surgery for each of these fracture types further emphasizes the importance of early, accurate operative management of even the most straightforward acetabular fractures.

Annotated References

1. Aho AJ, Isberg UK, Katevuo VK: Acetabular posterior wall fracture: 38 cases followed for 5 years. *Acta Orthop Scand* 1986;57:101–105.

   Results were good in 17 of 18 patients with no sciatic nerve injury who were treated nonsurgically with successful closed manual reduction of the femoral head dislocation. Of the 20 patients who required surgical intervention because of persistent instability, six had poor results due to femoral head necrosis.

2. de Ridder VA, de Lange S, Kingma L, et al: Results of 75 consecutive patients with an acetabular fracture. *Clin Orthop* 1994;305:53–57.

3. Kiebaish AS, Roy A, Rennie W: Displaced acetabular fractures: Long-term follow-up. *J Trauma* 1991;31:1539-1542.

4. Letournel E, Judet R (eds): *Fractures of the Acetabulum*, ed 2. Berlin, Germany, Springer-Verlag, 1993.

   The authors provide a thorough review of acetabular fracture evaluation and treatment. Radiographic and anatomic descriptions of each of the three fracture types discussed in this chapter are provided, along with surgical approaches and management. A large series of fractures with long-term follow-up is presented in detail. Good results correlated with accurate fracture reduction.

5. Matta JM: Operative treatment of acetabular fractures through the ilioinguinal approach: A 10-year perspective. *Clin Orthop* 1994;305:10–19.

   Twenty of the 422 patients treated in this series had transverse fractures. The ilioinguinal approach was used in 14 of these patients. Successful reduction of transverse fractures can be achieved by an experienced acetabular surgeon while limiting the risks of ectopic ossification and sciatic nerve palsy associated with posterior surgical approaches.

6. Matta JM, Merritt PO: Displaced acetabular fractures. *Clin Orthop* 1988;230:83–97.

   A prospective study of the first 121 displaced acetabular fractures in this series. The rate of satisfactory reduction improved gradually over the first 50 cases in this series, reflecting a well-documented surgical learning curve. Overall, clinical results were satisfactory in 80% of patients.

7. Mayo KA: Open reduction and internal fixation of fractures of the acetabulum: Results in 163 fractures. *Clin Orthop* 1994;305:31–37.

8. Pantazopoulos T, Mousafiris C: Surgical treatment of central acetabular fractures. *Clin Orthop* 1989;246:57–64.

9. Helfet DL, Schmeling GJ: Management of complex acetabular fractures through single nonextensile exposures. *Clin Orthop* 1994;305:58–68.

10. Roffi RP, Matta JM: Unrecognized posterior dislocation of the hip associated with transverse and T-type fractures of the acetabulum. *J Orthop Trauma* 1993;7:23–27.

    The authors describe five patients with displaced transverse or T-type fractures who were transferred with unrecognized posterior dislocation of the hip. Although the dislocation was recognizable on the anteroposterior pelvic radiograph, oblique views and CT made the diagnosis obvious. The authors stress that appropriate initial radiographic evaluation is imperative.

11. Vailas JC, Hurwitz S, Wiesel SW: Posterior acetabular fracture-dislocations: Fragment size, joint capsule, and stability. *J Trauma* 1989;29:1494–1496.

12. Calkins MS, Zych G, Latta L, et al: Computed tomography evaluation of stability in posterior fracture dislocation of the hip. *Clin Orthop* 1988;227:152–163.

    CT measurements of the percentage of remaining posterior acetabulum in posterior fracture dislocations of the hip were evaluated to determine the stability of the hip. All hips with less than 34% of the posterior acetabulum remaining were unstable, whereas hips with more than 55% of the posterior acetabulum remaining were stable.

13. Brumback RJ, Holt ES, McBride MS, et al: Acetabular depression fracture accompanying posterior fracture dislocation of the hip. *J Orthop Trauma* 1990;4:42–48.

    The authors provide a retrospective review of 75 posterior fracture dislocations of the hip. Marginal impaction fractures were found in 17 cases (23%). The diagnosis could be made preoperatively from CT scans. The assessment, protocols, surgical management, and postoperative management are discussed.

14. Anglen JO, DiPasquale T: The reliability of detecting screw penetration of the acetabulum by interoperative auscultation. *J Orthop Trauma* 1994;8:404–408.

15. Goulet JA, Rouleau JP, Mason DJ, et al: Comminuted fractures of the posterior wall of the acetabulum: A biomechanical evaluation of fixation methods. *J Bone Joint Surg* 1994;76A:1457–1463.

    This biomechanical study supports clinical observations that, for transversely comminuted fractures, fixation with a buttress plate is stronger than fixation with screws alone. Supplementary fixation with spring plates was also shown to help prevent redisplacement of concentrically comminuted fractures of the posterior wall of the acetabulum.

16. Johnson EE, Matta JM, Mast JW, et al: Delayed reconstruction of acetabular fractures 21–120 days following injury. *Clin Orthop* 1994;305:20–30.

    Delayed reconstruction of acetabular fractures was undertaken between 21 and 120 days following injury in 207 patients. Good to excellent results were achieved in 89% of posterior column fractures and in 69% of transverse fractures, but in only 51% of posterior wall fractures. Surgical reconstruction of acetabular fractures following this delay is difficult and requires considerable experience. The higher rate of failure associated with delayed surgical management, especially for posterior wall fractures, is further evidence of the importance of early recognition and surgical management of these fractures.

17. Mayo KA, Letournel E, Matta JM, et al: Surgical revision of malreduced acetabular fractures. *Clin Orthop* 1994;305:47–52.

    Reoperation in 64 patients with malreduction of acetabular fractures was evaluated in this multicenter study. Twenty-two patients had posterior wall fractures, and 45% of this group achieved good or excellent results. Although these results compare unfavorably to results in large series of singly operated acute fractures, early recognition and repeat surgical intervention seem warranted when malreduction of posterior wall fractures is recognized.

18. Johnson EE, Eckardt JJ, Letournel E: Extrinsic femoral artery occlusion following internal fixation of an acetabular fracture: A case report. *Clin Orthop* 1987;217:209-213.

    One case is reported in which a posterior to anterior lag screw was malpositioned, leading to penetration of the superior pubic ramus adjacent to the superficial femoral artery. Extrinsic compression of the vessel was relieved by removal of the screw. Guidelines for screw placement are suggested.

19. Routt ML Jr, Swiontkowski MF: Operative treatment of complex acetabular fractures: Combined anterior and posterior exposures during the same procedure. *J Bone Joint Surg* 1990;72A:897-904.

    Twenty-four patients were treated with combined anterior and posterior approaches. Eleven had transverse fractures alone or associated with other fracture types. An anatomic reduction was achieved in 10 of the 11 fractures. Dual approaches offer an alternative to extensile approaches for reduction and fixation of transverse acetabular fractures in which anatomic reduction cannot be achieved by one approach alone.

20. Letournel E: The treatment of acetabular fractures through the ilioinguinal approach. *Clin Orthop* 1993;292:62-76.

21. Dickinson WH, Duwelius PJ, Colville MR: Muscle strength testing following surgery for acetabular fractures. *J Orthop Trauma* 1993;7:39-46.

    A retrospective clinical analysis of muscle strength performed on 30 patients who were treated surgically for acetabular fractures. The average deficit in abduction strength was 50%. The loss of abduction strength was significantly greater for patients operated on through a Kocher-Langenbeck approach.

22. McLaren AC: Prophylaxis with indomethacin for heterotopic bone after open reduction of fractures of the acetabulum. *J Bone Joint Surg* 1990;72A:245-247.

    Forty-four fractures of the acetabulum requiring dissection through the gluteal muscles were reviewed radiographically to record the development of ectopic bone. Brooker class II ectopic ossification was decreased from 50% to 5.5% in the patients who were treated with indomethacin.

23. Moed BR, Maxey JW: The effect of indomethacin on heterotopic ossification following acetabular fracture surgery. *J Orthop Trauma* 1993;7:33-38.

    Sixty-six fractures of the acetabulum requiring dissection through the gluteal muscles were reviewed radiographically to record the development of ectopic bone. The incidence of severe heterotopic ossification (Brooker class III and class IV) was significantly reduced in the patients given indomethacin.

24. Fassler PR, Swiontkowski MF, Kilroy AW, et al: Injury of the sciatic nerve associated with acetabular fracture. *J Bone Joint Surg* 1993;75A:1157-1166.

    Fourteen patients, three with iatrogenic injuries, were studied. Seven patients who had an injury of both the tibial and peroneal components of the sciatic nerve recovered complete or nearly complete motor and sensory function of the tibial component. Mild involvement of the peroneal nerve had a favorable prognosis, whereas patients with severe injury of the peroneal component did not recover good function. Clinical data and functional outcomes are correlated with electromyographic abnormalities.

25. Calder HB, Mast J, Johnstone C: Intraoperative evoked potential monitoring in acetabular surgery. *Clin Orthop* 1994;305:160-167.

26. Helfet DL, Hissa EA, Sergay S, et al: Somatosensory evoked potential monitoring in the surgical management of acute acetabular fractures. *J Orthop Trauma* 1991;5:161-166.

    Fifty patients underwent intraoperative somatosensory-evoked potential (SSEP) monitoring in association with acetabular fracture surgery. Iatrogenic sciatic or peroneal neurapraxia occurred in one patient (2%), a rate that compares favorably to the 5% to 20% rate reported in the literature. Intraoperative SSEP changes occurred more often in the group of patients in whom the sciatic nerve was impaired preoperatively. SSEP monitoring may be of most use for the fractures described in this chapter, since the sciatic nerve is at greatest risk with the posterior approaches required by these fractures.

27
Complex Fractures of the Acetabulum

Introduction

Over the last 10 years, our ability to recognize complex, or associated, acetabular fractures has improved, primarily because of the availability of, and advances in, computed tomography (CT). Early recognition and referral to experienced acetabular surgeons is now possible. Modification of the standard surgical approaches has been necessary to allow fixation of these more difficult fractures. A variety of modified, combined, or enlarged approaches now exist through which stable fixation may be achieved. It is difficult to assess the results of the improved evaluation, approaches, and fixation because of the preliminary nature of much of the literature from the United States.

Definition of Injury/Classification of Injury

The five basic types of fractures of the acetabulum are the posterior wall, posterior column, anterior wall, anterior column, and transverse fractures.[1] The five associated, or complex, fractures of the acetabulum are either combinations of these five basic fractures or are basic fractures with an additional fracture line or lines: (1) posterior column with posterior wall, (2) transverse with posterior wall, (3) T-shaped, (4) anterior wall or column with posterior hemitransverse, and (5) associated both columns (Fig. 1). In all of these patterns, with the exception of the posterior column with posterior wall, fracture lines involve both columns of the acetabulum.

The posterior column with posterior wall fracture type is a combination of the two basic fractures and can be associated with posterior dislocation or subluxation. Some authors prefer to group this pattern with the five basic fractures as only the posterior column is involved and one simple (posterior) approach usually can be used.[2]

The transverse with posterior wall type of fracture combines the two basic patterns. Dislocation or subluxation can occur either centrally or posteriorly. Early recognition and reduction of posterior dislocations are important to minimize complications, such as osteonecrosis, nerve injury, and femoral head damage.[3]

A T-shaped fracture type combines a transverse fracture with an additional vertical fracture. The transverse fracture divides the acetabulum into two components: an iliac, or superior, fragment and an ischiopubic, or inferior, fragment. The vertical fracture then divides the ischiopubic fragment into two separate fragments. The vertical fracture line often traverses the thin bone of the cotyloid fossa and then exits the obturator foramen in a variable position. Recognition of this vertical component, and therefore making the diagnosis of the "T," is critical in planning surgical approaches. A single simple approach may not afford adequate exposure to all three fragments if displaced or comminuted, and a combined or extensile approach may be necessary.

The anterior and posterior hemitransverse fracture type involves both columns. Anteriorly, either a wall or column fracture is present. The fracture in the posterior column corresponds to a transverse fracture. The degree of displacement of the hemitransverse component is important in determining approach. For example, a minimally displaced transverse component with a displaced anterior column fracture could be approached anteriorly. With displacement of the hemitransverse component, access to the posterior column becomes necessary.[4]

Associated both-column fractures, also known as the "floating acetabulum," occur when no portion of the acetabular articular surface is in continuity with the intact ilium. The "spur sign," seen best on the obturator oblique view, is pathognomonic for a both-column fracture. It represents the intact ilium protruding beyond the medially displaced acetabulum. Fracture lines into the joint then may follow any of the previously mentioned fracture patterns. Because none of the joint fragments are tethered to the intact ilium, an acceptable reduction may possibly be achieved in traction. This reduction is characterized by displacement or gaps without step-offs and is called secondary congruence.

Evaluation of Injury

The physical diagnosis and radiographic evaluation of the patient with a complex acetabular fracture should follow previously mentioned guidelines (chapter 22). In addition, the physical examination should include careful assessment of the skin for the presence of abrasions or hematoma. The presence of skin pathology must be considered when planning the surgical approach. A degloving injury of the skin over the abductors, termed a Morel-Lavalle lesion,

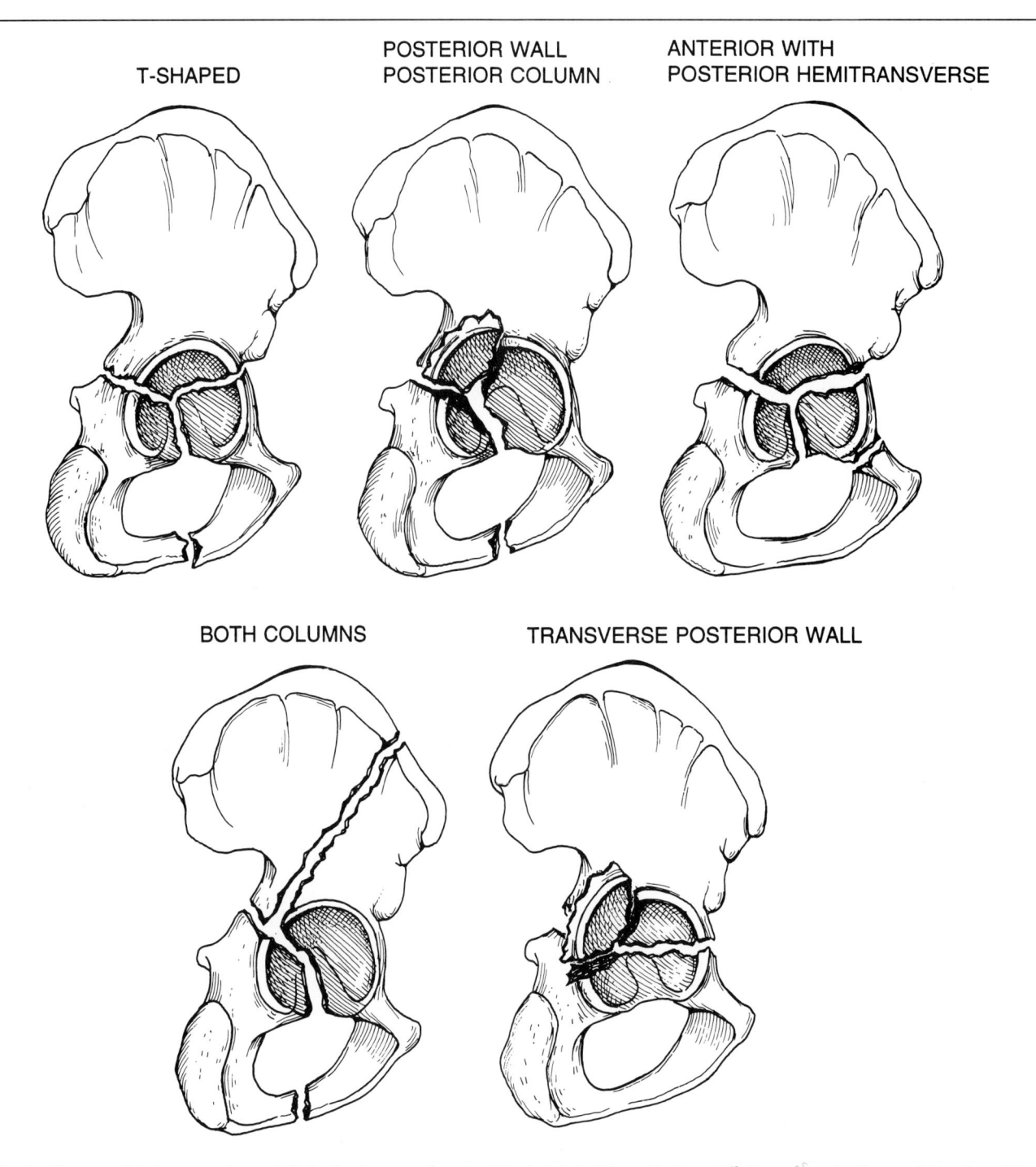

Fig. 1 The associated or complex acetabular fractures as described by Judet, Judet, and Letournel.[19] (Reproduced with permission from Mayo KA: Fractures of the acetabulum. *Orthop Clin North Am* 1987;18:43-57.)

may be associated with an increased risk for infection or skin breakdown,[5] particularly with approaches outside the pelvis, such as the extended iliofemoral or triradiate. The radiographic evaluation should include angiography in cases of hemodynamic instability and when an extensile exposure is planned. Angiography should be performed in the hemodynamically unstable patient with a complex acetabular fracture if other causes of shock have been ruled out, particularly if a fracture line involves the sciatic notch. This pattern indicates potential damage to the superior gluteal artery, which may require embolization to control bleeding.[6] The extended iliofemoral approach of Letournel[1] and the modified extensile iliofemoral approach of Reinert and associates[7] both create flaps based on the superior gluteal artery (SGA). Preexisting injury to the SGA may result in ischemic necrosis of the abductors.[6] A cadaveric angiographic study in which the SGA was ligated showed absence of flow to the abductors after extended iliofemoral, triradiate, and modified extensile approaches.[8] Flow remained intact after a combined ilioinguinal and Kocher-Langenbeck approach despite SGA ligation.

Treatment Options and Results of Treatment

Overview

After adequate physical and radiographic evaluation, dislocations should be immediately reduced, and femoral or tibial skeletal traction should be placed. Skeletal traction affords some immobilization and pain control. Timely transfer to a referral center should occur if the primary orthopaedic surgeon is not comfortable with the diagnosis and surgery of complex acetabular fractures. In one study, the authors showed that the referring orthopaedic surgeon's diagnosis was incorrect or incomplete in 40% of cases.[9] Delay in transfer and delay in surgical intervention worsen the prognosis.[3,10]

Some complex acetabular fractures can be treated nonsurgically with acceptable results. In general, if a stable and congruent reduction of the weightbearing dome can be obtained in traction, nonsurgical treatment is an option. The roof arc angles have been described as a method of quantifying the intact weightbearing dome.[11] The medial, anterior, and posterior roof arc angles are measured on the anteroposterior (AP), obturator oblique, and iliac oblique radiographs, respectively. An adequate weightbearing dome (fracture lines outside the weightbearing dome) is presumed when the medial roof arc is greater than or equal to 30°, the anterior roof arc is greater than or equal to 40°, and the posterior roof arc is greater than or equal to 50°. A "high" or transtectal transverse fracture line would correspond to roof arc angles below the guidelines, indicating a fracture across the weightbearing dome and a tendency for the head and ischiopubic fragment to displace medially. Conversely, a "low" or infratectal transverse fracture line would have roof arc measurements greater than the guidelines, would not involve the weightbearing dome, and would be unlikely to displace medially.

The roof arc measurements are only a guideline. The femoral head must also remain congruently reduced with traction removed for nonsurgical treatment to be an option. Adequate roof arc measurements, or the presence of secondary congruence in a both-column fracture as described above, plus femoral head congruity out of traction are considered requirements and indications for nonsurgical treatment.

Using these indications, some T-shaped and both-column fractures can be treated successfully in traction.[12,13]

Less frequently, transverse fractures with posterior wall involvement and anterior fractures with posterior hemitransverse involvement may be treated nonsurgically.

Posterior column with posterior wall fractures are usually very unstable. Gravity tends to displace these fractures, even in traction. Unless nondisplaced, this fracture pattern should be considered an indication for surgical intervention.

Closed reduction plus traction is rarely successful in achieving or maintaining a reduction in displaced fractures of the dome as in high transverse or T-shaped fractures.[9] In these cases, traction is considered a temporizing measure that affords some immobilization and some pain control prior to definitive treatment.

Traction as definitive treatment requires serial radiographs throughout the course, because further displacement of fractures while in traction may occur.[14] Traction for less than 6 weeks is probably inadequate for healing.[13] Failure to achieve congruency in fractures across the weightbearing dome leads to poor results in patients treated nonsurgically.[11,12]

The systemic complications of immobilization are well documented. The presence of multiple trauma, adult respiratory distress syndrome, and trauma to the ipsilateral limb are considered indications for rapid transfer to an appropriate facility for surgical management. A small number of patients with displaced complex acetabular fractures may not be candidates for either extended traction or a major surgical procedure. Multiple trauma with established adult respiratory distress syndrome, skin lesions, burns, or a patient's refusal to accept blood transfusions because of religious beliefs, for example, may preclude open reduction. CT-guided percutaneous fixation[15] and external fixation[16] may be options for a very small, carefully selected group of patients. These procedures, investigational at present, may provide enough provisional fixation to mobilize the patient, avoiding the potentially disastrous complications of both surgical and nonsurgical standard treatment regimens.

Surgical Approaches

If surgical treatment is chosen, the approach should be carefully selected based on fracture pattern, displacement, and need for access to the joint. Controversy remains regarding the optimal exposure for complex fracture patterns involving the anterior and posterior columns.[2]

Simple Approaches There are many options for surgical treatment, including the Kocher-Langenbeck, ilioinguinal, and extended iliofemoral approaches.[1] Each has specific advantages and disadvantages. The Kocher-Langenbeck, or posterior, approach allows access to the posterior wall and column, the articular surface, the lateral wall of the ilium, and the posterior aspect of the quadrilateral plate by palpation. Osteotomy of the greater trochanter can increase access to the lateral ilium.[17] Potential drawbacks are risk to the sciatic nerve, heterotopic ossification, and inability to reduce or achieve fixation of the anterior column.

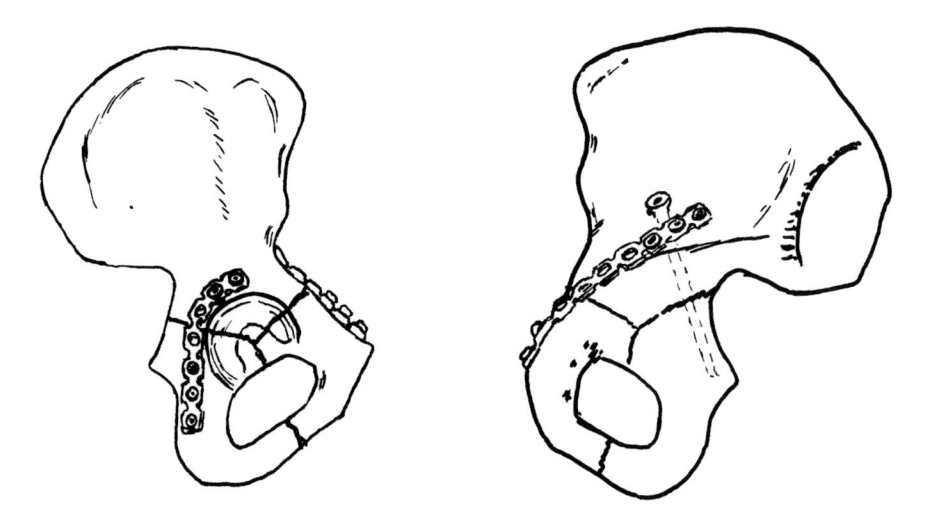

Fig. 2 Example of standard internal fixation techniques for a T-shaped fractures with posterior column lag screw, anterior column plate, and posterior column plate.

The ilioinguinal approach[4] provides access to the anterior wall, the anterior column, and the internal surface of the ilium. The posterior column is accessible only by palpation along the quadrilateral plate, and the articular surface is not visualized. Benefits of the ilioinguinal approach over the posterior approach include lower rates of heterotopic ossification,[18,19] earlier muscular rehabilitation, and less loss of abductor strength than posterior approaches.[20] It is not, however, without complications. Inguinal hernias[2] and injuries to the vas deferens,[20] external iliac artery,[4] or external iliac vein[19] have been reported.

The ilioinguinal approach can be applied to selected complex fractures, such as an anterior with posterior hemitransverse fracture, a T-shaped fracture, or some both-column fractures, but it is not adequate for all types of both-column fractures (Fig. 2).[18] It is specifically indicated in fractures stabilized less than 15 to 20 days postinjury, when the posterior column is one major fragment, or when there is an associated small posterior inferior wall fragment that may be neglected.

Extensile Approaches Letournel[18] considered a substantial delay in surgical intervention (more than 15 to 20 days) and two-column fractures with extensive involvement of the posterior column and wall as contraindications to the use of the ilioinguinal approach. For these fractures, the extended iliofemoral approach was developed. An inverted "J" skin incision along the iliac crest is followed by elevation of the abductors off the external iliac fossa, creating a flap based on the pedicle of the superior gluteal artery. The internal iliac fossa is also exposed. The extended iliofemoral incision allows access to the ilium, the articular surface, and the anterior column to the level of the iliopectineal eminence. Disadvantages include a high rate of heterotopic ossification (57% to 86 %),[4,21,22] and a high rate of infection (3% to 10%).[13,23]

Reinert and associates[7] chose to modify Letournel's extended iliofemoral exposure. They cited as disadvantages the possible conflict between the exposure's skin incision and that for subsequent arthroplasty, the difficulty mobilizing the abductor musculature in large patients, and the relative weakness of the soft-tissue repair of the abductor origin and insertion. The skin incision for the modified extensile iliofemoral approach is T-shaped: a vertical limb that can be used for later total hip arthroplasty and a horizontal limb along the iliac crest. Osteotomies, as opposed to soft-tissue incision, are used to mobilize the abductor origin, the greater trochanter, and the anterior superior iliac spine. Careful ligation of the ascending branch of the lateral femoral circumflex artery is performed for possible reanastomosis in the event of injury to the SGA. The exposure allows access to the acetabulum similar to the extended iliofemoral. The high incidence of Brooker types 3 and 4 heterotopic ossification (20%) in patients without prophylaxis is a disadvantage.

The triradiate incision for complex acetabular fractures was created by adding an anterosuperior extension, extending from the greater trochanter to the anterior superior iliac spine, to the Kocher-Langenbeck approach.[24] With further anteromedial extension, the deep dissection of the ilioinguinal approach can be performed. The approach affords access similar to that of the extended iliofemoral, with the exception that the external iliac fossa is not completely exposed. The surgeon can begin with the Kocher-Langenbeck approach and proceed to the triradiate intraoperatively if further exposure is needed.

The extended iliofemoral approach, the modified extensile iliofemoral approach, and the triradiate incision all afford excellent access to the joint for reduction of complex acetabular fractures. In one study of two extensile approaches, the triradiate and the extended iliofemoral, all reductions were displaced less than 2 mm. Complication rates were similar with two exceptions. The overall rate of heterotopic ossification was 86% in the extended iliofemoral group and 53% in the triradiate group ($p = 0.011$). Triradiate incisions made with the superior angle less than 120 degrees were at risk for superficial skin slough.[21]

Alternatives to Extensile Approaches The complications that accompany the extensile approaches have lead some authors to prefer simple exposures for complex fractures.[2] Other authors report difficulty obtaining reduction with T-shaped or both-column fractures when a single approach is used.[19] In particular, rotation of the transverse component can be difficult.[25] Helfet and Schmeling,[2] however, obtained a satisfactory reduction in 90.5% of complex fractures treated with a strict protocol of a single approach, indirect reduction of the nonexposed column using a Judet table or femoral distractor, and radiographic guidance. There were no infections and only 2% developed significant heterotopic ossification.

The combined anterior and posterior approach is another alternative to the extensile exposures and their potential problems.[26] This method can be performed during the same[26] or subsequent[4] procedures. In one study, anatomic reductions were reported in 88% of complex fractures treated with the combined approach.[26] Symptomatic heterotopic ossification occurred in 8%. A possible benefit to the combined approach is retention of abductor muscle power.

Instead of combining the ilioinguinal and the posterior approach, other authors have chosen to modify the ilioinguinal approach, taking advantage of its benefits while improving ease of reduction of complex fractures. An extended ilioinguinal approach has been developed for specific both column fractures with involvement of the sciatic buttress or sacroiliac joint,[5] considered a potential contraindication for the ilioinguinal approach.[18] Access to the posterior external iliac surface is obtained through a posterolateral extension. This approach does not violate a Morel-Lavalle lesion and leaves the anterior circumflex artery anastomosis intact, theoretically decreasing risk of infection and of ischemia to the abductors.

Lateral extension of the ilioinguinal approach, with dissection along a limited portion of the outer table of the ilium, has also been described.[27] This may permit passage of a cerclage wire or aid reduction of fractures extending into the sciatic notch.

A modified Stoppa approach has been developed[28] as another alternative approach to the extensile and ilioinguinal approaches for complex acetabular fractures. This approach is similar to the ilioanterior approach described by Hirvensalo for fixation of pelvic and acetabular fractures.[29] Dissection proceeds from the midline subperiosteally deep to the femoral vessels and iliopsoas. It allows access to the pubis, obturator foramen, quadrilateral plate, and pelvic brim. This approach was developed to avoid the consequences of stripping the abductors off the ilium during the extensile exposures, namely heterotopic ossification and infection, the consequences of heterotopic ossification prophylaxis (radiation and indomethacin), and the potential neurovascular hazards of the ilioinguinal approach. In one series,[28] 89% of the clinical and radiographic results were satisfactory in a consecutive series of 55 fractures (complex or anterior wall or column types).

Reduction and Fixation

The surgical approaches required for complex acetabular fractures are demanding and require practice on cadavers as well as experienced supervision on patients. Similarly, the reduction techniques require considerable practice, education, assistance and equipment. At least two experienced surgeons and one surgical assistant are required. The average operating times are between 4.5 to 5.2 hours.[2,21] Average blood loss ranges from 1,150 to 1,300 cc, justifying the use of red blood cell retrieval and autotransfusion systems.

Lateral trochanteric traction pins combined with manual traction or the femoral distractor are helpful in reducing central dislocations. The effect of gravity accentuates the tendency for the femoral head to displace medially when the patient is in the lateral decubitus position. The affected limb may be placed in skeletal traction to assist reduction in the lateral decubitus position. The femoral distractor may be used in any position to aid in reduction. The fracture table or Judet table is an excellent adjunct to reduction.[30] Trochanteric traction may be applied through attachments to the table. Drawbacks are that it forces the choice of a single approach,[23] and has inherent risks. Two pudendal nerve palsies, one pubic ramus fracture and one soft-tissue injury of the labia majora resulting in skin slough, have been reported as complications of use of the fracture table.[2]

Abdominal retractors, self-retaining retractors, and extra long drills, taps, and screwdrivers are required. Provisional reduction can be maintained by standard reduction clamps, pelvic reduction clamps, K-wires, a variety of specially developed reduction clamps,[19] or cerclage wires.[27] Reduction techniques for most types and variants of acetabular fractures have been described.[4] The translation and rotation of each fracture reduction must be assessed and accepted. The use of image intensification may help the intraoperative assessment of reduction.

Rigid internal fixation is accomplished with lag screws and contoured pelvic reconstruction plates. Small-diameter (3.5 to 4.0 mm) screws of greater lengths than those required for extremity fixation (> 50 mm) must be available. Lag screw fixation follows the general principles of internal fixation, however, the three-dimensional anatomy and the direction of the fracture lines must be taken into consideration.

Lag screws must be supplemented with buttress plates. Careful contouring of pelvic reduction plates is required to prevent redisplacement and deformity. It is not necessary to fill all holes, and those adjacent to the joint should be deliberately left empty. Because of the complex three-dimensional anatomy, it is not always possible to put the buttress plate in the most biomechanically appropriate posi-

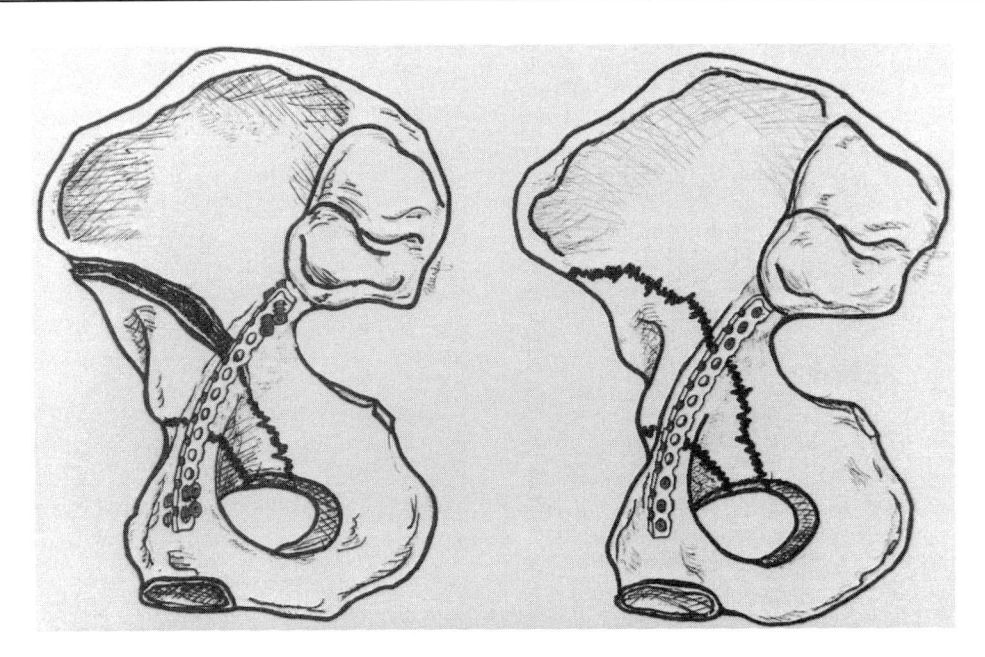

Fig. 3 Anterior column fracture reduced via modified Stoppa intrapelvic approach with pelvic brim plate. (Reproduced with permission from Cole JD, Bolhofner BR: Acetabular fixation via a modified Stoppa intrapelvic approach. *Clin Orthop* 1994;305:112-123.)

tion. For this reason, fixation of fractures involving the quadrilateral plate can sometimes be difficult to maintain. Contoured spring plates placed along the pelvic brim and extending inferiorly to buttress the quadrilateral plate, or fixation from the medial aspect using the modified Stoppa or ilioanterior approach may supplement standard fixation (Fig. 3).[28,29]

A postoperative CT scan of the acetabulum is always necessary. The reduction can be assessed and complications, such as intra-articular screws or bony fragments, can be visualized.

Results

Fractures with involvement of both of the acetabular columns, and specifically T-shaped fractures, have a worse prognosis than basic fractures.[31] Failures are generally more common in complex fractures.[32] The role of reduction of the weightbearing dome and restoration of femoral head congruence in achieving good results is well documented.[13]

Some difficulty comparing clinical results exists because of the lack of a standardized functional grading system. The Harris Hip Scale and D'Aubigne and Postel rating systems were originally developed for total hip arthroplasty patients and may underestimate the functional deficits in the younger population sustaining acetabular fractures. Matta's modification of the D'Aubigne and Postel rating system[11] has made this system more stringent, and it is currently the most widely used system. Good to excellent clinical results are obtained in 78% of complex fractures and 84% of basic fractures treated surgically.[4]

Radiographic results are even less standardized throughout the literature. The reader must discern what was considered an acceptable reduction before the results can be interpreted. It is very difficult to compare series. Three radiographic scoring systems have been developed that appear to be reproducible and which may help clarify this issue if applied.[4,30] Given this lack of standardization, "satisfactory" radiographic results (variably described as less than 2 mm of step-off, less than 3 mm of step-off, "nearly" anatomic, or secondary congruence) have been achieved in 66% to 100% of surgically treated complex acetabular fractures.[21,33]

Anatomic reductions (as opposed to satisfactory) have been achieved in 67% to 88% of surgically treated complex acetabular fractures.[25,26] In one study in which the ilioinguinal incision was used, the author obtained perfect reductions in 73% of both-column fractures, 85% of anterior with posterior hemitransverse, and 67% of T-shaped fractures.[18] Further analysis of all exposures showed perfect reductions in 61% of both-column fractures, 68% of anterior with posterior hemitransverse fractures, 70% of T-shaped fractures, 67.5% of transverse with posterior wall fractures, and 90% of posterior column with posterior wall fractures.[4]

Regardless of treatment method, most authors report a strong correlation of anatomic or satisfactory reduction with good to excellent clinical results.[34] Several studies, however, have pointed out that good to excellent reductions may not guarantee good clinical results, and other factors may be important.[30,35] Dislocation, osteonecrosis and femoral head damage may lead to poor outcome despite adequate surgical intervention.[33]

Surgical stabilization may achieve more than 80% good to excellent results if stabilization occurs within 14 days.[4] Delay beyond this time has been associated with poorer results in small series.[3] In one study of 188 fractures in 187 patients reconstructed 21 to 120 days after injury, good to excellent clinical results were achieved in only 65%, related to the difficulty in obtaining an anatomic reduction.[10] In addition, perfect reduction resulted in a very good or excellent clinical result only 67% of the time as opposed to more than 87% of the time in the series by Letournel and Judet,[4] probably related to cartilage damage, femoral head erosion, and osteonecrosis caused by the delay. Risk of failure was increased for posterior wall, transverse with posterior wall, and T-shaped fractures.

Inexperience on the part of the surgeon also increases the risk of failure. Virtually all reported series have found a "learning curve" phenomenon in which earliest cases had worse outcomes.[13] The experience of the surgical team has a bearing on the results. One series with nine surgeons sharing responsibility for acetabular fracture care, thereby decreasing the surgical experience of each surgeon, reported worse results and more complications than the series of experienced surgeons.[35] The results of another study showed that inexperienced surgeons were less likely than experienced acetabular surgeons to choose surgical treatment (37% of cases versus 72%) or achieve anatomic results (46% of cases versus 77%).[9]

Failure to select the appropriate surgical approach may result in malreduction, suboptimal fixation, or malpositioned intra-articular hardware. In one study, surgical malreduction was secondary to incorrect choice of approach in 12 of 64 cases requiring revision.[36] Loss of fixation with displacement of the fracture poses the acetabular surgeon with a similar problem. Reoperation is technically more difficult because of scar, soft-tissue contracture, and heterotopic ossification. Near anatomic radiographic results have been achieved in 36 of 64 revisions (56%) in one study.[36] Adequate reduction became more difficult to achieve with longer delay between injury and revision. The overall clinical outcome was good or excellent in 42%, but was also correlated to delay in revision. If revision occurred less than 3 after injury, 57% had good or excellent results. This figure dropped to 37% in those revised at 3 to 12 weeks from injury and to 29% in those revised 12 weeks or more after injury. A substantial number of patients with malreduction or loss of fixation can benefit from surgical revision performed by experienced acetabular surgeons.

Patient selection is a critical factor and can be somewhat controversial. The presence of severe comminution or osteoporosis may preclude rigid internal fixation. Immunosuppressed patients and the morbidly obese are at risk for infectious complications, which preclude secondary reconstruction with total hip arthroplasty. The need for mobilization must always be weighed carefully against the risks of surgical intervention. Less invasive surgical procedures with indirect reduction techniques[2] may possibly play a role in the future for patients at risk. Although it has been possible to achieve anatomic reductions in the majority of complex acetabular fractures treated by experienced surgeons, questions remain as to which patients should receive major surgical intervention. Future work in acetabular surgery should be directed at minimizing surgical complications, identifying patients with poor prognosis, and developing appropriate treatment alternatives for these patients.

Conclusions

The treatment of associated or complex acetabular fractures is difficult and demanding. A "learning curve" phenomenon demonstrated in many studies underscores the time, effort, and experience necessary to achieve good results. Early referral to specialists in acetabular surgery has been shown to improve the outcome. The literature reports good and excellent results in close to 80% of displaced complex acetabular fractures.[4] Approach selection is controversial at this time. The extensile approaches, while affording excellent access, can be associated with a high rate of complications. Minimizing surgical dissection, use of less extensile approaches, use of image intensification, and indirect reduction techniques may help to reduce postsurgical complications.[2] Poor results correlate most often with poor reduction. Delay in reduction of dislocation and failure to implement appropriate traction may place the femoral head at risk for erosion and osteonecrosis, also leading to failures of treatment. Accurate diagnosis, timely reduction of dislocations, traction, and early surgical intervention for unstable or incongruous reductions can lead to satisfactory results in the hands of experienced surgeons.

Annotated References

1. Judet R, Judet J, Letournel E: Fractures of the acetabulum: Classification and surgical approaches for open reduction: Preliminary report. *J Bone Joint Surg* 1964;46A:1615-1646.

2. Helfet DL, Schmeling GJ: Management of complex acetabular fractures through single nonextensile exposures. *Clin Orthop* 1994;305:58-68.

   Eighty-four displaced complex acetabular fractures were treated either through the Kocher-Langenbeck (33) or the ilioinguinal (51) approaches. Satisfactory reduction was achieved in 90.5%, with a low complication rate.

3. Roffi RP, Matta JM: Unrecognized posterior dislocation of the hip associated with transverse and T-type fractures of the acetabulum. *J Orthop Trauma* 1993;7:23-27.

   Five cases of T-type or transverse with posterior wall fractures were transferred to the authors 3 to 5 days after injury, with undiagnosed posterior dislocations of the hip. All were originally interpreted on the basis of a single AP film as a central fracture-dislocation of the acetabulum. Failure to recognize the posterior hip dislocation may increase the incidence of sciatic nerve injury (80%), osteonecrosis of the femoral head (40%), and femoral head damage.

4. Letournel E, Judet R (eds): *Fractures of the Acetabulum*, ed 2. Berlin, Germany, Springer-Verlag, 1993.

5. Weber TG, Mast JW: The extended ilioinguinal approach for specific both column fractures. *Clin Orthop* 1994;305:106-111.

   The approach, a combination of the ilioinguinal and the posterior approach to the sacroiliac joint, is described. It is recommended as an alternative to the extensile iliofemoral approach for both column fractures, specifically when the fracture involves the sciatic buttress or the sacroiliac joint.

6. Bosse MJ, Poka A, Reinert CM, et al: Preoperative angiographic assessment of the superior gluteal artery in acetabular fractures requiring extensile surgical exposures. *J Orthop Trauma* 1988;2:303-307.

   Eight patients with complex acetabular fractures involving the sciatic notch and requiring extensile surgical exposure were studied with preoperative angiography and were found to have injuries to the superior gluteal artery.

7. Reinert CM, Bosse MJ, Poka A, et al: A modified extensile exposure for the treatment of complex or malunited acetabular fractures. *J Bone Joint Surg* 1988;70A:329-337.

8. Juliano PJ, Bosse MJ, Edwards KJ: The superior gluteal artery in complex acetabular procedures: A cadaveric angiographic study. *J Bone Joint Surg* 1994;76A:244-248.

   A cadaveric angiographic study in which the SGA was ligated showed absence of flow to the abductors after extended iliofemoral, triradiate, and modified extensile approaches. Flow remained intact after combined ilioinguinal and Kocher-Langenbeck approach despite SGA ligation.

9. Kebaish AS, Roy A, Rennie W: Displaced acetabular fractures: Long-term follow-up. *J Trauma* 1991;31:1539-1542.

10. Johnson EE, Matta JM, Mast JW, et al: Delayed reconstruction of acetabular fractures 21-120 days following injury. *Clin Orthop* 1994;305:20-30.

    Results of 188 acetabular fractures surgically treated 21 to 120 days after injury are reported. Good and excellent results were more difficult to achieve (65%), and anatomic reduction was less likely to correlate with a good to excellent clinical result (67%) than those reported in the literature. Failures were common (26%). Posterior wall, transverse with posterior wall and T-shaped fractures have an increased risk of failure when treated in this time frame.

11. Matta JM, Anderson LM, Epstein HC, et al: Fractures of the acetabulum: A retrospective analysis. *Clin Orthop* 1986;205:230-240.

12. Heeg M, Oostvogel HJ, Klasen HJ: Conservative treatment of acetabular fractures: The role of the weight-bearing dome and anatomic reduction in the ultimate results. *J Trauma* 1987;27:555-559.

13. Matta JM, Mehne DK, Roffi R: Fractures of the acetabulum: Early results of a prospective study. *Clin Orthop* 1986;205:241-250.

    Matta's criteria for nonsurgical treatment, applied prospectively, are supported. Improved surgical results, primarily due to improved surgical reduction, are reported.

14. Spencer RF: Acetabular fractures in older patients. *J Bone Joint Surg* 1989;71B:774-776.

15. Gay SB, Sistrom C, Wang GJ, et al: Percutaneous screw fixation of acetabular fractures with CT guidance: Preliminary results of a new technique. *AJR Am J Roentgenol* 1992;158:819-822.

16. Vaatainen U, Makela A: Treatment of a central fracture-dislocation of the hip using external fixation with iliofemoral distraction. *J Orthop Trauma* 1993;7:521-524.

17. Bray TJ, Esser M, Fulkerson L: Osteotomy of the trochanter in open reduction and internal fixation of acetabular fractures. *J Bone Joint Surg* 1987;69A:711-717.

18. Letournel E: The treatment of acetabular fractures through the ilioinguinal approach. *Clin Orthop* 1993;292:62-76.

    The approach is described and its indications, contraindications, and fixation techniques are discussed. Perfect reductions were obtained in 73% of all cases, 73% of both columns, 85% of anterior with posterior hemitransverse, and 67% of atypical T-shaped fractures.

19. Matta JM: Operative treatment of acetabular fractures through the ilioinguinal approach: A 10 year perspective. *Clin Orthop* 1994;305:10-19.

    The ilioinguinal approach was used for anterior wall and column, associated anterior and posterior hemitransverse, and certain both column and T-shaped fractures. The incision and some reduction techniques, as well as some potential problems with reduction are described. Good and excellent clinical results were achieved in 84% with low complication rates.

20. Dickinson WH, Duwelius PJ, Colville MR: Muscle strength testing following surgery for acetabular fractures. *J Orthop Trauma* 1993;7:39-46.

21. Alonso JE, Davila R, Bradley E: Extended iliofemoral versus triradiate approaches in management of associated acetabular fractures. *Clin Orthop* 1994;305:81-87.

    The authors report on the use of the extended iliofemoral or triradiate approaches for associated acetabular fractures. No significant differences were found between the two groups with respect to reductions or intraoperative complications. The extended iliofemoral approach had a significantly higher rate of heterotopic ossification. Triradiate incisions with a superior angle of less than 120° were at risk for superficial wound infection and skin slough.

22. Ghalambor N, Matta JM, Bernstein L: Heterotopic ossification following operative treatment of acetabular fractures: An analysis of risk factors. *Clin Orthop* 1994;305:96-105.

23. Goulet JA, Bray TJ: Complex acetabular fractures. *Clin Orthop* 1989;240:9-20.

    The results of 31 complex acetabular fractures are presented. Specific options for internal fixation of each type are described.

24. Mears DC, Rubash HE (eds): *Pelvic and Acetabular Fractures*. Thorofare, NJ, Slack, 1986.

25. de Ridder VA, de Lange S, Kingma L, et al: Results of 75 consecutive patients with an acetabular fracture. *Clin Orthop* 1994;305:53-57.

26. Routt ML Jr, Swiontkowski MF: Operative treatment of complex acetabular fractures: Combined anterior and posterior exposures during the same procedure. *J Bone Joint Surg* 1990;72A:897-904.

    Twenty-four patients with complex acetabular fractures were

surgically stabilized by combined anterior (iliofemoral or ilioinguinal) and posterior (Kocher-Langenbeck) approaches. Anatomic reduction was achieved in 88%. There were no infections and no permanent iatrogenic nerve injuries.

27. Schopfer A, Willett K, Powell J, et al: Cerclage wiring in internal fixation of acetabular fractures. *J Orthop Trauma* 1993;7:236-241.

28. Cole JD, Bolhofner BR: Acetabular fracture fixation via a modified Stoppa limited intrapelvic approach: Description of operative technique and preliminary treatment results. *Clin Orthop* 1994;305:112-123.

   The modified Stoppa approach for access to the anterior column, quadrilateral plate, and pelvic ring is described. Indications were displaced anterior wall or column, transverse, T-shaped, both column, or anterior plus posterior hemitransverse. New plating options are afforded, which may have a mechanical advantage over existing techniques.

29. Hirvensalo E, Lindahl J, Bostman O: A new approach to the internal fixation of unstable pelvic fractures. *Clin Orthop* 1993;297:28-32.

30. Ruesch PD, Holdener H, Ciaramitaro M, et al: A prospective study of surgically treated acetabular fractures. *Clin Orthop* 1994;305:38-46.

   A prospective study of 91 fractures (74 associated) treated surgically according to a protocol. A strict radiographic assessment tool and clinical assessment score are presented and used. Radiographic and clinical results were satisfactory in 81% and 81%, respectively. Adequate reduction did not correlate with good clinical results.

31. Pennal GF, Davidson J, Garside H, et al: Results of treatment of acetabular fractures. *Clin Orthop* 1980;151:115-123.

32. Ylinen P, Santavirta S, Slatis P: Outcome of acetabular fractures: A 7-year follow-up. *J Trauma* 1989;29:19-24.

33. Oransky M, Sanguinetti C: Surgical treatment of displaced acetabular fractures: Results of 50 consecutive cases. *J Orthop Trauma* 1993;7:28-32.

34. Letournel E: Acetabulum fractures: Classification and management. *Clin Orthop* 1980;151:81-107.

35. Kaempffe FA, Bone LB, Border JR: Open reduction and internal fixation of acetabular fractures: Heterotopic ossification and other complications of treatment. *J Orthop Trauma* 1991;5:439-445.

   The results of 49 patients treated surgically by 9 surgeons over a 10-year period are presented. Complication rates were very high. Forty percent had poor radiographic results; 38% had poor clinical results.

36. Mayo KA, Letournel E, Matta JM, et al: Surgical revision of malreduced acetabular fractures. *Clin Orthop* 1994;305:47-52.

   Sixty-four patients with malreduced (52) fractures or loss of reduction (12) underwent surgical revision. Good to excellent clinical results were achieved in 42%. Results were most favorable when revision occurred less than 3 weeks after injury. A significant number of patients may benefit from reoperation.

28
Acetabular Fractures: Postoperative Management and Complications

There exists general agreement that to obtain satisfactory long-term results in the treatment of acetabular fractures, an anatomic reduction of the weightbearing articular surface and a congruent reduction of the hip must be obtained. To achieve these goals, surgical treatment is often necessary. Management of these patients in the early postoperative period significantly affects the long-term results of surgery. It is critical to carefully assess the long-term functional outcomes as well as the potential complications that may result from surgical treatment of acetabular fractures to make appropriate decisions in patient care.

Postoperative Management

Acetabular fracture surgery often involves long anesthesia and surgical times as well as significant blood loss and fluid replacement. Accordingly, these patients require close postoperative monitoring of their pulmonary status and hemodynamic stability. The monitoring must be individualized based on the patient's preoperative medical status, associated injuries, and the complexity of the surgery. Intravenous antibiotics (cephalosporins) are administered for 24 to 48 hours postoperatively, with the first dose given before surgery.

Physical therapy is begun on the first postoperative day to begin passive or active/conserted motion of the hip and extremity, and to teach the patient an active exercise program to perform while in bed. Continuous passive motion (CPM) is used at some institutions but has not proved to be more effective than passive motion performed by a physical therapist. In patients with a comminuted posterior wall fracture it may be appropriate to limit hip flexion. Mobilization is begun as early as pain permits, and patients begin gait training with the physical therapist usually by the second postoperative day. The patient is initially allowed only touch-down weightbearing on the affected extremity with the use of a walker or crutches. Full weightbearing is not allowed until 8 to 12 weeks postoperatively. Patients with injuries of the opposite extremity that do not allow weightbearing are taught bed-to-chair transfers. Progressive resistance exercises to increase hip strength, particularly hip abduction, are encouraged from the time of full weightbearing and continued on a long-term basis. Significant muscle weaknesses have been demonstrated at greater than 2 years postoperatively, most notably in patients whose surgery was performed through a Kocher-Langenbeck approach.[1] Anteroposterior (AP) and Judet view radiographs should be obtained postoperatively, and a follow-up AP pelvic radiograph should be obtained within the first 2 weeks postoperatively, after ambulation has begun, to assess for any secondary loss of reduction. Postoperative computed tomography (CT) is essential if there is any question from the plain radiographs of intra-articular hardware or concerns regarding the reduction. If reoperation for loss of reduction is needed, results have been better when the reoperation is performed within the first 3 weeks.[2]

Heterotopic ossification is a well-recognized complication of surgical treatment for acetabular fractures and can jeopardize the benefits of surgery. Many theories have been proposed as to the cause of heterotopic ossification, but none has been proved conclusively. Both local and systemic factors have been implicated. Heterotopic ossification occurs more commonly with stripping of the gluteal muscles from the external iliac fossa, and its incidence is therefore dependent on the surgical exposure used. It occurs most commonly following extensile exposures, including the extended iliofemoral, modified extensile exposure, triradiate exposure, and combined exposures. Overall rates of heterotopic ossification with these extensile exposures have been reported to be between 45% and 100%, with the rates of severe heterotopic ossification reported to be between 14% and 50% when no prophylaxis was used.[3-9] Kocher-Langenbeck exposures have also been associated with significant rates of heterotopic ossification, with overall rates of approximately 25% reported in large series when no prophylaxis was used.[3,10] Heterotopic ossification following the ilioinguinal approach for acetabular fractures is uncommon, and significant heterotopic ossification following ilioinguinal exposures is rare unless the exposure was extended onto the external iliac fossa.[3,11-15] A direct relationship between the severity of heterotopic ossification and loss of function has been demonstrated.[15,16] As such, routine prophylaxis against heterotopic ossification is recommended postoperatively for all patients who undergo extensile exposures or a Kocher-Langenbeck exposure. Prophylaxis after the ilioinguinal exposure is needed only if the exposure was extended onto the external iliac fossa. Current prophylactic methods that have proved effective include postoperative treatment with indomethacin and the use of low-dose irradiation. Indomethacin has been shown to decrease the occurrence of severe forms of heterotopic ossification and also to decrease the overall incidence of heterotopic ossification.[3,4,14,16] The recommended prophylactic dose of indomethacin is 25 mg three times a day, administered orally or by rectal suppository, beginning on the first postoperative day and continuing for 3 to 6 weeks postoperatively. Complication rates with this regimen of indomethacin have been low. Heterotopic ossification prophylaxis by means of low-dose irradiation has also been shown to decrease the severity and overall incidence of heterotopic ossification after acetabular fracture surgery.[3,5,14,17] The treatments must be started before the fourth postoperative day to be effective. Current regimens include 1,000 rad in divided doses, or 700 rad given in divided doses or as a single dose. The long-term effects of irradiation in this patient population are unknown, and the risk of radiation-induced malignant disease, sterility, and genetic alterations in offspring must be considered when the treatment is recommended. The combination of indomethacin and postoperative irradiation has also been reported recently (BR Moed, E Letournel, unpublished data).

Venous thromboembolic disease is a serious and frequent complication in patients with acetabular fractures and necessitates the routine use of deep vein thrombosis (DVT) prophylaxis in this patient population. Numerous treatment protocols, including anticoagulation, mechanical antithrombotic devices, vena caval filters, and serial screening programs, alone or in combination, have been advocated. Prophylaxis for DVT is discussed in more detail later in this chapter.

Complications

Complications can be divided into those that occur early and those that occur late. Early complications include death, infection, nerve injury, thromboembolism, vascular complications, intra-articular screw placement, and secondary fracture displacement. Late complications include nonunion, heterotopic ossification, osteonecrosis, and post-traumatic arthritis.

Early Complications

Death Perioperative mortality is reported at 0 to 2.5% in most large series of operatively treated acetabular fractures.[3,8,9,11,12,18,19] Massive pulmonary embolus (PE) is the most commonly reported cause of death in these patients. Myocardial infarction, cerebrovascular accident, and inadequate intraoperative and postoperative fluid resuscitation have also been reported. Acetabular fractures are usually secondary to high-energy trauma and are often associated with other significant injuries. These may include head injury, chest injury, intra-abdominal injury, long bone fractures, and associated pelvic ring injuries. Additionally, acetabular fractures with displacement at the sciatic notch may cause injury to the superior gluteal artery and lead to significant unrecognized retroperitoneal hemorrhage.[20] These associated injuries increase the morbidity and mortality in patients with acetabular fractures and must be properly assessed and treated before one considers operative treatment for the acetabulum. Age over 60 years has been associated with higher mortality rates; however, acceptable results have been reported with the surgical treatment of acetabular fractures in elderly patients.[21]

Infection In the absence of other associated injuries and with minimal soft-tissue injury, the incidence of infection after acetabular surgery should be no different from that seen after other types of hip surgery. However, most patients with acetabular fractures have other associated injuries or local soft-tissue injury, or both. These may include ipsilateral open fractures and visceral injuries. Additionally, nutritional compromise in polytrauma patients may lead to some degree of immunocompromise. Infection rates are generally reported to be between 2% and 5% in most large series of acetabular fractures.[3,8,9,11,12,18,19] The risk of infection is increased by associated urologic and gastrointestinal injuries, and the presence of suprapubic catheters and colostomies may necessitate changing the planned surgical approach. It is critical for the orthopaedic surgeon to be present with the general trauma surgeons at the time of laparotomy to help select appropriate sites for catheters and ostomies. Likewise, open wounds and open fractures of the ipsilateral lower extremity may increase the incidence of wound infection. When treating fractures of the ipsilateral lower extremity, the surgeon should avoid making incisions that may later compromise surgical treatment of the acetabular fracture. Local soft-tissue injuries, including lacerations, abrasions, and closed degloving injuries (Morel-Lavale lesion), may also increase infection rates and may lead to a change in the surgical approach. Severe deep muscle injury from local trauma often leads to nonviable muscle and, unless debrided at the time of open reduction and internal fixation, may lead to higher infection rates. Obesity has also been associated with higher postoperative infection rates. Perioperative intravenous antibiotics, adequate debridement of nonviable tissue at the time of surgery, and careful surgical techniques should be employed to help decrease the incidence of infection. If deep infection does occur, early surgical treatment is required.

Nerve Injury Sciatic nerve injury that mainly involves the peroneal branch is the most common iatrogenic nerve injury following acetabular surgery. It is usually secondary to prolonged or vigorous retraction of the sciatic nerve and occurs most commonly during Kocher-Langenbeck approaches, but it is also seen following extensile exposures to the acetabulum. Preoperative sciatic nerve injury has been reported in approximately 12% of acetabular fractures but has been reported in up to 25% in some smaller series.[3,6,22] It has also been suggested that patients with preexisting sciatic nerve damage are at increased risk for iatrogenic nerve palsy following operative treatment.[23] It is helpful to keep the hip in full extension and the knee flexed at least 60° to decrease the tension on the sciatic nerve during Kocher-Langenbeck and extensile exposures. Intraoperative somatosensory-evoked potential monitoring has been reported with stimulation of the posterior tibial nerve only and more recently with stimulation of the posterior tibial nerve and the peroneal nerve.[23-25] In these series, a low incidence of postoperative iatrogenic sciatic nerve injuries was reported (2%); however, the role of intraoperative somatosensory-evoked potential monitoring has yet to be clearly established. Overall, in most large series of acetabular fractures an incidence of postoperative sciatic nerve injury of approximately 2% to 6% is reported.[3,8,9,12,18,19] Late occurring sciatic nerve injuries have also been reported but are uncommon.[3,26] They are thought to occur secondary to entrapment of the nerve in heterotopic bone or fibrous tissue, and have been reported to respond to neurolysis. The prognosis for recovery from sciatic nerve palsies has been shown to be related to the severity of the initial clinical deficit of the nerve. The tibial component, when involved, has an excellent prognosis for functional recovery, while recovery of the peroneal component is dependent on the severity of the initial deficit. Satisfactory functional recovery of the nerve has been reported in 30% to 65% of patients and may occur as early as 3 months or over a period that can extend up to 3 years.[3,27] Carbamazepine has been reported to provide effective relief of neurogenic pain secondary to peripheral injury of the nerve when dysesthesias and hyperesthesias are present.[27]

Damage to the lateral femoral cutaneous nerve of the thigh and femoral nerve palsies have been reported after anterior approaches to the acetabulum. If the lateral femoral cutaneous nerve has been severely damaged during the exposure, a decision may be made to sacrifice the nerve and bury the ends of the nerve beneath the surrounding muscle to avoid a painful neuroma. Letournel and Judet[3] reported a 12% incidence of symptomatic neuralgia of the lateral femoral cutaneous nerve following anterior approaches and reported two cases of femoral nerve palsy following ilioinguinal approaches that resolved over 1 year. The inferior gluteal nerve may be injured if the gluteus maximus is split too far medially, and the superior gluteal nerve may be injured by excessive retraction of the gluteus medius. Injury to these nerves will lead to significant persistent gait abnormalities and atrophy of the gluteal muscle mass. If the nerves remain in continuity, the prognosis for functional recovery is good.

Thromboembolism The exact incidence of DVT associated with acetabular fractures and acetabular surgery is unknown. Reports vary, depending on the screening methods used, the type of prophylaxis used, the presence and nature of associated injuries, and the patient population. Letournel reported a 6% incidence of DVT or PE in a series of 569 fractures operated on within 21 days of injury.[3]

Seven incidents occurred early in the series, before the authors routinely used anticoagulant prophylaxis, and the other 22 occurred with varying anticoagulant prophylaxis regimens. The Consensus Development Conference of the National Institutes of Health reported the incidence of DVT to be approximately 20% in young polytrauma patients.[28] In a recent prospective study that used serial duplex ultrasound (US) screening in patients with a major fracture of the pelvis, the incidence of DVT was 15%.[29] Seventy percent of the patients in the study received some form of prophylaxis for DVT during their treatment. In a recent prospective randomized study the incidence of thromboembolic events in untreated patients with a pelvic fracture was 11%. There was an 8% rate of DVT and a 3% rate of PE.[30] In another recently reported prospective study of patients admitted to a trauma unit with injury severity scores greater than 9, the incidence of DVT in patients who received no prophylaxis was determined by venography. The overall incidence of DVT in this group of patients was 54%, and thrombi were detected in 61% of patients with a pelvic fracture. Only 1.5% of the patients in this study with DVT had clinical characteristics suggestive of thrombosis before the diagnosis was made by venography.[31]

Commonly used screening methods for DVT include ascending venography, duplex US, fibrinogen scans, and impedance plethysmography. All of these techniques have advantages and disadvantages, but venography remains the reference standard. Pelvic DVT is difficult to demonstrate by any of these methods and may go undetected.

Owing to the frequency of DVT in this patient population, DVT prophylaxis with an effective regimen should be considered the standard in all patients with acetabular fractures. The goal of DVT prophylaxis is to prevent the long-term morbidity associated with DVT and, more important, to avoid the potentially fatal complication of PE. The incidence of PE in these patients is reported to be between 0.5% and 10%. No consensus exists as to the most effective protocol for DVT prophylaxis in patients with acetabular fractures. Adjusted-dose heparin, Dextran 40, sodium warfarin (Coumadin), and low molecular weight heparin have all been shown to be effective in patients undergoing hip surgery. Pneumatic leg-compression devices used in combination with one of the other agents listed has also been shown to be an effective treatment. Greenfield filters are an effective means of preventing fatal PE in patients found to have DVT or PE preoperatively and in patients with a contraindication to anticoagulation who are thought to be at high risk for a thromboembolic event or who have had a documented thromboembolic event.[32,33] Noninvasive screening with duplex US should be performed preoperatively in patients transferred from an outside facility or in patients in whom there is a long delay from admission to surgery. If the results of duplex US are equivocal, then venography should be performed. Serial screening of these patients for DVT is ineffective in decreasing the incidence of clinically significant and fatal PE. An effective protocol was reported recently in 203 patients, 148 with an acetabular fracture and 55 with pelvic fracture. All patients underwent duplex US on transfer to the treating hospital. If DVT was detected, a Greenfield filter was placed preoperatively, and postoperatively the patients were treated with heparin for 4 to 5 days, beginning after the removal of the Hemovac drains. Warfarin therapy was instituted and continued for 12 weeks postoperatively in these patients. Patients with a negative duplex US study preoperatively were treated with pneumatic leg-compression devices preoperatively, and those devices were used continually during the surgical procedure and postoperatively. Warfarin was started 48 to 72 hours postoperatively, when the Hemovac drains were removed, and continued for 3 weeks. The prothrombin time was maintained at 1.3 to 1.4 times control. This protocol resulted in an overall incidence of DVT of 3%. There was a 2% incidence of proximal DVT and a 1% incidence of calf DVT. Nonfatal PE occurred in 1% of the patients, and there were no postoperative fatal PE.[34] Many of the other regimens include the use of heparin in the preoperative period and in the early postoperative period. Patients being treated with heparin must have their partial thromboplastin time carefully monitored. They must also have serial blood counts performed to watch for a drop in hemoglobin and to allow for early detection of thrombocytopenia, which may occur secondary to the use of heparin. Rates of hematoma formation postoperatively have been maintained low with careful monitoring in these patients.

Vascular Complications Vascular complications, including femoral artery thrombosis, femoral artery laceration, and femoral vein laceration, have been described with ilioinguinal approaches. Such complications have been reported in 0.8% to 2.0% of large series of ilioinguinal exposures.[3,11,12] Additionally, dissection too near the external iliac vessels can lead to division of the lymph channels and chronic lymphedema of the lower extremities. Failure to recognize and ligate anastomotic vessels between the external iliac or inferior epigastric arteries and the obturator artery (corona mortis), which occurs in up to 82.5% of cases, can lead to significant blood loss (D Teague and associates, unpublished data). Lag screws placed into the anterior column from the outer surface of the iliac wing that penetrate the superior pubic ramus at a point adjacent to the superficial femoral artery can lead to extrinsic compression of the artery.[35] Injury to the superior gluteal artery and vein at the greater sciatic notch during posterior column exposure can lead to significant blood loss and in extensile exposures can lead to gluteal muscle necrosis.[3,12,36]

Intra-articular Screw Penetration Erroneous placement of intra-articular screws is reported even by experienced acetabular surgeons. Auscultation with an esophageal stethoscope along the quadrilateral surface and the lateral ilium intraoperatively[37] and the intraoperative use of C-arm radiography have been used to attempt to detect intra-articular screws prior to wound closure. A thorough understanding of three-dimensional pelvic anatomy also decreases the

Table 1. Radiographic classification of heterotopic ossification

Class	Description
0	No heterotopic bone
I	Islands of bone within the soft tissues about the hip
II	Bone spurs from the pelvis or proximal end of the femur, leaving at least 1 cm between opposing bone surfaces
III	Bone spurs from the pelvis or proximal end of the femur, reducing the space between opposing bone surfaces to less than 1 cm
IV	Apparent bony ankylosis of the hip

risk of intra-articular screw placement. Postoperative radiographs, to include an AP pelvis view, Judet views, and a lateral pelvic view should be carefully assessed for any evidence of intra-articular hardware. If these radiographs do not conclusively rule out intra-articular screw placement, a postoperative CT scan is required to accurately determine screw position. If an intra-articular screw is identified, it should be removed as soon as feasible to avoid abrading the articular surface of the femoral head.

Secondary Fracture Displacement Secondary fracture displacement is seen in approximately 1% of cases. It may occur secondary to patient noncompliance, a second traumatic event, or inadequate stabilization of the fracture primarily. When loss of satisfactory reduction is identified on follow-up radiographs, a difficult decision must be made concerning the wisdom of reoperation. In a report on 64 patients with surgical malreduction or secondary loss of reduction, reoperation resulted in reconstruction within 2 mm of being anatomic in 56% of the patients, and 42% of patients obtained good or excellent functional results. In this series a delay to reoperation had an adverse affect on the surgical result.[2] These results do not compare favorably with results obtained on singly operated fractures and lead to an increased complication rate. However, reoperation can salvage some failed open reductions. Reoperation should only be considered by very experienced acetabular fracture surgeons and only after appropriate counseling of the patient on the expected results and possible complications.

Late Complications

Nonunion Nonunion following open reduction and internal fixation of acetabular fractures is uncommon and reported in less than 1% of cases. Letournel and Judet[3] reported four nonunions in 569 patients operated on within 21 days of sustaining an acetabular fracture. Nonunion has been reported more commonly with complex acetabular fractures that had imperfect reductions postoperatively and in patients treated with delayed acetabular reconstruction.

Heterotopic Ossification Heterotopic ossification and its prophylaxis were previously described in this chapter. The degree of heterotopic ossification is most commonly reported by the use of the Brooker classification, which is based on the AP pelvic radiograph (Table 1).[38] In many recent reports this has been modified to include Judet views as well as the AP pelvic radiograph in an attempt to more accurately define the degree and location of the heterotopic ossification. Although heterotopic ossification remains very common after acetabular fracture surgery, it rarely requires surgical excision. Surgical excision should be considered only when heterotopic bone formation severely reduces hip mobility. A preoperative CT scan is helpful in planning surgery for the excision of heterotopic bone, and surgery should be delayed until the heterotopic ossification is mature (usually a minimum of 6 to 12 months). Bone excision can usually be accomplished through the original surgical incision. The sciatic nerve and superior gluteal neurovascular bundle may be encased in bone, and great care must be used in dissecting these structures. Excision of heterotopic ossification following acetabular fracture surgery will yield an improved range of motion postoperatively.[15]

Osteonecrosis Osteonecrosis of the femoral head occurs in approximately 3% to 4% of acetabular fractures and is most commonly associated with those that have associated posterior hip dislocations and less commonly with those that have an anterior or central hip dislocation. Ipsilateral femoral neck fractures have also been associated with a higher risk of osteonecrosis of the femoral head. Femoral head collapse will be apparent radiographically in less than 2 years in the great majority of cases. The majority of these patients have a poor result. Osteonecrosis of segments of the acetabulum has also been described and is usually the result of extensive stripping of bone fragments. It has been described for a portion of the anterior column and for posterior wall fragments as well. This may lead to overlying chondrolysis.

Posttraumatic Arthritis Posttraumatic arthritis may result from imperfect reductions, chondral injuries to the acetabulum, femoral head lesions, unrecognized intra-articular screw placement, and preexisting arthritis. It is important to note significant chondral injuries and femoral head lesions at the time of surgery for long-term prognostic significance. Many of these patients will require further surgery because of severe hip pain and functional limitations. Hip arthrodesis and total hip replacement arthroplasty are the most common salvage procedures in this group of patients. Total hip replacement has been shown to have higher rates of component loosening and failure when performed after an acetabular fracture as compared to results in age-matched controls.[39]

Controversies in Management

The most effective means of DVT prophylaxis and the length of time it is needed remain areas of controversy in acetabular fracture surgery. Because of the low overall incidence of clinically significant PE and the clinical diversity of this patient population, large numbers of patients are needed when comparing forms of treatment. This has made much of the literature on this topic of questionable benefit.

Another area of controversy in the treatment of acetabular fracture is the need for primary total hip arthroplasty at the time of fracture treatment. Primary total hip arthroplasty at the time of open treatment of acetabular fractures has been performed in special circumstances, when the expected outcome was dismal. It has been considered in an attempt to decrease the overall long-term disability of the patient as well as to gain a more satisfactory long-term clinical outcome. Results of total hip arthroplasty after a failed open reduction and internal fixation of acetabular fractures are not as good as would be expected for age-matched controls.[39] A primary total hip arthroplasty might be considered in a patient with a severe femoral head lesion noted preoperatively on CT scans and at the time of surgery. Primary total hip arthroplasty might also be considered in a patient with a severely comminuted ipsilateral femoral neck fracture, as results of treatment of this injury have been poor. Presently there is little information available in the literature to help with this decision-making process.

Acetabular fractures are severe injuries that carry significant morbidity and often long-term disability, even with appropriate treatment. Recovery is prolonged, and persistent muscle weakness and gait abnormalities are the norm. Muscle testing more than 2 years after injury has shown that significant muscle weakness persists. Up to 30% of patients have been reported not to return to work, and the average time to return to work has been reported to be more than 7 months. The modified D'Aubigne Postel and Harris hip scores have been commonly used to assess functional outcomes after surgery for acetabular fractures. These scores may not adequately correlate with the objective and subjective functional outcomes of the patient. New functional outcome assessment instruments are being evaluated and validated in ongoing studies. These outcome assessments will be necessary to give further insight into the true functional outcome that these patients can expect.

Annotated References

1. Dickinson WH, Duwelius PJ, Colville MR: Muscle strength testing following surgery for acetabular fractures. *J Orthop Trauma* 1993;7:39–46.

   A retrospective clinical analysis and muscle strength testing were performed on 30 patients who had undergone surgery for acetabular fractures. At an average of 21 months of follow-up, only 14 patients had a normal gait. The overall strength deficit was 27% and the average strength deficit for abduction was 50%. Abduction strength loss was statistically greater in patients operated on through posterior approaches.

2. Mayo KA, Letournel E, Matta JM, et al: Surgical revision of malreduced acetabular fractures. *Clin Orthop* 1994;305:47–52.

   A retrospective evaluation (average follow-up, 4.2 years) of the success of reoperation in 64 patients with surgical malreduction or secondary loss of reduction showed that 56% of patients had reconstruction to within 2 mm of being anatomic, and 42% of patients had good or excellent outcomes. The perioperative complication rate was 19%.

3. Letournel E, Judet R (eds): *Fractures of the Acetabulum*, ed 2. Berlin, Germany, Springer-Verlag, 1993.

   The authors present a comprehensive description of the evaluation and treatment of patients with acetabular fractures. The results of treatment of a large series of acetabular fractures are given, with detailed descriptions of complications and postoperative management.

4. McLaren AC: Prophylaxis with indomethacin for heterotopic bone after open reduction of fractures of the acetabulum. *J Bone Joint Surg* 1990;72A:245–247.

   The article provides a retrospective review of 44 patients with acetabular fractures, of whom 18 received indomethacin, 25 mg orally three times a day, and 26 received no heterotopic ossification prophylaxis. Brooker grade 2 or more severe heterotopic ossification developed in 50% of patients who received no prophylaxis but in only 5.5% of patients treated with indomethacin.

5. Bosse MJ, Poka A, Reinert CM, et al: Heterotopic ossification as a complication of acetabular fracture: Prophylaxis with low-dose irradiation. *J Bone Joint Surg* 1988;70A:1231–1237.

   The article is a retrospective review of 37 patients who underwent surgery for 38 complex acetabular fractures through an extended iliofemoral or a modified extended iliofemoral incision. Prophylactic irradiation (1,000 rad in 200-rad increments, starting on the third postoperative day) was administered to 18 of the patients. The group of patients treated with prophylactic irradiation had a lower overall incidence of heterotopic ossification and a lower incidence of severe heterotopic ossification.

6. Routt ML Jr, Swiontkowski MF: Operative treatment of complex acetabular fractures: Combined anterior and posterior exposures during the same procedure. *J Bone Joint Surg* 1990;72A:897–904.

7. Reinert CM, Bosse MJ, Poka A, et al: A modified extensile approach for the treatment of complex or malunited acetabular fractures. *J Bone Joint Surg* 1988;70A:329–337.

8. Mears DC, Rubash HE: Extensile exposure of the pelvis. *Contemp Orthop* 1983;6:21–32.

9. Matta JM, Mehne DK, Roffi R: Fractures of the acetabulum: Early results of a prospective study. *Clin Orthop* 1986;205:241–250.

10. Oransky M, Sanguinetti C: Surgical treatment of displaced acetabular fractures: Results of 50 consecutive cases. *J Orthop Trauma* 1993;7:28–32.

11. Matta JM: Operative treatment of acetabular fractures through the ilioinguinal approach: A 10-year perspective. *Clin Orthop* 1994;305:10–19.

    On review of 119 acetabular fractures treated through the ilioinguinal approach, at an average of 3 years of follow-up, 84% of patients had good or excellent clinical results. Complications included wound infections in 3%, iatrogenic nerve palsy in 2%, significant heterotopic ossification in 1%, and death from PE in 1%. This approach offers the advantages of low complication rates, rapid recovery of muscle function, and improved cosmesis.

12. Mayo KA: Open reduction and internal fixation of fractures of the acetabulum: Results in 163 fractures. *Clin Orthop* 1994;305:31–37.

13. Helfet DL, Schmeling GJ: Management of complex acetabular fractures through single nonextensile exposures. *Clin Orthop* 1994;305:58–68.

    The article presents a retrospective review of 84 complex acetabular fractures operated on through a single nonextensile exposure. Indirect reduction was obtained with use of either the Judet table, lateral trochanteric traction, or a femoral distractor. Satisfactory reduction was obtained in 90.5% of the cases, with a decreased complication rate.

14. Johnson EE, Kay RM, Dorey FJ: Heterotopic ossification prophylaxis following operative treatment of acetabular fracture. *Clin Orthop* 1994;305:88–95.

    On retrospective review of 87 patients surgically treated for 88 acetabular fractures, heterotopic ossification prophylaxis with indomethacin resulted in a statistically significant reduction in the rate of heterotopic ossification in patients operated on through the extended iliofemoral approach but not in patients operated on through the Kocher-Langenbeck approach. The incidence of heterotopic ossification in patients who underwent ilioinguinal approaches was extremely low.

15. Ghalambor N, Matta JM, Bernstein L: Heterotopic ossification following operative treatment of acetabular fracture: An analysis of risk factors. *Clin Orthop* 1994;305:96–105.

    The authors analyzed outcomes in 237 patients surgically treated for acetabular fractures to identify risk factors predisposing to the development of heterotopic ossification. Factors that correlated with the formation of significant heterotopic ossification were the iliofemoral surgical approach, associated injuries of the abdomen and chest, multiple operative findings, and T-type fractures. The clinical significance of heterotopic ossification and the results of excision are also reviewed.

16. Moed BR, Maxey JW: The effect of indomethacin on heterotopic ossification following acetabular fracture surgery. *J Orthop Trauma* 1993;7:33–38.

    The article presents a retrospective review of 66 patients with acetabular fractures operated on through a posterior or an extensile surgical approach. Prophylactic indomethacin decreased the incidence of severe heterotopic ossification. Statistical analysis revealed that male sex and an extensile operative approach were significant risk factors for heterotopic ossification formation.

17. Slawson RG, Poka A, Bathon H, et al: The role of postoperative radiation in the prevention of heterotopic ossification in patients with post-traumatic acetabular fracture. *Int J Radiol Oncol Biol Phys* 1989;17:669–672.

18. Matta JM, Merritt PO: Displaced acetabular fractures. *Clin Orthop* 1988;230:83–97.

19. Matta JM, Anderson LM, Epstein HC, et al: Fractures of the acetabulum: A retrospective analysis. *Clin Orthop* 1986;205:230–240.

20. Bosse MJ, Poka A, Reinert CM, et al: Preoperative angiographic assessment of the superior gluteal artery in acetabular fractures requiring extensile surgical exposures. *J Orthop Trauma* 1988;2:303–307.

21. Helfet, DL, Borrelli J Jr, DiPasquale T, et al: Stabilization of acetabular fractures in elderly patients. *J Bone Joint Surg* 1992;74A:753–765.

On retrospective review of 18 patients, 60 years or older, who were treated surgically for an acetabular fracture, complications included two postoperative nonfatal PE and one secondary loss of reduction. Treatment was thought to have failed in only one patient.

22. Wright R, Barrett K, Christie MJ, et al: Acetabular fractures: Long-term follow-up of open reduction and internal fixation. *J Orthop Trauma* 1994;8:397–403.

23. Moed BR, Maxey JW, Minster GJ: Intraoperative somatosensory evoked potential monitoring of the sciatic nerve: An animal model. *J Orthop Trauma* 1992;6:59–65.

The authors studied spinal and cortical somatosensory-evoked potential monitoring in 18 cat hind limbs. Significant waveform changes immediately preceded postoperative peripheral nerve deficits, and loss of motor function may be avoided by immediate response to the changes. The authors recommend stimulating both the peroneal and tibial nerves while obtaining individual (not simultaneous) recordings for each nerve.

24. Helfet DL, Hissa EA, Sergay S, et al: Somatosensory evoked potential monitoring in the surgical management of acute acetabular fractures. *J Orthop Trauma* 1991;5:161–166.

This article is a review of 50 patients who underwent acetabular fracture surgery with the use of somatosensory-evoked potential (SSEP) monitoring. Twenty-six percent of the patients developed significant SSEP changes intraoperatively. When the nerve was involved preoperatively, SSEP changes developed in 60% of the patients. There was a 2% rate of iatrogenic sciatic nerve injury. The authors recommend use of SSEP monitoring for acetabular fracture surgery.

25. Calder HB, Mast J, Johnstone C: Intraoperative evoked potential monitoring in acetabular surgery. *Clin Orthop* 1994;305:160–167.

The authors review 88 patients who underwent intraoperative somatosensory-evoked potential (SSEP) monitoring with stimulation of the peroneal and posterior tibial nerve. The results indicate that SSEP responses are an effective means of indicating intraoperative changes in sciatic nerve physiology, but they do not necessarily predict functional outcome. Iatrogenic sciatic nerve palsies occurred in 2% of their patients.

26. Ruesch PD, Holdener H, Ciaramitaro M, et al: A prospective study of surgically treated acetabular fractures. *Clin Orthop* 1994;305:38–46.

27. Fassler PR, Swiontkowski MF, Kilroy AW, et al: Injury of the sciatic nerve associated with acetabular fracture. *J Bone Joint Surg* 1993;75A:1157–1166.

The authors review treatment results in 14 patients with a sciatic nerve palsy associated with a displaced acetabular fracture. Eleven of the 14 patients had residual neurologic sequelae. The peroneal division was involved in every case, and its recovery was dependent on the severity of the initial deficit. When the tibial nerve was also involved, the involvement of the peroneal nerve was more severe, and the recovery of the tibial nerve occurred earlier and was more complete.

28. National Institute of Health Consensus Development: Prevention of venous thrombosis and pulmonary embolism. *JAMA* 1986;256:744–749.

29. White RH, Goulet JA, Bray TJ, et al: Deep-vein thrombosis after fracture of the pelvis: Assessment with serial duplex-ultrasound screening. *J Bone Joint Surg* 1990;72A:495–500.

Serial duplex US screening was performed on 42 patients who had a major fracture of the pelvis. Some form of prophylactic agent was used at some point during hospitalization in 70% of these patients. DVT was found in 15% of the patients. Older age and a higher modified injury severity score were weakly associated with the development of DVT but were not statistically significant.

30. Fisher CG, Blachut PA, Salvian AJ, et al: Effectiveness of pneumatic leg compression devices for the prevention of thromboembolic disease in orthopaedic trauma patients: A prospective, randomized study of compression alone versus no prophylaxis. *J Orthop Trauma* 1995;9:1–7.

A prospective randomized clinical trial in 304 patients with hip and pelvic fractures compared pneumatic sequential compression devices (PSLCD) and no prophylaxis for prevention of DVT. PSLCD was effective in reducing DVT in patients with hip fractures but not in patients with a pelvic fracture. A thromboembolic event occurred in 11% of patients who received no prophylaxis.

31. Geerts WH, Code KI, Jay RM, et al: A prospective study of venous thromboembolism after major trauma. *N Engl J Med* 1994;331:1601–1606.

Consecutive patients admitted to the trauma unit at Sunnybrook Health Science Center with an Injury Severity Score of 9 or greater were evaluated with venography to determine the incidence of DVT. No DVT prophylaxis was used in these patients. The overall incidence was 54%. DVT was detected in 61% of patients with pelvic fracture. Risk factors were identified and discussed.

32. Collins DN, Barnes CL, McCowan TC, et al: Vena caval filter use in orthopaedic trauma patients with recognized preoperative venous thromboembolic disease. *J Orthop Trauma* 1992;6:135–138.

This article reviews a protocol for treatment of 35 patients with pelvic or lower extremity fractures requiring surgery who also had documented significant acute DVT. Patients were treated with low-dose Coumadin and vena caval filters inserted prophylactically prior to surgery. There were no PEs and no complications from filter insertion.

33. Webb LX, Rush PT, Fuller SB, et al: Greenfield filter prophylaxis of pulmonary embolism in patients undergoing surgery for acetabular fracture. *J Orthop Trauma* 1992;6:139–145.

34. Fishmann AJ, Greeno RA, Brooks LR, et al: Prevention of deep vein thrombosis and pulmonary embolism in acetabular and pelvic fracture surgery. *Clin Orthop* 1994;305:133–137.

    A prospective study was conducted to evaluate a protocol for DVT and PE in patients with operatively treated fractures of the pelvis and acetabulum. The protocol involved preoperative noninvasive screening, intraoperative and postoperative mechanical antithrombotic devices, and postoperative Coumadin. The protocol was thought to be effective.

35. Johnson EE, Eckardt JJ, Letournel E: Extrinsic femoral artery occlusion following internal fixation of an acetabular fracture: A case report. *Clin Orthop* 1987;217:209–213.

36. Juliano PJ, Bosse MJ, Edwards KJ: The superior gluteal artery in complex acetabular procedures: A cadaveric angiographic study. *J Bone Joint Surg* 1994;76A:244–248.

    A cadaveric study was performed to assess collateral circulation to the abductor muscle flap created by extensile acetabular exposures in the presence of ipsilateral superior gluteal artery occlusion. Angiography and a microfil injection study was performed. The authors recommend preoperative angiographic studies to assess the superior gluteal artery in patients who are candidates for an extensile exposure.

37. Anglen JO, DiPasquale T: The reliability of detecting screw penetration of the acetabulum by intraoperative auscultation. *J Orthop Trauma* 1994;8:404–408.

    A dog and cadaveric study was performed to assess the reliability of detecting intra-articular screws by auscultation along the lateral ilium with an esophageal stethoscope. This technique was thought to be simple, accurate, and reliable. Once heard, the sound of a screw in the joint was said to be memorable.

38. Brooker AF, Bowerman JW, Robinson, RA, et al: Ectopic ossification following total hip replacement: Incidence and a method of classification. *J Bone Joint Surg* 1973;55A:1629–1632.

39. Romness DW, Lewallen DG: Total hip arthroplasty after fracture of the acetabulum: Long-term results. *J Bone Joint Surg* 1990;72B:761–764.

    This article presents a retrospective review of 55 primary total hip arthroplasties performed in 53 patients with a previous acetabular fracture and an average follow-up of 7.5 years. The incidence of radiographic loosening of the acetabular component was 52.9%, and there was a 13.7% revision rate. These rates are four to five times higher than in other series matched for age.

29
Hip Dislocations and Fractures of the Femoral Head

Hip Dislocations

A simple dislocation of the hip without associated fractures of the acetabulum or femoral head or neck is a relatively uncommon but devastating injury. This section will cover the pertinent anatomy, diagnostic evaluation, decision-making, treatment, and results for simple dislocations of the hip.

Anatomy

The hip joint is an extremely stable anatomic structure because of the relationship between the femoral head, acetabulum, and its labrum.[1] This situation ensures that at least 70% of the femoral head is covered by any part of the acetabular complex during any position of hip motion. This is supplemented by a very strong capsular complex, which, in association with the powerful muscles about the hip joint, provides secondary restraints to prevent dislocation. The blood supply to the femoral head is particularly important with regard to the long-term consequence of a simple hip dislocation. An extracapsular vascular ring formed from the medial circumflex and lateral circumflex arteries gives rise to ascending arteries, which pierce the hip joint at its capsular insertion along the trochanteric region posteriorly. These arteries ascend along the posterior aspect of the femoral neck and perforate the femoral head at the junction of the articular cartilage inferiorly. This arrangement does not allow significant displacement from the normal anatomic position.

Consequently, during a dislocation of the hip significant tension is placed on the arterial and venous circulation, temporarily interrupting blood supply to the femoral head. This will lead to the development of osteonecrosis.

The sciatic nerve lies in very close relationship to the femoral head posteriorly. It is at extreme risk in any posterior dislocation.

Diagnostic Assessment

An understanding of the mechanism of hip dislocations is important in order to appreciate and interpret the history of the injury. Because of the extraordinary stability of the hip joint, high energy is required to dislocate the hip once it is in the appropriate abnormal position. In order for a simple dislocation to occur, the hip must have reached one of its extremes in range of motion. Therefore, a posterior dislocation will occur with the hip adducted, flexed to approximately 90°, and internally rotated. A force driven along the femoral shaft will dislocate the hip rather than fracturing the posterior acetabular wall. Similarly, if the hip becomes flexed to 90°, and is externally rotated, it will tend to be levered out of the hip joint. Depending on rotation, the hip will be dislocated either anteroinferiorly in the obturator foramen or superiorly over the pubic ramus. Thus, the position of the patient's lower limb at time of impact, along with the physical examination, give important clinical information as to the type of hip dislocation.

The classic posterior dislocation is flexed, adducted, and internally rotated; the classic anterior dislocation is flexed, externally rotated, and abducted. Some superior dislocations may simply be shortened and severely externally rotated as the hip is sitting out over the top of the acetabulum. Other significant injuries are associated with these dislocations, particularly where the force has been applied at the level of the knee. There may be knee dislocations, posterior cruciate injuries, and vascular injuries. An anterosuperior dislocation of the femoral head can lead to femoral artery or vein compromise. A posterior dislocation can cause impingement and compression or contusion of the sciatic nerve, leading to sciatic nerve palsy, this is most commonly seen in the peroneal nerve branch. Total assessment of the trauma patient must be carried out as advised by the Advanced Trauma Life Support® protocol to avoid missing other injuries secondary to the high-energy trauma that causes the dislocated hip.

Radiographic investigation must include an anteroposterior (AP) radiograph of the pelvis on which both hips are seen. Even in the most subtle dislocations, if the normal hip is compared to the abnormal hip with regard to joint space, medial clear space (the space between the teardrop and the femoral head), definition of the lesser trochanteric profile, and associated acetabular fractures, a hip dislocation should be evident. With a femoral shaft fracture, the AP pelvic radiograph is imperative because the associated shaft fracture may mask the physical findings of a dislocation.

Further plain radiographic evaluation is best accomplished through the use of the Judet views of the pelvis. If a large cassette is used to include the complete pelvis, the normal hip can be used for comparison. The most appropriate view for determining a posterior dislocation with any kind of posterior wall injury is the obturator oblique view. The iliac oblique view can be used to assess the associated anterior wall fracture for anterior dislocations.

At this point, the diagnosis of a simple hip dislocation is made. Further radiographic investigations are not required. Prompt reduction of the hip is more important.

Treatment

Prompt reduction of the simple dislocated hip is imperative. The earlier the reduction within the context of the patient's overall physical condition, the better the results should be. Reduction after 24 hours is correlated with a higher incidence of osteonecrosis and posttraumatic arthritis. Within the first 24 hours, there has been no statistical correlation with improved results the quicker the hip is reduced.[2-6]

The dislocated hip is reduced by longitudinal traction in the position of deformity to overcome any muscular spasm, subsequent repositioning of the hip by recreating the deformity, and then repositioning of the dislocated components.

The reduction must be performed gently, requiring that the patient be relaxed. Depending on the patient's condition, it may be appropriate to use intravenous anesthetics in the emergency department. However, if the reduction cannot be accomplished by this method after one attempt, the patient should be taken to the operating room, where reduction can be performed with general anesthesia, including muscle relaxation. Following closed reduction, the hip must be tested for stability. It should be gently tested through a full range of motion to see whether it may redislocate. At the same time, careful auditory and tactile evaluation for crepitus in the hip joint must be undertaken. This will help determine further follow-up and surgical intervention.

At this point, a plain radiograph of the pelvis, including both hips, is performed. Assessment of the dislocated hip with respect to the normal hip is carried out to determine the adequacy of joint space, intactness of Shenton's line, the profile of the lesser trochanter, the position of the femoral shaft, and the presence of any incongruity. If not obtained before reduction, it may be appropriate at this point to obtain the Judet oblique views. Computed tomography (CT) is only needed to evaluate a simple dislocation if there is a concern that the reduction is incongruent, that there is an associated acetabular fracture, or if there is an associated femoral head fracture.

At this point, if the hip is stable with full range of motion, there is no evidence of crepitus during joint motion and the AP radiograph and Judet views show a concentric reduction, no further radiographic investigations are indicated. The patient is usually placed in skin or boot traction.

If the hip cannot be reduced closed, open reduction is mandatory through a posterior approach.

Postreduction treatment of the dislocated hip consists of early ambulation with weightbearing as tolerated by the patient's hip discomfort. There is no proof that delayed weightbearing beyond that which is required for the relief of pain has any influence on the outcome of the simple hip dislocation.

Protected weightbearing is carried out until the patient is free of pain, which usually occurs between 10 days and 2 weeks. At this point, walking aids are discarded and the patient is gradually allowed increased activities. Between 4 and 6 weeks the patient will be able to resume most preinjury activities. It may take up to 3 months for full recovery of muscle power and strength. If there has been a sciatic nerve injury, appropriate splinting of the lower extremity must be undertaken to maintain the plantigrade position of the foot. Appropriate management of causalgic pain is important.

Patient follow-up must continue for a minimum of a year. The patient is warned about the risk of osteonecrosis and posttraumatic arthritis that may occur over the ensuing 2 to 5 years following this injury.

Classification of Injury

The classification of simple dislocations of the hip fall into two categories: posterior or anterior. Anterior injuries can be looked upon as being obturator or over the pubic ramus. This simple classification is probably all that is needed for simple dislocations of the hip.

Complications

Irreducible Dislocation of the Hip Occasionally a simple hip dislocation will be irreducible. This is usually caused by entrapment of either a tendon or capsular structure or an unrecognized osteochondral fracture fragment that is blocking reduction. These impediments can usually be recognized in two ways. First, the hip will not reduce, no matter how much muscle relaxation is available. This can best be ascertained by using an image intensifier to watch the reduction if there have been previous problems with closed technique. Second, the hip will appear to reduce with a palpable clunk but through any range of motion will start to sublux and feel unstable. This is usually related to an incarcerated fragment or potential hip joint instability due to avulsion of the labrum. It is obvious that if the hip cannot be held in joint, an open reduction must be performed emergently. However, if the hip can be kept reduced and maintained by traction, further investigations using CT scans may be worthwhile to define the injury. However, the most important determinant of whether further surgical intervention is needed for an irreducible hip will be the potential for long-term instability. If the orthopaedic surgeon believes that the hip is unstable and there is no incarcerated fragment, then exploration and repair of the capsular and labral structures is probably indicated in the first several days. Delay makes repair difficult at 6 to 8 weeks if instability still exists.

Osteonecrosis Osteonecrosis of the femoral head has been reported in 1% to 17% of these injuries. At present all that can be stated about the timing of reduction is that it appears that the earlier it occurs, the less the potential chance for this entity to occur. The break point appears to be 24 hours. However, because the cause of osteonecrosis is uncertain for hip dislocations, the treatment becomes uncertain with regard to the promptness of reduction. This will completely depend on the associated injuries and the condition of the patients.[2-4,6]

Traumatic Arthritis Traumatic arthritis is probably the most frequent long-term complication. It is probably related to the severity of the injury. As this is a high-energy injury, there is significant damage to the articular surface of the femoral head and acetabulum.

Unappreciated damage at the time of injury probably occurs in a significant number of patients, which leads to arthritis. Some evidence of occupational hazard, in particular heavy labor, may predispose those with dislocations of the hip to increased osteoarthritis.[4,7,8]

Recurrent Dislocation Recurrent dislocation is an exceedingly rare complication. The majority of these patients have had some form of capsular defect associated with a posterosuperior labial detachment. Repair involves closing of capsular defect and buttressing of this either through soft-tissue or bony repairs.

Missed Dislocations A missed dislocation up to approximately 3 to 4 months may still be salvaged by an open reduction.

Preoperative traction may be indicated to bring the femoral head down to the appropriate acetabular level, followed by open reduction to replace the femoral head in the acetabulum. In young individuals this may be a very appropriate approach, whereas in older patients, hip arthroplasty may be indicated and might be considered a more cost-effective treatment.

Sciatic Nerve Injury Sciatic nerve injuries occur in 8% to 19% of hip dislocations; 40% to 50% will recover full function. While recovery is occurring, the appropriate positioning, physical therapy, range of motion, and mobility of an extremity must be carried out.

Results

It has usually been assumed that a simple dislocation of the hip has carried with it an excellent prognosis. It appears, however, that in the recent literature this may not be true. A large series of 74 patients from Britain has shown that the results of treatment were considered excellent or good in 56 and unsatisfactory in 18. This was correlated with the development of radiographically evident osteoarthritis.

Even in the satisfactory group, patients complained of discomfort after prolonged walking or exercise. This study also suggested that both the etiology and the patient's occupation can affect the ultimate outcome.[7]

Patients whose occupations involve heavy labor seem to be at risk for developing arthritis following hip dislocation. These results have been confirmed in a study in Germany, which involved 50 isolated or simple traumatic dislocations in adults. This study showed poor outcomes in 16 of 30 posterior dislocations and three of 12 anterior dislocations. A correlation between the overall severity of injuries and the direction of dislocation was found in this series. The delay in reduction showed no correlation because all reductions were done within 12 hours.[4]

Summary

With simple dislocations of the hip, accurate diagnosis is easily accomplished through clinical evaluation and plain radiographs. Prompt reduction of the hip is usually accomplished, and treatment is easily instituted with protected weightbearing until comfortable, followed by return to activities as determined by muscle function and recovery. However, results are probably not as good as has been predicted and the patient should be warned that early development of osteoarthritis is a potential complication from this injury. Osteonecrosis has yet to be correlated with time of reduction, although it appears that any reduction within the first 24 hours is probably satisfactory, preferably earlier, if possible, depending on the patient's condition.

Fractures of the Femoral Head

Fractures of the femoral head represent one segment of complex hip dislocations. The majority of complex dislocations of the hip are associated with acetabular fractures. The end result of femoral head fractures is related to the relative anatomy and pathology of the hip dislocation.

Relevant Anatomy

Approximately 70% of the articular surface of the femoral head is responsible for load transfer. Damage to the articular surface related to a femoral head fracture thus decreases the total surface available for load transfer. This change in the force per unit area on articular cartilage can lead to significant changes in the joint surface and, hence, posttraumatic osteoarthritis. Areas of depression or impaction through the femoral head will also lead to crushing of the articular cartilage matrix and damage to the cells. A congruent relationship between the femoral head and the acetabulum is particularly important for normal hip joint function. Any change in this relationship, such as a loss of a fragment of femoral head, will allow noncongruent motion to occur within the hip joint. This will lead to posttraumatic arthritis.

Diagnostic Evaluation

It is important to recognize that femoral head fractures are associated with hip dislocations. Posterior dislocations, which are the most common, are associated with approximately a 7% incidence of femoral head fracture. Therefore, when reviewing the radiographs of the posterior dislocation, it is imperative that the empty acetabulum be studied for any evidence of a femoral head fracture. Radiographs of the femoral head may show a fracture.

In anterior dislocations, a higher incidence of associated femoral head fractures is seen (10% to 68%), although most of these are related to impaction lesions because the hip is levered out over the anterior aspect of the acetabulum.[9] Clinically, the same history and physical features are seen with this as with dislocations. Radiographic diagnostic techniques first involve an AP pelvic radiograph of both hips. This radiograph must be reviewed carefully to determine whether or not there has been a femoral head fracture. The femoral neck should also be evaluated with regard to any femoral neck fractures that may change the technique of reduction. If there is any question, it is very helpful to obtain the Judet views of the acetabulum, which can often show a femoral head fracture that was missed on the AP view.

Unless the patient has had an emergent CT scan for another reason, there is no need for any further radiographic intervention at this time. What should be accomplished at this time is a prompt reduction of the hip. The same criteria exist here as with hip dislocations. The reduction must be done as quickly and as gently as possible. If a closed reduction without general anesthetic is unsuccessful once, the patient should then be placed under general anesthetic with muscle relaxation and the hip reduced. Following closed reduction, confirmation of the reduction must be carried out by a plain AP radiograph of the pelvis. This will confirm reduction, but for more precise detail, a CT scan will be required.

Classification

Pipkin[10] has provided the most widely used classification to date. His classification divides the femoral head fracture at the fovea. A type I fracture occurs below the fovea; a type II fracture occurs above the fovea. Consequently, a type II fracture potentially still has a blood supply through the foveal artery and may have a better prognosis; however, this fracture involves the superior weightbearing dome. Type III and IV fractures are femoral head fractures associated with a femoral neck injury or an acetabular fracture, respectively. Osteochondral or transchondral shear fractures of the weightbearing surface of the femoral head or depression fractures of the superolateral weightbearing surface are not included in this, but have been included in a classification by Brumback and associates.[11] All the procedure types are included in the comprehensive classification used by Mueller.

However, the importance of the classification system is to recognize where the fracture has occurred, as well as what the blood supply and morphology are to better determine the treatment options and prognosis.

Treatment

As mentioned, emergent gentle closed reduction is first performed. If reduction is successful, further treatment is based on a description of the fracture fragment.

With an isolated shear fracture below the fovea (Pipkin type I) and an anatomic reduction with less than 1 mm of stepoff, closed treatment following reduction is recommended. Usually 4 weeks of light skin traction or skeletal traction followed by touchdown weightbearing on crutches for a further 4 weeks will provide for healing. If reduction is inadequate, a Smith-Petersen approach to the hip joint should be carried out and the fracture fragment fixed using interfragmental compression screw fixation. It is imperative that the screw heads be buried beneath the articular cartilage of the femoral head.

With fractures above the fovea or involving the superior weightbearing dome (Pipkin type II), anatomic reduction is mandatory. If this is not achieved through a closed reduction and confirmed by CT, open reduction is carried out through a Smith-Petersen anterior approach to the hip. Stabilization of the fracture through interfragmental screw compression techniques is required.

Age will have some role to play. In patients for whom total hip arthroplasty is more suitable because of age or activity levels, this may be the appropriate choice.

With fractures involving the femoral neck, the prognosis is related to the femoral neck injury and its degree of displacement. In younger, active patients, emergent open reduction and internal fixation is required. This is probably best done either through a Watson-Jones anterolateral approach or a Smith-Petersen approach to the hip. If the fracture is not amenable to internal fixation, arthroplasty is probably indicated. Femoral head fractures associated with acetabular injuries are again dealt with at time of acetabular fracture surgery. This will probably significantly affect the long-term results of the acetabular fracture.

Femoral head fractures associated with anterior dislocations are extremely difficult to manage. Transchondral or osteochondral shear injuries that lead to a noncongruent reduction are potentially unstable and should be either excised or fixed internally, depending on the size and location of the fracture fragment. For large fractures that involve the weightbearing position, internal fixation is needed.

The choice of approach will be determined by the location of the fracture based on CT. Anterior fracture fragments are approached anteriorly, and posterior fractures are approached posteriorly. Elevation of depression injuries to the femoral head at present has no data to support its use. Excision of the fragments may be used with severe comminution or if small femoral head fragments are between the femoral head and acetabulum. Occasionally, excision may be necessary at the time of open treatment of an irreducible hip dislocation fracture if it is impossible to fix the associated femoral head fracture.

IV
Spine

Paul A. Anderson, MD
Section Editor

30
Patient Assessment in Spinal Injury

Care of the patient with a spinal injury begins at the scene of the accident. Emergency medical technicians assess and stabilize the patient before removal to a hospital facility. Potential spinal injury must be assumed, but airway management and circulatory stabilization are the most urgent concerns.[1,2]

The diagnosis and acute management of potential spinal injury may be divided into six separate phases: (1) initial assessment, immobilization, and transportation; (2) medical management; (3) radiologic diagnosis; (4) anatomic alignment; (5) surgical decompression; and (6) stabilization.

Assessment and treatment begin at the accident scene or prehospital phase and continue on arrival in the emergency room. At the scene, the patient is placed in a neutral position, with maintenance of airway and circulation a priority. The cervical spine may be immobilized in a variety of ways. A study reported that improper extrication and immobilization of the cervical spine at the accident scene could lead to further neurologic compromise and also suggested that the spinal cord was most susceptible to injury with flexion and extension movements and that immobilization with sandbags, tape, or spine board was superior to immobilization with a collar alone.[3] A recent investigation that compared extrication collars found the cervical spine was adequately immobilized by the rigid collars most often used today by emergency medical techniques.[4] Because multilevel fractures occur in 15% to 20% of these patients, transport should be on a spine board.[5] The Ferno-Washington stretcher may be used as an adjunct to the spine board in the transportation and stabilization of patients with suspected thoracic and lumbar fractures.[6] Access to the oropharynx must be available to maintain airway and prevent aspiration.

On arrival in the emergency room the patient is stabilized according to the standard principles of airway maintenance, breathing, and circulation. An initial radiographic trauma profile consisting of lateral cervical spine, chest, and pelvic radiographs is obtained, and then a thorough physical examination must be done. Documentation of findings on the initial examination is extremely important, with careful attention to distal motor function and sacral sparing, because these are important prognostic indicators of future neurologic recovery.[7,8] In polytrauma patients, strict adherence to principles of airway maintenance, breathing, and circulation take precedence over correction of bony injury.

In individuals with a spinal cord injury above C5, the ability to breathe may be significantly impaired, and respiratory compromise may result.

Patient assessment begins with the history from the patient and the observations of the investigating officer and paramedical personnel involved in treating the patient. Information should include the circumstances of the accident, the position in which the patient was found, whether or not a seat belt or restraining device was used, initial examination results at the scene, and the type of treatment provided at the scene of the accident.

Physical Examination

The physical examination begins with inspection of the patient. Clothing should be carefully removed so that a systematic visual evaluation can be performed. Areas of tissue abrasions, contusions, lacerations, and limb asymmetry should be meticulously documented. Abnormal chest expansion or paradoxical breathing may indicate possible pulmonary and cardiac injury. Extremities and joints are carefully evaluated for crepitus, abnormal motion, and malalignment. Abnormal or asymmetric pulses may indicate arterial damage secondary to lacerations, transections, or intimal tears. Decreased blood pressure with an elevated heart rate indicates a decreased circulating blood volume, whereas low blood pressure with a decreased pulse rate may be indicative of a sympathectomy from a spinal cord injury rather than hypovolemic shock.

The abdomen is examined for possible peritoneal signs, indicating damaged viscera. In the event of spinal cord injury, the abdominal examination is negative and a peritoneal lavage may be required to rule out visceral damage. Lap belt injuries can cause bowel rupture or major vessel, liver, spleen, and urologic injury.[9]

In evaluating the chest, each rib must be carefully palpated for continuity or crepitus. Subcutaneous emphysema indicates severe pulmonary trauma. The pelvis is evaluated for abnormal widening of the symphysis pubis or asymmetry of the iliac wings.

After a complete evaluation of the extremities, the spine is examined in a systematic manner. The anterior aspect of the cervical collar is carefully removed and the neck is inspected visually for bruises, abrasions, or lacerations.

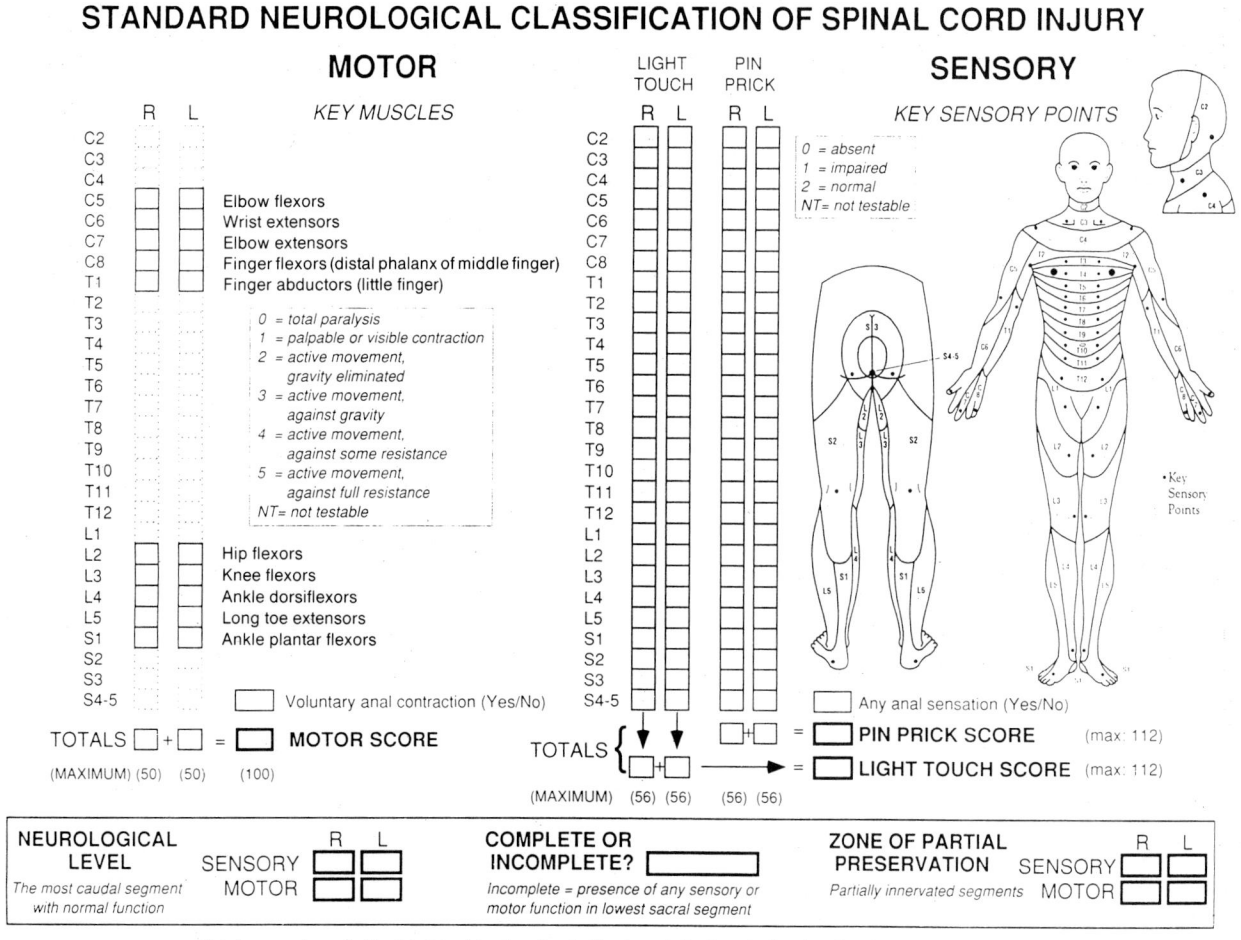

STANDARD NEUROLOGICAL CLASSIFICATION OF SPINAL CORD INJURY

Fig. 1 The diagram distributed by the American Spinal Injury Association facilitates accurate documentation of initial neurologic status and provides a means of monitoring changes as they occur with time following the injury, which assists in determining the prognosis of spinal injuries. (Reproduced with permission from the American Spinal Injury Association.)

Venous congestion is evidenced by distended jugular veins. The carotid pulses are palpated carefully and the trachea is evaluated for any deviation from the midline. The collar is then replaced and the patient is carefully rolled to allow palpation of the entire spine from occiput to sacrum. Great care must be exercised with the log roll maneuver, because an unstable spine can displace and possibly lead to neural compromise.[6] Each spinous process should be palpated, with the examiner noting tenderness, alignment, fascial defects, asymmetry, or interspinous widening indicating possible unstable spine injuries. The sacroiliac joints are then evaluated for longitudinal migration or instabilities in lateral compression. The patient is then carefully rolled back to the supine position and a thorough neurologic examination is performed.

Neurologic Evaluation

The neurologic examination consists of evaluation of motor, sensory, and reflex portions of the nervous system. Strict attention must be directed to sharp/dull discrimination, reaction to changes in temperature, and the ability to distinguish between light and deep pressure. Evaluation of motor function must include not only the presence or absence of function, but also grades of strength (Fig. 1).

Sensory Evaluation

The sensory level in each patient should be carefully tested using an alcohol wipe to distinguish temperature changes, a sterile needle to evaluate pain sensation, and light touch to evaluate ability to detect changes in pressure. These are functions of the spinothalamic tract, whose fibers reside in the anterolateral portion of the spinal cord. Posterior column function of the spinal cord can be tested using a tuning fork to detect vibration or the position of the limb in space. The muscles are enervated by the neural tissues in the corticospinal tracts that are positioned in the anterior lateral aspect of the spinal cord. The sensory and motor examination must be performed in a sequential and systematic manner.

Evaluation of sensation begins with the cervical region and proceeds distally to assess specific dermatomal regions (Table 1). Unrestricted access to the patient is mandatory. C1 and C2 roots provide sensation from the occipital region to the nape of the neck. C3 and C4 provide sensation in a cape distribution from the neck and shoulders posteriorly to the anterior chest just inferior to the clavicles.

The thoracic region and abdomen receive sensory enervation from the thoracic nerve roots, with significant sensory overlap in this area owing to the dual enervation of the skin. Anatomically, the skin in this area receives input from the fibers of three different spinal nerve levels. Localizing sensory levels in this region are the nipple line, which represents a T5 level, and the umbilicus, representing the T10 level. The inguinal region receives input from the lower thoracic and upper lumbar regions.

The lower extremity and perineum are enervated by the roots composing the lumbosacral plexus. L1 and L2 enervate the skin just below the inguinal ligament and the inner thigh. L3 and L4 provide sensation to the anterior, anterolateral thigh and knee area; L5 provides sensation to the lateral aspect of the calf and the dorsomedial skin of the foot and ankle; and S1 provides sensation to the posterior calf and the lateral and plantar aspects of the foot.

The perineum is enervated by the sacral nerves S2 through S5 and is important as a prognostic indicator for functional recovery in patients with a spinal cord injury.[7,8]

Motor Evaluation

After a thorough assessment of sensory function, the muscles are evaluated and the observations regarding functional strength are carefully recorded (Table 2). C1 and C2 enervate the musculature of the suboccipital triangle. C3 and C4, in conjunction with the intercostal nerves, provide respiratory function via the diaphragm. Patients with lower cervical and thoracic spinal cord injuries often present with paradoxical respiration. The cord injury renders the intercostal and abdominal musculature nonfunctional. The diaphragm contracts with inspiration, which displaces the abdominal contents inferiorly and results in abdominal distention rather than the flattening of the abdomen and expansion of the chest that normally occur with inspiration in neurologically intact patients. Should the C3 and C4 roots be nonfunctional, the diaphragm will be paralyzed and severe respiratory compromise may result. Muscles enervated by C5 include the deltoid, the internal and external shoulder rotators, and the biceps. Muscles enervated by C6 include the biceps, brachioradialis, and the wrist extensors. Function of the triceps, wrist flexors, and finger extensors is provided by C7. Finger flexors and hand intrinsics are enervated by the C8 root, and interossei function is provided by the T1 root.

Thoracic roots enervate the intercostal, abdominal, and paraspinal muscles. Upper abdominal contraction without lower abdominal contraction results in the upward migration of the umbilicus (Beevor's sign) and is indicative of paralysis below T10. L1–L3 function is tested by evaluating hip flexors and adductors. L4 function involves the quadriceps femoris and anterior tibialis. L5 enervates the hip abductors, the hamstring group, and the extensor hallucis longus. S1 function encompasses the hip extensors, the lateral hamstring group, and the gastrocnemius-soleus complex. S2–S5 roots enervate the sphincter muscles of the perineum.

Table 1. Major sensory levels

Nerve root	Enervates
C4	Clavicle
C5	Deltoid region
C6	Radial forearm and thumb
C7	Middle finger
C8	Fifth finger
T1	Medial, proximal arm
T5	Nipples
T7	Costal margins
T10	Umbilicus
T12	Inguinal ligament
L3	Anterior thigh
L4	Medial aspect of knee
L5	Lateral calf, dorsum of foot, great toe
S1	Lateral foot, fifth toe
S2	Posterior thighs
S3–S4	Buttocks, perianal region

Table 2. Major motor levels

Level	Muscle group	Action	Deep tendon reflex
C5	Deltoid, shoulder rotators	Abduction of shoulder, external rotation of arm	Biceps jerk (C5–C6)
C6	Biceps, brachialis, wrist extensors	Flexion of elbow	Brachio-radialis jerk (C5–C6)
C7	Triceps, wrist flexors	Extension of elbow, wrist	Triceps jerk
C8	Intrinsic hand muscles	Abduction, adduction of fingers	
L2–L3	Iliopsoas	Hip flexion	
L4	Quadriceps	Extension of knee	Knee jerk
L5	Tibialis anterior and posterior, extensor hallucis longus	Dorsiflexion of foot and great toe	
S1	Gastrocnemius	Plantar flexion of foot	Ankle jerk
S4–S5	Anal sphincter	Voluntary contraction of anal sphincter	

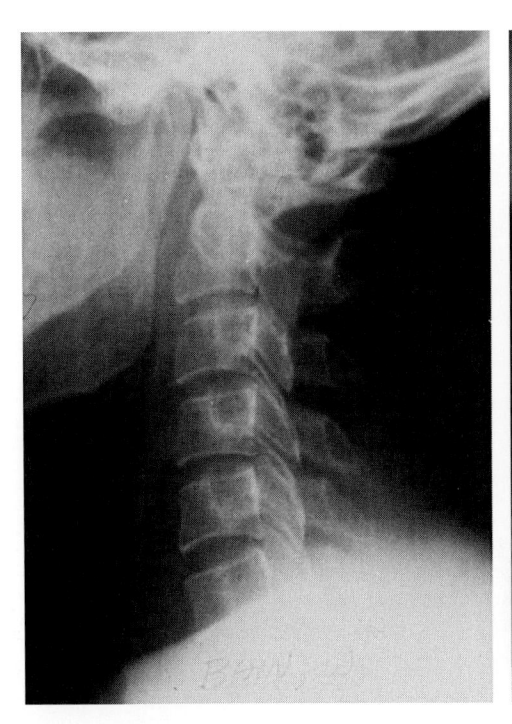

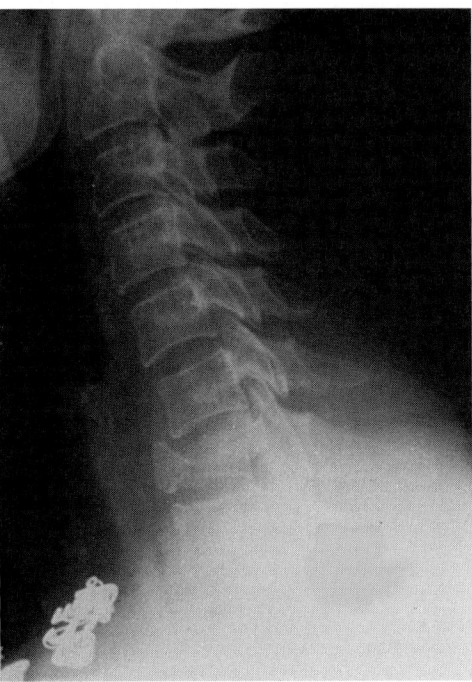

Fig. 2 Left, This lateral cervical radiograph is not acceptable because it does not show the cervicothoracic junction. Only six cervical vertebrae can be seen. Therefore, the cervical spine cannot be cleared with this radiograph. **Right,** When the entire cervical spine is thoroughly evaluated, with visualization of the cervicothoracic junction, a teardrop fracture of the C7 vertebra is noted. All seven cervical vertebrae must be visualized, as well as the cervicothoracic junction, before the cervical spine can be adequately evaluated and cleared.

Table 3. Segmental reflexes

Reflex	Level
Biceps	C5
Brachioradialis	C6
Triceps	C7
Upper abdominal*	T7–T10
Lower abdominal*	T10–T12
Cremasteric*	L1
Knee jerk	L4
Posterior tibial jerk	L5
Ankle jerk	S1
Bulbocavernosus†	S2–S4
Anocutaneous‡	S4–S5

* Cutaneous reflexes decreased in upper motor neuron lesion
† Contraction of bulbocavernosus muscle after stimulation of glans penis
‡ Contraction of anal sphincter after perineal skin is stroked

Reflex Evaluation

After a thorough muscle evaluation, the reflex function is tested (Table 3). The biceps reflex evaluates C5 function; the brachioradialis, C6 function; and the triceps reflex, C7 function. Important reflex functions in the lower extremity include the L4 quadriceps reflex (knee jerk) and the Achilles reflex, which evaluates the S1 function. These deep tendon reflexes are mediated through the anterior horn cells. The cerebral cortex provides an inhibitory function to prevent excessive reaction to stimulation. Inability to elicit a reflex can be caused by peripheral nerve damage that interrupts the reflex loop as well as from central damage resulting in spinal shock.

The abdominal and cremasteric reflexes are upper motor neuron tests that require superficial stimulation of the skin and are mediated through the central nervous system. The superficial abdominal reflex is elicited by stroking the skin in each quadrant of the abdomen and noting whether the umbilicus is drawn toward the stimulated area. Enervation of the abdominal musculature is segmental in nature, with the upper musculature enervated by T7–T10 and the lower muscles by T10–L1. Asymmetric loss of this reflex may indicate a localized lower motor neuron lesion.

The superficial cremasteric reflex is elicited by stroking the skin of the inner thigh. In the male patient, the scrotum will be drawn upward by the cremasteric muscle if the reflex is intact. Absence of the reflex is indicative of an upper motor lesion, and unilateral absence suggests a lower motor lesion. Anatomically, this reflex involves T12 through L2. Loss of superficial reflexes and an exaggerated response of the deep tendon reflexes due to loss of cerebral inhibition are indicative of upper motor neuron pathology.

Pathologic reflexes are significant because their presence indicates an upper motor neuron lesion. The Babinski test is performed by stroking the skin on the lateral plantar surface with a sharp object, such as a key or the reflex hammer handle. A positive (pathologic) response is indi-

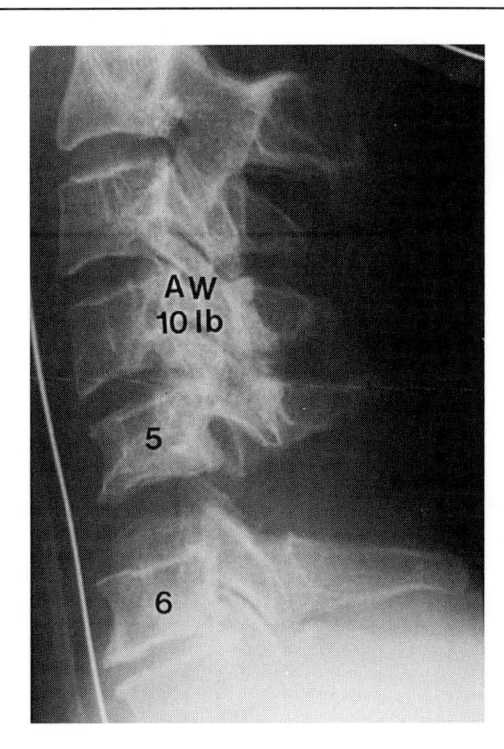

Fig. 3 In performing the stretch test, minimal weight must be applied initially and strict attention to detail must be given to prevent overdistraction of the grossly unstable spine.

cated by extension of the great toe with flexion and splaying of the other toes. The Oppenheim test is done in a similar manner. The fingernail or hammer handle can be drawn along the tibial crest, with a positive test indicated by the same response as in the Babinski test.

The presence or absence of sacral sparing is extremely important in the evaluation of spinal trauma patients. This provides an indicator for prognosis of functional recovery. Sphincter function is tested by inserting a gloved finger into the rectum and noting resting tone. The patient is then asked to voluntarily contract the sphincter. Sensation to light touch and pinprick are also evaluated at this time. Stimulating the skin around the anus elicits the superficial anal reflex and contraction of the anal sphincter. This reflex involves S2–S4 function. During the rectal examination in males, the position of the prostate should be noted. Abnormal position is indicative of a possible urethral tear and warrants further evaluation. Special care must be exercised during Foley catheter insertion in these patients.

Individuals presenting with a neurologic deficit must be evaluated for spinal shock. Spinal shock is often present within 24 hours of injury and results from edema from the initial trauma to surrounding neural tissues. These patients will exhibit loss of motor, sensory, and reflex functions. Whether the neurologic deficit is complete or partial cannot be determined at this point.

The bulbocavernosus reflex is important in evaluation of the spinal injury patient because its presence signifies resolution of spinal shock and allows the examiner to determine whether a complete or incomplete neurologic deficit exists. This reflex is elicited by stimulation of the penis or clitoris by digital pressure or traction on the Foley catheter while a gloved finger is positioned in the rectum and a resulting contraction of the anal sphincter is noted. A positive response indicates resolution of spinal shock with return of the reflex arch.

Radiographic Evaluation

Once airway, circulation, and other system damage has been assessed, attention is directed toward radiographic evaluation of the spine. In anyone with suspected spinal injury, the entire spine should be evaluated in both the anteroposterior (AP) and lateral planes, looking for asymmetry of spinal alignment and soft tissue disruption. A cross-table lateral cervical spine radiograph will demonstrate 77% of the cervical pathology.[10] The addition of an AP and an open mouth odontoid view will increase accuracy to 84%. It is imperative to see all seven cervical vertebrae and the cervicothoracic junction before an adequate assessment can be made (Fig. 2). In patients with short necks, a transaxillary (swimmer's) view is helpful. If this is not acceptable, computed tomography (CT) of this area must be performed. Flexion and extension views are contraindicated in patients with neurologic deficits. The cervical collar must remain in position until the spine is shown radiographically to be uninvolved, as determined by a qualified evaluator. Once the lateral view has been verified to be normal and the patient is alert, conscious, and neurologically intact, flexion-extension radiographs may be obtained. These must be done under strict physician control and the patient must be able to actively flex and extend the neck in a voluntary manner. One should look for subluxation, abnormal disk space widening, or an asymmetric widening of the spinous processes with this study.

Some 3% to 5% of comatose patients will have an associated neck injury. In patients who are alert, conscious, and neurologically intact, with no overt fracture or dislocation visualized radiographically, a distraction or stretch test can be performed.[11] This must be done under *strict physician control* as the weight is added. Traction is applied through secure skeletal fixation or a head halter. Minimum weight is placed initially to minimize the risk of severe displacement, and the radiograph is obtained (Fig. 3). Weight is added to the longitudinal traction in 5- to 10-lb increments, and lateral radiographs are obtained after each addition of weight. It is important to allow at least 5 minutes between incremental weight applications to allow for neurologic examination and creep of the viscolastic structures involved. A positive test is indicated by any asymmetric widening of the disk space, increased intraspinous gap, sagittal rotation, or a change in neurologic status. As soon as injury is discovered, Gardner-Wells tongs should be placed to stabilize the spine and protect the neural tissues.

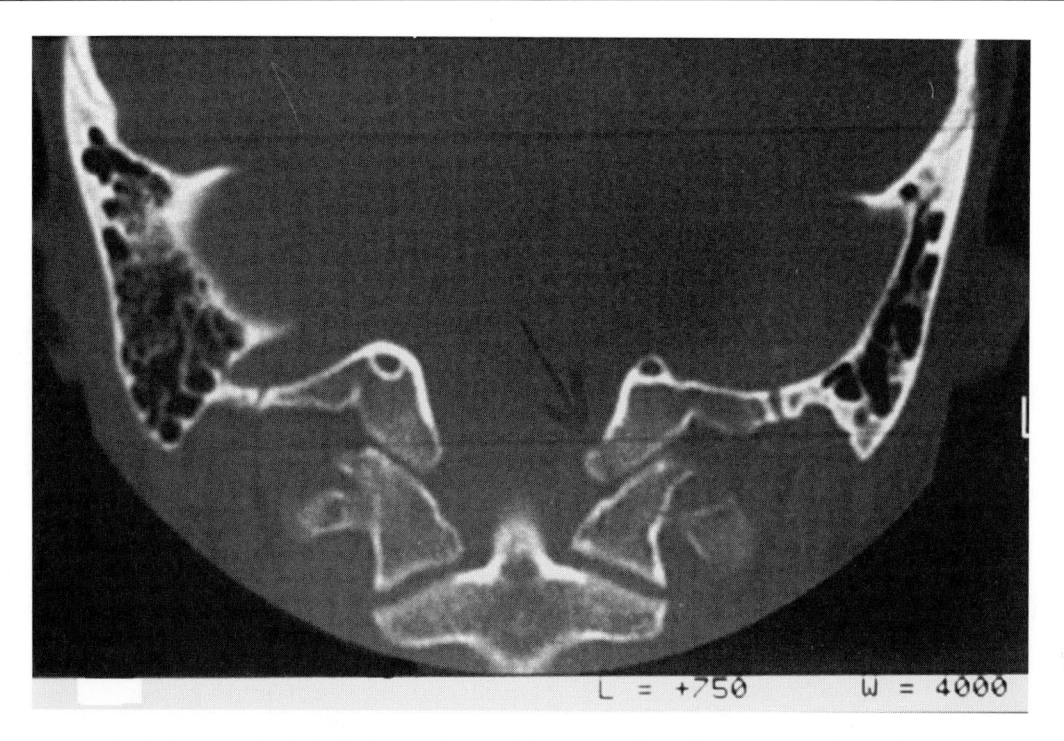

Fig. 4 CT is extremely helpful in cases in which the fracture is not obvious on routine radiographic evaluation. This scan shows a fracture of the occipital condyle in a patient who continued to complain of significant occipitocervical pain, although the radiographs were read as normal.

CT is helpful in diagnosing occult fractures of the cervical spine.[12] Using thin section tomography, the authors of one study demonstrated fractures in 70% of a group of patients whose spinal radiographs revealed no obvious fracture in the standard three views (Fig. 4).[10]

The use of magnetic resonance imaging (MRI) has greatly augmented the evaluation of spinal trauma.[13-15] MRI enhances soft tissue visualization, allowing intramedullary contusions, hematomas, ligament tears, disk herniations, and fluid accumulation to be seen (Fig. 5). Fat suppression studies provide an excellent method of evaluating soft tissue disruptions in the cervical end of the central cord.

When evaluating MRI results in individuals in traction devices for spinal stabilization, critical analysis is important, because these devices can cause image artifacts and compromise the ability to obtain valid information. These artifacts can often be eliminated by disrupting the electrical continuity of the supporting frame of the device.[16] After radiographic evaluation of the spine, stability criteria can be assessed using the grading schemes set forth by White and associates.[11] Although not scientifically validated, this scheme provides guidelines that use both the physical examination and the radiographic evaluation to ascertain potential problem areas that may require surgical stabilization. Once specific problem areas are identified within the spine, appropriate treatment regimens can be instituted.

Spinal Cord Injury

The experimental evidence that the spinal cord undergoes progressive changes after injury and that the changes are less in myelinated axonal tracts than in gray matter has important therapeutic implications. These progressive changes have been termed *secondary injury*.[17] Although initially the secondary injury was thought to have been caused by ischemia, other biochemical events have been implicated.

Following injury, adenosine triphosphate (ATP) storages are depleted, causing failure of calcium-dependent enzymes and membrane transport systems.[17,18] Under these conditions, uncontrolled intracellular influx of calcium is observed. The mitochondrial calcium pump is overloaded, uncoupling oxidative phosphorylation and further decreasing production of ATP. Calcium-dependent phospholipase A_2 is activated, which breaks down membranes and releases arachidonic acid. Arachidonic acid is metabolized into a variety of substances that can decrease local spinal cord blood flow, cause release of lysosomal enzymes, mediate platelet aggregation, and generate peroxide free radicals. The peroxide free radicals are released into the cytosol, where they can break down cellular membranes, creating more free radicals. Disruption of cellular membranes by peroxidation and hydrolytic enzymes is thought to be an important component of the secondary injury following

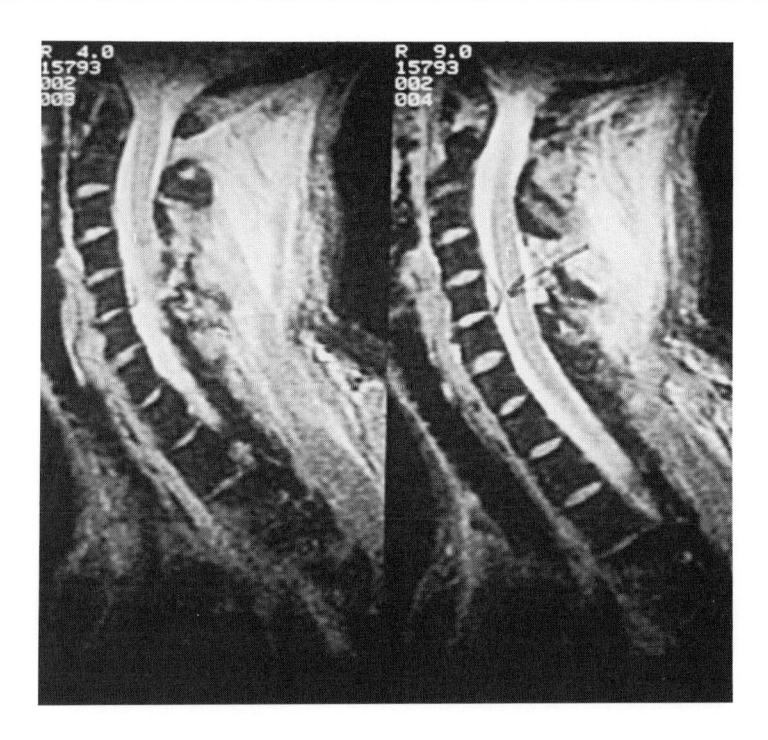

Fig. 5 Sagittal MRI of the cervical spine showing significant soft tissue disruption posteriorly and a disk herniation at C5–6. Knowledge of disk material in the canal will allow this situation to be properly addressed, minimizing the risk of neurologic compromise should a reduction maneuver be required.

spinal cord trauma. Recently, researchers have focused on pharmacologic techniques to limit lipid peroxidation and thereby decrease the secondary injury.

Experimental Treatment of Spinal Cord Injuries

Methylprednisolone succinate is a corticosteroid that has a significantly greater effect on decreasing lipid peroxidation than dexamethasone. Animal studies confirm that methylprednisolone given in high doses decreases lipid peroxidation, preserves the integrity of neuronal structures, and improves outcome following experimental spinal cord injuries. Large doses (30 mg/kg) of the drug are required and must be administered within 8 hours of injury. The efficacy of methylprednisolone in humans has been confirmed by the National Spinal Cord Injury Study 2 (NSCIS 2).[19] This double-blind, randomized study of 476 patients compared placebo, naloxone, and methylprednisolone in patients with spinal cord injuries. Statistically significant improvement in motor and sensory scores occurred in the groups given methylprednisolone, compared to those given placebo or naloxone. However, the degree of overall motor improvement was small. Actual functional recovery was not measured in this study. Patients with incomplete as well as complete spinal cord injuries benefited if the drug was given within 8 hours of injury. Complications such as wound infection and gastrointestinal bleeding were greater in the methylprednisolone group but not to a level of statistical significance. Lesions of the conus medullaris and cauda equina were not evaluated.

Triliazoid is an aminosteroid that does not have glucocorticoid activity but is a potent inhibitor of lipid peroxidation. This drug has been demonstrated to promote functional recovery in experimental spinal cord injury models. It is currently being investigated in the NSCIS 3 investigation.

Gangliosides are large glycolipid molecules that are found on the outer surface of most cell membranes. They are thought to be involved in immunologic processes and other cellular membrane properties such as binding and transport. Gangliosides are highly concentrated in neural tissues. In cell culture, they induce nerve cytogenesis and have a trophic effect on nerve cells. In experimental traumatic brain injuries, they have been shown to reduce cerebral edema and speed recovery. The authors of one study reported a statistically significant increase in functional recovery in spinal cord–injured patients given GM-1 ganglioside compared to placebo.[20] Unlike methylprednisolone, this drug can be administered effectively up to 3 days after injury. Although the results are encouraging, gangliosides are considered experimental and are currently undergoing a multicenter investigation.

Summary

Critical factors such as spinal stability and neurologic compromise become important issues in planning treatment regimens in polytrauma patients. In individuals who sustain a neurologic deficit as a result of spinal trauma, the extent of the deficit and its improvement over time become extremely important in counseling the patient and family members regarding the prognosis. An accurate, documented physical examination and a thorough radiographic assessment are essential in the evaluation of patients with spinal injuries.

References

1. Garfin SR, Shackford SR, Marshall LF, et al: Care of the multiply injured patient with cervical spine injury. *Clin Orthop* 1989;239:19-29.

2. Green BA, Eismont FJ, O'Heir JT: Spinal cord injury: A systems approach. Prevention, emergency medical services, and emergency room management. *Crit Care Clin* 1987;3:471-493.

3. Podolsky S, Baraff LJ, Simon RR, et al: Efficacy of cervical spine immobilization methods. *J Trauma* 1983;23:461-465.

4. McGuire RA, Degnan G, Amundson GM: Evaluation of current extrication orthoses in immobilization of the unstable cervical spine. *Spine* 1990;15:1064-1067.

5. Vaccaro AR, An HS, Lin S, et al: Noncontiguous injuries of the spine. *J Spinal Disord* 1992;5:320-329.

6. McGuire RA, Neville S, Green BA, et al: Spinal instability and the log-rolling maneuver. *J Trauma* 1987;27:525-531.

7. Stauffer ES: Neurologic recovery following injuries to the cervical spinal cord and nerve roots. *Spine* 1984;9:532-534.

8. Stauffer ES: Spinal cord injury syndromes. *Semin Spine Surg* 1991;3:87-90.

9. Gertzbein SD, Court-Brown CM: Flexion-distraction injuries of the lumbar spine: Mechanisms of injury and classification. *Clin Orthop* 1988;227:52-60.

10. Streitwieser DR, Knopp R, Wales LR, et al: Accuracy of standard radiographic views in detecting cervical spine fractures. *Ann Emerg Med* 1983;12:538-542.

11. White AA, Southwick WO, Panjabi MM: Clinical instability in the lower cervical spine: A review of past and current concepts. *Spine* 1976;1:15-27.

12. Post MJ, Green BA: The use of computed tomography in spinal trauma. *Radiol Clin North Am* 1983;21:327-375.

13. Beers GJ, Raque GH, Wagner GG, et al: MR imaging in acute cervical spine trauma. *J Comput Assist Tomogr* 1988;12:755-761.

14. Schaefer DM, Flanders A, Northrup BE, et al: Magnetic resonance imaging of acute cervical spine trauma: Correlation with severity of neurologic injury. *Spine* 1989;14:1090-1095.

15. Kerslake RW, Jaspan T, Worthington BS: Magnetic resonance imaging of spinal trauma. *Br J Radiol* 1991;64:386-402.

16. Malko JA, Hoffman JC Jr, Jarrett PJ: Eddy-current-induced artifacts caused by an ''MR-compatible'' halo device. *Radiology* 1989;173:563-564.

17. Young W: Secondary injury mechanisms in acute spinal cord injury. *J Emerg Med* 1993;11(suppl 1):S13-S22.

18. Janssen L, Hansebout RR: Pathogenesis of spinal cord injury and newer treatments: A review. *Spine* 1989;14:23-32.

19. Bracken MB, Shepard MJ, Collins WF, et al: A randomized controlled trial of methylprednisolone or naloxone in the treatment of acute spinal-cord injury: Results of the Second National Acute Spinal Cord Injury Study. *N Engl J Med* 1990;322:1405-1411.

20. Geisler FH, Dorsey FC, Coleman WP: Recovery of motor function after spinal-cord injury: A randomized, placebo-controlled trial with GM-1 ganglioside. *N Engl J Med* 1991;324:1829-1838.

31
Pathophysiology and Experimental Treatment of Spinal Cord Injury

Introduction

Numerous historical accounts testify to the devastating nature of spinal cord injury (SCI). Harvey Cushing, as a military surgeon during World War I, noted that approximately 80% of all patients with spinal cord injury died within 2 weeks.[1] Ancient Egyptian physicians described spinal cord injury as "a disease not to be treated."[2] This lamentable situation persisted until World War II with the advent of powerful antibiotics, better understanding of treatment of some of the systemic consequences of SCI, and the opening of centers specializing in treating spinal cord injury, such as the Stoke-Mandeville Center.[3] However, the success of interventions targeted at restoring neurologic function has been notably dismal. Descriptions of surgical approaches to SCI include direct reanastomosis of the injured segment and grafting cadaver spinal cord into the injured site, decompressive laminectomy, dural expansion, and midline myelotomy. All attempts have failed until recently, with promising reports of fetal tissue grafting into experimental models of SCI. For the most part, better rehabilitation has played the important role in improving outcome for these patients. Contemporary research on the pathophysiologic processes that occur after an injury to the central nervous system has supported rational drug treatment strategies that have definitively improved neurologic function after SCI in humans.

This chapter will focus on the pathophysiologic events that take place after SCI and treatments that are clinically useful or are in the midst of clinical trials.

Pathophysiologic Consequences of Spinal Cord Injury

The pathology of SCI can be divided temporally (acute versus chronic) and structurally (primary versus secondary injury). These divisions intertwine; primary and secondary injury have both acute and chronic phases. Primary injury results from the transfer of kinetic energy to the substance of the spinal cord, disrupting axons, damaging nerve cells, and rupturing blood vessels. In the acute stages (defined here as the first 8 hours), hemorrhage and necrosis occur in the central gray matter in the first hour after injury, followed by edema and hemorrhage in the white matter in the next 7 hours (Fig. 1). Later, inflammatory cells migrate to the injury site along with glial proliferation. Scar and cyst formation occur within 1 to 4 weeks (Fig. 2). Secondary injury results from ischemia caused by reduced blood flow to the damaged segment. The reduction in blood flow may be caused by a compromised spinal canal, significant spinal cord hemorrhage and edema, or reduced systemic blood pressure. Generally, all three events occur simultaneously in the setting of traumatic SCI. In the acute stages, ischemia sets up a chain of biochemical reactions that result in membrane disruption and cell death. These series of well-described, universal reactions have proven to be the basis for the success of pharmacologic interventions to date. Later, in the chronic phase, neurons may attempt repair by axon and dendritic outgrowth, but these repair processes are aborted and inhibited by intrinsic and extrinsic signals.

Primary Injury: Acute Structural and Physiologic Disruption of Axons

The fiber tracts of the spinal cord are typically not physically severed as a result of nonpenetrating trauma (Fig. 3). In a series of postmortem examinations, anatomic separation was observed in five of six cases of SCI due to gunshot wound, but this finding was present in only three of 15 cases when SCI was caused by motor vehicle accident or fall.[4] The separation of axons is a gradual process, occurring at the site of injury over a period of days after the injury. It generally is a result of a series of pathologic events rather than immediate physical separation. Axonal separation is caused by damage to the axon membrane and internal cytoskeleton proteins.[5] As a consequence of interruption of the continuity of the axon, retrograde degeneration, known as Wallerian degeneration, occurs to the remaining axon and nerve cell body. At the injury site, inflammatory cells respond to parenchymal hemorrhage, with early infiltration of neutrophils followed later by microglia and mac-

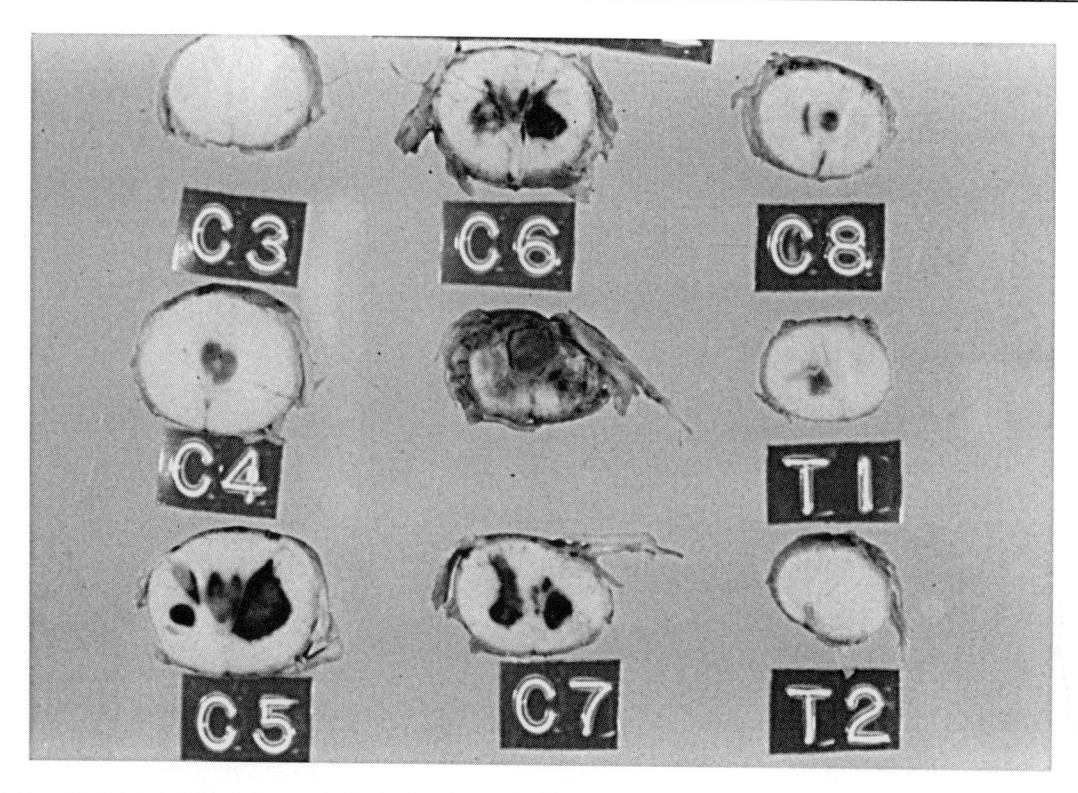

Fig. 1 Multiple sections taken through the cervical spinal cord of an individual with spinal cord injury. These sections demonstrate the rostrocaudal extent of hematomyelia and its predilection for the gray matter. The injury occurred at the C6 level, and more extensive damage is apparent within the white matter.

rophages. Within 1 to 4 weeks, there is astrocyte proliferation and hypertrophy, causing a glial scar.

There is a physiologic disruption of information transmitted through the axon, caused immediately by the kinetic energy of the injury. This may be due to an immediate depolarization of the axonal membrane associated with failure to repolarize that results as potassium is leaked from the axon.[6] Alternatively, the recognized hypoperfusion of the spinal cord that occurs within hours of injury may create ischemic conditions at the injury site, resulting in failure of conduction. Finally, the process of remyelination of undisrupted axons after injury may occur aberrantly, if at all, causing either inadequate or a complete absence of conduction through the injury site even though the axons may be physically present.

Secondary Injury: Ischemia at the Injury Site

SCI is characteristically associated with immediate hemorrhage and edema within the gray matter.[7-10] Within the first minute of SCI, petechial hemorrhages form in the central gray matter. These hemorrhages coalesce over the next 30 to 60 minutes, resulting in the familiar hemorrhagic central necrosis. Over the next 4 to 8 hours, the hemorrhage may extend to include the white matter. Extension of hemorrhage may be a result of hypoperfusion. Experiments in animal models have universally shown a reduction in blood flow at the injured site that persists for a number of hours afterward.[11] The reduction in blood flow may lead to death of cells and axons that were initially not irreversibly injured and may lead to ischemia and death beyond that of the injury site.[12] It is in this arena that significant pharmacologic efforts have been focused, based on information derived from study of neuronal response to ischemia throughout the CNS.

Ischemic changes throughout the central nervous system are characterized by a large influx of Ca^{2+} into the cell.[13] Calcium influx is primarily through channels that are opened by excitatory amino acids, such as glutamate. This specific channel is known as the N-methyl, D-aspartate (NMDA) channel. This channel is not blocked by commonly used Ca^{2+} channel blockers, such as nimodipine, rather by drugs such as MK-801 or ketamine that specifically block the NMDA channel. A number of metabolic reactions result, including failure of mitochondria and activation of phospholipases, proteases, and ATPases. The result is a loss of energy stores and breakdown of the cell membrane. Membrane breakdown is also mediated through the generation of free radicals and activation of membrane phospholipases and lipases. Free radical formation is promoted by the failure of the cell to convert oxygen completely to carbon dioxide and water, and results in lipid peroxidation and subsequent failure of the cell membrane.[14-16] Drugs such as methylprednisolone or the 21-aminosteroid tirilizad mesylate inhibit membrane peroxidation.[17]

Chronic Changes: Cystic Cavitation and Scar Formation

Over a period of weeks, a glial scar is formed at the site of injury. This glial scar inhibits axonal regrowth not only physically but perhaps also through the release of growth-inhibiting proteins produced by oligodendrocytes. Small cysts are seen at the site as a result of necrosis. Infrequently, these may coalesce and extend to form a posttraumatic syrinx that will compromise residual neurologic function.

Experimental Treatment

Animal model systems have been developed to replicate some or all of the early pathophysiologic events of traumatic SCI in humans.[18] Studies using these models have led to clinical pharmacologic trials that have focused on early secondary injury events.[12] To date, there is no convincing evidence that surgical intervention on the human spinal cord itself improves neurologic outcome after injury. Stabilization of the bony and ligamentous elements of the spine or removal of disk or bone fragments that cause compression may prevent further injury to the damaged spinal cord, thereby improving long-term neurologic outcome. There is promising evidence from the laboratory that anatomic and functional restoration can occur after SCI using fetal tissue grafts. However, there is no definitive proof that surgical strategies, such as laminectomy, opening of the dura for cord decompression, or grafting of tissues (such as omentum), improve neurologic function. Proposed surgical strategies should be subjected to prospective and randomized clinical trials to compare the role of surgery to current medical treatment. Although the surgeon may be reluctant to consider such a trial for ethical reasons, multiple carotid endarterectomy trials and the extracranial-intracranial bypass study were performed under just such conditions, and were invaluable in clearly defining the role of these surgical procedures.

Corticosteroids are recognized to reduce edema from tumors in the CNS, and have been repeatedly used in the treatment of SCI. Corticosteroids have multiple effects that are dose dependent, and include membrane stabilization, modification of electric activity, and lysosomal inhibition. Basic science investigation throughout the 1980s and be-

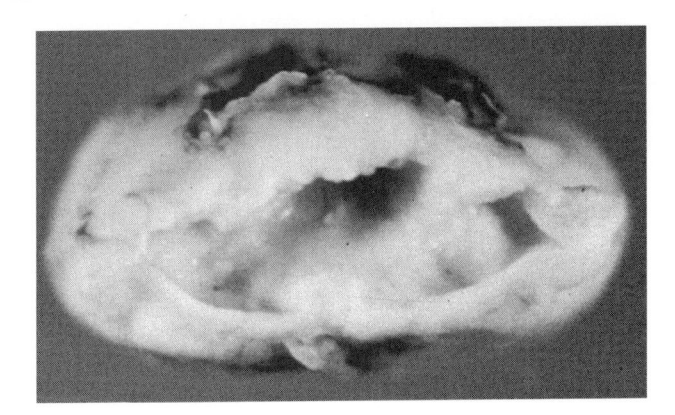

Fig. 2 Cystic cavity within the cervical spinal cord in an individual who died 2 years after spinal cord injury. The outermost tracts of white matter are preserved, but were not functional in this individual.

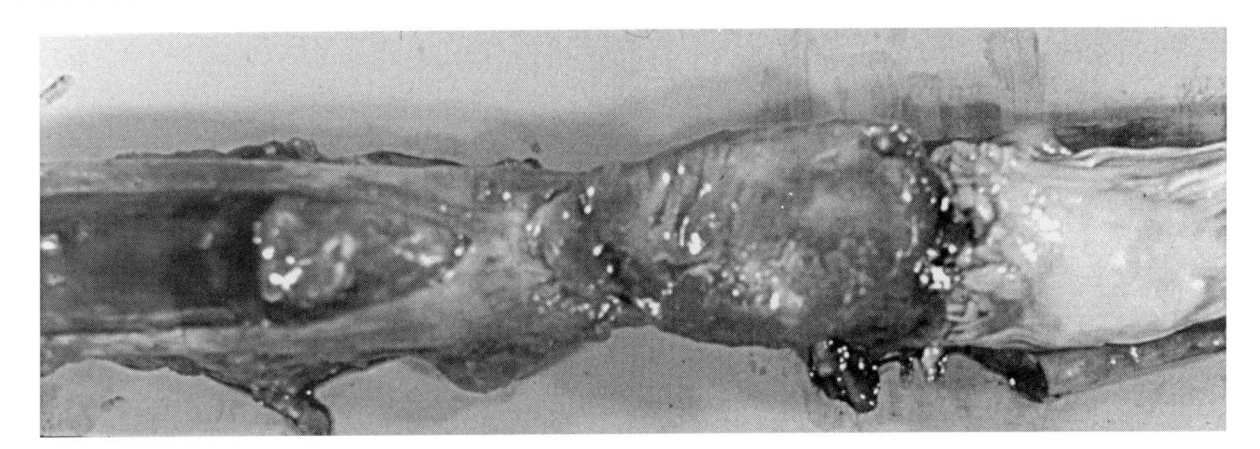

Fig. 3 Acute spinal cord injury close to the level of the cauda equina, following a flexion-distraction injury at the T12-L1 level. Hemorrhage is present rostrally (to the left on the specimen) but there is not physical transection.

yond has better defined the critical role that steroids play in ischemic injury, namely, acting as antioxidant agents to scavenge free radicals and prevent lipid membrane breakdown. These effects in the laboratory led to a multicenter trial of the glucocorticoid methylprednisolone in the treatment of acute SCI in the early 1980s.

The National Spinal Cord Injury Study (NASCIS 1) compared low-dose methylprednisolone (100 mg bolus followed by 100 mg/day) to high-dose drug (1,000 mg bolus and 1,000 mg/day) for 10 days in a prospective, double-blind, randomized study.[19] Because the practice at the time of the study was to administer steroids, a placebo arm was unavailable. Patients were enrolled within the first 48 hours after injury. The results showed no improvement in outcome with steroids and an increase in morbidity associated with high-dose methylprednisolone due to infections. However, laboratory evidence during the time of the study indicated that a significant dose-response curve existed, showing that even the high-dose group was at 50% below the optimal dose.[20,21] Furthermore, timing of drug administration was also critical, with few benefits demonstrated in animals given the drug 8 hours or more after injury. Finally, methylprednisolone had its major effect within the first 24 hours of administration.

The evidence from these basic science studies prompted a second study in the late 1980s, this time examining very-high-dose methylprednisolone, naloxone, or placebo given within 8 hours of injury for a 24-hour period in a double-blind, randomized study (NASCIS 2).[22-24] Results from this study were far more encouraging for use of methylprednisolone, compared to naloxone or placebo. Methylprednisolone given within 8 hours of injury at a loading dose of 30 mg/kg and then continued with a constant infusion of 5.4 mg/kg for 23 hours improved motor and sensory outcome in both complete and incomplete spinal cord injury. These results were not demonstrated in patients entered in the naloxone arm of the trial, with outcome in these patients being essentially the same as placebo. No significant increase was found in morbidity or mortality with any of the drugs. Consequently, methylprednisolone is routinely given to patients with traumatic SCI under the parameters defined by this study.

Two important pharmacologic clinical trials were underway as of 1995. The results of the NASCIS 2 study ethically prohibit the use of placebo for future drug trials, so the NASCIS 3 study is comparing the efficacy of methylprednisolone to Tirilazad mesylate in a multicenter, randomized, double-blind trial. Patients are entered within 8 hours of injury, given the bolus dose of methylprednisolone, then randomized into the two treatment arms. Tirilazad mesylate is one of the class of compounds known as 21-aminosteroids, or lazaroids.[25] This drug scavenges free radicals effectively without such adverse consequences of high-dose glucocorticoids as immunosuppression.

A second multicenter, randomized, double-blind trial is comparing outcome of SCI after the administration of monosialotetrahexosylganglioside (GM-1). This study was begun after a promising initial study.[26] Gangliosides are glycolipid molecules found in very high concentrations in normal brain cell membranes. The mechanism of action of gangliosides is unclear, and may be related more to stimulation of dendritic outgrowth and neuronal recovery than to inhibition of specific biochemical processes that occur as a result of ischemia. In this trial, patients are given methylprednisolone and then divided into two arms, one set of patients given GM-1 and the other given placebo. Timing of administration of GM-1 appears to be less critical than with methylprednisolone and patients are enrolled within 3 days of injury. GM-1 is continued for several weeks. Clearly, there may be a role for combined drug treatment, that is, to reduce the effects of ischemia and promote intrinsic neuronal recovery processes.

References

1. United States Surgeon-General's Office: Care of head injuries and injuries to the spine and peripheral nerves in forward hospitals, in *The Medical Department of the U.S. Army in the World War.* Washington, DC, Government Printing Office, 1927, pp 755-758.

2. Smith E: *The Edwin Smith Surgical Papyrus.* Chicago, IL, University of Chicago Press, 1930, pp 323-332.

3. Watson DO, Skerritt PW, Kerr M: Medical care and restoration, in Bedbrook G (ed): *Lifetime Care of the Paraplegic Patient.* Edinburgh, Scotland, Churchill Livingstone, 1985, p 7-21.

4. Bunge RP, Puckett WR, Becerra JL, et al: Observations on the pathology of human spinal cord injury: A review and classification of 22 new cases with details in from a case of chronic cord compression with extensive focal demyelination. *Adv Neurol* 1993;59:75-89.

5. Povlishock J: Traumatically induced axonal injury: Pathogenesis and pathobiological implications. *Brain Pathol* 1992;2:1-12.

6. Kakulas BA: Pathology of spinal injuries. *Cent Nerv Sys Trauma* 1985;1:117-129.

7. Guttmann L (ed): *Spinal Cord Injuries: Comprehensive Management and Research.* Oxford, UK, Blackwell Scientific Publishers, 1973.

8. Hughes J: Pathology of spinal cord damage in spinal injuries, in Feiring EH, Abler C (eds): *Brock's Injuries of the Brain*

and *Spinal Cord and Their Coverings*, ed 5. New York, NY, Springer-Verlag, 1974.

9. Hughes JT (ed): Trauma to the spinal cord, in *Pathology of the Spinal Cord*, ed 2. London, UK, Lloyd-Luke, 1978, pp 91-104.

10. Jellinger K: Neuropathology of cord injuries, in Vinken PJ, Bruyn GW, Braakman R (eds): *Handbook of Clinical Neurology: Injuries of the Spine and Spinal Cord. Part 1.* Amsterdam, The Netherlands, North Holland Publishers, 1976, vol 25, pp 43-121.

11. Young W: Blood flow, metabolic and neurophysiological mechanisms in spinal cord injury, in Becker DP, Povlishock JT (eds): *Central Nervous System Trauma: Status Report.* Bethesda, MD, NINCDS, 1985, p 463.

12. Nockels R, Young W: Pharmacologic strategies in the treatment of experimental spinal cord injury. *J Neurotrauma* 1992;9(suppl 1):S221-S227.

13. Balentine JD, Hogan EL, Banik NL, et al: Calcium and the pathogenesis of spinal cord injury, in Dacey RG Jr, Winn HR, Rimel RW, et al (eds): *Trauma of the Central Nervous System.* New York, NY, Raven Press, 1985, pp 285-295.

14. Anderson DK, Means ED: Pathophysiological mechanisms in acute spinal cord trauma: Effects of decompartmentalized iron on cell membranes, in Dacey RG Jr, Winn HR, Rimel RW, et al (eds): *Trauma of the Central Nervous System.* New York, NY, Raven Press, 1985, pp 297-308.

15. Anderson DK, Hall ED: Pathophysiology of spinal cord trauma. *Ann Emerg Med* 1993;22:987-992.

16. Hall ED, Braughler JM: Role of lipid peroxidation in post-traumatic spinal cord degeneration: A review. *Cent Nerv Sys Trauma* 1986;3:281-294.

17. Hall ED, Braughler JM: Glucocorticoid mechanisms in acute spinal cord injury: A review and therapeutic rationale. *Surg Neurol* 1982;18:320-327.

18. Young W, Ransohoff J: Injuries to the cervical cord: Acute spinal cord injuries: Experimental therapy, pathophysiological mechanisms, and recovery of function, in *The Cervical Spine*, ed 2. Philadelphia, PA, JB Lippincott, 1989, pp 464-495.

19. Bracken MB, Collins WF, Freeman DF, et al: Efficacy of methylprednisolone in acute spinal cord injury. *JAMA* 1984;251:45-52.

20. Braughler JM, Hall ED: Pharmacokinetics of methylprednisolone in cat plasma and spinal cord following a single intravenous dose of the sodium succinate ester. *Drug Metab Dispos Biol Fate Chem* 1982;10:551-552.

21. Hall ED, Braughler JM: Effects of intravenous methylprednisolone on spinal cord lipid peroxidation and (NA^+K^+)-: ATPase activity. Dose-response analysis during 1st hour after contusion injury in the cat. *J Neurosurg* 1982;57:247-253.

22. Bracken MB: Treatment of acute spinal cord injury with methylprednisolone: Results of a multicenter, randomized clinical trial. *J Neurotrauma* 1991;8(suppl 1):S47-S52.

23. Bracken MB, Shepard MJ, Collins WF, et al: A randomized, controlled trial of methylprednisolone or naloxone in the treatment of acute spinal-cord injury: Results of the Second National Acute Spinal Cord Injury Study. *N Engl J Med* 1990;322:1405-1411.

24. Bracken MB, Shepard MJ, Collins WF Jr, et al: Methylprednisolone or naloxone treatment after acute spinal cord injury: 1-year follow-up data. Results of the Second National Acute Spinal Cord Injury Study. *J Neurosurg* 1992;76:23-31.

25. Anderson DK, Braughler JM, Hall ED, et al: Effects of treatment with U-74006F on neurological outcome following experimental spinal cord injury. *J Neurosurg* 1988;69:562-567.

26. Geisler FH, Dorsey FC, Coleman WP: Recovery of motor function after spinal-cord injury: A randomized, placebo-controlled trial with GM-1 ganglioside. *N Engl J Med* 1991;324:1829-1838.

32
Prognosis of Spinal Cord Injuries

Prognostication of outcome following spinal cord injury (SCI) is based on clinical information obtained by neurologic examination. In the past, there was no universally accepted classification system for measuring the severity of SCI. Not only was it difficult to compare outcomes of different published series, since different definitions and testing procedures were employed, but it was difficult for physicians to communicate with one another or to accurately track a patient's progress.

The Frankel score or modified Frankel score was the most commonly used classification system.[1] Patients were assigned to one of five broad categories, based on the results of motor and sensory examination. Although helpful, this system was insensitive to changes within each category and depended on broad categories that were not well defined. Thus, for more than 25 years the international community in SCI recognized the need for improved measures of injury severity.

To respond to the need for more reliable methods of clinically assessing the extent of SCI, the American Spinal Injury Association (ASIA) in 1982 developed standards for the neurologic classification of SCI. Recognizing the need to develop standards that would have worldwide acceptance, the ASIA sought input from representatives of diverse medical specialties and professional societies and, in 1992, published revised standards.[2] These standards were endorsed by the International Medical Society of Paraplegia, in Barcelona, and became known as the International Standards.

The International Standards provide a more accurate means of quantifying motor recovery than the Frankel system. They represent the most valid, precise, and reliable minimum data set to assess SCI and are being used by the National Model System Spinal Cord Injury data base. The prognostic information presented in this chapter is primarily based on studies that follow these standards.

This chapter reviews the International Standards, summarizes outcome studies conducted using the International Standards, and describes the use of electrophysiologic, radiologic, and hemodynamic studies to predict neurologic recovery.

International Standards

The International Standards are based on a systematic neurologic examination of key dermatomes and myotomes representing the key neurologic segments of the spinal cord. They differ from the original ASIA standards published in 1982 in several important respects. First, the definition of the completeness of spinal cord injury was changed to a definition based on the presence or absence of sacral sparing. Second, sensation is recorded at a specific point within each dermatome to improve reliability.

Neurologic Level

Neurologic level of injury refers to the most caudal segment of the spinal cord with normal motor and sensory function on both sides of the body. Because the segments at which there is normal function frequently differ by side and in terms of sensory versus motor testing, four different components may be identified in determining the neurologic level: right sensory level, left sensory level, right motor level, and left motor level. (A diagram distributed by the American Spinal Injury Association facilitates accurate documentation of initial neurologic status. A copy of this diagram can be found in the chapter, *Patient Assessment in Spinal Injury*.)

Completeness of SCI

Immediately after SCI, a state of spinal shock develops that may result in areflexia for varying time periods. A patient with no motor or sensory function below the neurologic level of injury during this time may still regain excellent function. However, as the length of time after injury increases, the persistence of a complete injury progressively reduces the chance for significant motor and sensory recovery.

The International Standards' definition of completeness of injury has recently been redefined. Incomplete injury is defined as partial preservation of sensory and/or motor functions below the neurologic level and includes the lowest sacral segment. Sacral sensation includes sensation at the anal mucocutaneous junction as well as deep anal sensation. The test of motor function is the presence of voluntary anal sphincter contraction upon digital examination. Complete injury is defined by the absence of sensory and motor function in the lowest sacral segment.[3]

In the acute phase it is often difficult to perform an accurate motor or sensory examination because the patient is undergoing acute medical stabilization or surgery, may be sedated, intoxicated, confused, or in pain, or may have the limbs restricted by intravenous lines or splints. Additionally, regardless of when the first accurate examination is performed, neurologic recovery or deterioration may have occurred between the injury and the time of the initial examination. In one study, examinations conducted between 72 hours and 1 week after injury more accurately predicted short-term (up to 3 months) functional muscle recovery than examinations conducted within the first 24 hours after injury.[4] Electrophysiologic, hemodynamic, and radiologic studies add little predictive power to the 1-month neurologic examination, which reliably prognosticates neurologic recovery. Further technical refinement of these studies may, however, be helpful in assessing spinal cord status in the earlier, acute phase, when findings on neurologic examination may be unreliable.

Sensory and Motor Scores

Calculation of motor and sensory scores provides a convenient way of monitoring changes in neurologic status based on serial neurologic examinations. However, these scores must be carefully interpreted. Because the motor score is derived from the bilateral manual muscle strength grades of key muscles representing isolated neurologic segments, recovery of these key muscles implies an accurate indication of segmental recovery. Each of these muscles, however, is enervated by several segments. Also, the total score of these key muscles assumes that they are representative of all muscles and functions of the extremities. Further, the relationship between a muscle's manual muscle test grade to contractile strength is nonlinear, and there is considerable variation in muscle strength among individuals because of different body size and level of physical conditioning.

Cord Syndromes

Several clinical syndromes have been identified that exhibit characteristic patterns of neurologic loss, depending on the anatomic lesions within the cord. A central cord syndrome occurs primarily in the cervical region and results in sacral sparing and greater motor loss in the upper extremities than in the lower extremities. The hands often demonstrate a more pronounced motor deficit than the upper arms, with full functional recovery rare. In a Brown-Séquard lesion, hemisection of the cord produces ipsilateral loss of motor function and proprioception and contralateral loss of pain and temperature sensation. Patients with Brown-Séquard injuries often make a good functional recovery and frequently become ambulators. A significant problem is residual spasticity. In an anterior cord syndrome there is preservation of proprioception with variable loss of motor function and pain sensation. In a posterior cord injury, motor function, pain, and light touch sensation are preserved but proprioceptive function is lost. This type of cord syndrome is extremely rare. Injury of the cord at the sacral level produces the conus medullaris syndrome, which usually results in areflexia of the bowel, bladder, and lower extremities. In a cauda equina lesion, the lumbosacral nerve roots within the spinal canal are injured, resulting in areflexia of the bladder, bowel, and lower extremities.

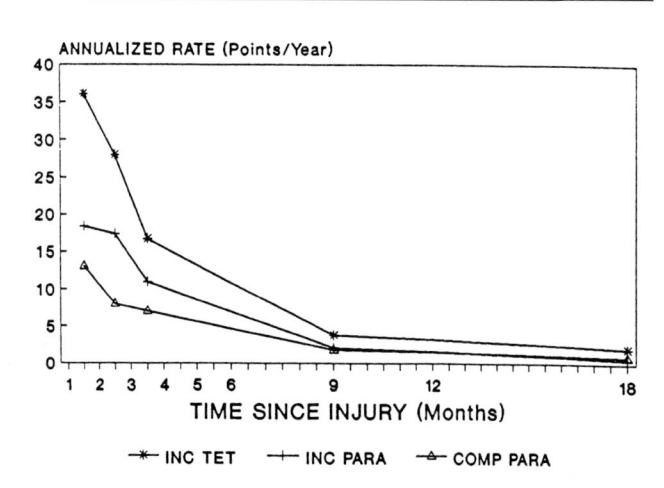

Fig. 1 Annualized recovery rate of lower extremity motor score for complete paraplegia, incomplete paraplegia, and incomplete tetraplegia.[6,15,17]

Recovery

Rate of Recovery

Changes in the motor and sensory scores between examinations may be used to quantify rates of recovery. The annualized rate of recovery is determined by dividing the change in scores for two successive examinations by the time interval (in days) between the examinations to quantify the amount of recovery per day. This figure is then multiplied by 365 days to express the rate of recovery during a particular interval that would have been expected if it were to have continued over the course of a year (Figs. 1 and 2). Patients with incomplete injuries have higher initial motor recovery rates than those with complete injuries. This is true in both the upper and lower extremities. The rate of recovery for both complete and incomplete SCI declines rapidly in the first 6 months after injury, and the rate of recovery after 1 year is minimal. The rate of decline in the sensory scores parallels the decline in motor recovery. Optimal recovery of motor function is dependent upon appropriate management of the patient in the initial postinjury phase.

Motor Recovery After Complete Paraplegia

Of 142 patients with complete paraplegia 1 month after injury, none with an initial neurologic level of injury above T9 had regained any lower extremity motor function 1 year after injury.[5] Thirty-eight percent of patients with an

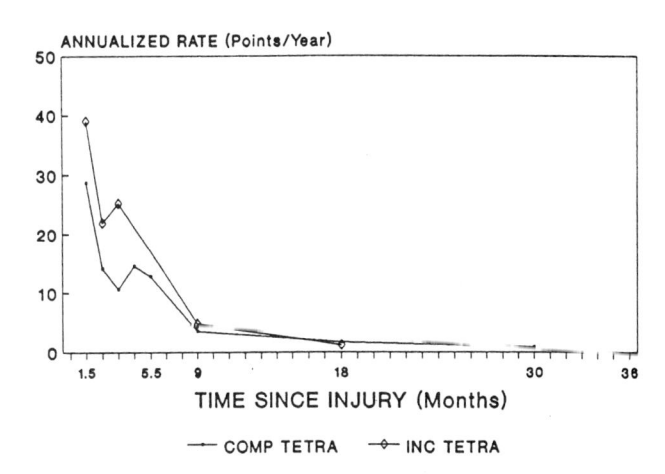

Fig. 2 Annualized recovery rate of upper extremity motor score for complete tetraplegia and incomplete tetraplegia.[6,16]

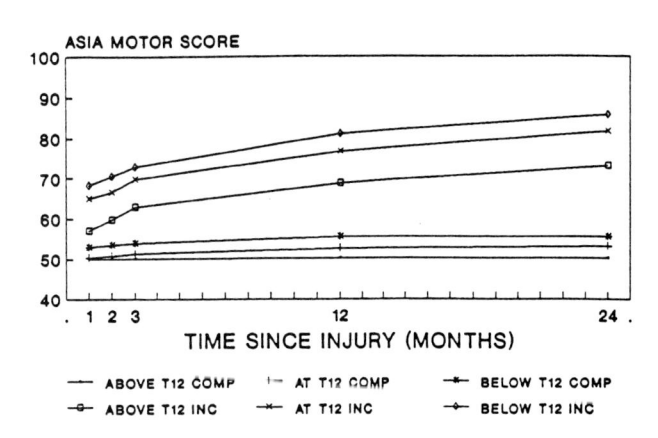

Fig. 3 Recovery of ASIA motor score after complete and incomplete paraplegia by level.[15,17]

initial neurologic level of injury at or below T9 had some return of lower extremity motor function, primarily in the hip flexors and knee extensors. Only 5% of patients recovered sufficient hip and knee extension to reciprocally ambulate using conventional orthoses and crutches. All of the latter group had initial neurologic levels of injury at or below T12. Four percent of patients who had complete injuries on admission to rehabilitation (average, 21 days) converted from complete SCI to incomplete SCI. Half of the patients who experienced late conversion regained control of bladder and bowel function, consistent with the fact that the definition of incomplete injury is based on sacral sparing and recovery of sacral function. One third of patients who experienced late conversion to incomplete SCI and who had levels of injury at L1 and L2 were able to ambulate with a reciprocal gait pattern at 1 year following injury.

There is a significant difference in the recovery of motor function between individuals with complete SCI and those with cauda equina lesions. Individuals with cauda equina lesions generally have incomplete lesions and have areflexia in the lower extremities. The incidence of complete injuries, however, decreases as the vertebral injury descends to the more caudal regions of the spine. Figure 3 shows the different rates of motor recovery based on initial neurologic levels of injury.

Motor Recovery After Incomplete Paraplegia

Fifty-four individuals underwent serial prospective examinations after incomplete paraplegia.[6] Patients were divided into three groups based on the neurologic level of injury 1 month after injury (above T12, at T12, or below T12). These groups were based on anatomic differences corresponding to the expansion of the spinal cord and the formation of the conus at T10, the emergence of the lumbar roots at T12, and the location of the cauda equina. At 1 month those with an initial neurologic level of injury above T12 had the lowest mean lower extremity motor score and those with a neurologic level of injury below T12 had the highest (Fig. 3). Between 1 month and 1 year, there was a significant change in the lower extremity motor score across all three groups, averaging 12 points. The motor recovery curves were parallel, and the differences between the three groups remained approximately constant throughout follow-up, indicating that the rate of recovery was the same (Fig. 3). Seventy-six percent of patients had sufficient recovery of lower extremity muscles to ambulate with a reciprocal gait and achieve community ambulation status.

Motor Recovery After Complete Tetraplegia

Sixty-one individuals admitted with a diagnosis of complete tetraplegia underwent prospective examinations for motor and sensory recovery.[17] At 1 month after injury, the average ASIA motor score (AMS) progressively increased for those with neurologic levels of injury from C4 to C8. The amount of motor recovery was independent of the initial neurologic level of injury for levels between C4 and C8. In the interval between 1 month and 1 year after injury the AMS increased an average of 9 points. The ASIA motor score is plotted in Figure 4 as a function of time since injury for patients grouped according to their motor level of injury at 1 month. Motor recovery followed similar patterns at the C4, C5, C6, and C7 levels.

Motor Recovery After Incomplete Tetraplegia

Recovery of the upper extremity motor score and lower extremity motor score in 50 patients with incomplete tetraplegia is depicted in Figure 5. The motor recovery curves of the upper and lower extremities were approximately the same. Forty-six percent of patients were able to ambulate in the community at 1-year follow-up using a reciprocal gait.

If axonal regeneration of descending corticospinal tracts played a major role in motor recovery in patients with

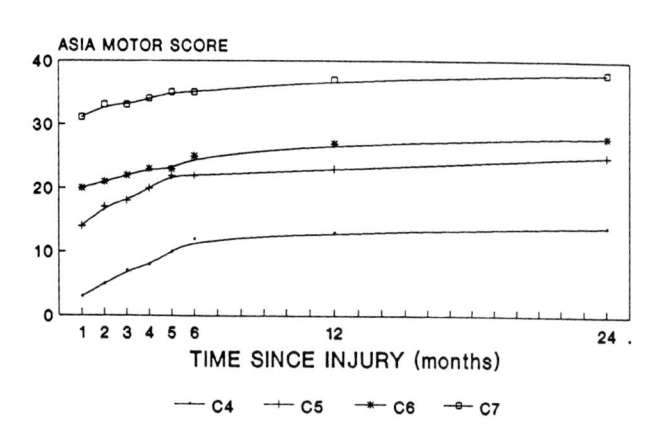

Fig. 4 Recovery of upper extremity motor score after complete tetraplegia, by level of SCI.[16]

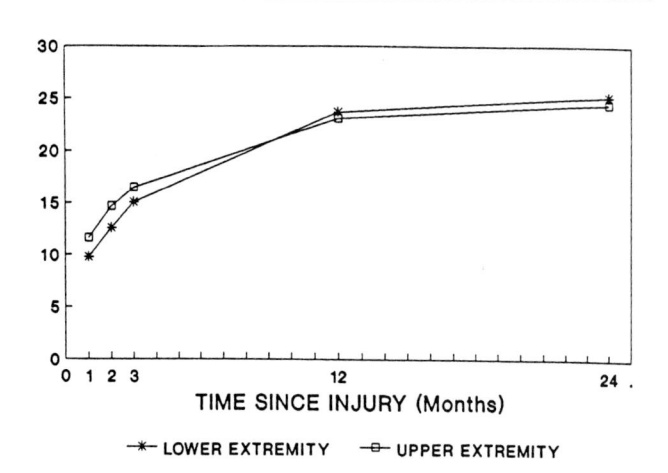

Fig. 5 Upper and lower extremity motor score recovery.[6]

incomplete tetraplegia, upper extremity motor score recovery would precede lower extremity motor score recovery and lower extremity motor score recovery could be delayed 1 or more years after injury. However, the timing of both upper and lower extremity motor score recovery was the same, with the most rapid recovery occurring in the first months after injury (Fig. 5). From this observation, we conclude that upper motor neuron regeneration did not play a major role in the observed lower extremity motor score recovery.

In a study of 27 patients with incomplete tetraplegia and anterior cord syndrome who were initially motor complete, patients with sacral pin sensation had a significantly better prognosis for lower extremity motor recovery than those patients who were incomplete on the basis of light touch only.[8] These findings were confirmed in a study that found that patients having bilateral sacral pin sensation but no lower extremity motor function at 1 month had regained an average of 12 motor points at 1 year.[9]

Brown-Séquard injuries constitute a subset of incomplete SCI. The prognosis after Brown-Séquard-like injuries is generally favorable, although few patients have the classic syndrome. Most patients have a Brown-Séquard-plus syndrome consisting of a mixed type with asymmetric paresis, with hypalgesia more marked on the less paretic side. In a review of 39 patients with Brown-Séquard and Brown-Séquard-plus syndromes, 75% ambulated independently at discharge and nearly all achieved bladder and bowel continence.[10]

Functional Recovery

Because individuals with incomplete SCI have such variable motor and sensory function, it is difficult to predict function based on the neurologic level of injury. Guidelines for expected levels of function have been developed for individuals with complete paraplegia and tetraplegia. Using a patient's neurologic level of injury, predictions about mobility, transfers, self-care, and equipment needs can be made (Tables 1 and 2).

In a study of the relationship between the Motor Index Score (MIS) and functional status in both tetraplegics and paraplegics, the initial MIS was correlated with overall functional outcome in patients with tetraplegia but not in individuals with paraplegia.[11] Also, the initial MIS correlated with both the MIS and overall functional outcomes at discharge from rehabilitation in patients with complete injuries but not in those with incomplete lesions.

Motor Recovery and Injury Pattern

To determine whether type of fracture or gunshot injury correlated with extent of motor impairment at 1 month and/or amount of motor recovery between 1 month and 1 year, prospective neurologic examinations were performed on 278 patients with traumatic SCI.[12] Fractures were classified by the Allen system (cervical spine) or the Denis system (thoracic and lumbar spine). Gunshot injuries were classified based on trajectory and bullet location. When controlling for level (paraplegia versus tetraplegia) and completeness of SCI, there were no significant differences in motor recovery based on type of injury (penetrating versus nonpenetrating), type of fracture, or bullet location. Injuries severely disruptive of the spinal canal were more likely to result in complete SCI. Flexion-rotation injuries in the thoracic and lumbar spine, bilateral facet dislocations in the cervical spine, and gunshot wounds in which the bullet passed through the canal were more likely to be complete. Incomplete injuries were more common among patients with preexisting cervical spondylosis who had fallen and patients with gunshot wounds in which the bullet did not penetrate the spinal canal.

Specific Muscle Recovery

In a multicenter evaluation of upper extremity motor recovery, motor recovery to grade 3/5 in the elbow flexors, elbow extensors, and wrist extensors was found to be more likely in patients who had some voluntary motor function

Table 1. Expected function according to level of injury complete tetraplegia

Neurologic Level	Muscles Present	Mobility	Transfers	Self-care
C1-C3	Limited neck muscles Respirator dependent	Possible candidate for electric wheelchair with portable respirator and tongue switch/breath control	Dependent transfers requiring a lift	Dependent
C4	Neck, trapezius Functional diaphragm	Electric wheelchair with chin or tongue control	Dependent transfers requiring a lift	Dependent
C5	Same as above and biceps	Electric wheelchair with hand control or possibly manual wheelchair with handrim projections (pegs)	Dependent transfers	Assisted with light hygiene and self feeding with proper equipment
C6	Same as above and wrist extensors	Manual wheelchair with friction surface handrims May require electric wheelchair for use in community	Independent transfers with sliding board and proper equipment	Independent in upper extremity activities with proper equipment Independent-assisted with lower extremity dressing and bowel/bladder management
C7	Same as above and triceps	Manual wheelchair may require friction surface handrims	Independent transfers with sliding board	Independent with proper equipment
C8	Same as above and finger flexors	Manual wheelchair may require friction surface handrims	Independent transfers	Independent
T1	Same as above and hand Intrinsics	Manual wheelchair with standard handrims	Independent transfers	Independent

Table 2. Expected function according to level of injury complete paraplegia

Neurologic Level	Muscles Present	Mobility	Transfers	Self-care
T1-T8	Hand intrinsics chest	Manual wheelchair with standard handrims	Independent	Independent
T9-T12	Same as above and trunk muscles	Manual wheelchair Some T12 may ambulate	Independent	Independent
L1-T2	Same as above and hip flexors	Manual wheelchair May be household or limited community ambulator with crutches and orthoses	Independent	Independent
L3-T5	Same as above and knee extensors	May be community ambulator with proper equipment and training	Independent	Independent

1 week after injury.[13] Similar findings have been reported for all upper and lower extremity muscles in complete and incomplete SCI. The strength of a muscle at 1 month is highly predictive of recovery to functional (grade 3) recovery. Tables 3 and 4 cross-tabulate the strength of muscles at 1 month and 1 year for upper and lower extremity muscles after complete and incomplete SCI.

Ambulation

A direct relationship has been reported between motor power and walking ability.[13] Patients who were able to walk in the community had pelvic control with at least fair hip flexor strength and at least fair extensor strength in one knee so that no more than one knee-ankle-foot orthosis was required, enabling the patient to achieve a reciprocal gait pattern. The ability to walk with a reciprocal gait pattern is primarily determined by the strength of the hip flexors, which enable a forward step and reciprocation, and the quadriceps, which provide knee stability and the ability to ambulate without the aid of a knee-ankle-foot orthosis. A strong correlation has been found between the lower extremity motor score, physiologic energy expenditure, and gait performance.[14] All patients with a lower extremity motor score greater or equal to 30 points were community ambulators, walked with a reciprocal gait pattern, and did not routinely use a wheelchair. Energy expenditure rose rapidly and gait performance fell markedly as the lower extremity motor score progressively decreased below 30 points. This explained why many patients with increasing paralysis preferred a wheelchair, which required less energy expenditure. No patients with lower extremity motor scores less than 20 points were community ambulators.

At 1-year follow-up, 47% of individuals with incomplete tetraplegia had recovered sufficient lower extremity strength to use a reciprocal gait pattern with conventional orthoses and/or crutches as their primary mode of ambulation in the community. In contrast, 76% of patients with

Table 3. Prediction of lower extremity motor recovery[6,15,17]

Manual Muscle Strength at One Month*	Percent with Functional 3/5 Strength or More at 1 Year		
	Complete Paraplegia	Incomplete Paraplegia	Incomplete Tetraplegia
0/5	5%	26%	24%
1/5, 2/5	64%	85%	82%

* ASIA key muscles

Table 4. Prediction of upper extremity motor recovery[6,15,17]

Manual Muscle Strength at One Month*	Percent with Functional 3/5 Strength or More at 1 Year	
	Complete Tetraplegia	Incomplete Tetraplegia
0/5	20%	54%
1/5	90%	73%
2/5	100%	100%

* ASIA key muscles

Table 5. 1-Year follow-up ambulation status[6,15,17]

Lower Extremity Asia Motor Score (1 Month)	Community Ambulation Status (1 Year)		
	Complete Paraplegia	Incomplete Paraplegia	Incomplete Tetraplegia
0	<1%	33%	0%
1–10	45%	70%	21%
11–20		100%	63%
> 20		100%	100%
Total	5%	76%	47%

incomplete paraplegia achieved community ambulation status 1 year after injury (Table 5). Even though the mean lower extremity motor score of patients with incomplete tetraplegia may be the same as that for patients with incomplete paraplegia, the associated upper limb and trunk paralysis in the former group limits the use of upper extremity assist devices, accounting for the lower rate of community ambulation.[9]

Lower extremity motor score at 1 month is predictive of further motor recovery and achievement of community ambulation status at 1 year. Table 5 cross-tabulates the lower extremity motor score at 1 month and the percent of patients achieving ambulation in the community at 1 year. The majority of patients with a lower extremity motor score greater than 10 points achieved community ambulation status at 1 year.

Mortality and Morbidity

As both acute and long-term rehabilitative care have improved over the past four decades, the life expectancy of an individual with SCI has approached that of able-bodied individuals. The median years of survival for individuals injured before 30 years of age, between 30 and 50 years, and after 50 years are 43, 24, and 11 years, respectively.

The most common causes of death among individuals with SCI are renal failure and respiratory system diseases.

Tests Predicting Neurologic Recovery

Electrophysiologic Predictors

Somatosensory-evoked potentials (SEPs) offer a noninvasive means of assessing spinal cord integrity. They may be useful in predicting neurologic recovery in patients with SCI. In patients undergoing surgical decompression for myelopathy, early recovery of SEPs predicted a better clinical result, and the presence of recognizable SEPs immediately after injury is considered an encouraging prognostic feature. Studies have shown that complete absence of SEPs correlates with a complete lesion and poor prognosis. SEPs do not, however, appear to add much prognostic information to the initial physical examination findings in patients with SCI.

The limitations of SEPs in predicting motor recovery may be due to the fact that the signal is transmitted via the dorsal columns (proprioception), therefore bypassing an anterior cord lesion and motor pathways.

Motor-evoked potentials may provide better data for prognostication of motor recovery after SCI. However, the test is invasive, requiring direct stimulation of the spinal cord. Further investigation of motor-evoked potentials is necessary to determine the prognostic potential of this technique.

Hemodynamic Predictors

Experimental data suggest that improving spinal cord blood flow by increasing blood pressure can improve outcome in SCI. In analyzing the hemodynamic parameters of 50 patients with acute cervical SCI, a differentiation could not be made between complete and incomplete lesions or between patients with functional improvement and those without.[15] It appeared that severe hemodynamic deficits in the patient with acute cervical SCI were associated with a poor prognosis but that normal hemodynamics did not necessarily dictate neurologic recovery.

Radiologic Correlation

There appears to be poor correlation between radiographic findings and neurologic recovery. In cervical spine injuries there is poor correlation between plain radiographic findings and the type of SCI.[16] The mechanism of injury also appears to be unrelated to prognosis. This may be due to the fact that the bony elements of the spine often recoil from a more dislocated position after injury. Thus, plain radiographs frequently do not demonstrate the severity of the original bony injury and therefore may not be representative of the degree of trauma to the cord. As in the cervical spine, there is poor correlation between canal compromise and neurologic compromise in the thoracolumbar spine. Also, there is no correlation between neurologic recovery and the final spinal canal dimensions.

With its excellent soft-tissue imaging capabilities, magnetic resonance imaging (MRI) has proved invaluable in the direct visualization of injury to the spinal cord and in offering the clinician information regarding the prognosis of such injuries. Several investigators have found a correlation between the pattern of spinal cord injury on T2-weighted images performed acutely after injury and neurologic recovery. The appearance of the spinal cord could be classified as normal or as falling into one of three general injury patterns. Type I injuries produced a central area of hypointensity consistent with acute intraspinal hemorrhage. Type II injuries were associated with a bright signal with cord enlargement consistent with cord edema. The less frequent Type III injuries produced a mixed pattern of central hypointensity surrounded by hyperintensity. Patients with type I injuries (cord hemorrhage) exhibited little or no improvement in Frankel classification and MIS and usually developed intracordal cysts on follow-up MRI. In type II injuries, recovery was variable and correlated with findings on the initial physical examination. All patients with type III injuries had good neurologic recovery, as did those with normal MRIs.

Presently, a detailed neurologic examination performed approximately 1 month after SCI provides the most reliable prognostic information for outcome. With continued refinement and investigation, hemodynamic, imaging, and electrophysiologic studies may provide earlier prognosis than results of the 1-month neurologic examination.

Complications Related to Neurologic Recovery

There are basically two trends related to neurologic deterioration in an individual with SCI. The first relates to deterioration during the acute care management of the patient. In one study, the conditions of 14 of 283 individuals with SCI deteriorated during acute hospitalization.[17] In 12 of the cases that deteriorated, a specific management event was identified as precipitating the neurologic decline. The second basic trend relating to neurologic deterioration involves posttraumatic syrinx formation. With the advent of more sensitive diagnostic tools, the incidence of posttraumatic syrinx has increased. Any patient presenting with a late decline in neurologic function should be evaluated for a posttraumatic syrinx.

Annotated References

1. Frankel HL, Hancock DO, Hyslop G, et al: The value of postural reduction in the initial management of closed injuries of the spine with paraplegia and tetraplegia. *Paraplegia* 1969;7:179-192.

2. American Spinal Injury Association: *Standards for Neurological and Functional Classification of Spinal Cord Injury.* Chicago, IL, American Spinal Injury Association, 1992.

3. Waters RL, Adkins RH, Yakura JS: Definition of complete spinal cord injury. *Paraplegia* 1991;29:573-581.

4. Brown PJ, Marino RJ, Herbison GJ, et al: The 72-hour examination as a predictor of recovery in motor complete quadriplegia. *Arch Phys Med Rehabil* 1991;72:546-548.

5. Waters RL, Yakura JS, Adkins RH, et al: Recovery following complete paraplegia. *Arch Phys Med Rehabil* 1992;73:784-789.

    This prospective study of 148 individuals demonstrated no motor recovery in subjects with initial neurological level of injury above T9. Twenty percent of individuals with levels of injury at or below T12 were able to ambulate in the community using orthoses and/or crutches.

6. Waters RL, Adkins RH, Yakura JS, et al: Motor and sensory recovery following incomplete paraplegia. *Arch Phys Med Rehabil* 1994;75:67-72.

    In 54 subjects, motor recovery was independent of level of injury.

    The lower extremity ASIA motor score increased an average of 11.8 points between admission and the annual exam.

7. Waters RL, Adkins RH, Yakura JS, et al: Motor and sensory recovery following complete tetraplegia. *Arch Phys Med Rehabil* 1993;74:242-247.

    Motor recovery was independent of level of injury between C4 and C8. Rate of motor recovery decreased rapidly in the first six months following injury and then plateaued.

8. Crozier KS, Graziani V, Ditunno JF Jr, et al: Spinal cord injury: Prognosis for ambulation based on sensory examination in patients who are initially motor complete. *Arch Phys Med Rehabil* 1991;72:119-121.

9. Waters RL, Adkins RH, Yakura JS, et al: Motor and sensory recovery following incomplete tetraplegia. *Arch Phys Med Rehabil* 1994;75:306-311.

10. Roth EJ, Park T, Pang T, et al: Traumatic cervical Brown-Séquard and Brown-Séquard-plus syndromes: The spectrum of presentations and outcomes. *Paraplegia* 1991;29:582-589.

11. Lazar RB, Yarkony GM, Ortolano D, et al: Prediction of functional outcome by motor capability after spinal cord injury. *Arch Phys Med Rehabil* 1989;70:819-822.

12. Waters RL, Sie I, Adkins RH, et al: Injury pattern effect on motor recovery after traumatic spinal cord injury. *Arch Phys Med Rehabil* 1995;76:440-443.

13. Ditunno JF Jr, Stover SL, Freed MM, et al: Motor recovery of the upper extremities in traumatic quadriplegia: A multicenter study. *Arch Phys Med Rehabil* 1992;73:431-436.

14. Waters RL, Adkins R, Yakura J, et al: Prediction of ambulatory performance based on motor scores derived from standards of the American Spinal Injury Association. *Arch Phys Med Rehabil* 1994;75:756-760.

    This comparison of biomechanical parameters of walking and strength as assessed by the ASIA motor score indicates that the ASIA motor score correlates strongly with ability to walk.

15. Levi L, Wolf A, Belzberg H: Hemodynamic parameters in patients with acute cervical cord trauma: Description, intervention, and prediction of outcome. *Neurosurgery* 1993;33:1007-1017.

16. Scher AT: Is the pattern of neurological damage of diagnostic value in the radiological assessment of acute cervical spine injury? *Paraplegia* 1981;19:248-252.

17. Marshall LF, Knowlton S, Garfin SR et al: Deterioration following spinal cord injury: A multicenter study. *J Neurosurg* 1987;66:400-404.

33
Occipital Cranial Injuries

Traumatic injuries to the occipitocervical complex are infrequent. The close proximity of the brain stem and spinal cord to the surrounding bony ligamentous structures usually makes neurologic deficits associated with this type of injury fatal. A better understanding of the bony and ligamentous anatomy and a high index of suspicion for these injuries seem to be associated with increasing reports of survival.

Bony Anatomy

The foramen magnum is a large hole in the occipital bone at the base of the skull through which the spinal cord passes. The anterior rim of the foramen magnum is called the basion, and the posterior rim is called the opisthion. Two occipital condyles are situated on the inferior surface of the occipital bone along the anterior lateral edge of the foramen magnum.

The first cervical vertebra supports "the globe of the head" and thus is called the atlas. The atlas is a ring of bone with an anterior and posterior arch and two large lateral masses. The concave superior surface of the lateral masses articulates with the occipital condyles, allowing the head to flex and extend. The inferior aspect of the lateral masses is concave and oval. It articulates with the flat convex superior facet of C2, which allows rotation of C1 on C2. The atlas is an unusual vertebra, having no vertebral body or spinous process. Functionally, it acts like a bony meniscus or bushing between the occiput and C2.

The axis, or C2, is a more conventional vertebra with a body, lamina, and spinous process. It is distinguished by the fact that it has a superior bony projection from the body, called the odontoid process or dens. Embryologically, the dens represents the body of the atlas that separated and united with the axis. The axis pivots or rotates around the odontoid process. The articular processes of the axis are in different planes. The convex superior facets are anterior along the odontoid, allowing rotation. The inferior facets of the axis are posterior and obliquely oriented, similar to the lower cervical facet joints.

Ligamentous Anatomy

The morphology of the craniocervical articulations accounts for the wide range in neck motion. The internal cranial cervical ligaments include the tectorial membranes, the transverse ligaments, and the alar and apical ligaments. The internal cranial cervical ligaments provide significant biomechanical stability.[1,2] Posterior to the dens, limiting anterior atlantoaxial translation, are the tectorial membrane and the transverse ligament. The tectorial membrane is the cranial prolongation of the posterior longitudinal ligament. This thin, flat ligament is located behind the dens, attaches to the foramen magnum anteriorly, and acts to check extension of the occiput on the axis. Conversely, flexion is limited by impingement of the anterior arch of the atlas on the basion. The transverse ligament attaches to the lateral masses of the atlas medially. The alar ligaments run obliquely, from the tip of the dens to the inner aspect of the occipital condyles. These two strong bands limit lateral flexion and rotation. On lateral flexion, the contralateral alar ligament tightens, which limits flexion. With moderate cervical rotation, the ipsilateral alar ligament tightens initially, then shortens and winds around the dens on extreme rotation, allowing the contralateral ligament to tighten and limit further rotation. The tectorial membrane and alar ligament restrict distraction of the occiput on C1 or C1 on C2. The apical ligament is a vestigial structure located between the tip of the dens and the anterior midpoint of the foramen magnum.

The external cranial cervical ligaments include the ligamentum nuchae, ligamentous flavum, and the anterior and posterior atlanto-occipital membranes, as well as the atlantoaxial membrane. They have little effect on stability.

Kinematics

The upper cervical spine, or cervicocranium, is uniquely adapted and functionally distinct from the subaxial cervical spine. The osseous structures include the base of the skull with its occipital condyles, the atlas vertebra, and the axis vertebra. The atlanto-occipital and atlantoaxial joints are inherently unstable joints; they depend on complex ligaments for stability. Though each provides some degree of flexion/extension, rotation, and lateral bending, each joint has a primary motion. The atlanto-occipital provides primarily flexion and extension and the atlantoaxial joints (C1–2) provide 50% of the rotation in the cervical spine. Another unique anatomic feature is the large space available for the spinal cord (SAC) at this level. Between the posterior aspect of the odontoid process (dens) and the posterior arch of the atlas, the diameter of the sagittal canal is at least twice the diameter of the spinal cord at this level, providing more room for the cord than at any other level of the cervical spine. This feature is in part responsible for infrequent spinal cord injuries associated with atlas injuries.

Occipital Condyle Fractures

Fractures of the occipital condyles are commonly overlooked and not evident on plain radiographs. Frequently, diagnosis requires a high index of suspicion, particularly in patients with loss of consciousness, cranial nerve injuries, or occipital headaches following a direct blow to the head. The diagnosis is verified with computed tomography (CT), with coronal reconstruction or tomography. The suspected mechanism of injury is sudden cranial deceleration or a direct blow, which are common in patients with atlanto-occipital ligamentous instability. Occipital condyle fractures have been classified into three types (Fig. 1).[3] A type I injury is a unilateral, undisplaced, comminuted fracture that is the result of impaction of the skull on the atlas, similar to a Jefferson fracture. The injury compromises the functional integrity of the ipsilateral alar ligament, but stability is maintained by the contralateral alar ligament and tectatorial membrane.

A type II occipital condyle fracture occurs as part of a basilar skull fracture. The fracture line may enter the foramen magnum or the condyle may break off. These stable injuries occur from a direct blow to the skull.

A type III injury is an alar ligament avulsion fracture of the occipital condyles (Fig. 2). It is caused by either cervical lateral flexion or cervical rotation, or by a combination of the two mechanisms. These injuries are potentially unstable inasmuch as the alar ligament represents one of the primary restraints to occipital cervical rotation and lateral flexion.

Because type I and type II injuries are stable, they can be treated in a cervical orthosis for 6 to 8 weeks, followed by flexion-extension radiographs to confirm healing. Type III injuries are potentially unstable. Treatment includes 12 weeks of halo or rigid cervical orthosis. If postimmobilization stress radiographs determine incomplete healing or instability, an occipitocervical fusion is recommended. Patients with type III injuries and associated atlanto-occipital instability should be treated by primary occipitocervical fusion.

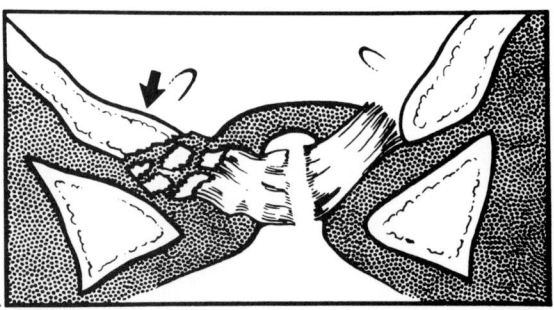

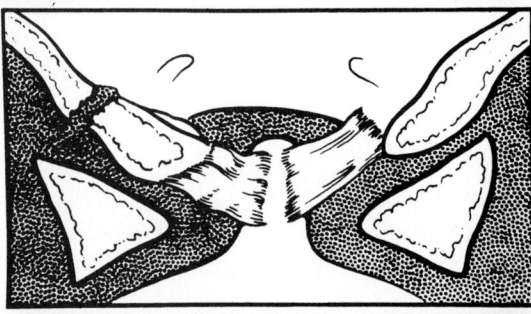

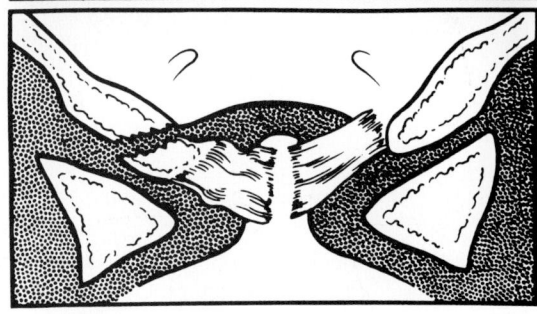

Fig. 1 Classification of occipital condyle fractures. **Top,** Type I impacted occipital condyle fracture. **Center,** Type II basilar skull type occipital condyle fracture. **Bottom,** Type III avulsion-type occipital condyle fracture. (Reproduced with permission from Anderson PA, Montesano PX: Injuries to the occipitocervical articulation, in Chapman M, Madison M (eds): *Chapman's Operative Orthopaedics,* ed 2. Philadelphia, PA, JB Lippincott, 1993.)

Occipitocervical Instability

Forensic reports show that atlanto-occipital dislocations are frequently identified following motor vehicle accidents. The suspected mechanism of injury is hyperextension and distraction. Patients rarely survive the dislocation. In spite of better emergency on-site resuscitation and transportation, there are still delays in diagnosis and treatment for the majority of patients who do survive. Associated head injuries, noncontiguous spinal fractures, and inadequate understanding of the bony anatomy of plain radiographs are responsible for the delay in diagnosis.

The radiographic findings in atlanto-occipital dislocations are listed in Outline 1.

Routine plain lateral cervical radiographs do not clearly demonstrate the atlanto-occipital joint because the joint atlanto-occipital dislocations. These dislocations are most common in nonfatal injuries, involve rupture of all major ligaments, and are highly unstable. Type II injuries occur when there is vertical displacement between either the occiput and C1 or between C1 and C2. Vertical displacement of the occiput on C1 is normally less than 2 mm.[1] More than 2 mm of distraction suggests rupture of the tectorial membrane and the alar ligaments. When vertical displacement occurs between C1 and C2, the atlanto-axial joint capsules and membranes are involved rather than those that connect the occiput to the atlas. In this pattern, the tectorial membrane and alar ligaments are also disrupted. Injuries to the transverse ligament of the axis have been shown to be associated with atlanto-occipital instability.[5] When the atlanto-dens interval exceeds 7 to 10 mm, secondary damage to the alar ligaments and tectorial membrane occurs. These combined injuries are grossly unstable and require a posterior occipitocervical fusion. Type III injuries in which the occiput dislocates posterior to the atlas are, theoretically, fatal. The patient may survive if the posterior arch of C1 is fractured and moves backward with the spinal cord and brain stem.

Treatment of Occipitocervical Instability

If a patient survives an occipitocervical dislocation, treatment is potentially life saving but extreme caution is warranted. All supporting ligaments are torn, therefore making reduction with cranial traction risky. Only 2 to 5 lbs of cranial traction can be used. Occasionally traction for other cervical injuries may demonstrate undetected C1–2 facet subluxations or mild vertical displacements.

An important consideration in management is the relative position of the head and neck. With anterior displacements, the thorax is elevated with blanket rolls, allowing the occiput to translate posteriorly. Conversely, posterior dislocations may be reduced by placing towels behind the occiput to bring the cranium forward on the cervical spine. Simple elevation of the head of the bed may allow gravity to reduce a vertical translation.

Following a successful closed reduction of the injury, the patient is placed in a halo vest. Supine and upright radiographs must be repeated. Angulation and translation has been shown to occur, particularly between the occiput and C1, in patients rigidly immobilized in a halo vest.[6] The catastrophic risk of a loss of reduction and the uncertainty that the pure ligamentous disruptions will heal with closed treatment make aggressive surgical treatment warranted. A posterior occipitocervical fusion is indicated for long-term stability, despite the expected loss of range of motion.

Occipitocervical Fusions

The injured patient immobilized in a halo vest is brought to the operating room. A fiberoptic nasotracheal intubation

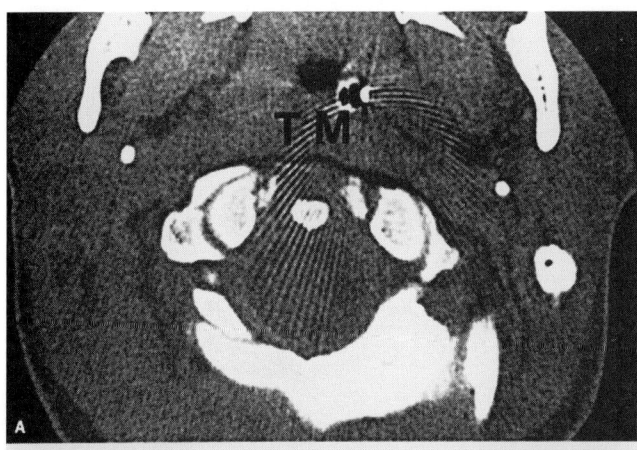

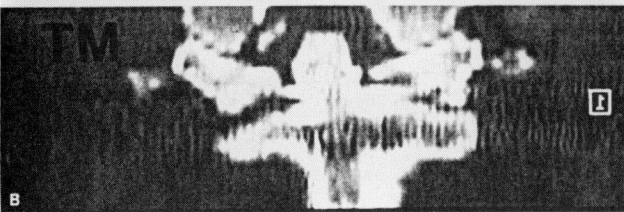

Fig. 2 A 20-year-old female involved in a motor vehicle accident in which she suffered a closed head injury and bilateral occipital condyle fractures. Plain cervical radiographs were negative. **Top,** CT reveals bilateral type III occipital condyle fracture. **Bottom,** CT shows medial displacement of the occipital condyle fracture. (Reproduced with permission from Anderson PA, Montesano PX: Injuries to the occipitocervical articulation, in Chapman M, Madison M (eds): *Chapman's Operative Orthopaedics,* ed 2. Philadelphia, PA, JB Lippincott, 1993.)

Outline 1. Radiologic signs of atlanto-occipital injuries

Prevertebral soft-tissue swelling

Basion to dens distance > 5 mm

Clivus not pointing to dens tip

Mastoid not overlying dens

Powers ratio > 1.0

lies oblique to the X-ray beam and is obscured by the mastoid process and cranium. An important landmark is the basion, which may be difficult to distinguish. The clivus, a bony plateau between the sella turcica and the basion, is easy to identify and points directly to the dens in normal situations. CT with 1.5-mm slices and midplane reconstructions are the most useful diagnostic studies for this injury. Diastasis of the joints greater than 2 mm indicates vertical instability. Occipital condyle fractures are present in 50% of cases of atlanto-occipital dislocation.

Occipitocervical instability has been classified according to the primary direction of displacement of the occipital condyle to the atlas (Fig. 3).[4] Type I injuries are anterior

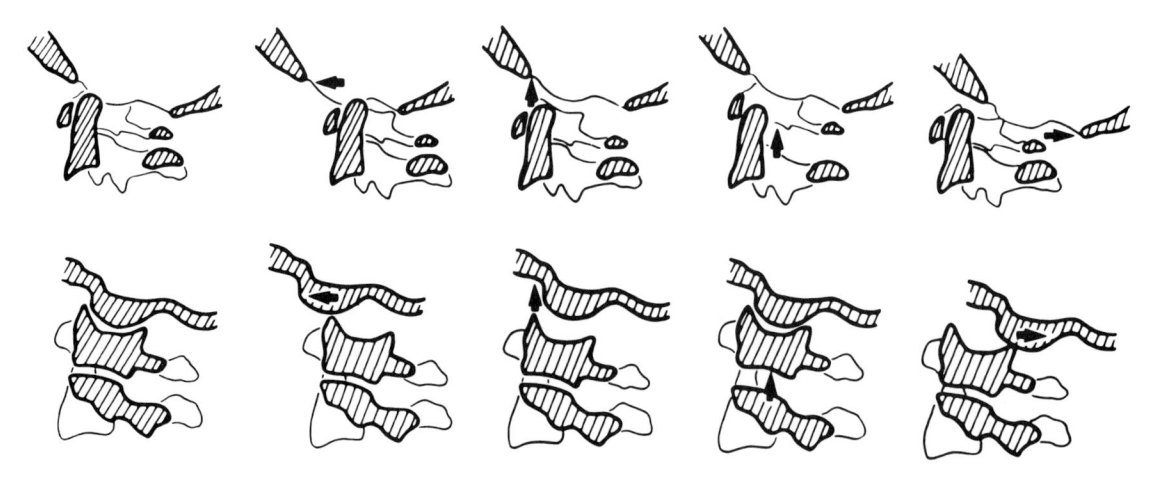

Fig. 3 Classification of occipitocervical instability. **Left** to **right**, Normal, anterior, vertical occiput C1; vertical C1–C2; posterior. (Reproduced with permission from Anderson PA, Montesano PX: Injuries to the occipitocervical articulation, in Chapman M, Madison M (eds): *Chapmans' Operative Orthopaedics,* ed 2. Philadelphia, PA, JB Lippincott, 1993.)

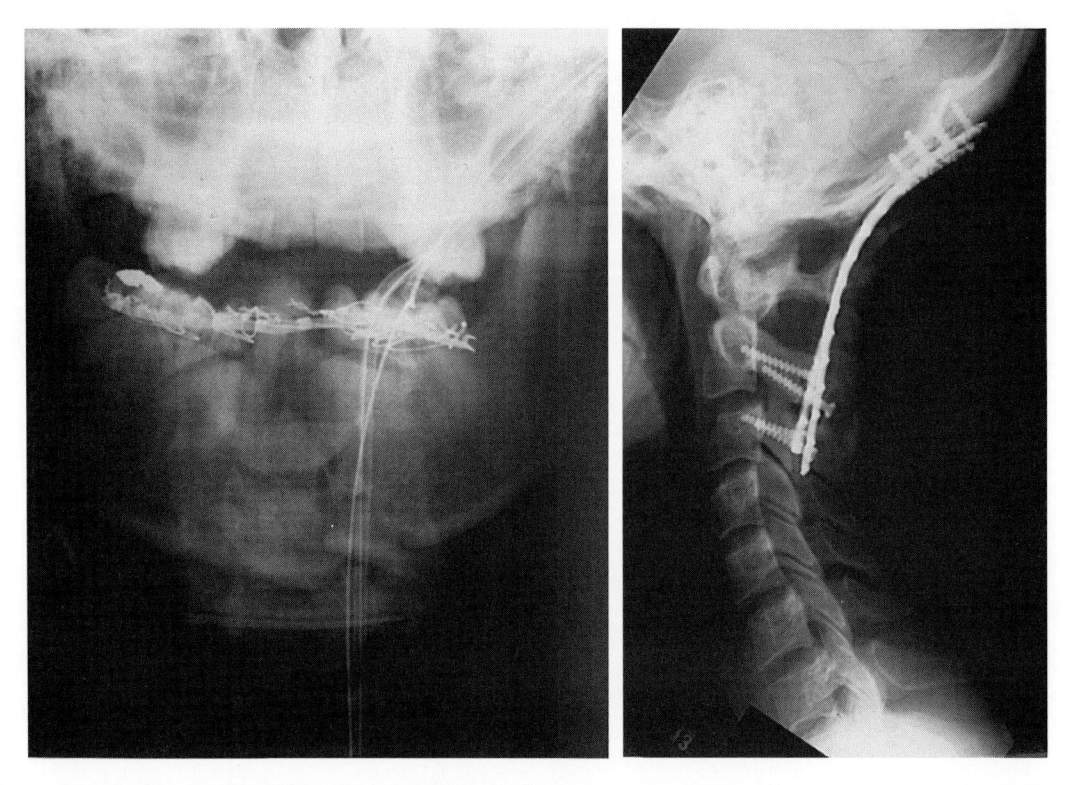

Fig. 4 A 28-year-old male after a motor vehicle accident. **Left**, The patient sustained occipital cervical dislocation, vertical occiput. The patient was quadraplegic on admission. **Right**, Early open reduction with internal fixation led to complete resolution of neurologic injury. (Courtesy of Daniel R. Benson, MD.)

is performed with the patient awake. The patient is then turned prone in the halo vest. A neurologic examination is repeated and a lateral radiograph is obtained to assure proper alignment. A general anesthetic is given and the halo vest is kept in place.

In the past 60 years, numerous occipitocervical fusion techniques have been reported. Onlay grafts wired to the occiput and cervical spine have been described. Others have reported in situ techniques with postoperative immobilization by traction or halo vest. The technique described by Bohlman, which avoids intracranial placement of wires, is perhaps the simplest and most widely used. Two corticocancellous iliac strips are secured to the occiput through a midline extracranial tunnel, to C1 with a sublaminar wire, and to C2 with a wire through a hole in the base of the spinous process. Recently, more rigid instrumentation has been employed to provide immediate stability and avoid long-term postoperative immobilization. Ranford and Itoh have championed the use of a contoured Luque rectangle with occipital intracranial attachment and sublaminal cervical wires. Roy-Camille developed an angled plate fixed to the occiput with screws and secured to C3 and C4 with screws through the plate into the lateral masses. This technique has been modified with the use of AO 3.5-mm reconstruction plates, similarly secured and bent to fit the bony shape of the occipitocervical segment (Fig. 4). The more stable reconstruction (using plates and screws) of these highly unstable injuries allows earlier mobilization and rehabilitation.

Conclusion

Occipitocranial injuries are extremely unstable and frequently cause severe neurologic deficits or death. Occipitocervical injuries must be considered and ruled out in patients injured during a high-energy motor vehicle accident, patients with head injury and impaired consciousness, pedestrians struck by cars, patients deteriorating neurologically during hospitalization, and patients with palsies of the sixth, eleventh, and twelfth cranial nerves.[7] The diagnosis is usually delayed because understanding of the bony anatomy on plain radiographs is inadequate. When the diagnosis is suspected, CT with multiplane reformation usually accurately depicts the injury. Type I and type II occipital condyle fractures are stable and can be treated with immobilization. Type III occipital condyle fractures and all occipitocervical ligamentous injuries are highly unstable and require aggressive posterior occipitocervical arthrodesis.

Annotated References

1. Werne S: Studies in spontaneous atlas dislocation. *Acta Orthop Scand* 1957;239(suppl):5–150.
   This is the most comprehensive work on normal and pathologic upper cervical spine anatomy.

2. Dvorak J, Panjabi MM: Functional anatomy of the alar ligaments. *Spine* 1987;12:183-189.
   This is the most recent and complete review of the anatomy and physiology of the alar ligaments.

3. Anderson PA, Montesano PX: Morphology and treatment of occipital condyle fractures. *Spine* 1988;13:731–736.
   The authors present the largest series of occipital condyle fractures and they present a clinically relevant classification.

4. Traynelis VC, Marano GD, Dunker RO, et al: Traumatic atlanto-occipital dislocation: Case report. *J Neurosurg* 1986;65:863–870.

5. Anderson PA: Occipital cervical instability associated with traumatic tears of the transverse ligament of the atlas. *Orthop Trans* 1988;12:41.

6. McAfee PC, Cassidy JR, Davis RF, et al: Fusion of the occiput to the upper cervical spine. A review of 37 cases. *Spine* 1991;16(suppl 10):S490–S494.

7. Schliack H, Schaefer P: Hypoglossal and accessory nerve paralysis in a fracture of the occipital condyle. *Nervenarzt* 1965;36:362–364.

34

The Atlas Vertebra: Fractures and Ligamentous Injuries

Introduction

The cervicocranium is at increased risk for injury. High-energy forces, such as those generated in motor vehicle accidents or falls, can impart large injuring forces to the head. Because of the mass of the head and its position relative to the trunk, the atlas and axis and their associated joints are at relatively increased risk for injury. The highly specific motions of these two joints further enhance their susceptibility to injury.

Fractures of the Atlas

Atlas fractures comprise 10% of all cervical spine fractures and 2% of all spine fractures. Most importantly, 50% of all atlas fractures are associated with other spinal fractures, most frequently in the cervical spine. The most common associated fractures are of the odontoid process or hangman's fractures. Neurologic deficits are rarely associated with atlas fractures because of the large canal diameters and space available for the cord (SAC) at C1. The presence of a spinal cord injury should prompt a diligent search for the associated fracture(s). Twenty-five percent of atlas fractures are associated with significant craniofacial trauma, including closed head injuries.

Radiology

In most circumstances injuries to the atlas may be readily diagnosed from plain radiographs. A lateral view may be used to identify fractures of the posterior arch, a widened atlanto-dens interval, segmental malrotation, or abnormal soft-tissue contours. Anterior soft-tissue thicknesses greater than 10 mm at the anterior C1 arch, or greater than 5 mm at the inferior corner of C2 are beyond the upper limits of normal and may indicate the presence of an anterior arch fracture or a ligamentous instability. The open-mouth odontoid view is useful for evaluating the relative position of the articular masses of the atlas to the articular masses of the axis. Bursting fractures of the atlas or rotatory instabilities may be identified with this view. Fracture lines through the anterior or posterior arches may only be inferred because they are poorly seen on this view. Impaction fractures of the atlas, on the other hand, may be identified. Lateral flexion/extension views may be useful in ruling out ligamentous instabilities.

Computed tomography (CT) is invaluable because it provides a highly detailed understanding of fracture patterns. When CT is used to evaluate suspected cervicocranial trauma, it is crucial that the scans be performed with thin slices (1.5- to 2-mm thick) and that the gantry angle be aligned parallel to the equator of the atlas vertebra. If the images are made out of the plane of the vertebra, fractures may be overlooked. Sagittal and coronal reformations will provide additional information regarding fractures of the articular masses, odontoid process, and the overall alignment of the occipito-atlantal and atlantoaxial articulations. Anteroposterior (AP) and lateral tomography may be useful in some circumstances if doubt remains about certain injuries following CT. In general CT is more readily available and is likely to be obtained for evaluation of suspected head, chest, or abdominal injuries in the patient with blunt trauma. Adding a properly prescribed CT scan of the cervical spine adds little time to the evaluation but considerable sensitivity and specificity.

Classification

Fractures of the atlas vertebra may be classified according to their location and treatment requirements. Fractures of the arches may be of two types. Fractures may be isolated to a single arch, anterior or posterior, or may occur simultaneously to both arches, also called "bursting" fractures (eg, Jefferson fractures). Bursting fractures disrupt the integrity of the ring, permitting lateral mass subluxation and possibly failure of the transverse ligament. Lateral mass fractures have two variants: impaction fractures, in which the integrity of the ring is preserved, and more complex lateral mass fractures, which may be comminuted, separating the lateral mass from the anterior and posterior arches. These fractures have the same potential for subluxation and transverse ligament injury as other burst fractures.

Anterior Arch Fractures If only a single arch is fractured, two fracture lines must be present. In the case of the anterior

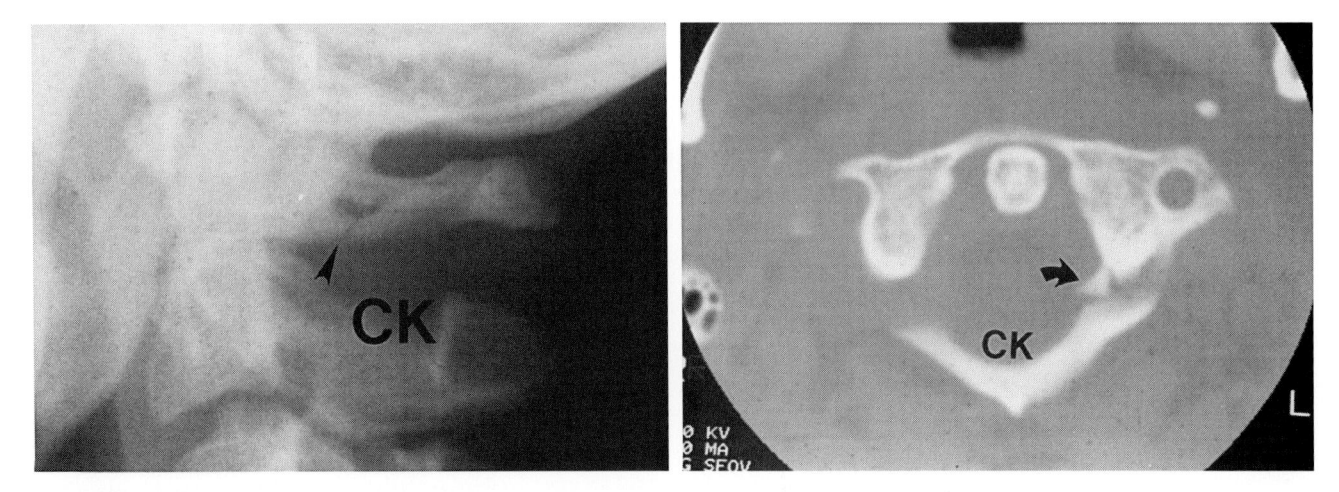

Fig. 1 Left, Lateral radiograph of the cervicocranium illustrating a posterior arch fracture (arrowhead) of the atlas. **Right,** An axial CT of the same patient indicating the fracture through the left side of the arch (curved arrow) at its weakest point, the vascular groove for the vertebral artery. The fracture of the right arch is out of the plane of the image but should not be overlooked.

arch, fractures usually are found at the junction of the anterior arches and the articular masses. This generally is a stable fracture of little consequence; however, an extension instability may exist if there is sufficient disruption of the anterior atlanto-dens joint. Flexion/extension views can exclude such instabilities. The presence of a fracture should be suspected when soft-tissue swelling is visible on the lateral cervical spine film. Anterior arch fractures may also occur as avulsions of the insertion of the longus coli or as horizontal cleavage fractures through the anterior arch. These fractures are rarely of clinical significance; however, they may be a sign of vertical instability of the occipito-atlantal joint. Anterior arch fractures in the absence of instability are typically treated symptomatically with a rigid collar. If the application of skull tong traction is being contemplated, and such anterior arch fractures are present, then the initial traction should be of low weight and radiographs should be taken immediately following application of the traction to look for overdistraction of the cervicocranium and subsequent spinal cord injury.

Posterior Arch Fractures Isolated posterior arch fractures are usually the result of a combined hyperextension and axial load. The arch fails at its weakest point, the vascular grooves where the vertebral arteries traverse the arch just behind the articular masses (Fig. 1). Patients most often complain of upper neck pain or occipital pain. Occasionally, paresthesias are noted in the distribution of the greater occipital and/or lesser occipital nerves. Hypesthesia may be identified if sought. The fractures may be seen on the lateral cervical spine film. Anterior soft-tissue swelling is unlikely and the articular masses will be noted in their normal relationship on the odontoid view. When either of the latter findings are present, a Jefferson or bursting fracture of the atlas should be suspected. The isolated posterior arch fracture is treated symptomatically with a rigid collar or as dictated by other associated fractures of the cervical spine.

Lateral Mass Fractures Impaction and complex lateral mass fractures are the two principal variants of lateral mass fractures. They generally are the result of asymmetric axial loads applied through the head to the upper cervical spine. Impaction fractures result in loss of articular mass height, but the integrity of the ring is preserved. Atlantoaxial subluxation is unusual. With the complex lateral mass fracture, in addition to loss of height of the articular mass, there are fractures of the arches separating the arches from the articular mass and allowing subluxation. Comminution is quite frequent. Bony avulsion of the insertion transverse ligament may also occur. Patients will complain of largely unilateral neck pain, especially with motion, particularly rotation. The fractures are not visualized on the lateral cervical spine view but may be seen on the open-mouth odontoid. Decreased height of the lateral mass on the affected side or an asymmetric degree of displacement of the lateral mass may be found. Anterior soft-tissue swelling may be present. These fractures are treated in the same way as a bursting fracture of the atlas. Patients often have decreased lateral rotation following fracture healing, presumably due to articular fibrosis.

Burst Fractures of the Atlas (Jefferson Fractures) These fractures result from a combination of an axial load applied through the vertex of the skull and the unique articular geometry of the cervicocranium (Fig. 2). The ring of the atlas fails in tension through both the anterior and posterior arches. At least one fracture line is present through each arch, but as many as two or three many be found. The

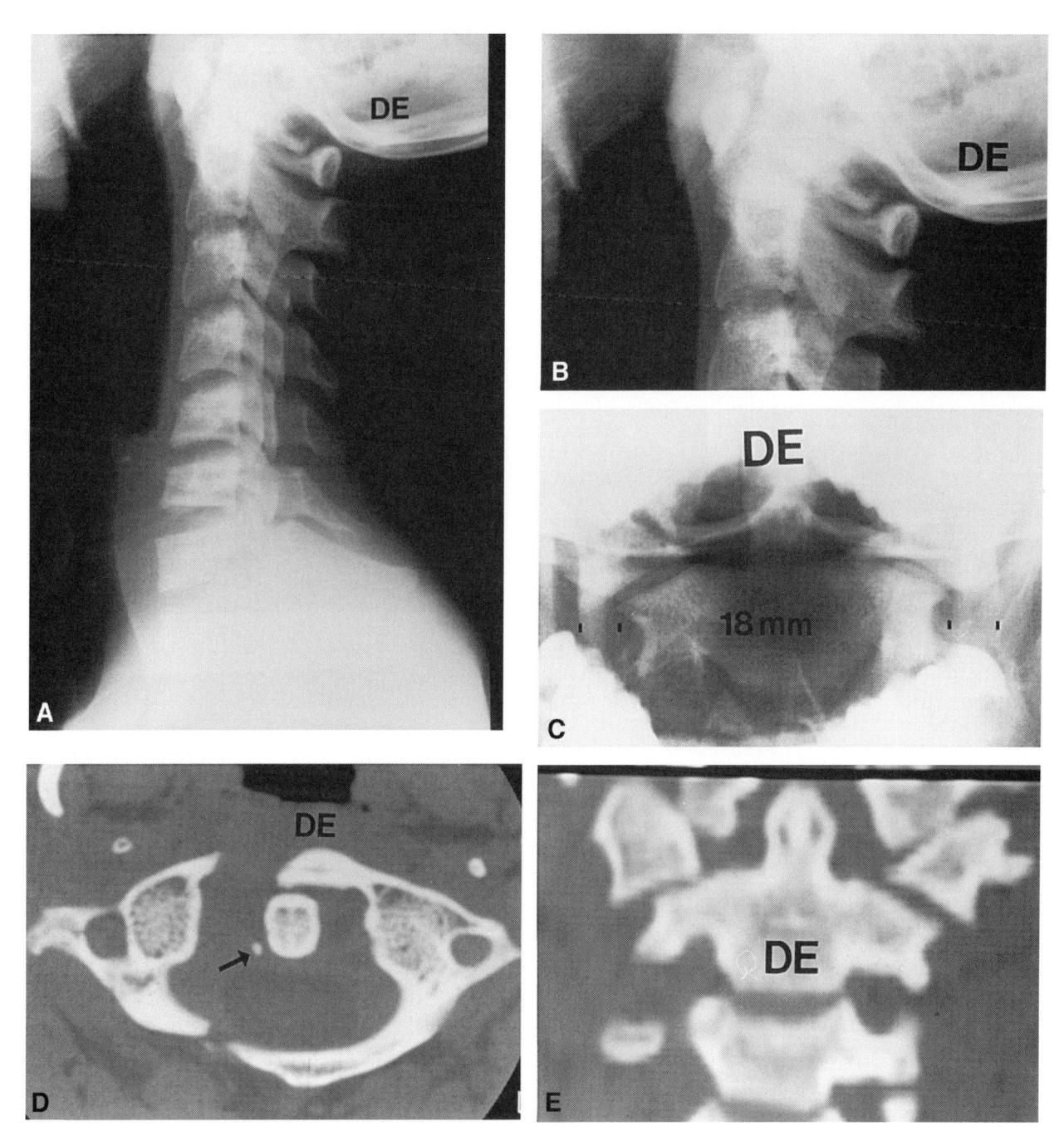

Fig. 2 A, Lateral cervical radiograph following a football collision and complaints of neck pain. Note the posterior arch fracture of the atlas and the associated C5 compression fracture. **B,** Close-up view of posterior arch fracture of the atlas. **C,** The open-mouth odontoid view reveals 18 mm of lateral mass subluxation associated with a bursting fracture of the atlas. Rupture of the transverse ligament should be inferred, which is supported further by the axial CT image (**D**). The transverse ligament has failed by bone avulsion (arrow) at its insertion. A coronal CT reformation (**E**) clearly demonstrates the lateral mass subluxation, as well as the articular geometry that leads to this type of fracture.

fracture permits lateral subluxation of the articular masses of C1 relative to C2, which is easily quantified on the open-mouth odontoid view. Both anterior soft-tissue swelling and a posterior arch fracture are usually present on the lateral cervical spine film. These films should be scrutinized carefully to identify other fractures of the cervical spine, particularly those of the axis vertebrae. Fifty percent of all such fractures have an associated fracture elsewhere in the spine, particularly the cervical spine (Fig. 2, A). Because the fracture fragments displace outward and the SAC is large, these injuries are rarely associated with spinal cord injuries. The presence of neurologic deficits should prompt a repeated search for other spinal fractures or closed head injuries. Separation of the lateral masses places the transverse ligament at risk for rupture. Anatomic separation of the lateral mass greater than 6.9 mm, or greater than 8.0 mm (as measured on the open-mouth odontoid view), implies rupture of the transverse ligament (Fig. 2, C). Typically, the ligament fails by avulsion at its bony insertion rather than as a midsubstance tear (Fig. 2, D). Thin-section CT sections will demonstrate all of the necessary fracture anatomy and may even identify the bony ossicle avulsed with the transverse ligament.

The treatment of these fractures is still under debate. The issue is whether to treat all such fractures with immediate halo vest application or to treat a certain subset with a period of skeletal traction. Those fractures with more than 7 mm of lateral mass separation are treated with traction for 4 to 6 weeks until a stable reduction is achieved. A halo vest is then applied until the fracture(s) are completely healed. Unfortunately, it is not clear whether this reduction improves the ultimate functional outcome or reduces the rate of nonunion.

Nonsurgical treatment of these fractures is generally the rule. Surgical treatment is indicated if a halo vest is contraindicated by associated injuries, such as skull fractures, severe chest trauma, and burns. Additionally, other fractures may be present in the cervical spine, for which the optimal treatment is surgical intervention. If this is the case, surgical treatment of the atlas fracture may be relatively indicated. Alternatively, surgical treatment of the other cervical fracture may be followed by immobilization in a halo vest. In general, it is the associated fracture that dictates the treatment method used. However, halo vest immobilization frequently will suffice for these other fractures, such as odontoid fractures or hangman's fractures. If a halo vest is contraindicated and surgical intervention is required, C1-C2 arthrodesis is the treatment of choice, provided the surgeon has sufficient experience with posterior transarticular screw fixation. If the surgeon is not familiar with this technique, occipito-cervical fusion should be performed.

Contrary to previous recommendations, transverse ligament failure inferred by excessive lateral mass separation is not an indication for acute surgical intervention. Although previously termed "unstable," clinical experience has demonstrated that residual atlantoaxial instability is quite rare in spite of the degree of lateral mass separation noted on the odontoid view. It is not necessary to proceed with early surgical intervention in such circumstances. If follow-up lateral flexion/extension views indicate atlantoaxial instability following the removal of the halo vest, C1-C2 fusion should be performed. If the posterior arch of the atlas is intact, conventional posterior wiring techniques may be employed, provided ample space is available for the safe passage of wire. Alternatively, the C1-C2 transarticular screw fixation technique of Magerl provides excellent immediate stability with a high rate of fusion. Although technically more demanding, this procedure is quite helpful in the presence of deficient posterior arches, nonunions, combined fractures of the atlas and axis, and abnormal canal diameters where wire passage risks spinal cord injury. Patients should be advised at the time of their injury that up to 80% of patients with these fractures will have some degree of symptoms in the upper cervical spine. Limited rotation is to be expected. Nonetheless, the functional outcome is favorable.

Ligament Injuries and Instabilities About the Axis

Transverse Ligament Failure Without Fracture

Traumatic rupture of the transverse ligament in the absence of an atlas fracture is quite rare. The injury is presumed to result from a combined flexion/anterior translation force. Neurologic injuries vary in their incidence and type, but are more likely to be present when this injury is associated with an intact odontoid process. Patients vary from having no spinal cord deficit to a Brown-Sequard syndrome to pentaplegia. The latter is incompatible with life unless ventilatory support is immediately available at the time of injury. The diagnosis is made by observing an anterior atlanto-dens interval (ADI) greater than 3 mm in adults or 4.5 mm in children. If the lateral cervical spine film is taken with the atlantoaxial joint in the reduced position, the ADI will be normal. Awake, cooperative patients should have supervised active flexion and extension views performed to exclude the possibility of transverse ligament rupture. Anterior soft-tissue swelling should heighten one's suspicion for such an injury. A CT scan through this area may show bony avulsion of the insertion of the transverse ligament, because this is the more common mode of failure. Ligamentous healing is unreliable, hence treatment requires C1-C2 arthrodesis.

Transverse Ligament Rupture Due to Atlas Fractures

Rupture of the transverse ligament is commonly associated with bursting fractures of the atlas. It may be inferred when the total lateral mass separation seen on the open-mouth odontoid view is greater than 8 mm (Fig. 2, C). Nonetheless, residual atlantoaxial instability following healing of the atlas fracture is rare. Early surgical intervention is not indicated. Lateral flexion/extension views should be obtained following removal of the halo vest.

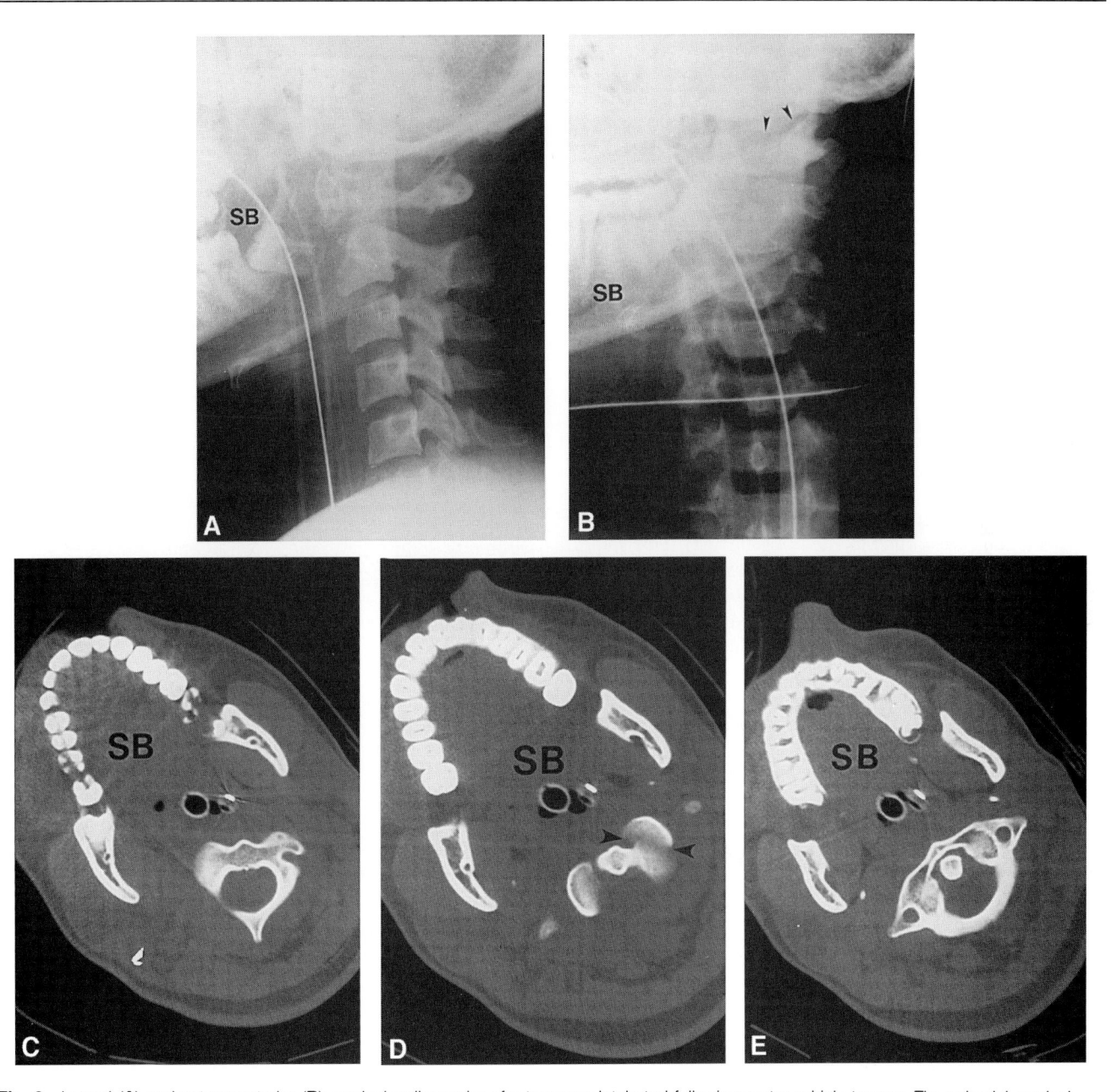

Fig. 3 Lateral (**A**) and anteroposterior (**B**) cervical radiographs of a teenager intubated following motor vehicle trauma. The subaxial cervical spine is seen in "true" lateral and AP images, whereas the skull and atlas appear bizarre. Combined malrotation of the skull and atlas upon C2 is responsible for this unusual appearance, suggesting the diagnosis of traumatic atlantoaxial rotatory subluxation. The sequential axial CT images (**C-E**) confirm the diagnosis. **D,** The left C1 articular mass subluxed anterior to the C2 articular surface is demonstrated.

Atlantoaxial Rotatory Fixation (RF)

The diagnosis of atlantoaxial rotatory fixation is difficult and often delayed. One clue may be the observation of torticollis or the "Cock-Robin" position. The lateral cervical spine film may also offer a clue. If it is a true lateral view of the cervical spine from C2-T1 while C1 looks bizarre, the observer should look further. The bizarre appearance of C1 may be an indication of rotation (Fig. 3).

Further inspection of the angles of the mandibles, the teeth, the sella turcica, and occipital condyles may confirm the presence of rotation above C2. Normally, these structures should all superimpose. The next view requested should be a "true lateral of the skull." In this case, a true lateral of the skull with superimposition of the structures mentioned above as well as a true lateral of C1 will be present. The fixed rotation at the atlantoaxial joint will then impart a malrotated appearance to C2 and below. The ADI may be readily quantified on this view.

The open-mouth odontoid view may provide additional clues for the diagnosis. The lateral mass that is subluxed anteriorly is larger and shifted closer to the midline than the opposite lateral mass. Hence, the clear space between the dens and the articular mass will be asymmetric. One might also observe the "wink" sign on the affected side. This consists of the disappearance of the normally visible articular cartilage space at the atlantoaxial joint on the side that is subluxed. The joint space should be visible on the opposite side. Identification of the position of the spinous processes of C2 relative to the midline of the skull may also be an indicator of malrotation.

CT may be useful when properly performed. Thin cuts with sagittal and coronal reformations will demonstrate the relationship of the articular masses and help exclude the presence of associated fractures. Dynamic CT can also confirm the fixed position of the articular masses if necessary.

Early diagnosis is the key to successful treatment. Skull tong traction is instituted to attempt reduction. This should be closely supervised to avoid overdistraction of the cervical spine either at the level of the injury or from other associated injuries. If such indirect reduction techniques are not successful, awake transoral manipulation may be performed, although the need for this is rare. Once the articular masses are reduced, atlantoaxial stability should be assessed with physician-supervised active flexion/extension views. An abnormal ADI is diagnostic of transverse ligament failure and indicates the need for C1-C2 arthrodesis. All other patients are immobilized in a rigid collar.

Complications

The most frequent complication of atlas fractures or instabilities is failure to diagnose them. The radiographic findings may be subtle. A high level of suspicion must be maintained, especially in the setting of head-injured patients, because of the increased frequency of cervicocranial injuries in these hosts. The possibility of occult occipito-atlantal instabilities associated with these fractures must be excluded. Nonunions may occur, although they are rare and most often occur with delayed or inadequate treatment of the original fracture. A high percentage of patients complain of mild to moderate pain and stiffness following atlas fractures. Periarticular fibrosis and joint incongruity probably contribute to these complaints. Furthermore, it is not clear whether these complaints are due to changes at the atlantoaxial or occipito-atlantal joints, or both. Fusion is rarely indicated. Occipital neuralgias may be seen in association with C1 fractures and subluxations.

Bibliography

Dvorak J, Panjabi MM: Functional anatomy of the alar ligaments. *Spine* 1987;12:183-189.

Dvorak J, Schneider E, Saldinger P, et al: Biomechanics of the craniocervical region: The alar and transverse ligaments. *J Orthop Res* 1988;6:452-461.

Hadley MN, Dickman CA, Browner CM, et al: Acute traumatic atlas fractures: Management and long term outcome. *Neurosurgery* 1988;23:31-35.

Heller JG, Viroslav S, Hudson T: Jefferson fractures: The role of magnification artifact in assessing transverse ligament integrity. *J Spinal Disord* 1993;6:392-396.

Landells CD, Van Peteghem PK: Fractures of the atlas: Classification, treatment and morbidity. *Spine* 1988;13:450-452.

Levine AM, Edwards CC: Fractures of the atlas. *J Bone Joint Surg* 1991;73A:680-691.

Levine AM, Edwards CC: Traumatic lesions of the occipitoatlantoaxial complex. *Clin Orthop* 1989;239:53-68.

Monu J, Bohrer SP, Howard G: Some upper cervical spine norms. *Spine* 1987;12:515-519.

Penning L, Wilmink JT: Rotation of the cervical spine: A CT study in normal subjects. *Spine* 1987;12:732-738.

Segal LS, Grimm JO, Stauffer ES: Non-union of fractures of the atlas. *J Bone Joint Surg* 1987;69A:1423-1434.

35
Fractures of the Axis

The typical fracture patterns of the second cervical vertebrae involve fractures of the odontoid process, traumatic spondylolisthesis, and miscellaneous fractures. Management of odontoid fractures continues to evoke the most controversy.

Odontoid Fractures

Anatomy

The axis has four ossification centers: the odontoid process, the axis body, and the two neural arches. These ossification centers are joined to one another by cartilaginous plates or synchondroses rather than by epiphyseal plates and are fused by age 7. The transverse synchondrosis that joins the odontoid to the C2 body lies inferior to the junction of the odontoid and the body in the adult[1] and can predispose to a type III fracture before its fusion. The odontoid process is a well-vascularized structure and loss of blood supply due to injury is not a likely cause of nonunion. A rich arterial network, including branches from the vertebral internal and external carotid arteries, anastomose and supply the odontoid process from base to tip.[2,3]

The odontoid process and atlas with the associated ligamentous structures are the key to stability of the atlantoaxial complex.[4] The transverse ligament, which arises from the lateral masses of the atlas and passes directly behind the odontoid process, prevents anterior dislocation of the atlas on the axis. The anterior arch of C1 prevents posterior displacement of the atlas on the axis. Little intrinsic stability is gained from the facet joints because they lie in the horizontal plane and are designed to facilitate rotation. The paired accessory ligaments arise from the lateral masses of the atlas and attach to the base of the odontoid on each side. The paired alar ligaments attach the occipital condyles to the superior aspect of the odontoid process.[4,5] The apical ligament attaches the foramen magnum to the tip of the odontoid. The majority of odontoid factures occur below the attachment of these ligaments to the proximal fragment, which explains the unstable nature of these injuries.[1,4,5]

The recent interest in the use of odontoid screw fixation has led to investigations into the bony morphology of the odontoid process. The dens is a conical structure that is thickest at its base. It projects an average of 15 mm from the body of the second vertebra. The size of the odontoid process does not correlate with the height or weight of the specimen.[6,7]

Evaluation

Odontoid fractures account for approximately 15% of all cervical spine fractures.[8–10] Over the last few decades, the most common mechanism of injury producing an odontoid fracture has been motor vehicle accidents.[5,8,11] The average age of persons sustaining an odontoid fracture is approximately 40 years of age,[5,8,11] with a wide range from the very young to the very old. In fact, the odontoid fracture is the most common individual cervical spine fracture in people younger than 8 years of age and older than 70 years of age.[12,13]

The typical high-energy injury pattern is not always seen in the very young and very old patient population. Apparently low-energy injuries, such as falls from short distances, are often responsible. Thus, a high index of suspicion is needed for a diagnosis of odontoid fractures, regardless of the mode of injury.[9,14] Odontoid fractures are among the most commonly missed spinal injuries.

Odontoid fractures are produced by flexion and extension moments with rotation probably also being a factor. Flexion causes anterior displacement of the odontoid process after it has fractured; extension produces posterior displacement. Knowledge of this may be helpful in fracture reduction. Anterior displacement is usually more common than posterior displacement, but posterior displacement may be more common in the elderly.[9,11,13,15]

Odontoid fractures are among the most commonly missed spinal injuries. In spite of this, the majority of odontoid fractures can be diagnosed from plain radiographs. In one study, 94% of odontoid fractures were diagnosed with combined lateral anteroposterior (AP) open mouth and oblique radiographs.[16] If these initial studies do not show the odontoid well or if a high index of suspicion persists despite normal radiographs, additional studies are warranted. Tomography or thin section computed tomography (CT) with sagittal and coronal refiguration may be helpful.[17]

Classification

The classification proposed by Anderson and D'Alonzo[5] is still universally accepted and useful in determining pro-

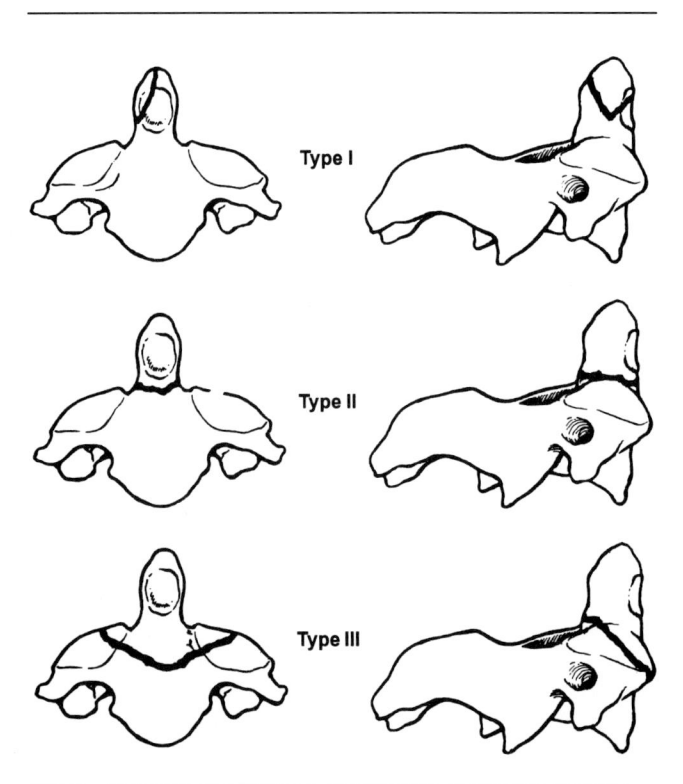

Fig. 1 Anderson and D'Alonzo classification of odontoid fractures, types I, II, and III. (Reproduced with permission from Anderson LD, D'Alonzo RT: Fractures of the odontoid process of the axis. *J Bone Joint Surg* 1974;56A:1663–1674.)

grams and directing treatment (Fig. 1). The type I fracture is an oblique fracture through the apex of the dens, which probably represents an avulsion of the alar ligaments.[4,5] The type I fracture is extremely rare, but may be associated with atlanto-occipital dislocation.[11,18] The type II fracture, the most common fracture, occurs at the base of the odontoid at its junction with the body of the axis. The type III fracture extends downward through the body of the axis.[5]

Treatment

Prognosis may be dictated by associated fractures, which are seen in up to 20% of patients. Type I fractures may be treated symptomatically in a collar or brace and should heal uneventfully.[5] Their association with atlanto-occipital dislocation has been established.[11,18] Type III fractures have also been typically thought of as being benign-type fractures that heal readily when properly diagnosed and immobilized. Clark and White's[11] multicenter study drew attention to a 13% nonunion rate with these fractures. The mode of treatment from the various centers ranged from no treatment at all to the use of halo immobilization. The authors found no statistically significant relation between union and displacement or angulation but noted a trend for nonunion with displacement greater than 5 mm and angulation greater than 10° for these type III fractures. Thus, these authors recommended halo immobilization until healed (8 or 12 weeks) for type III fractures, with the understanding that surgery could be required for especially unstable fractures.

Type II Fractures Significant controversy still exists as to the proper management of type II odontoid fractures. The literature varies with respect to the rate of nonunion with nonsurgical management of these fractures. Rates noted range from 10% to 67%.[5,8–11,13,19,20] There are several predictors of nonunion; amount of initial displacement (more than 5 to 6 mm), direction of displacement (nonunion more likely for posterior than for anterior), angulation (greater than 10°), age (more than 60 years), smoking, time to diagnosis, and method of treatment.[5,8–11,13,19,20] To further cast doubt on the validity of nonsurgical management of type II fractures, one series showed the union rate for primary posterior cervical fusion to be 96%, and thus the authors recommended considering primary fusion for patients with significant displacement, angulation, or both.[11] In this same study, however, all fractures that failed to unite by primary nonsurgical management united after delayed surgical fusions.[11] Other authors have documented similar results after delayed fusions.[8,21]

It seems wise then, as Anderson and D'Alonzo recommended 20 years ago,[5] to educate the patient as to the possibility of nonunion and the need for delayed fusion after several months of halo immobilization versus primary fusion with the inherent risks of surgery in this area. Should nonsurgical management fail, the results from secondary fusion seem to be as good as those from primary fusion.[8,11,21] The proper nonsurgical management includes reduction of displaced fractures and then serial monitoring with halo immobilization until healing occurs, usually in 12 weeks.[8,10,11] If traction fails to achieve stable alignment, or if displacement recurs with halo immobilization, surgical intervention is warranted.

The Elderly Patient The management of odontoid fractures in older patients deserves special mention. Dens fractures in persons older than 60 years of age are frequently delayed in diagnosis, are often the result of low-energy trauma, are posteriorly displaced, and have a high likelihood of nonunion.[9,11,13] The clinical outcome in patients with nonunion may not be unsatisfactory, however, and thus may not warrant aggressive treatment, such as surgery with its inherent risks. Several authors have reported that halo immobilization should always be considered, but is not necessarily needed for a successful outcome.[9,13] Late myelopathy or other neurologic deficit from nonunion has not been seen.[9,13]

Recent Surgical Advances The recent popularity of anterior screw fixation of odontoid fractures deserves mention. Proponents cite the advantage that it allows direct fracture control in unstable type II fractures and some "shallow" type III fractures, and that the loss of motion (rotation) seen with the typical C1–C2 posterior fusion is not found with anterior stabilization procedures.[22–25] Limited neck motion has been documented after C1–C2 posterior fusion, but it was rarely of clinical concern to the patients.[11] Anterior screw fixation can be considered with a type II odontoid fracture associated with a C1 ring fracture (which may occur in up to 16% of patients with type II odontoid fractures).[22–24] However, other authors state that it is appropriate to treat concomitant C1 ring fractures with type II odontoid fractures in halo fixation for a time sufficient to allow the atlas fracture to heal. If the odontoid fracture does not heal, a posterior C1–C2 fusion is indicated.[10,26]

If the decision to use anterior screw fixation is made, controversy exists as to the number of screws needed to stabilize the fractured odontoid. Two screws have been advocated by some authors[22,24] while single screw fixation has been successful for others.[23,27,28] It has been shown biomechanically that one screw may suffice.[29]

The rate of union for anterior fixation is similar to posterior C1–C2 fusion[22,25] but the complication rate may be higher.[22] Because of the potential for complications with this relatively new technique, it cannot yet be recommended in the routine management of odontoid fractures.

Traumatic Spondylolisthesis of the Axis

Anatomy
The relevant anatomy with respect to odontoid fractures is discussed above. Further expanding upon this, the second cervical vertebra may be thought of as a transitional unit (including the head, atlas, odontoid process, and body of the axis cephalad) with the typical subaxial vertebrae below. The critical area is in the region of the pars interarticularis of the axis, which is the focal point of the forces that are typically encountered in this injury.[1,30–32]

Classification
The mechanism most often cited as producing the typical injury is one of extension combined with an axial load.[1,26,30,33] These combined forces, typically seen in motor vehicle accidents when the face strikes the windshield or in falls, produce a bilateral fracture through the pars region. The amount of displacement, seen in the form of anterior displacement of the body of C2 on C3, and angular deformity relate to the degree of loading initially seen as well as secondary forces apparent in acceleration-deceleration injury patterns.[1,26,33] The association of this injury pattern to the historic hangman's fracture is mentioned here to eliminate confusion. The typical "hangman's fracture" is produced by an extension-distraction force[31,32,34–37] and is rarely seen today except when certain patterns of traumatic spondylolisthesis are treated with overzealous traction as will be discussed in the following section.

This classification was modified in 1985 by Levine and is currently the one most often quoted.[33] It consists of four types of fracture patterns (Fig. 2). A biomechanical explanation of each injury pattern has been proposed and is useful in planning treatment and prognosis. The classification is based on the configuration of the fracture on a lateral radiograph. Type I injuries result from a hyperextension-axial load mechanism, as has been previously discussed. These injuries include all nondisplaced fractures and those with up to 3 mm of displacement with no angulation.[26,33] Type II injuries show C2–C3 displacement as well as angulation resulting from initial hyperextension-axial loading with the addition of "rebound flexion."[26–33] Type IIA injuries show moderate degrees of displacement combined with severe angulation. Levine[33] reported this in 5% of patients studied and recognized this pattern as including a different mechanism of injury: flexion-distraction. It is in these patients that excessive traction with attempted reduction may produce radiographs typically of the "hangman's fracture," representing, in fact, an iatrogenic hanging of sorts.[35,36] Type III injuries are also rare but are very difficult to treat. These represent unilateral or bilateral facet dislocations in addition to the bilateral posterior element fractures and result from a flexion-compression mechanism.[26,33]

Treatment
Neurologic deficits are rarely produced by the typical injury patterns and can be explained by the fact that these fractures typically produce a widened canal in an area of the spine that already has ample room for the spinal cord.[30,32] Most neurologic deficits can be explained by the associated injuries to the head and spine, especially in the cervical region. Associated cervical injuries are seen in 14% to 30% of patients, and the great majority of these are in the upper three cervical segments.[31–33,37] Therefore, once the initial diagnosis is made, a search for other injuries is critical.[31,32,37,38]

Type I injuries are stable and may be treated with a cervical collar for 8 to 12 weeks.[26,30,33] Levine has shown in long-term follow up that type I injuries may be more problematic than type II fractures. Type I injuries rarely produce a spontaneous fusion anteriorly between C2 and C3, as seen with type II fractures. The lack of fusion allows mobility at the C2–C3 facet joint, which, combined with the original axial loading injury, can produce degenerative arthritis in 30% of patients with type I injuries.[39] Type II injuries with severe displacement are treated in traction initially with slight extension of the neck. The reduction that is gained is typically lost after application of the halo-vest because the traction cannot be maintained with halo immobilization. This is usually of no consequence, however, because of the rare association with neurologic injury and the high likelihood of achieving union with these fractures. If displacement is great enough (more than 6 mm), it may be necessary to treat in traction for several weeks to maintain alignment.[8,26,30,33] Halo immobilization typically lasts 10 to 12 weeks. The rare nonunion can be treated with anterior C2–C3 fusion. C1–C3 posterior fusion also can be attempted, but is less desirable because an additional intact level is added to the arthrodesis.[39]

Type IIA fractures should be treated initially with halo immobilization with some degree of compression and extension in order to counteract the injury-producing

Type I   Type II

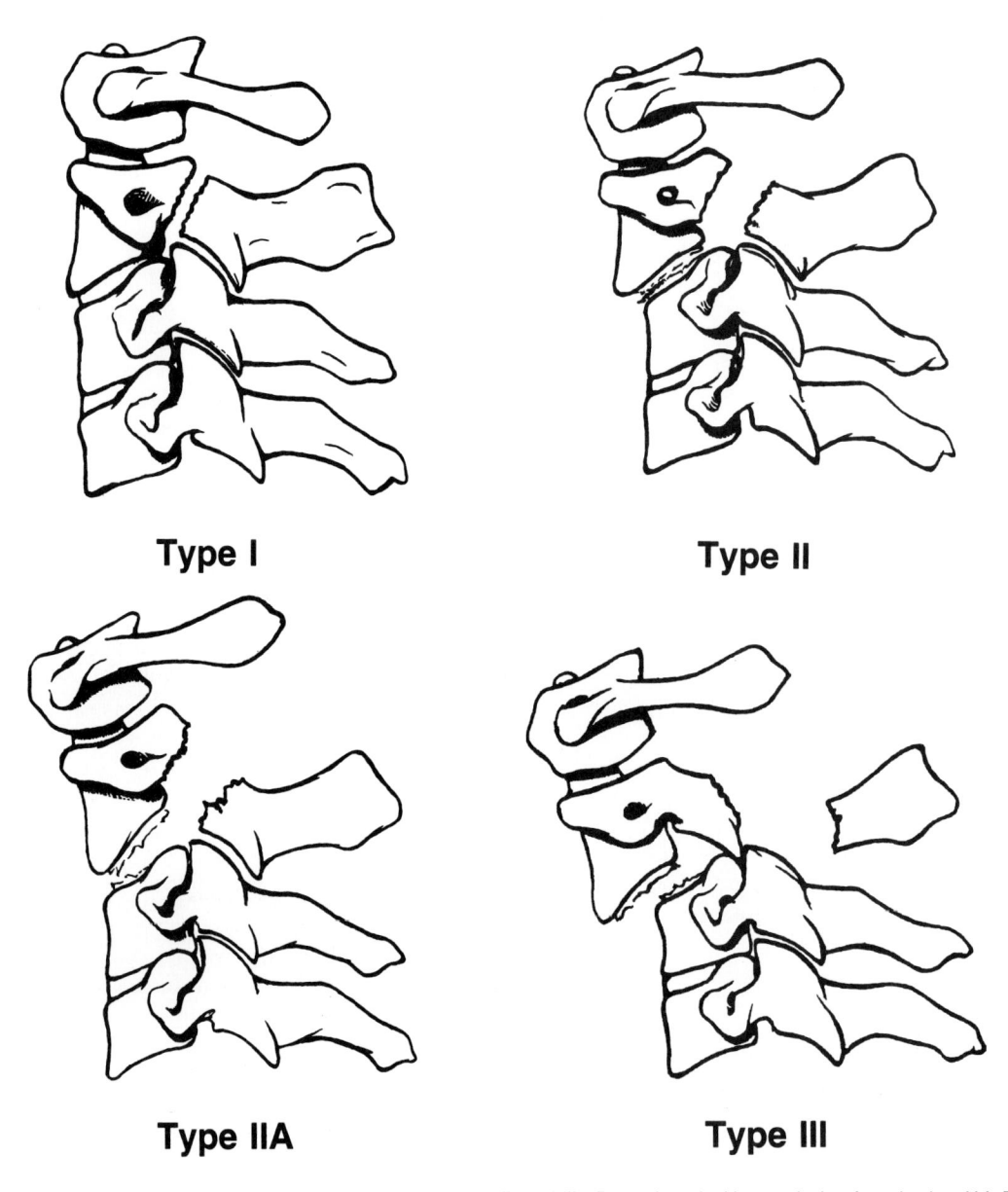

Type IIA   Type III

Fig. 2 Classification of traumatic spondylolisthesis of the axis, types I, II, and III. (Reproduced with permission from Levine AM, Edwards CC: The management of traumatic spondylolisthesis of the axis. *J Bone Joint Surg* 1985;67A:217–226.)

force.[26,33] This fracture pattern is likely to distract with the application of traction. The rare type III fracture pattern has an associated unilateral or bilateral facet dislocation at C2–C3 in addition to angulation and displacement anteriorly. This pattern is associated with neurologic deficits and is the only pattern in which surgical intervention is typically needed.[26,30,33] Attempted closed reduction of the facet dislocation is usually unsuccessful. Surgical stabilization of the facet joint(s) is often needed even if closed reduction is successful. The neural arch fracture is then managed by closed means with halo immobilization.[26,33]

Miscellaneous Axis Fractures

In addition to the typical odontoid fracture and traumatic spondylolisthesis injury to the axis, other fractures are seen, albeit less commonly. These include C2 vertebral body fractures, lateral mass fractures, lamina fractures, and spinous process fractures. As one might suspect, there are no reports of large series with specific recommendations for managing these fractures. Traction has been recommended for displaced vertebral body fractures of C2. Residual translation is tolerated and usually will heal with halo immobilization. Angulation of the C2 vertebral body may not be as well tolerated because this may narrow the spinal cord via the odontoid process.[8,26] Less severe injuries can be treated with a rigid collar.

Annotated References

1. The Cervical Spine Research Society Editorial Committee: *The Cervical Spine*, ed 2. Philadelphia, PA, JB Lippincott, 1989.

2. Althoff B, Goldie IF: The arterial supply of the odontoid process of the axis. *Acta Orthop Scand* 1977;48:622–629.

3. Schiff DC, Parke WW: The arterial supply of the odontoid process. *J Bone Joint Surg* 1973;55A:1450–1456.

4. Schatzker J, Rorabeck CH, Waddell JP: Fractures of the dens (odontoid process): An analysis of thirty-seven cases. *J Bone Joint Surg* 1971;53B:392–405.

5. Anderson LD, D'Alonzo RT: Fractures of the odontoid process of the axis. *J Bone Joint Surg* 1974;56A:1663–1674.

    This classification is useful in determining prognosis and directing treatment. It is universally accepted and is the classification system most often quoted in the literature to date.

6. Schaffler MB, Alson MD, Heller JG, et al: Morphology of the dens: A quantitative study. *Spine* 1992;17:738–743.

7. Heller JG, Alson MD, Schaffler MB, et al: Quantitative internal dens morphology. *Spine* 1992;17:861–866.

8. Hadley MN, Browner C, Sonntag VK: Axis fractures: A comprehensive review of management and treatment in 107 cases. *Neurosurgery* 1985;17:281–290.

9. Pepin JW, Bourne RB, Hawkins RJ: Odontoid fractures with special reference to the elderly patient. *Clin Orthop* 1985;193:178–183.

10. Rizzolo SJ, Cotler JM: Unstable cervical spine injuries: Specific treatment approaches. *J Am Acad Orthop Surg* 1993;1:57–66.

11. Clark CR, White AA: Fractures of the dens: A multicenter study. *J Bone Joint Surg* 1985;67A:1340–1348.

    This multicenter study included 144 patients. The results confirmed the validity of the classification by Anderson and D'Alonzo. The authors also emphasized the potential difficulty in treating type II fractures with the degree of angulation and amount of displacement being important criteria in guiding management.

12. Crawford AH: Operative treatment of spine fractures in children. *Orthop Clin North Am* 1990;21:325–339.

13. Ryan MD, Taylor TK: Odontoid fractures in the elderly. *J Spinal Disord* 1993;6:397–401.

14. Seimon LP: Fracture of the odontoid process in young children. *J Bone Joint Surg* 1977;59A:943–948.

15. Southwick WO: Management of fractures of the dens (odontoid process). *J Bone Joint Surg* 1980;62A:482–486.

16. Ehara S, el-Khoury GY, Clark CR: Radiologic evaluation of dens fractures: Role of plain radiography and tomography. *Spine* 1992;17:475–479.

17. Sutterlin CE, Gutentag I, Martinez CR, et al: False-positive diagnosis of an odontoid fracture by CT scan. *J Orthop Trauma* 1989;3:348–351.

    CT of acute cervical spine trauma has a role but not for the diagnosis of type II odontoid fractures. Conventional polytomography is superior to CT as an adjunct to plain films in the diagnosis of odontoid fractures, according to the authors.

18. Pedersen AK, Kostuik JP: Complete fracture-dislocation of the atlantoaxial complex: Case report and recommendations for a new classification of dens fractures. *J Spinal Disord* 1994;7:350–355.

19. Lind B, Nordwall A, Sihlbom H: Odontoid fractures treated with halo-vest. *Spine* 1987;12:173–177.

20. Schweigel JF: Management of the fractured odontoid with halo-thoracic bracing. *Spine* 1987;12:838–839.

21. Apuzzo ML, Heiden JS, Weiss MH, et al: Acute fractures of the odontoid process: An analysis of 45 cases. *J Neurosurg* 1978;48:85–91.

22. Aebi M, Etter C, Coscia M: Fractures of the odontoid process: Treatment with anterior screw fixation. *Spine* 1989;14:1065–1070.

23. Esses SI, Bednar DA: Screw fixation of odontoid fractures and nonunions. *Spine* 1991;16(suppl 10):S483–S485.

24. Etter C, Coscia M, Jaberg H, et al: Direct anterior fixation of dens fractures with a cannulated screw system. *Spine* 1991;16(suppl):S25–S32.

25. Montesano PX, Anderson PA, Schlehr F, et al: Odontoid fractures treated by anterior odontoid screw fixation. *Spine* 1991;16:S33–S37.

26. Levine AM, Edwards CC: Treatment of injuries in the C1–C2 complex. *Orthop Clin North Am* 1986;17:31–44.

27. Borne GM, Bedou GL, Pinaudeau M, et al: Odontoid process fracture osteosynthesis with a direct screw fixation technique in nine consecutive cases. *J Neurosurg* 1988;68:223–226.

28. Chang KW, Liu YW, Cheng PG, et al: One Herbert double-threaded compression screw fixation of displaced type II odontoid fractures. *J Spinal Disord* 1994;7:62–69.

29. Sasso R, Doherty BJ, Crawford MJ, et al: Biomechanics of odontoid fracture fixation: Comparison of one- and two-screw technique. *Spine* 1993;18:1950–1953.

30. White AA III, Panjabi MM (eds): *Clinical Biomechanics of the Spine,* ed 2. Philadelphia, PA, JB Lippincott, 1990.

31. Effendi B, Roy D, Cornish B, et al: Fractures of the ring of the axis: A classification based on the analysis of 131 cases. *J Bone Joint Surg* 1981;63B:319–327.

32. Francis WR, Fielding JW, Hawkins RJ, et al: Traumatic spondylolisthesis of the axis. *J Bone Joint Surg* 1981;63B:313–318.

33. Levine AM, Edwards CC: The management of traumatic spondylolisthesis of the axis. *J Bone Joint Surg* 1985;67A:217–226.

    Fifty-two patients were studied in this retrospective analysis and a classification relating fracture type to mechanism of injury was developed.

34. Roda JM, Castro A, Blazquez MG: Hangman's fracture with complete dislocation of C2 on C3: Case report. *J Neurosurg* 1984;60:633–635.

35. Schneider RC, Livingston KE, Cave AJE, et al: "Hangman's fracture" of the cervical spine. *J Neurosurg* 1965;22:141–154.

36. Sherk HH, Howard T: Clinical and pathologic correlations in traumatic spondylolisthesis of the axis. *Clin Orthop* 1983;174:122–126.

37. Fielding JW, Francis WR Jr, Hawkins RJ, et al: Traumatic spondylolisthesis of the axis. *Clin Orthop* 1989;239:47–52.

38. Garfin SR, Shackford SR, Marshall LF, et al: care of the multiply injured patient with cervical spine injury. *Clin Orthop* 1989;239:19–29.

39. Levine AM, Rhyne AL: Traumatic spondylolisthesis of the axis. *Semin Spine Surg* 1991;3:47–60.

36
Lower Cervical Injuries: Classification and Initial Management

Classification of lower cervical spine injuries requires a clear understanding of the anatomy of the cervical spine and the mechanism of injury.[1] There is no universally accepted osteoligamentous classification of lower cervical spine fractures and dislocations, although many types of classifications have been described. A frequently noted classification, that of Allen and Ferguson, is based on a study of 165 cervical spine injuries categorized into six phylogenes based on the mechanism of injury.[1] The forces involved are categorized as distraction, extension, extension-compression, compression, flexion-compression, flexion, and distraction-flexion. In addition, these phylogenes are also broken into stages according to the severity of injury, ie, stage I, causing only mild anatomic disruption, and stages III, IV, and V, causing severe anatomic disruption. In general, the severity of neurologic injury increases with the increase in anatomic disruption.[2]

An important concept in understanding cervical spine trauma is that of cervical instability. White and Panjabi[3] have defined clinical instability as a loss of the ability of the spinal elements to maintain a relationship between the vertebral segments under physiologic loads. This instability may lead to damage of the spinal cord or nerve roots and may lead to immediate or late deformity or pain. Stability is primarily determined by radiographic assessment. Table 1 delineates the radiographic assessment of stability and assigns a point value to various anatomic changes. A total point score of five or more suggests an unstable cervical spine. Instability is indicated if a vertebra translates more than 3.5 mm or angulates greater than 11° between segments.

In general, low-energy injuries to the cervical spine that do not involve significant disruption of the posterior tensile or anterior loadbearing structures are stable. On the contrary, those injuries with substantial disruption of anterior or posterior elements, loss of anterior loadbearing capacity, compromise of the spinal canal, or facet joint subluxation, dislocation, or fracture should be considered unstable.[4]

A commonly used classification of cervical spine injuries involves a mechanistic anatomic description of the cervical injury. The six categories include (1) minor compression and avulsion fractures; (2) facet injuries (occult ligamentous, unilateral or bilateral subluxation or dislocation, and facet fractures); (3) vertebral body compression fractures; (4) burst-type fractures; (5) teardrop fracture-dislocations; and (6) extension injuries, including laminar, facet, and lateral mass fractures.

Minor Compression and Avulsion Fractures

A mild compression fracture involves loss of the anterior vertebral height of less than 25%. Generally, the posterior vertebral wall remains intact. If the anterior compression is more than 50%, the posterior ligaments may be unstable and this would no longer be a minor fracture. Most of these minor compression fractures can be treated with a rigid collar until solid, usually 6 to 8 weeks.

A fracture of the spinous process, commonly known as "clay-shoveler's fracture," is most frequent at the C7 level. flexion-extension radiographs should be done to check for instability. Symptomatic treatment is generally all that is necessary.

Specific Injuries

Occult Facet Subluxation

This cervical injury generally presents with a tender, painful posterior cervical spine with normal plain radiographs. The injury can frequently be missed unless flexion-extension radiographs are made in the first 7 to 14 days. High quality magnetic resonance imaging (MRI) may be helpful in diagnosing the ligamentous disruption of the posterior elements. Minimal subluxation on flexion-extension radiographs can be treated with a rigid collar for 6 to 8 weeks. Follow-up flexion-extension radiographs are necessary to avoid progressive subluxation. Progressive subluxation or continued painful subluxation requires a posterior fusion with iliac crest graft.

Unilateral Facet Dislocation

Unilateral facet dislocation is commonly missed on original cervical spine radiographs. The patient may clinically pres-

Table 1. Checklist for the diagnosis of clinical instability in the lower cervical spine*

Element	Point Value
Anterior elements destroyed or unable to function	2
Posterior elements destroyed or unable to function	2
Relative sagittal plane translation > 3.5 mm	2
Relative sagittal plane rotation > 11°	2
Positive stretch test	2
Spinal cord damage	2
Nerve root damage	1
Abnormal disc narrowing	1
Dangerous loading anticipated	1

* Total of 5 or more = unstable
(Reproduced with permission from White AA III, Panjabi MM (eds): *Clinical Biomechanics of the Spine*, ed 2. Philadelphia, PA, JB Lippincott, 1990.)

ent with torticollis, with the chin rotated to the contralateral side and the neck bent to the injured side (Fig. 1). As the inferior facet dislocates anterior to the superior facet, the vertebral bodies subluxate approximately 25%. Frequently, the lateral radiograph gives a "bow-tie sign." The anteroposterior radiograph generally shows the spinous process deviated toward the dislocated facet. Oblique radiographs clearly show the dislocated facet (Fig. 2). Nerve root compression or spinal cord injury is not unusual with unilateral facet dislocation. In a report of 24 cases of unilateral cervical locked facets, the author noted that 70% had radiculopathy, 20% were normal, and 10% had spinal cord injuries.[5]

Most agree that reduction of a unilateral facet dislocation reduced postinjury pain and gives the best chance of neurologic improvement, but that the method of obtaining reduction of the dislocated facet is controversial.[6] Attempted closed reduction by skeletal traction is recommended by most. If skeletal traction is not successful in reducing the facet dislocation, open reduction is recommended with a posterior cervical fusion of the injured levels. Closed reduction by manipulation under anesthesia has been described but should be considered with caution. Following successful closed reduction of a unilateral facet injury, treatment using the halo vest has been advocated by some, although a high failure rate has been shown with halo treatment of these injuries.[7,8] Surgical intervention has been suggested to provide the greatest probability of achieving and maintaining anatomic reduction and appears to eliminate chances of late symptoms.[9,10] Because this is primarily a ligamentous injury, spontaneous bony fusion of the facet or vertebral bodies may not occur with conservative brace treatment. Posterior cervical fusion appears to be the treatment of choice for most unilateral facet injuries.

Bilateral Facet Dislocations

This severe cervical injury involves disruption of all posterior ligaments and the disk. The upper vertebral body is displaced 50% anterior to the lower vertebral body (Fig. 3). Severe injury to the spinal cord is common in bilateral facet dislocations.

Considerable attention over the past several years has focused on the diagnosis of disk disruption associated with bilateral facet dislocations. Several reports of neurologic

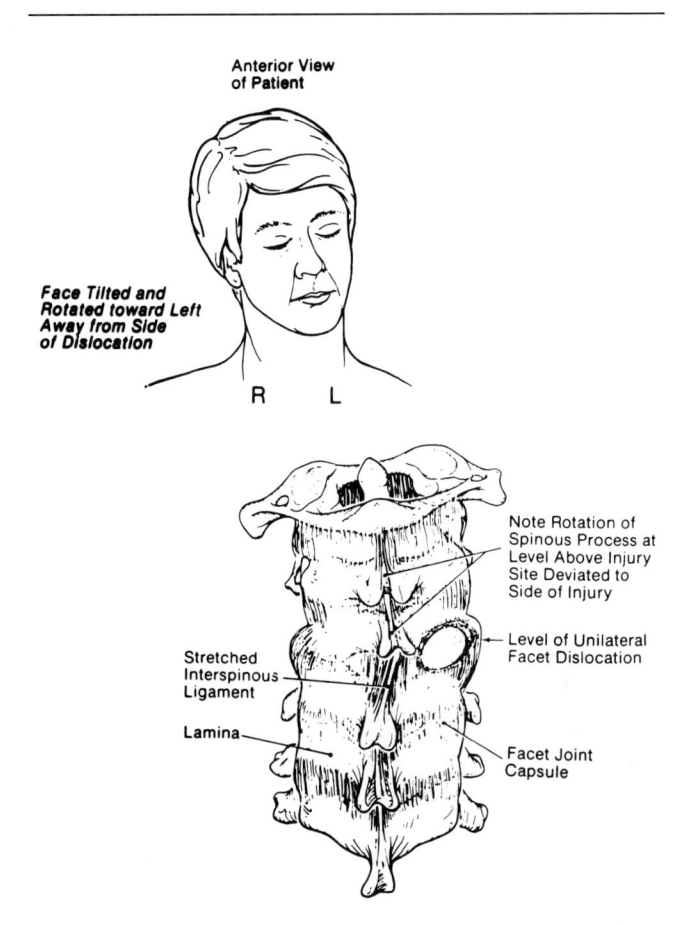

Fig. 1 Unilateral facet dislocation. Note that the face tilts away from the side of dislocation and the spinous process of the level above injury deviates to the side of injury. (Reproduced with permission from White AA III, Panjabi MM (eds): *Clinical Biomechanics of the Spine*, ed 2. Philadelphia, PA, JB Lippincott, 1990.)

deficit associated with reduction of a bilateral facet dislocation have shown the importance of determining the position of the disk in this injury.[11-13] In a study of 68 patients with cervical facet dislocation or subluxation, the authors reported a 9% incidence of herniated disk material into the canal.[12] A significant reduction in disk space height may suggest disk herniation into the spinal canal. In a neurologically normal patient with a bilateral facet dislocation, it is prudent to obtain an MRI study or myelogram/computed tomogram to determine the position of the disk. Some cases may require anterior diskectomy before spinal realignment.

Initial management of bilateral facet dislocations generally involves placement of Gardner-Wells tongs and skeletal traction in the attempt to obtain reduction. Skeletal traction must be performed in the presence of a physician with close monitoring of the radiographic and neurologic status. Appropriate sedation with muscle-relaxing agents is helpful in obtaining reduction. Skeletal traction is begun with 10 to 15 pounds and weight is added in 5-pound increments with a lateral radiograph obtained following

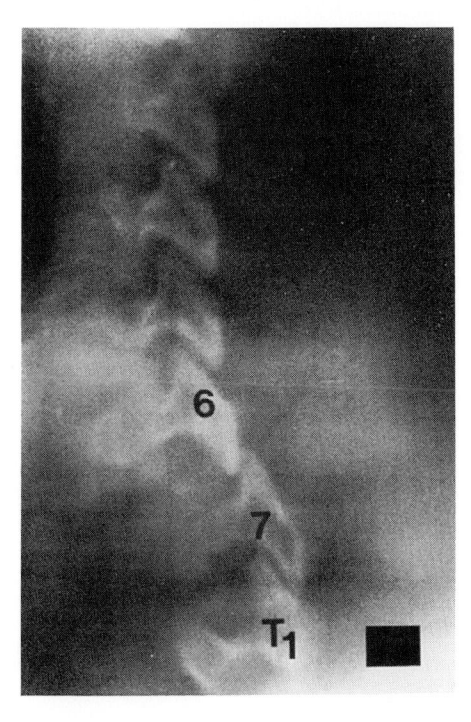

Fig. 2 Unilateral facet dislocation. Lateral tomogram reveals the C6 inferior facet dislocated anterior to the C7 superior facet. (Reproduced with permission from White AA III, Panjabi MM (eds): *Clinical Biomechanics of the Spine*, ed 2. Philadelphia, PA, JB Lippincott, 1990.)

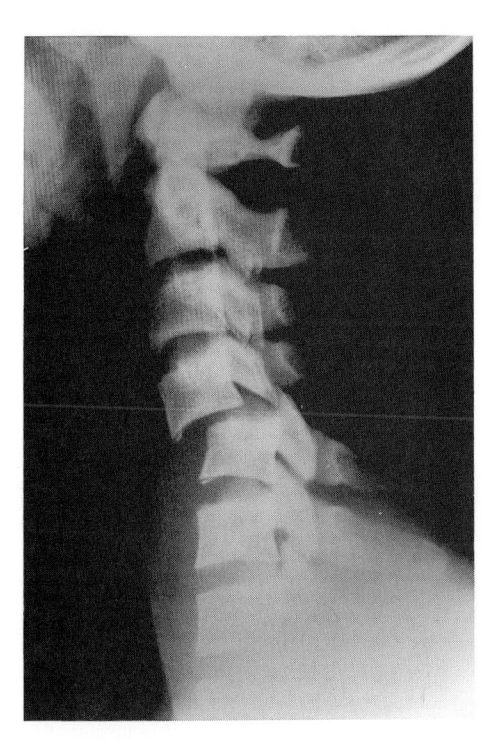

Fig. 3 Bilateral facet dislocation. Note the 50% vertebral body subluxation of C4 anterior to C5. Also note the C4 inferior facets "locked" anterior to superior facets of C5.

each change of weight until reduction is accomplished. The amount of weight needed is variable, with up to one third of body weight recommended. Sixty to 75 pounds of traction have been reported. Neurologic improvement may occur with realignment. Following successful reduction, the patient is kept in traction until a posterior cervical arthrodesis with either spinous process wiring or lateral mass plates can be accomplished. Attempts at closed reduction should be terminated if the patient's neurologic status deteriorates, if greater than 1 cm of distraction occurs at any level, or once reduction is successful.

Halo vest management after closed reduction of bilateral facet dislocation has been reported to have a high failure rate, including recurrent facet dislocation or subluxation.[14,15]

The timing for reduction of these cervical injuries with spinal cord injury is controversial, but recent evidence suggests that there may be a window of opportunity in the first 1 to 2 hours following a cervical injury during which some element of spinal cord injury may be reversible if spinal cord compression is removed. In an animal model (beagle dogs) of spinal cord injury, 50% constriction of the spinal cord produced complete paraplegia.[16] Six dogs were decompressed immediately following compression, six dogs were decompressed 1 hour following compression, six dogs at 6 hours, six at 24 hours, and six at 1 week following compression. Daily neurologic evaluations and somatosensory-evoked potentials were performed. Six weeks following decompression, neurohistologic analysis, including electron microscopy, was performed. The dogs decompressed immediately and at 1 hour following the spinal cord injury had significant neurologic improvement, were able to ambulate, and obtained substantial recovery of somatosensory-evoked potentials. The dogs decompressed 6 hours or more after spinal cord injury remained with complete paraplegia. In the clinical arena, there have been multiple anecdotal reports of recovery of complete quadriplegia from immediate reduction of bilateral facet dislocations.

In a report of 68 patients with cervical facet fracture-dislocation, the authors noted 78% improved with rapid closed reduction.[17] They suggested that the timing of decompression realignment appeared to be the most important variable in neurologic improvement. This evidence suggests that in patients with fracture-dislocations and spinal cord injury early reduction should be attempted at least by skeletal traction, if possible. If there is compression of neural tissue, vertebral fractures or dislocations must be reduced to minimize eschemia, edema formation, and allow for spinal cord recovery.

Vertebral Body Fractures

Vertebral body fractures occur from an axial compressive load. They may occur with or without the involvement of the posterior lamina and facet joints. Vertebral body fractures include compression fractures, sagittal plane fractures, burst-type fractures, and teardrop fracture-dislocations.

Vertebral body compression fractures are the result of a flexion-compression force and may be mild with less than 25% compression of the anterior vertebral body. Such injuries are generally stable and may require simple orthotic treatment. More severe compression forces will further compress the vertebral body; if more than 50% of the anterior body is compressed, this typically disrupts the posterior ligamentous elements and may lead to an unstable injury. Generally, severe axial compression injuries are unstable and require stabilization. It is difficult to control kyphosis if a significant compression fracture with posterior ligamentous disruption is treated in a rigid orthosis. Initial management includes skeletal traction for spinal realignment.

Because halo vests do not provide significant resistance to axial compressive loads, many of the severe compression fractures require either posterior or anterior stabilization. In a review of 64 consecutive C3 to C7 spinal injuries, the authors classified these according to the presence of severe ligamentous injury or severe vertebral body injury.[18] They suggest that only injuries without severe ligamentous or severe vertebral body injury can be successfully stabilized by a cervical orthosis.

Sagittal plane fractures also occur from an axial compressive load, and the hallmark, a midsagittal fracture plane extending from one vertebral endplate to the other, is commonly seen on an anteriopsterior radiograph and/or computed tomography. The lateral radiograph may appear normal. This fracture may be associated with posterior element disruption such as laminar or facet fractures. Severe spinal cord change is not unusual with sagittal plane fractures. Simple nondisplaced sagittal plane vertebral body fractures without posterior element involvement may heal in a halo vest. Serial radiographs are necessary to ensure maintenance of anatomic alignment. When significant vertebral body displacement is evident, with or without posterior element involvement, initial traction will help reduce and align the fracture and surgical stabilization is usually necessary.

Vertebral body burst fractures occur with axial compressive forces that retropulse bony fragments into the spinal canal. These fragments are generally from the superior endplate of the lower vertebrae. Initial management requires skeletal traction in an attempt to realign the spinal canal and, occasionally, to decompress the spinal cord. In patients with spinal cord injury, if skeletal traction does not successfully provide neural decompression, then an anterior vertebrectomy and fusion is required. An anterior cervical plate may also be considered. A burst fracture is generally an unstable injury and, because a halo vest does not provide significant resistance to axial compressive loads, these burst-type fractures are generally not amenable to nonsurgical care.

The final vertebral body fracture is the teardrop fracture-dislocation. Originally described by Schneider and Kahn, this fracture-dislocation consists of a characteristic triangular or quadrilateral fragment from the anterior inferior margin of the vertebral body with posterior dislocation of the spine at the level of fracture (Fig. 4). This severely unstable injury involves a high-energy compressive force. This injury frequently involves posterior element disruption. Displacement of a teardrop fracture-dislocation denotes complete failure through the motion segment. Initial management for teardrop fracture-dislocations includes skeletal traction, although care must be taken to avoid overdistraction. In a report of five cases of overdistraction by skull traction, the authors note that injuries with disruption of both anterior and posterior elements are specifically vulnerable to overdistraction with skull traction.[19] These severe injuries are generally not amenable to conservative orthotic care and routinely require anterior vertebrectomy and strut-graft fusion with anterior plating. There is controversy as to whether an anterior plate has sufficient biomechanical support for these highly unstable injuries and occasionally posterior fusion with either wiring or lateral mass plates may be necessary to accompany the anterior vertebrectomy and fusion.

Extension Injuries

Extension injuries of the cervical spine include unilateral/bilateral laminar fractures, unilateral/bilateral facet fractures, and lateral mass pedicle fractures. These injuries are

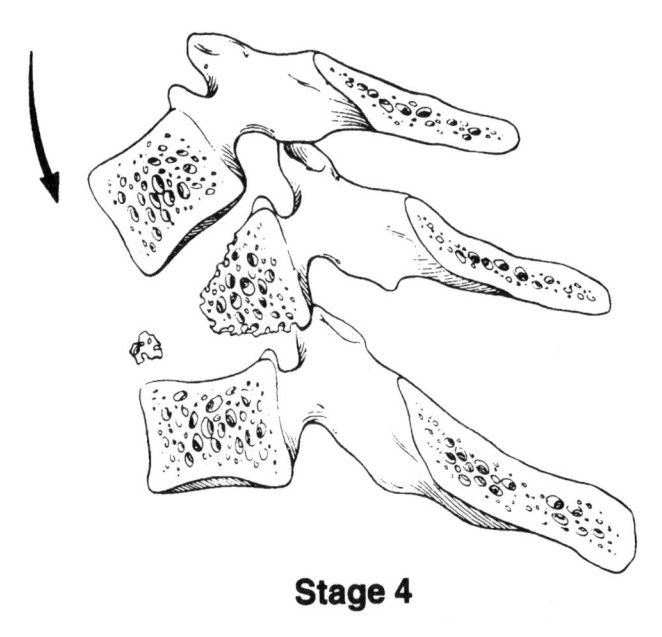

Fig. 4 Teardrop fracture-dislocation. Note that the characteristic fragment of bone from the anterior inferior margin of the vertebral body with posterior dislocation of the spine at the level of fracture.

generally the result of a compressive force with the neck in an extended position. They may be associated with any of the vertebral body fractures. Hyperextension injuries in the elderly spondylitic spine are frequently associated with a central cord injury. The simplest extension fracture is a teardrop avulsion fracture, which is quite different and much less severe than the previously described teardrop fracture-dislocation. The teardrop avulsion fracture involves a small fracture of the anterior inferior corner of the vertebral body. Flexion/extension radiographs are needed to rule out instability. Without hypermobility, this fracture can be treated with a neck orthosis for 6 to 8 weeks. Disk degeneration at the inferior disk space is not uncommon.

A unilateral laminar fracture is unusual unless associated with ipsilateral facet injury and/or pedicle fracture. Bilateral laminar fractures generally are associated with significant vertebral body fractures, including burst or teardrop fracture-dislocations. When associated with vertebral body fractures, they suggest a high-energy, severely unstable lesion. When posterior fusion surgery is performed, extreme care must be used in patients with posterior element fractures. Extension of a posterior fusion to a normal posterior element segment may be necessary with either posterior wiring or lateral mass plates. A unilateral laminar fracture with an ipsilateral pedicle fracture produces a "floating lateral mass fracture." The entire lateral mass is completely detached from the vertebral body and contralateral posterior elements. This is associated with severe vertebral body fractures and is generally highly unstable and internal fixation tends to be the treatment of choice.[20]

Ankylosing Spondylitis

Many recent reports of fractures of the cervical spine in patients with ankylosing spondylitis continue to show the high rate of spinal cord injury with these fractures. In one study, 11 such cases were reported and the authors noted that the injury was most often secondary to a minor trauma or a motor vehicle accident and that the level of vertebral involvement was most frequently between C5 and T1.[21] Axial traction as initial management followed by early cervical stabilization in patients with ankylosing spondylitis is recommended. Traction and subsequent cervical fusion should be applied and fixed in the direction of the pre-existing deformity because attempts to correct the pre-existing cervical thoracic kyphotic deformity may lead to neurologic deterioration.

Gunshot Wounds to the Cervical Spine

Gunshot wounds to the cervical spine are becoming more common with the increase in gang warfare. In general, decompressive surgery following gunshot wounds is based on the presence or absence of compressive pathology. A multicenter study has recently revealed that bullet removal does not improve neurologic recovery for thoracic spine injuries. This is most likely true for cervical injuries as well. Although severe osteoligamentous injury is rare following gunshot wounds, occasionally a severe instability will require surgical stabilization. In general, a rigid orthosis will suffice. Lead poisoning has not been shown to be a significant problem. Initial management includes a cervical orthosis and broad-spectrum antibiotics. There have been rare reports of cerebrospinal fluid leaks out of a wound or into the pleural cavity, but there is a greater risk of cerebrospinal fluid leaks following surgical removal of the bullet.

Annotated References

1. Allen BL Jr, Ferguson RL, Lehmann TR, et al: A mechanistic classification of closed, indirect fractures and dislocations of the lower cervical spine. *Spine* 1982;7:1-27.

2. McAfee PC: Cervical spine trauma, in Frymoyer JW, Ducker TB, Hadler NM, et al (eds): *The Adult Spine: Principles and Practice*. New York, NY, Raven Press, 1991, vol 2, pp 1063-1106.

3. White AA III, Panjabi MM (eds): *Clinical Biomechanics of the Spine*, ed 2. Philadelphia, PA, JB Lippincott, 1990.

4. Stauffer ES: Subaxial injuries. *Clin Orthop* 1989;239:30-39.

5. Shapiro SA: Management of unilateral locked facet of the cervical spine. *Neurosurgery* 1993;33:832-837.

6. Rizzolo SJ, Vaccaro AR, Cotler JM: Cervical spine trauma. *Spine* 1994;19:2288-2298.

7. Beyer CA, Cabanela ME, Berquist TH: Unilateral facet dislocations and fracture-dislocations of the cervical spine. *J Bone Joint Surg* 1991;73B:977-981.

   Thirty-six patients were treated with unilateral facet locations or fracture dislocations. Ten had open reduction and posterior fusion and 24 had nonoperative halo or collar management. Anatomic reduction was achieved more frequently in the operative group (60% compared to 25%). Only 36% of those treated with halo traction achieved or maintained any degree of reduction.

8. Bucci MN, Dauser RC, Manard FA, et al: Management of post-traumatic cervical spine instability: Operative fusion vs halo vest immobilization. Analysis of 49 cases. *J Trauma* 1988;28:1001-1006.

   Of 49 patients with traumatic cervical instability, 20 patients were treated with initial halo vest immobilization. Forty percent (8 of 20) of these went on to radiographic instability. Two of eight had progressive neurologic deficits due to loss of reduction while immobilized. This study indicates that halo vests do not protect patients with cervical instability from neurologic injury, nor does it absolutely immobilize the cervical spine.

9. Rockswold GL, Bergman TA, Ford SE: Halo immobilization and surgical fusion: Relative indications and effectiveness in the treatment of 140 cervical spine injuries. *J Trauma* 1990;30:893-898.

10. Sears W, Fazl M: Prediction of stability of cervical spine fracture managed in the halo vest and indications for surgical intervention. *J Neurosurg* 1990;72:426-432.

11. Mahale YJ, Silver JR, Henderson NJ: Neurological complications of the reduction of cervical spine dislocations. *J Bone Joint Surg* 1993;75B:403-409.

    Sixteen patients with cervical dislocations deteriorated neurologically during or after reduction. The dislocations were reduced by skull traction in four patients, by manipulation in four and operation in seven. Concominant disk herniation and a narrow canal are risk factors. Pre-reduction MRI or CT myelography is recommended.

12. Eismont FJ, Arena MJ, Green BA: Extrusion of an intervertebral disc associated with traumatic subluxation or dislocation of cervical facets: Case report. *J Bone Joint Surg* 1991;73A:1555-1560.

13. Robertson PA, Ryan MD: Neurological deterioration after reduction of cervical subluxation: Mechanical compression by disc tissue. *J Bone Joint Surg* 1992;74B:224-227.

14. Anderson PA, Budorick TE, Easton KB, et al: Failure of halo vest to prevent in vivo motion in patients with injured cervical spines. *Spine* 1991;16(suppl 10):S501-S505.

15. Whitehill R, Richman JA, Glaser JA: Failure of immobilization of the cervical spine by the halo vest: A report of five cases. *J Bone Joint Surg* 1986;68A:326-332.

16. Delamarter RB, Sherman J, Carr J: Pathophysiology of spinal cord damage: Recovery following immediate delayed decompression. *J Bone Joint Surg*, in press.

17. Hadley MN, Fitzpatrick BC, Sonntag VK, et al: Facet fracture-dislocation injuries of the cervical spine. *Neurosurgery* 1992;30:661-666.

18. Lemons VR, Wagner FC: Stabilization of subaxial cervical spinal injuries. *Surg Neurol* 1993;39:511-518.

19. Jeanneret B, Magerl F, Ward JC: Overdistraction: A hazard of skull traction in the management of acute injuries of the cervical spine. *Arch Orthop Trauma Surg* 1991;110:242-245.

20. Yablon IG, Palumbo M, Spatz E, et al: Nerve root recovery in complete injuries of the cervical spine. *Spine* 1991;10(suppl):S518-S521.

    Thirty-six patients with complete quadriplegia from cervical fracture dislocations were reviewed. Twenty-two underwent surgical decompression and fusion and 14 had halo vest treatment only. Of those treated with surgery 32% improved one level and 18% two levels. Without surgery, only one patient improved one level. A better functional outcome is suggested with surgical intervention.

21. Detwiler KN, Loftus CM, Godersky JC, et al: Management of cervical spine injuries in patients with ankylosing spondylitis. *J Neurosurg* 1990;72:210-215.

    Eleven patients with ankylosing spondylitis and traumatic cervical fracture/dislocation were reviewed. Three patients died shortly after admission due to pulmonary complications. The authors recommend initial axial traction followed by early surgical stabilization.

37
Lower Cervical Spine Injuries: Surgical Management

Introduction

Indications for the surgical management of lower cervical spine injuries are dependent on the clinical or radiographic determination of neurologic deficit, spinal malalignment, or spinal instability.[1] The presence of, or risk for, any of these conditions suggests that conservative measures alone (ie, brace, traction, halo vest) may be insufficient. Therefore, the objective of any surgical treatment would be to decompress neural elements, re-establish adequate cervical alignment, or restore stability to the cervical spine.[2]

The initial workup, classification, and management of lower cervical spine injuries was present in the preceding chapter and consists of immediate immobilization, neurologic evaluation, and a minimum of three radiographic views of the cervical spine (anteroposterior [AP], lateral, open mouth odontoid). The combination of neurologic assessment and radiographic documentation of cervical injury should allow the physician to begin formulating treatment. Usually additional imaging studies, such as computed tomography, magnetic resonance imaging (MRI), or lateral flexion/extension voluntary stress radiographs, will provide more detailed information on the extent of pathology and assist in planning appropriate treatment.

Upon the completion of radiographic and clinical assessment, the malaligned cervical spine should be placed in tong traction in an attempt to indirectly realign the spine. The neck can be slightly flexed or extended in reverse of the direction of injury. Traction is initiated with 5 to 10 pounds of weight, with incremental increases in weight of 5 pounds applied every 15 to 30 minutes until reduction has been achieved. The maximum weight for cervical traction is highly controversial, and recommendations range from 40 pounds to as much as 70% of the patient's body weight. Likewise, manipulative maneuvers to achieve reduction are also highly controversial and, if performed, limited to the conscious or alert patient without existing neurologic deficit. After the neck has been realigned, traction weight should be decreased to 5 to 10 pounds. If traction is unsuccessful, surgery is warranted to obtain reduction.

The general principles of surgical management in lower cervical spine injuries are to improve and/or protect the patient's neurologic function while establishing a normally aligned, stable, yet mobile and painless spine.[3] The neurologic component of injury warrants neural decompression which can be achieved by either spinal realignment (traction or surgery), or surgical excision. Spinal stability can be restored indirectly by halo vest or directly by surgical fixation. Open reduction and internal stabilization can be achieved anteriorly, posteriorly, or as a combination of the two. The clinical decision of anterior versus posterior stabilization is dependent on the pattern of injury and the location (anterior versus posterior) of the principal lesion to be addressed.[4]

Classification

The lower cervical spine injury classifications presented in the preceding section are determined radiographically and by the mechanism and anatomic region of injury, and they can be either major or minor in their complexity. Minor fractures, injuries that are stable and rarely associated with neurologic deficit, are generally managed nonsurgically. Major injuries, however, are more unstable and at greater risk for neurologic compromise, and therefore warrant surgical management.

Posteriorly, simple injuries include spinous process fractures, ipsilateral facet fractures or dislocations, and ipsilateral articular process fractures. Simple anterior injuries consist of transverse process fractures, teardrop avulsion fractures from the anterior/inferior portion of the vertebral body (as the result of hyperextension), and wedge compression fractures secondary to hyperflexion and involving less than 50% of the anterior vertebral body height.

Complex fracture patterns, involving both anterior and posterior elements, are always major injuries and are best treated surgically. Spinal stability and alignment can be jeopardized by loss of bony axial support anteriorly and decreased ligament or bone resistance to tensile loads posteriorly. Often the spinal canal is subjected to anterior or posterior bone or soft-tissue encroachment. The complex fracture types include burst fractures, sagittal plane fracture (vertebral body compression fractures), or teardrop fracture-dislocation.

Surgical Techniques

Cervical spine injury requiring direct reduction decompression or stabilization can be surgically approached anteriorly, posteriorly, or both.[3] The optimal approach is determined by the region of the cervical spine exhibiting the greatest neural canal compromise or instability. Most cervical spine dislocations or burst fractures result in anterior neurologic compression; once spinal alignment has been re-established, posterior decompression is rarely of benefit.[5,6]

The technique for anterior decompression consists of thorough excision of retropulsed bone or disk at the level of spinal injury. After all fragments are cleared from the spinal canal, spinal realignment is restored and stability established with a tricortical iliac graft fitted between intact vertebrae. Until fusion occurs, stabilization options include halo vest, anterior plate fixation, posterior fixation, or a combination of these methods, depending on the pathology encountered.[7]

Halo vest immobilization for the extremely unstable spine has been plagued by numerous complications. Reported complications have been loss of reduction, bone graft extrusion, pin site infections, pin loosening, and pin perforation of the calvarium.[8] The halo vest is primarily indicated for major cervical injuries that are not amenable to internal fixation, noncompliant patients, or to augment tenuous internal fixation/grafting.

Plate fixation has recently become popular in establishing immediate anterior stability. It is employed in combination with a tricortical bone strut graft and requires only limited postoperative brace immobilization.[9] Two types of screws, unicortical and bicortical, have been used to obtain purchase in the vertebral body. Biomechanical studies demonstrate excellent restoration of flexion and extension stability with anterior plates, however, their rotational stability is poor and must be augmented posteriorly.[4,7] Initial clinical reports have been favorable, although this technique increases the risk of spinal cord damage (especially bicortical screws), esophageal perforation from prominent hardware, or potential hardware loosening and subsequent implant migration.

Traditionally, posterior fixation and fusion has been the most popular method of internally re-establishing cervical spine stability (Fig. 1). Stabilization usually consists of one of a variety of intersegmental wiring techniques that can incorporate the spinous process, lamina, and/or facet.[1] Clinical and in vitro studies demonstrate that interspinous wiring techniques are highly effective for most flexion ligamentous injuries, however, the prerequisite for any wiring procedure is the presence of intact posterior bony elements.[10] In addition, these techniques are inadequate for extension or rotation injuries.[11] In highly unstable flexion injuries, interspinous wiring alone may still permit rotatory subluxation, and many authors recommend supplemental oblique or "checkrein" wiring from the superior facet laterally to the midline inferior spinous process. Finally, instability secondary to multi-level laminectomies requires wiring of corticocancellous strut grafts placed longitudinally along the facet.[3]

As an alternate method of posterior fixation, posterior cervical lateral mass plating has achieved recent acclaim due, in part, to its applicability despite the presence of compromised posterior elements.[7,12] Screws are placed in the lateral mass divergent from the midline in the coronal plane to avoid vertebral artery or nerve root injury, and perpendicular or oblique in the sagittal plane to avoid the facet joint. Often lateral mass plating can preclude the need for supplemental anterior stabilization, especially in injuries with rotatory or axial instability.[11] The preliminary clinical experience has been favorable and associated neurovascular complications have been minimal.[11]

Surgical Management of Posterior Cervical Spine Injuries

Optimal treatment for posterior lower cervical injuries can be clearly nonsurgical, clearly surgical, or controversial. Nonsurgical treatment ranges from a cervical collar or brace to halo immobilization and is intended to provide symptomatic relief while limiting spinal mobility for the adequately aligned injury with some degree of inherent stability. Clearly nonsurgical injuries include isolated fractures of the spinous posterior process or the lamina. The treatment for simple flexion-rotation trauma with ipsilateral facet ligamentous injury but without fracture or gross displacement is controversial. Flexion-extension radiographs are recommended and, if the spine is stable, sufficient treatment consists of a brace or a halo vest with serial stress radiographs to confirm healing in acceptable alignment. When frank instability is documented, surgical treatment is preferable and consists of simple interspinous wiring.[10]

Facet dislocations, with or without fractures, are common but treatment remains highly controversial. Depending on the extent of cervical flexion, rotation, and subsequent bone or ligamentous disruption, varying degrees of instability can be present. In unilateral facet dislocations only one facet is displaced while the contralateral facet remains intact. Initial treatment employs cervical traction, which achieves reduction in approximately 70% to 90% of patients. Some authors advocate manipulation if traction alone is unsuccessful,[13] but this is extremely hazardous and should be approached cautiously. Most surgeons prefer open reduction and simple posterior interspinous wiring and fusion if closed methods fail.

When closed unilateral facet reduction can be obtained, the optimal method of maintaining alignment is unclear. Many authors advocate halo vest immobilization for several months followed by stress radiographs upon halo removal. This treatment can be complicated by residual pain, loss of alignment, or residual instability.[14] Routine posterior cervical fusion consisting of interspinous wiring, oblique

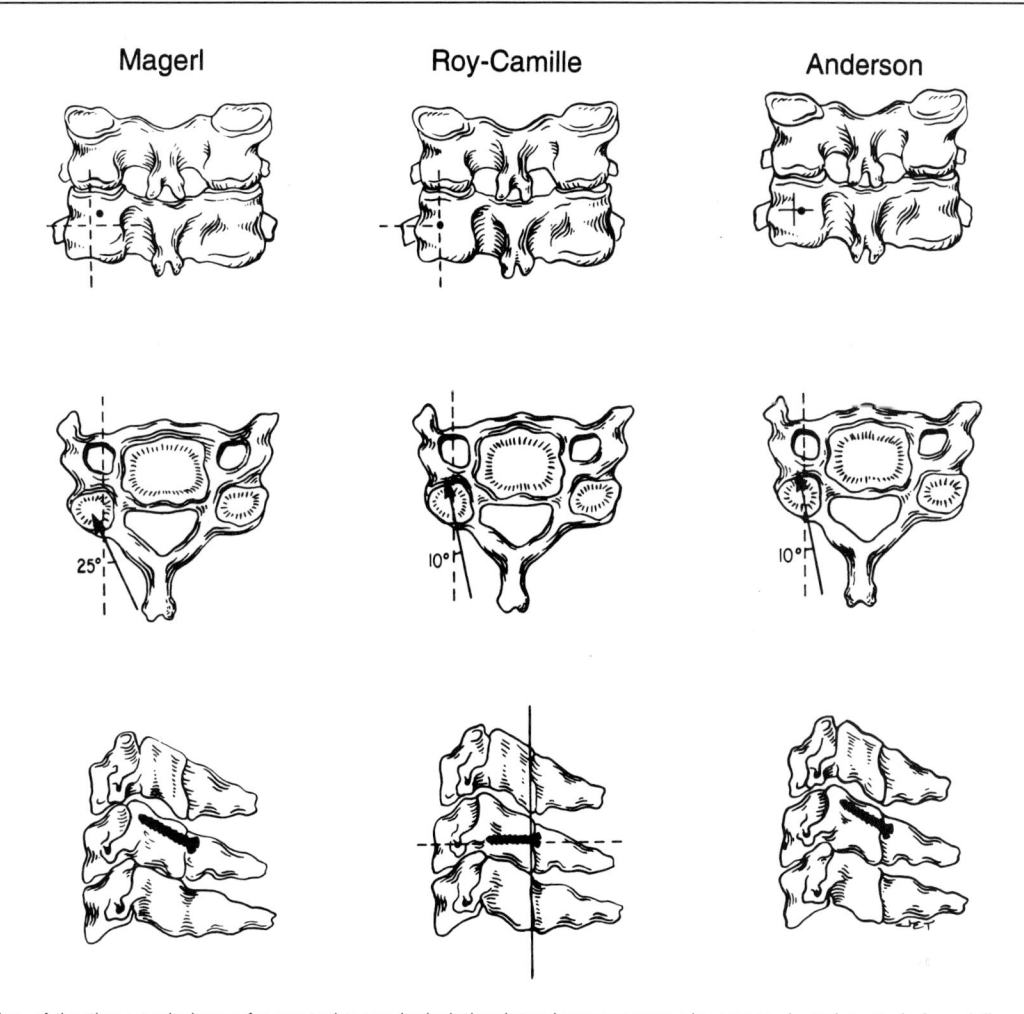

Fig. 1 Illustration of the three techniques for posterior cervical plating lateral mass screw placement viewed posteriorly, axially, and laterally.

wiring, or lateral mass plating has been recommended as the treatment of choice to ensure alignment and fusion of the compromised segment.

Bilateral facet dislocations occur secondary to severe ligamentous disruption and are, therefore, highly unstable. These injuries are also associated with a greater risk for neurologic deficit and are especially associated with disk herniation.[15] Initial radiographic assessment should always include MRI prior to attempting reduction. Extruded disk in the canal was noted in one study in which 7% of 68 patients had cervical facet injury. If the MRI is negative, initial treatment consists of tong traction, which is usually successful. Care must be taken not to apply excessive weight or to overdistract the injured segment.[15]

Following closed reduction, halo vest immobilization does not provide sufficient stabilization for the bilateral facet injury. Surgical stabilization is absolutely indicated and usually consists of posterior wiring or lateral mass plate fixation.[3] If an extruded disk is demonstrated by MRI, an anterior diskectomy should be performed prior to reduction, followed by bone grafting augmented with either an anterior plate or posterior wiring/fusion.[15]

Articular process fractures, whether they are unilateral or bilateral, are extremely unstable and also clearly require surgical treatment to maintain spinal alignment. This injury is often complicated if the clinician fails to appreciate that there is lateral mass separation and assumes that the patient has only a simple facet dislocation. Because of the loss of posterior element continuity, simple one-level interspinous wiring does not adequately control the significant rotational instability, and wiring must usually be extended one level to a normal segment.[16] These injuries represent the ideal indications for lateral mass plating, which provides greater torsional stability.[16,17]

Anterior Injuries

The appropriate treatment for anterior cervical injuries is also extremely variable and can be nonsurgical, surgical, or controversial. Anterior injuries that are clearly nonsurgical usually require a cervical collar for symptomatic relief only. Serial follow-up radiographs to include lateral flexion/extension voluntary stress views should be obtained to confirm that stability is maintained. Acute injuries demonstrating instability sufficient enough to warrant halo vest immobilization are more prudently managed by internal stabilization.

The anterior cervical injuries effectively treated nonsurgically include isolated fractures of the transverse process, avulsion teardrop (hyperextension) injuries, and compression fractures with decreased anterior body height not exceeding 50% of normal. Isolated transverse process fractures result from muscular avulsion injuries that do not affect spinal alignment or stability. Avulsion teardrop fractures may disrupt the disk in addition to the anterior/inferior bony aspect of the body; however, these injuries remain stable as long as the posterior longitudinal ligament and the posterior bony/ligamentous structures remain intact. Hyperextension voluntary stress lateral radiographs will confirm stability prior to application of a cervical orthosis. The principal long-term complication of this injury has been disk degeneration at the affected motion segment.

Anterior compression injuries with less than 50% loss of body height rarely disrupt the disk, middle column, posterior longitudinal ligament, or posterior stabilizing structures and are generally stable and warrant collar immobilization only. Seemingly mild compression fractures have occasionally demonstrated instability and progression of deformity and, therefore, should be followed closely.[18] If vertebral body compression exceeds 50% of the anterior height, the likelihood for posterior ligamentous disruption increases. Lateral flexion and extension stress radiographs should demonstrate increased interspinous separation or significant segment angulation. This more severe compression injury is most appropriately treated with a fusion achieved by either posterior interspinous wiring or anterior strut graft and plating if significant vertebral body height has been compromised.

Burst fractures usually demonstrate spinal canal compromise due to retropulsed bone from the superior endplate of the lower vertebra. Surgical management is clearly indicated for burst fractures that compromise neurologic function, encroach upon the spinal canal, or demonstrate gross instability. Burst fractures of the vertebral body threaten the ability of the spine to withstand axial load and can be complicated by significant angulation or loss of height. Among the more complex anterior fracture patterns are sagittal plane fractures, burst fractures limited to the anterior and middle spinal columns without posterior column disruption, or fracture-dislocation/teardrop fractures. Flexion-extension films are not recommended when the fracture configuration suggests obvious instability. Sagittal plane fractures may be associated with lamina or facet fractures, adjacent motion segment fractures, ligamentous disruption, and neural injury. Isolated nondisplaced sagittal plane fractures can be managed in a halo vest; however, injuries with body displacement are preferably treated with anterior decompression and fusion. Anterior fusion alone is contraindicated if anterior fracture stability is also associated with posterior description.[3] There may or may not be associated lamina or pedicle fractures in addition to the anterior bony description. Initial treatment consists of traction realignment and reduction of the bony fragments. As definitive fixation, a halo vest does not provide sufficient stability and these injuries are more appropriately managed by anterior decompression and bone strut anterior grafting.[19] Because of the significant associated posterior bony and ligamentous injuries, strut grafting alone is inadequate stabilization. Burst fractures should be augmented with anterior cervical plate, halo vest, or supplemental posterior fixation to maintain cervical alignment.[4]

Unlike the hyperextension injury, the cervical avulsion teardrop fracture-dislocation results from the combination of axial load and compression with a displaced triangular or quadrilateral fracture fragment from the anterior-inferior margin of the body and significant disruption of the ligamentous structures posteriorly. This injury is extremely unstable and frequently presents with gross malalignment and neurologic deficit. Loss of anterior bone and ligament continuity, in addition to the posterior instability, allows the posterior inferior position of the body to displace into the spinal canal. Tong traction should be carefully applied to avoid overdistraction but re-establish cervical alignment. Definitive treatment consists of corpectomy, strut grafting, and anterior plating with or without supplemental posterior fixation.[20]

Fractures of the vertebral body with lamina facet injuries usually represent three-column injuries and are highly unstable. These injuries require a combination of anterior surgical decompression, strut grafting, and plating in addition to posterior stabilization consisting of either wiring or plating for rotational stability.[3]

At the time of this writing, bone screws placed posteriorly into vertebral elements have not been cleared for general use in this specific manner by the Food and Drug Administration (FDA). These are Class III devices. This category includes screws placed transfacetally, within pedicles, or in articular, lateral masses. Some screws have been approved for use within the sacrum as Class II devices. Some companies have received Class II clearance for use of screws in lumbar pedicles specifically to supplement fusions in the treatment of grade III and IV spondylolisthesis with the proviso that these devices are removed after the arthrodesis has healed. Anterior vertebral body screws (cervical, thoracic, and lumbar) are Class II devices and can be used as labeled in vertebral bodies. Many of the posterior screw-based devices have been shown in laboratory and clinical testing to be useful and can be used in an off-label manner if the physician feels this is appropriate and important for the treatment of the patient. As with all surgeries, informed consent should explain the procedure and why a particular technique has been chosen, as well as its risks and benefits. The question of whether informed consent regarding pedicle screws must include a discussion of the device's FDA clearance status is currently being litigated in several jurisdictions.

References

1. White AA, Panjabi MM: The role of stabilization in the treatment of cervical spine injuries. *Spine* 1984;9:512–522.
2. Gill K, Paschal S, Corin J, et al: Posterior plating of the cervical spine: A biomechanical comparison of different posterior fusion techniques. *Spine* 1988;13:813–816.
3. Stauffer ES: Management of spine fractures C3-C7. *Orthop Clin North Am* 1986;17:45–53.
4. Stauffer ES, Kelly EG: Fracture-dislocations of the cervical spine: Instability and recurrent deformity following treatment by anterior interbody fusion. *J Bone Joint Surg* 1977;59A:45–48.
5. McAfee PC, Bohlman HH: One-stage anterior cervical decompression and posterior stabilization with circumferential arthrodesis. *J Bone Joint Surg* 1989;71A:78–88.
6. Bohlman HH: Acute fractures and dislocations of the cervical spine: An analysis of three hundred hospitalized patients and review of the literature. *J Bone Joint Surg* 1979;61A:1119–1142.
7. Montesano PX, Jauch EC, Anderson PA, et al: Biomechanics of cervical spine internal fixation. *Spine* 1991;16(suppl 3):S10–S16.
8. Garfin SR, Botte MJ, Waters RL, et al: Complications in the use of the halo dissection device. *J Bone Joint Surg* 1986;68A:320–325.
9. Ripa PR, Kowall MG, Meyer PR Jr, et al: Series of ninety-two traumatic cervical spine injuries stabilized with anterior ASIF plate fusion techniques. *Spine* 1991;16:S46-S55.
10. Coe JD, Warden KE, Sutterlin CE III, et al: Biomechanical evaluation of cervical spinal stabilization methods in a human cadaveric model. *Spine* 1989;14:1122–1131.
11. Cooper PR, Cohen A, Rosiello A, et al: Posterior stabilization of cervical spine fractures and subluxations using plates and screws. *Neurosurgery* 1988;23:300–306.
12. Ebraheim NA, Hoeflinger MJ, Salpietro B, et al: Anatomic considerations in posterior plating of the cervical spine. *J Orthop Trauma* 1991;5:196–199.
13. Cotler HB, Miller LS, DeLucia FA, et al: Closed reduction of cervical spine dislocations. *Clin Orthop* 1987;214:185–199.
14. Cheshire DJ: The stability of the cervical spine following conservative treatment of fractures and fracture-dislocations. *Paraplegia* 1969;7:193–203.
15. Avena MJ, Eismont FJ, Green BA: Intervertebral disc extrusion associated with cervical facet subluxation and dislocation. *J Bone Joint Surg* 1991;73A:1555–1560.
16. Levine MA, Mazel C, Roy-Camille R: Management of fracture separations of the articular mass using posterior cervical plating. *Spine* 1992;17(suppl 10):S447-S454.
17. Anderson PA, Henley MB, Grady MS, et al: Posterior cervical arthrodesis with AO reconstruction plates and bone graft. *Spine* 1991;16(suppl 3):S72–S79.
18. Mazur J, Stauffer S: Unrecognized spinal instability associated with seemingly simple cervical compression fractures. *Spine* 1983;8:687.
19. Bucci M, Dauser R, Maymond F, et al: Management of post-traumatic cervical spine instability: Operative fusion versus halo vest immobilization. Analysis of 49 cases. *J Trauma* 1988;28:1001.
20. Cybulski GR, Douglas RA, Meyer PR Jr, et al: Complications in three-column cervical spine injuries requiring anterior-posterior stabilization. *Spine* 1992;17:253–256.

38

Thoracolumbar Fractures: Injury Evaluation and Classification

Injury Evaluation

Detailed guidelines for extrication, immobilization, and initial evaluation of spinal injury victims have been described elsewhere in this text. During the injury evaluation phase, the thoracolumbar spine is protected and immobilized with long spinal boards and logrolling techniques. It is equally important to transfer the patient (especially one with sensory impairment) off of hard surfaces in a timely manner in order to prevent skin ischemia and the risk of pressure sores. The patient and/or rescue personnel should be questioned about the details of the accident (type of collision, whether the patient was ejected from vehicle, presence of windshield or steering column damage) as well as the presence of neurologic symptoms (transient and/or permanent). In motor vehicle accidents, knowledge about the restraint systems (ie, lap belt, lap and shoulder belt, air bag, etc) also may be helpful in understanding the spinal column injury.

The physical examination begins with inspection of the chest, abdomen, and back, noting any bruising and ecchymosis. Careful palpation along the spinal column is carried out, searching for point tenderness (either midline or paraspinal), spinous process widening, and rib or transverse process fractures. Detailed neurologic examination, including *mandatory* genitourinary and anal sensory and sphincter functional assessment, is completed and clearly documented in the patient's chart.

In unconscious patients or in those unable to cooperate with the physical examination, anteroposterior and lateral views of the entire spine must be obtained at the initial evaluation. In conscious and cooperative patients, radiographs should be obtained of any region where pain or tenderness is identified on examination. The decision to obtain additional radiographic studies, such as computed tomography (CT), magnetic resonance imaging (MRI), or myelography should be made on a case-by-case basis. Factors that would influence this decision would be presence of neurologic deficit, need to assess spinal stability, preoperative planning, and inadequate imaging with plain films alone (eg, cervicothoracic junction).

Cases in which the *complete neurologic deficit* or *incomplete neurologic deficit* clearly correlates with the level of injury (eg, L1 burst fracture) do not mandatorily require neuroradiologic (MRI, myelo-CT) evaluation. In this situation, a simple CT scan may provide sufficient information to guide either surgical or nonsurgical treatment planning. However, patients should undergo urgent MRI or myelo-CT evaluation if neurologic deficit (complete or incomplete) does not correlate with level of injury or if the deficit is shown to be progressing. In spinal column injuries, MRI holds an advantage by revealing bony compression on the neural elements, as well as directly imaging and discerning between hematomas or disk fragments in the canal.

Injuries in which spinal stability cannot be accurately assessed on plain radiographs also warrant additional studies. Thin slice CT images (3 mm or less) provide the best information on bony anatomy when coupled with sagittal or coronal reconstruction, subluxation or dislocation can also be accurately evaluated. MRI, although suboptimal on bony detail, can provide very useful information on soft-tissue/ligamentous injury, which may impact on overall spinal stability.

Somatosensory evoked potentials, cystometrogram, and electromyography are not typically indicated during the acute injury evaluation phase. These studies may be useful, however, in evaluating the extent and degree of the neurologic injury and the potential for long term recovery.

Classification

Thoracolumbar injuries can be classified using several different categories. The most commonly utilized categories have been based on fracture morphology, biomechanical force of injury, or spinal stability, or a combination of these parameters. Although categories and stratification may vary from one classification to another, the ultimate goal is to aid the clinician in diagnosis of the spinal column structural and neurologic injury and treatment planning.

A key issue in the evaluation and treatment of spinal trauma is that of spinal stability. Nicoll began by categorizing spinal injuries into stable and unstable groups. White and Panjabi proposed the currently accepted definition of clinical spinal instability as "the loss of the ability of the spine under physiologic loads to maintain its pattern of displacement so that there is no initial or additional neurologic deficit, no major deformity, and no incapacitating pain." Although most classifications address the issue of instability, the primary stratification of injuries is typically based on other parameters, such as fracture morphology or mechanism of injury.

After analyzing the biomechanical forces that produced spinal injury, Holdsworth categorized fractures into five basic types of violence (pure flexion, flexion and rotation, extension, vertical compression, and direct shearing). Recently, Gertzbein[1] presented the modified classification of Magerl and associates, which is also a mechanistic system with three broad categories: compression, distraction, and multidirectional translation (Fig. 1). This classification is then further subdivided on the basis of morphologic- or deformity-based categories with severity of injury, instability, and incidence of neurologic deficit increasing progressively with each subtype.[2]

Fracture morphology has also been commonly used as the primary parameter for categorizing injuries. Using data from plain films and CT, both Denis[3] and McAfee and associates[4] proposed classifications that were based on morphologic groups such as wedge/compression, burst fracture, Chance fracture, and fracture-dislocation. However, both of these classifications also incorporate nonmorphologic categories (seatbelt-type, flexion-distraction, translational) in their primary stratification.

In a review of a series of thoracic and thoracolumbar fractures managed with screw-plate instrumentation, Gaines and associates[5] proposed a novel classification that uses morphologic criteria. The "load sharing" classification (Fig. 2) recognizes the importance of anterior and middle column comminution and identifies injuries at high risk for pedicle screw failure. Between one and three points are assessed for comminution, displacement/apposition, and kyphotic deformity. This classification must be tested in a larger number of cases to support statistical validity. Furthermore, a spinal level-by-level analysis needs to be done to separate out the influence of regional sagittal alignment on screw fracture.

Holdsworth[6] and later Denis[3] also utilized the *spinal column* concept in stratifying their classifications. Denis described the three-column spine model (Fig. 3). The anterior column was defined as the anterior longitudinal ligament and the anterior half of the vertebral body with the associated disk and annulus. The middle column consists of the posterior longitudinal ligament and the posterior half of the vertebral body, disk, and annulus. The posterior column includes the bony neural arch as well as the associated ligamentous structures (facet capsules, ligamentum flavum, and inter spinous and supraspinous ligaments). Although the spinal columns have not been used as primary categories for classifying injuries, they are useful in subdividing certain fractures and in clarifying the extent and stability of any one particular injury (eg, two-column versus three-column disruption).

Thus far we have reviewed the basic units of a classification system. Other variables such as displacement, deformity, soft-tissue disruption, and neurologic deficit can also be used to further stratify injuries within a classification. The established classifications will not be reviewed in intimate detail in this text, but rather an overview of the most commonly encountered injury groups will be presented and pertinent points from the various classifications will be highlighted.

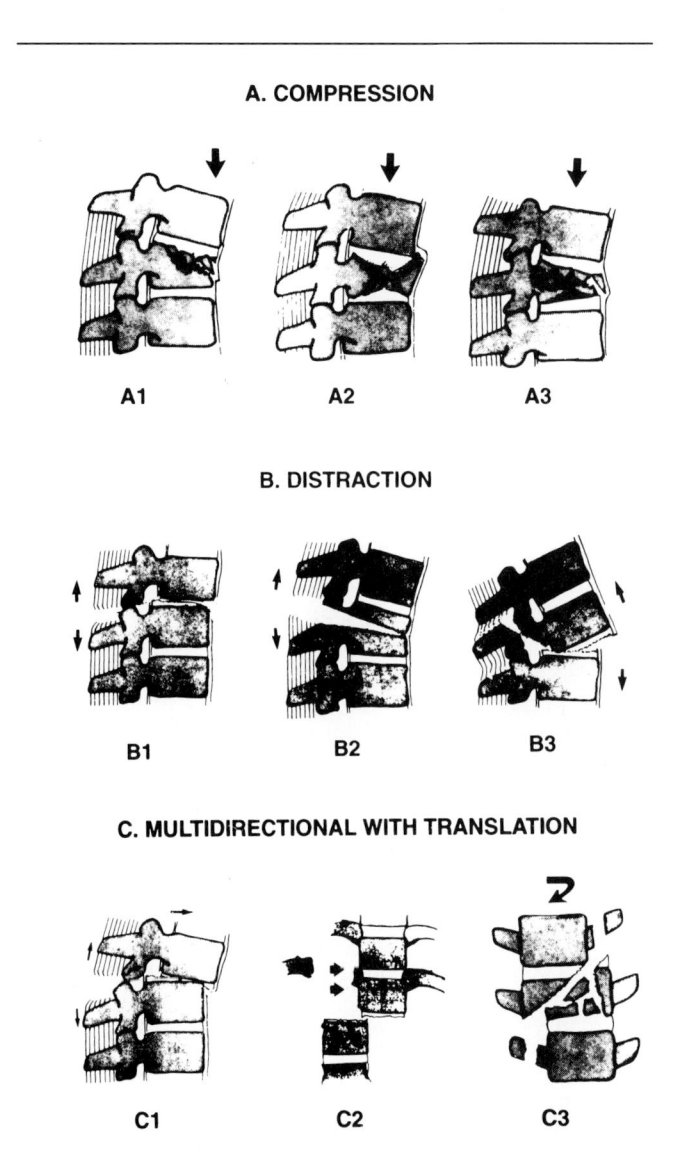

Fig. 1 The mechanistic classification of Magerl as modified by Gertzbein. This system takes into consideration both bony and ligamentous disruption with severity of injury progressively increasing from one category to the next. (Reproduced with permission from Gertzbein SD: Spine update: Classification of thoracic and lumbar fractures. *Spine* 1994;19:626–628.)

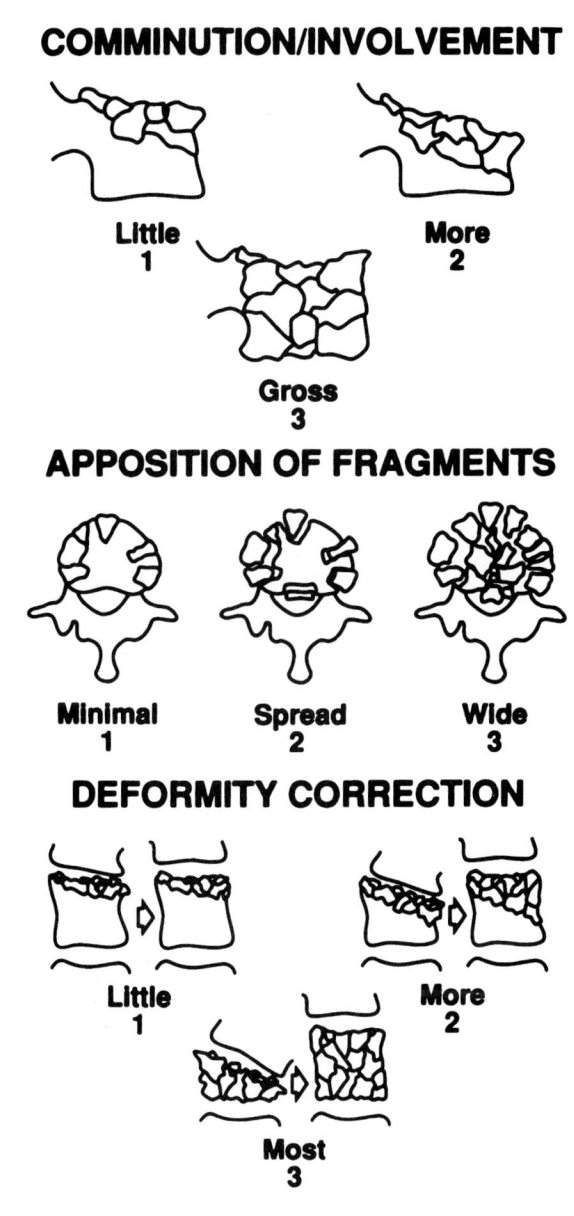

Fig. 2 The "load sharing" classification is based on fracture morphology and also takes into consideration postoperative alignment. This classification was designed to identify fractures that place pedicle screw instrumentation at high risk for failure. (Reproduced with permission from Stauffer ES (ed): *Thoracolumbar Spine Fractures Without Neurologic Deficit*. Rosemont, IL, American Academy of Orthopaedic Surgeons, 1993.)

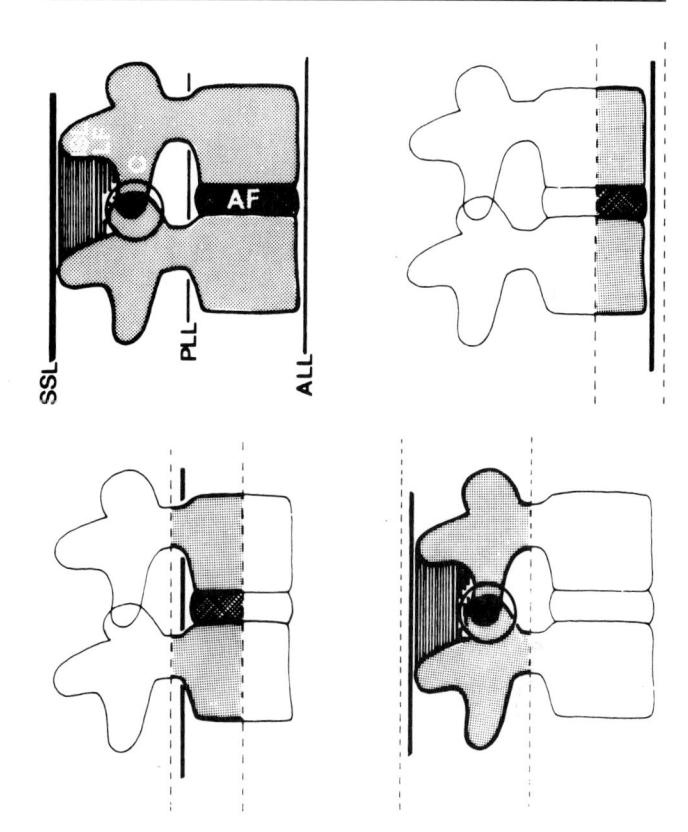

Fig. 3 The three-column spine model as described by Denis. The anterior column consists of the ALL and anterior one half of the body, disk, and annulus. The middle column contains the PLL and posterior one half of the body, disk, and annulus. The posterior column encompasses the bony neural arch and associated posterior soft-tissue stabilizers. (Reproduced with permission from Denis F: The three column spine and its significance in the classification of acute thoracolumbar spinal injuries. *Spine* 1983;8:817–831.)

Wedge/Compression Fractures

A wedge/compression fracture typically results from the application of a flexion moment (anterior flexion or lateral flexion) applied to the spine. Alternatively, axial loading to a kyphotic region can also produce compression fractures. By definition only the anterior column is involved, with accompanying loss of vertebral height; the middle and posterior columns remain intact. However, both Denis[3] and McAfee and associates[4] noted that with severe single level (ie, more than 50% anterior height loss) or multiple contiguous compression fractures, there may be an element of posterior column insufficiency with accompanying progressive deformity or neurologic injury.

Burst Fractures

These fractures are the result of axial loads applied to the spine. They occur most commonly at the thoracolumbar junction (T11-L2) with L1 being the most frequently involved level. The anterior and middle columns are always involved with a variable amount of retropulsion of middle column bone into the canal. Depending on the severity of the injury, the posterior column may not be involved or may be completely disrupted as well. Plain radiographs will reveal anterior height loss and middle column fracture with possible widening of the interpedicular distance on

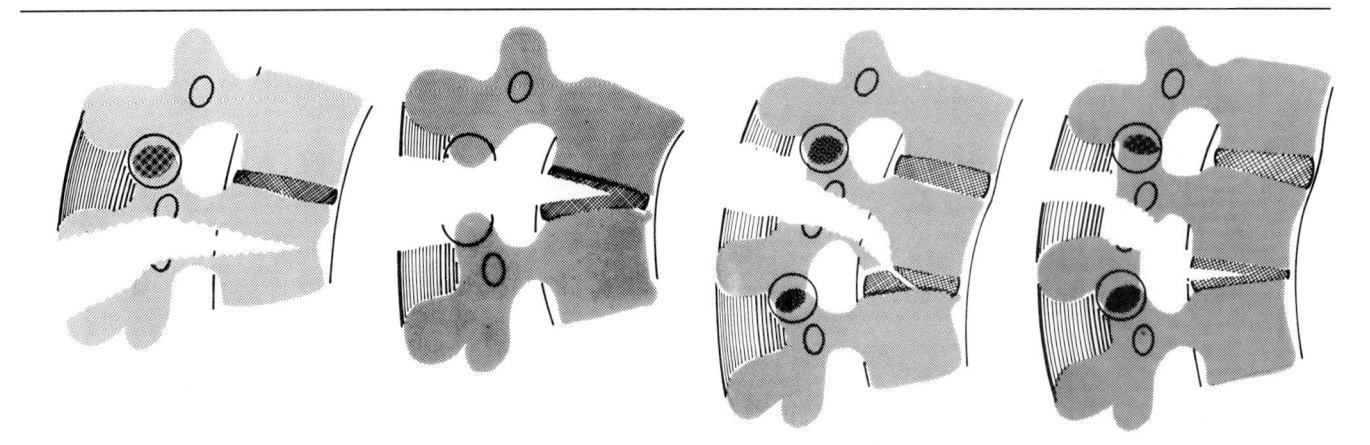

Fig. 4 Left, Flexion injury with fracture extending through bony elements of all three columns and limited to a single level. This is the fracture pattern described by Chance. **Center left, center right,** and **right,** Variants of the chance fracture with disruption through either bony or ligamentous structures and involvement of one or two adjacent segments. (Reproduced with permission from Denis F: The three column spine and its significance in the classification of acute thoracolumbar spinal injuries. *Spine* 1983;8:817–831.)

anteroposterior views. Posterior column damage is best assessed on thin slice CT images.

Burst fractures represent a broad spectrum of spinal column injury. Subdivision within this category, therefore, is helpful in both diagnosis and treatment planning. The subdivisions that have been used in the past separate fractures on the basis of either fracture morphology or spinal stability. Denis described five different types of burst fractures based on fracture morphology: Type A had superior and inferior end plate involvement; type B had only superior end plate fracture; type C had only inferior end plate disruption; type D burst fracture had three-column disruption with rotation, and Type E had significant lateral flexion. However, this subdivision does not clearly separate stable from unstable injuries.

Unstable Burst Fracture

McAfee and associates[4] separated burst fractures into stable and unstable groups. Unstable burst fractures were defined as having posterior column disruption in compression, lateral flexion, or rotation. Unstable burst fractures have a higher incidence of neurologic injury and usually have surgical stabilization. In addition to complete posterior column disruption (both bony and ligamentous), radiographic parameters such as greater than 15° to 25° of absolute kyphosis, greater than 50% anterior height loss, and more than 50% canal compromise have been used in defining an unstable burst fracture.

Stable Burst Fracture

Stable burst fractures are classified as those injuries with predominately anterior and middle column disruption without significant spinal deformity or canal compromise. Posterior column involvement may be present in the form of a vertical split through the spinolaminar complex. However, the posterior ligamentous structures remain intact, as does spinal stability. Stable burst fractures are often amenable to definitive management in a cast or total contact orthosis.

Flexion-Distraction Injuries

This group of injuries is characteristically caused by a primary flexion force acting on the spinal column with the fulcrum anterior to the vertebral body. A concomitant distraction force may also be present, further displacing the injury segments. Typically, all three columns are disrupted, however, as in burst fractures, there is a wide spectrum of injury. These injuries can also be subdivided on the basis of stability.

Stable Flexion Injuries

The flexion injury described by Chance involves transverse fracture through the bony elements of all three columns (Fig. 4). The fulcrum in this injury (eg, a seat belt) is positioned anterior to the anterior longitudinal ligament and the ligament remains intact. Although several variants of this injury have been described subsequently (Fig. 4), the key to classifying these as stable flexion injuries is that the anterior longitudinal ligament is preserved, there is no significant loss in anterior column height and there is no rotational, translational, or axial displacement.

Unstable Flexion-Distraction Injuries

The fulcrum, in this category of injuries, is typically within the middle column. The posterior column fails in tension/distraction while the anterior column fails in compression. Accordingly, there is a loss in anterior column height, possible anterior longitudinal ligament disruption, and posterior column disruption through bony, or ligamentous structures, or through a combination of posterior elements. As in the stable flexion injury, there is no rotational or translational displacement between the injured segments. The various different morphologic patterns of flexion distraction injuries have been reviewed in other classifications.[2,7]

Translational Injuries

Translational injuries are three-column injuries typically produced by a combination of forces acting simultaneously on the spinal column. Although different labels (fracture-dislocation, shear, multidirectional-translation) are used in the established classifications systems, there is unanimous agreement that this is the most unstable group of spinal injuries. All three columns are disrupted with possible anterior column height loss and typically rotational, axial, or translational displacement of the injured segments, resulting in spinal discontinuity. The combination of spinal column instability coupled with, nearly certain, complete neurologic deficit relegates these injuries to surgical stabilization.

Annotated References

1. Gertzbein SD, Court-Brown CM: Flexion-distraction injuries of the lumbar spine: Mechanisms of injury and classification. *Clin Orthop* 1988;227:52–60.

2. Gertzbein SD: Spine update: Classification of thoracic and lumbar fractures. *Spine* 1994;19:626–628.

   This classification stratifies injuries primarily on mechanism of injury and subdivides the categories based on fracture morphology. Progressing from type A1 through C3, there is increasing bony and soft-tissue injury with concomitantly increasing spinal instability and neurologic deficit.

3. Denis F: The three column spine and its significance in the classification of acute thoracolumbar spinal injuries. *Spine* 1983;8:817–831.

   The biomechanical concept of the three-column spine is presented along with a predominantly mechanistic classification system based on a retrospective review of 412 cases. The classification system is also correlated with neurologic deficit, spinal instability, and treatment rationale.

4. McAfee PC, Yuan HA, Fredrickson BE, et al: The value of computed tomography in thoracolumbar fractures: An analysis of one hundred consecutive cases and a new classification. *J Bone Joint Surg* 1983;65A:461–473.

   Along with a review of the entire spectrum of thoracolumbar fractures, the authors present criteria distinguishing between stable and unstable burst fractures.

5. Gaines RW Jr, Holt B, McCormack T: Abstract: A classification to predict screw breakage when using short segment instrumentation with pedicle screws: The load-sharing classification of spinal fractures. *Orthop Trans* 1994;18:103.

6. Holdsworth FW: Fractures, dislocations, and fracture: Dislocations of the spine. *J Bone Joint Surg* 1970;52A:1534–1551.

7. Gumley G, Taylor TK, Ryan MD: Distraction fractures of the lumbar spine. *J Bone Joint Surg* 1982;64B:520–525.

Bibliography

Buckholz RW, Gill K: Classification of injuries to the thoracolumbar spine. *Orthop Clin North Am* 1986;17:67–73.

Ferguson RL, Allen BL Jr: A mechanistic classification of thoracolumbar fractures. *Clin Orthop* 1984;189;77–88.

Willen JA, Gaekwad UH, Kakulas BA: Acute burst fractures: A comparative analysis of a modern fracture classification and pathologic findings. *Clin Orthop* 1992;276:169–175.

39

Thoracic and Lumbar Fractures: Nonsurgical Management

Introduction

Fractures of the thoracic and lumbar spine, with and without neurologic deficit, have been routinely treated nonsurgically until only the last few decades. The work of physicians such as Bedbrook[1] showed that these fractures could be treated either with bed rest or with various forms of cast immobilization and go on to successful uniting of the fracture and, neurologic improvement. The disadvantages of nonsurgical treatment are that it requires prolonged periods of bed rest with the associated nursing care and monetary costs. In most cases, the spinal deformity was only marginally improved.

The reports by Holdsworth and other surgeons in the 1940s and 1950s led to an increased interest in internal fixation of these fractures in an attempt to decrease the period of bed rest and degree of spinal deformity and to improve recovery of any neurologic deficit. At that time, the inadequacies of the available fixation devices deterred most physicians from using surgical techniques. A resurgence of interest in surgical correction of these traumatic spinal deformities occurred with the advent of the Harrington rod and the subsequent reports of many authors through the 1970s and 1980s.

The proper place of nonsurgical management of these fractures today is still being evaluated in light of the advances in internal fixation. Nonsurgical care today cannot be equated to nonsurgical care decades ago. In many cases today, the most conservative treatment regimen may well involve surgical intervention. This chapter will discuss only the nonsurgical treatment of fractures of the thoracic and lumbar spine and will try to review the current status and place of this form of treatment.

Nonsurgical treatment of injuries without neurologic deficit can be used for many cases. Injuries with associated neurologic loss are generally treated by surgical intervention to improve alignment and clear the spinal canal. This is in spite of conflicting reports correlating the degree of neurologic loss and the displacement and size of the spinal canal on initial radiographic studies.[2] Furthermore, the degree to which the canal has been restored postoperatively has no correlation with the postoperative neurologic status.[3] Most surgeons, however, continue to feel that if there is neurologic deficit, surgical intervention is usually appropriate.

Braces

Nonsurgical treatment of these injuries can consist of any combination of bed rest and external support. The period of bed rest recommended by most authors has steadily decreased. The type of braces available include simple corsets, three-point fixation devices, and total-contact orthoses.

Corsets cause only minimal restriction of motion. They do decrease the load on the spine both directly, by load sharing, and indirectly, by allowing some of the forces to be transmitted through the abdominal region.[4] Corsets and other forms of brace may increase the forces at the lumbar sacral junction and at the top of the brace. Simple corsets may also decrease the load applied to the spine because they remind the patient not to bend excessively and therefore will reduce the overall moment arm on the spinal segments. Corsets have no specific effect on intersegmental motion; the effect is rather more of a generalized decrease in motion.

Three-point fixation devices such as the Jewett brace may exert a force on the involved segments that is either flexion or extension.[5] The forces tend to be generally applied to the entire braced segment (T8 to L3) rather than to any specific intersegmental region. Three-point fixation devices share many of the same characteristics of the corsets plus they can apply a specific force—either flexion or extension. These devices are very poor at controlling rotation and side bending.

Total contact orthoses such as the TLSO do decrease motion in all three planes. They decrease the load on the spine directly by load sharing and indirectly by transferring forces through the abdominal cavity and also decreasing the moment arm. Total contact orthoses increase the forces at the lumbar sacral junction in a manner similar to that of corsets and three-point fixation devices.

Treatment

There are many fracture classification systems of spinal fractures, most of which are based on the three-column theory initially developed by Denis. Injury to any of the three columns as defined in the Denis classification may be osseous or ligamentous. The healing ability of these varying types of injuries needs to be appreciated. The initial degree of stability of a fracture and the subsequent late stability at 3 to 4 months may be totally different. Osseous injuries do tend to heal whereas ligamentous injuries may not. The maintenance of initial and late stability must be considered when assessing appropriate treatment, whether surgical or nonsurgical.

Certain general recommendations can be given with regard to the appropriateness of nonsurgical intervention over surgical intervention. Neurologic injury is generally regarded as an indication for surgical intervention. A single-column injury such as a small anterior compression fracture is usually appropriate for nonsurgical care. A two-column injury such as a burst fracture may at times be appropriate for either surgical or nonsurgical care. A three-column injury generally is not appropriate for nonsurgical care. There are exceptions to all rules and certainly there are some three-column injuries that can be managed nonsurgically.

Specific Fracture Patterns

Fractures of the lumbar spine in adolescents have several unique features. The fractures frequently involve the apophyseal end-plate and quite often are associated with neurologic deficit. These fractures will heal in most cases with nonsurgical methods. Neurologic involvement, however, must be addressed surgically.[6] There are isolated cases of these fractures without neurologic involvement and only minimal canal compromise that can be treated with a rigid orthosis.

Simple compression fractures of the anterior column are inherently stable. The goal of treatment is to decrease the moment arm across the area and allow healing to occur. This can be accomplished for thoracic fractures from T7 to the upper lumbar region with a hyperextension brace such as a Jewett. In this case, the brace is not used for load sharing but rather as a positional reminder to the patient not to bend and, therefore, increase the flexion moment across the injured segment of the vertebra. Cases that involve two or more vertebrae may be better treated with a TLSO. If the deformity is significant across multiple vertebrae, surgical intervention may be considered. This is particularly true of injuries to the upper thoracic spine. Bracing of this area is generally unsuccessful and surgical correction of these deformities is indicated. Single level compression fractures of over 50% involving the thoracic spine may present a similar pattern, requiring open reduction and internal fixation.

A two-column compression injury such as a burst fracture can be successfully managed nonsurgically. Many authors have established criteria for nonsurgical treatment:[7] generally, no neurologic deficit, a kyphotic angle of less than 25°, and less than 50% compromise of the spinal canal by the bony fragment. Various authors used serial computed tomography scans to show that the canal can be reconstituted over time without surgical intervention. This is particularly true in the younger individual. Late complications in this group of patients may occasionally be seen.[8] Denis documented a group of individuals who required late intervention because of progressive deformity and neurologic deficit.[9] Other authors such as Krompinger and associates[7] have not seen this problem. It would appear that by staying within those guidelines as developed by authors such as Krompinger, the possible need for late surgical intervention is probably less than 5%.

A three-column compressive injury, such as a three-column burst fracture, generally requires internal fixation. The same guidelines for two-column burst fractures can be applied, however, to the three-column injuries.[10] A patient who meets the general guidelines for nonsurgical care can be treated in a TLSO, but careful radiographic and neurologic follow-up must be carried out.

Flexion-distraction injuries of the so-called Chance type, if they are non-displaced, can be treated in a TLSO.[11] A Jewett brace should not be used because it cannot control the rotation and side bending forces sufficiently. Any displacement, whether angular or translational, should be addressed with internal fixation. General guidelines of approximately 15° of kyphosis and several millimeters or more of translation are generally considered to be indications for surgical intervention. A flexion-distraction injury that is predominant ligamentous should be considered for internal fixation and fusion because there may be late ligamentous instability even with adequate reduction.

Patients with fracture-dislocations of the thoracolumbar spine are best managed surgically. Bedbrook and others have demonstrated that gross deformities can be corrected with postural reduction in bed. However, surgical stabilization allows the rapid mobilization of these patients, which outweighs the surgical risks.[12]

Low lumbar burst fractures are different from other thoracolumbar burst fractures in several ways. First, the biomechanics are different because this segment of the spine is in lordosis. Second, any neurologic loss is in the root, not the cord. Several excellent reviews comparing nonsurgical to surgical treatment have been published. The general recommendation is to use surgical intervention if the fracture causes excessive kyphosis or neurologic loss.[13]

Nonsurgical immobilization requires immobilization of at least one hip.[14]

Conclusion

Nonsurgical treatment of fractures of the thoracolumbar spine is indicated for the majority of thoracic and lumbar injuries. Specific contraindications to nonsurgical care include polytrauma, excessive deformity, and/or neurologic deficit. Long periods of bed rest (ie, greater than 1 to 2 weeks) are not recommended by most authors today. Rapid mobilization in external devices such as Jewett hyperextension braces or TLSOs is generally the preferred method of treatment.

Two- and even some three-column burst fractures can be treated nonsurgically with good long-term results. Some flexion-distraction injuries can likewise be treated with an expected good long-term result. Fracture-dislocations and adolescent limbus fractures are generally best treated surgically.

Annotated References

1. Bedbrook GM: Spinal injuries with tetraplegia and paraplegia. *J Bone Joint Surg* 1979;61B:267–284.

   This is the classic article by Dr. Bedbrook describing his treatment techniques and results. The skilled nursing care required for this form of treatment must not be underappreciated.

2. Gertzbein SD: Scoliosis Research Society: Multi-center spine fracture study. *Spine* 1992;17:528–540.

   This is a multi-center study of over 1,000 fracture patients. A significant correlation was observed between the midsagittal diameter and cross sectional area and neurologic deficit at the level of the conus medullaris. No correlation could be seen at the cord level.

3. Crutcher JP Jr, Anderson DA, King HA, et al: Indirect spinal canal decompression in patients with thoracolumbar burst fractures treated by posterior distraction rods. *J Spinal Disord* 1991;4:39–48.

   Neurologic function at follow-up correlated with preoperative canal stenosis but did not correlate with residual stenosis after instrumentation.

4. Johnsson R: The use of orthoses in lumbar spine fusion. *Acta Orthop Scand* 1993;251(suppl):92–93.

5. Patwardhan AG, Li SP, Gavin T, et al: Orthotic stabilization of thoracolumbar injuries: A biomechanical analysis of the Jewett hyperextension orthosis. *Spine* 1990;15:654–661.

6. Epstein NE, Epstein JA: Limbus lumbar vertebral fractures in 27 adolescents and adults. *Spine* 1991;16:962–967.

7. Krompinger WJ, Frederickson BE, Mino DE, et al: Conservative treatment of fractures of the thoracic and lumbar spine. *Orthop Clin North Am* 1986;17:161–170.

   Guidelines established in this paper for conservative care have been carried through by most authors in the recent literature. The ability of the spinal canal to reconstitute itself, at times dramatically, is likewise illustrated.

8. McEvoy RD, Bradford DS: The management of burst fractures of the thoracic and lumbar spine: Experience in 53 patients. *Spine* 1986;10:631–637.

9. Denis F, Armstrong GW, Searls K, et al: Acute thoracolumbar burst fractures in the absence of neurologic deficit: A comparison between operative and nonoperative treatment. *Clin Orthop* 1984;189:142–149.

10. Knight RQ, Stornelli DP, Chan DP, et al: Comparison of operative versus nonoperative treatment of lumbar burst fractures. *Clin Orthop* 1993;293:112–121.

11. Gertzbein SD, Court-Brown CM: Rationale for the management of flexion-distraction injuries of the thoracolumbar spine based on a new classification. *J Spinal Disord* 1989;2:176–183.

12. Jacobs RR, Asher MA, Snider RK: Thoracolumbar spinal injuries: A comparative study of recumbent and operative treatment in 100 patients. *Spine* 1980;5:463–477.

13. An HS, Simpson JM, Ebraheim NA, et al: Low lumbar burst fractures: Comparison between conservative and surgical treatments. *Orthopedics* 1992;15:367–373.

14. Phelan ST, Jones DA, Bishay M: Conservative management of transverse fractures of the sacrum with neurological features: A report of four cases. *J Bone Joint Surg* 1991;73B:969–971.

40
Fractures of the Thoracolumbar Junction

Introduction

Treatment Goals

The evaluation and treatment of spinal fractures at the thoracolumbar junction involves an assessment of the patient's neurologic status and a recognition of the fracture pattern. The thoracolumbar junction is a transitional region in both the local biomechanics and neurologic tissues. The thoracolumbar junction is usually neutrally aligned between the kyphosis of the thoracic spine and the lordosis of the lumbar spine. The regional biomechanics change at the thoracolumbar junction from the more rigid thoracic spine to the mobile lumbar spine. The neural tissues within the spinal canal at the thoracolumbar junction also undergo significant changes. The spinal cord terminates with the conus medullaris and the cauda equina originates. The response of neurologic tissue to injury and its capacity to regenerate varies tremendously as the elements of the spinal cord make the transition into the peripheral nerve tissue of the cauda equina. The physician must understand the pattern of neurologic injury and the fracture pattern equally well to formulate an effective treatment plan.

The goals of treatment are to establish a balanced and painfree spinal column and to promote and maintain maximal neurologic function. Treatment must maximize and enhance neurologic recovery, prevent any neurologic damage, and prevent late neurologic deterioration. The restoration of normal spinal contours should include the immobilization and fusion of the fewest number of vertebrae possible, while providing adequate stability to enhance rehabilitation and to reduce the general complications associated with skeletal trauma.

The efficacy of the nonsurgical treatment of spinal fractures has been well established in the medical literature.[1-3] Postural reduction, bed rest, hyperextension casting, and bracing are effective means of treatment for certain fracture patterns in patients who are neurologically intact. Determining the need for surgical intervention involves a careful assessment of each patient's functional demands, rehabilitative needs, and other associated injuries. The surgical management of spinal fractures has been gaining acceptance. Patients who undergo surgery have easier rehabilitation, shorter hospital stays, fewer medical complications, and quicker return to their ultimate functional outcome than patients treated nonsurgically.[4-6] In patients with neurologic deficits associated with spinal injuries, several studies have demonstrated that reducing the angular spinal deformity and increasing the spinal canal clearance aid in neurologic recovery. Several studies have shown a neurologic recovery rate of more than 80% in patients with incomplete lesions who underwent surgical treatment compared with a recovery rate of only 60% to 70% in controls treated nonsurgically.[7-10]

Principles of Posterior Spinal Instrumentation

In the treatment of spinal fractures, posterior instrumentation can be used to correct the local deformity, to prevent the development of late deformity, to provide immediate stability, and to enhance healing at the fracture site. Posterior instrumentation can also be used to decompress the spinal canal by re-establishing the normal contours of the spinal column and by reduction of retropulsed fracture fragments through ligamentotaxis. Posterior spinal instrumentation can be used as a tension band, as an internal splint providing three-point fixation, or as a neutralization internal splint.[11]

Numerous types of spinal internal fixation devices are available. The four general categories of devices are compression implants, dual-hook rod constructs (Harrington) and multiple-hook rod constructs (Cotrel-Dubousset, Isola, TSRH), transpedicular implants, and segmental sublaminar wiring techniques (Luque).

Compression and neutralization implants are used in fracture patterns associated with failure of the posterior column under tension. The posterior compression construct functions as a tension band and restores tensile strength to the spinal motion segment. This construct does not improve the ability of the motion segment to withstand axial loading, rotation, lateral flexion, or shear forces. A posterior tension band only increases the resistance to flexion moments. Rod-hook montages in compression and spinous process wirings are commonly used posterior tension-band techniques. Pedicle screws provide a more rigid tension band that also increases the axial compression, rotational, and shear strength of the spinal motion segment.[12,13] The posterior tension band principle is most commonly used to treat flexion-distraction injuries. This construct is contraindicated in fracture patterns with disruption of the middle column (burst fractures) and transdiskal flexion distraction injuries. Compression alone in these injuries can increase the retropulsion of bone or disk fragments into the spinal canal.[14,15]

Internal splint constructs stabilize an injured spinal motion segment with three points of fixation. A contoured distraction rod or rod sleeves provide three points of fixation at the two hook sites and a third point of pressure over the injured spinal motion segment. This montage corrects the sagittal plane angulation and locks the spine into extension by tightening the anterior longitudinal ligament. Increasing the number of points of fixation increases the bending rigidity. Spinal constructs that provide segmental fixation through multiple hook placement (Cotrel-Dubousset, Isola, and TSRH (Texas Scottish Rite Hospital) give greater stability than a two-hook system (Harrington). Adequate contouring of the rod to provide close contact between the rod and spine is essential in improving the reduction and the stability of the montage. This construct cannot be used in fracture patterns associated with the destruction of the anterior longitudinal ligament; overdistraction of the injured motion segment will occur.

Neutralization constructs are used in patients who do not have an intact anterior longitudinal ligament. The three-point fixation technique depends on an intact anterior longitudinal ligament for its stability. If the ligament has been injured, overdistraction and destabilization at the fracture site can occur. Segmental spinal instrumentation that holds the spine in both flexion and extension is necessary for these injuries. These constructs are also used in flexion-distraction injuries that shear through the entire disk space. Reduction of these injuries with a posterior compression construct can cause the posterior portion of the disk space to compress, retropulsing disk material into the spinal canal.

Pedicle constructs provide segmental internal fixation of the spine. Pedicle fixation is particularly effective in patients in whom the posterior spinal elements are absent (laminectomy) or is unable to hold midline rod-hook instrumentation (multilevel lamina fractures). Pedicle fixation also permits short-segment construction that incorporates only the spinal motion segments involved in the fracture patterns. Short-segment pedicle constructs are effective for stabilizing posterior ligamentous injuries;[13,16] however, a short-segment construct provides less stability than an intact spinal motion segment in fracture patterns involving the anterior and middle columns (burst fractures).[17] Two-level pedicle constructs increase the axial and torsional stability of a spinal injury involving both the anterior and middle columns.[18] Pedicle constructs are most effectively used in fracture patterns involving the mid and lower lumbar spine. Lumbar spinal motion segment can be saved with short-segment constructs and the complications of hook placement in the lower lumbar spine are avoided.

Sublaminar wires help stabilize rod-hook constructs.[19,20] A Harrington distraction rod construct augmented with segmental sublaminar wires is a cost-effective montage; however, it has limited applications. The passage of sublaminar wires is associated with complications of dural laceration and neurologic injury during insertion and extraction. Luque rectangles and sublaminar wires have limited application in spinal fractures. Although the Luque construct is effective in resisting torsional forces, it does not resist axial compression forces.[21] It can be used in shear fracture-dislocations with minimal comminution in the anterior and middle columns. It should not be used in burst or other fracture-dislocation patterns in which there is a loss of the anterior column supporting elements.

Use of Posterior Instrumentation in Specific Fracture Patterns

Compression Fractures

Compression fractures result from axial loading of the anterior column.[14] The anterior portion of the vertebral body fractures and, importantly, the middle column remains intact and acts as a fulcrum. There is a variable injury to the posterior column. In compression fractures, the posterior column structures fail under tension, not axial loading. When the amount of vertebral body collapse approaches 50% of its height, the posterior ligamentous complex begins to fail under tension. The interspinous process distance increases proportionally to the amount of anterior wedging. Posterior instrumentation constructs are used in compression fractures to reduce the local kyphosis and re-establish anterior vertebral body height. Indications for posterior instrumentation in compression fractures may also include patients who will not tolerate bracing or a cast, progression of the deformity despite adequate external immobilization, and multiple adjacent compression fractures.

The posterior column deformity is reduced through compression; the anterior column deformity is reduced through distraction. A posterior tension band construct can reduce the posterior column injury but is rarely effective in restoring the anterior vertebral body height. A posterior rod-hook montage can reduce the local kyphosis and restore anterior vertebral height (Fig. 1). The rod must be bent into lordosis or rod sleeves must be used to correct the kyphosis.[22] The rod sleeves press against the intact lamina and facets and produce an anteriorly directed force vector that reduces the local kyphosis. Distraction between the hooks must be avoided because it will recreate the major injuring force and push the injured motion segment into kyphosis.

Pedicle instrumentation can also be used effectively to correct the injury pattern associated with compression fractures.[23]* In all compression injuries, the junction between the pedicle and vertebral body is intact. Screws can be inserted through the pedicle of the fractured vertebra and attached to a longitudinal posterior rod or plate. The pedicle screws can be manipulated with the fulcrum established at the rod-screw or plate-screw junction. The motion segment can then be brought out of kyphosis through distraction of the anterior column and compression of the posterior column.

All posterior constructs will fail unless the anterior column is adequately restored. If the anterior vertebral body height is not restored after posterior instrumentation is

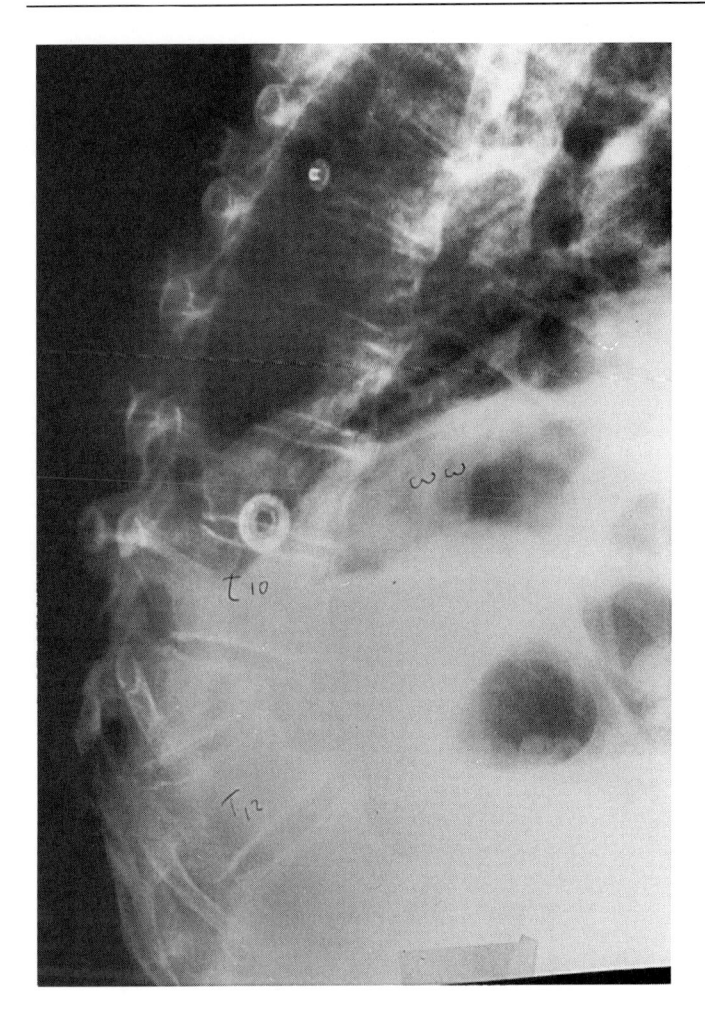

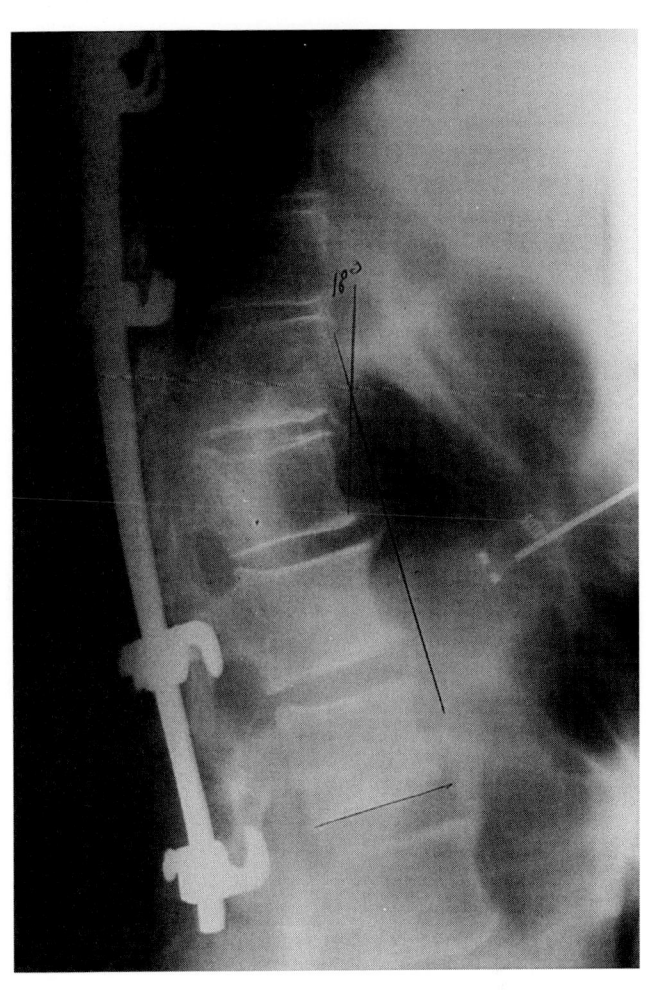

Fig. 1 Left, Lateral radiograph of the thoracolumbar junction of a 75-year-old man demonstrates a severe compression fracture of T11. The middle column is intact; there is more than 50% collapse of the anterior portion of the vertebral body, and the posterior elements are intact but splayed apart. The local kyphosis at the fracture site is 48°; the overall thoracic kyphosis was increased to more than 85°. **Right,** Lateral radiograph after posterior spinal fusion. A multilevel hook construct uses segmental instrumentation (Cotrel-Dubousset) to correct the deformity. A short compression montage was not used because of the magnitude of the deformity and the quality of the patient's bone.

applied, the anterior column may be successfully reconstituted through transpedicular bone grafting[24] (Fig. 2) or by an anterior interbody fusion.

Flexion-Distraction Injuries

Flexion-distraction injuries result from failure of the posterior and middle columns under tension forces generated by flexion of the spine.[14,25,26] There is variable injury to the anterior column, which acts as the fulcrum in this injury pattern. The anterior column may undergo a mild compression injury, however, the anterior longitudinal ligament remains intact. The disruption of the spinal columns may be through their ligamentous or bony components. The ability of these injuries to heal without surgery depends on the fracture pattern and the magnitude of the local kyphosis at the level of the injury. The local kyphosis after closed reduction of the injury should be within 10° of the normal sagittal spinal alignment. At the thoracolumbar junction, the kyphosis at the injury site should be reduced to neutral with no more than 10° of kyphosis being acceptable. Posterior bony arch injuries heal rapidly if the spine is properly aligned. Pure posterior ligamentous injuries necessitate open reduction and fusion.

The posterior instrumentation used to treat flexion-distraction injuries involves reduction of the kyphotic deformity through compression and maintenance of the reduction by a tension band principle. Single-level hook montages are the most commonly used constructs (Fig. 3). A single-level pedicle montage can also be used, however, the preoperative radiographs must be carefully inspected

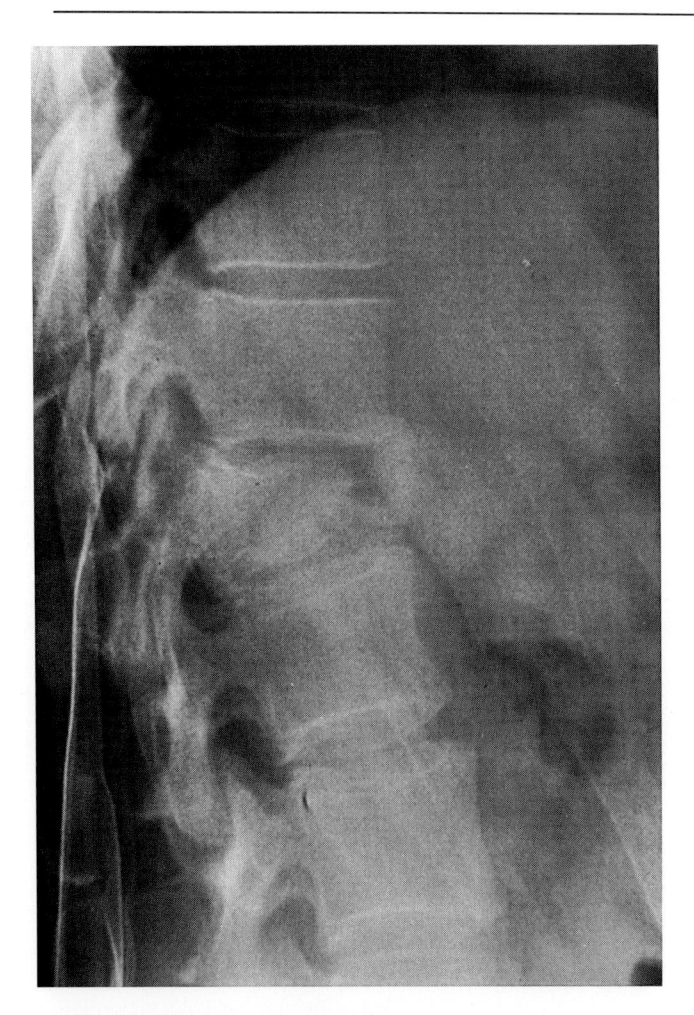

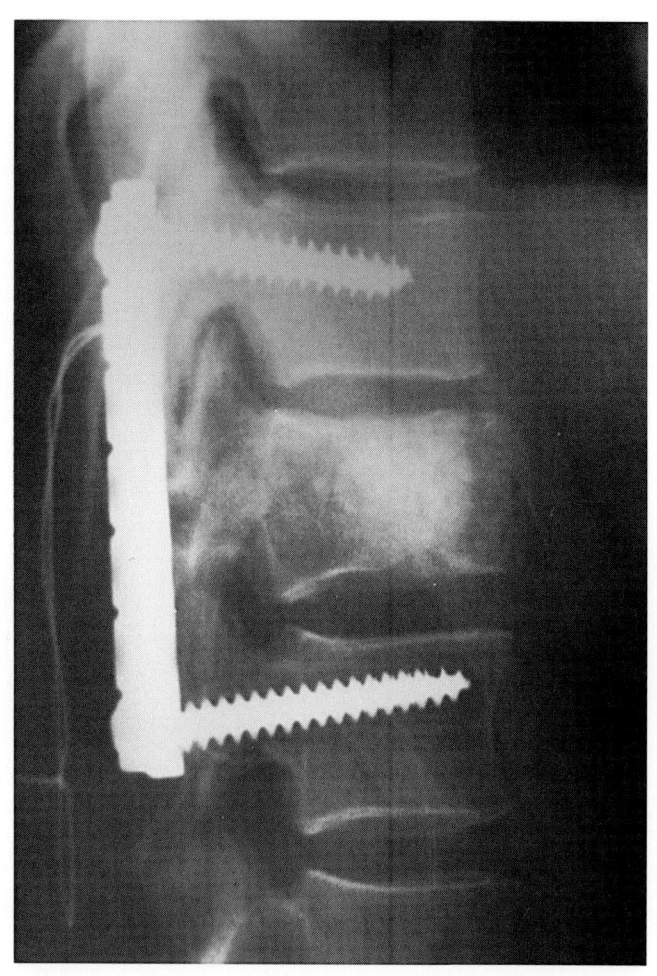

Fig. 2 Left, Lateral radiograph of the thoracolumbar junction shows a compression fracture of T12. There is more than 50% loss of anterior column height and the local sagittal angulation at the fracture site was 25°. **Right,** Postoperative lateral radiograph shows a short segment posterior compression instrumentation using pedicle screws. The anterior column was restored using a transpedicular bone grafting technique. The intravertebral bone graft is seen as the density in the midportion of the vertebral body.

to ensure that the pedicles are intact and not fractured. If the bony posterior elements of the injured spinal motion segment are disrupted and unable to hold a posterior spinal hook or pedicle screw, then the posterior construct should be extended one level beyond the fractured posterior elements. The posterolateral fusion does not need to include the uninjured spinal motion segment, and the instrumentation can be removed when the fusion is solid. Flexion-distraction injuries that involve the entire disk space may require a neutralization construct.[25,27] A posterior compression construct can significantly reduce the disk space height and promote retropulsion of disk material into the spinal canal.[15]

Lateral Distraction Injuries

Lateral distraction injuries are a variant of the lap-belt pattern.[28] Distraction occurs in the frontal plane. There is a unilateral opening of the disk space and subluxation of the facet joint. There is no sagittal plane translation. A posterior segmental compression montage on the side of the distraction injury can reduce the facet joint and realign the acute, angular scoliosis at the injured motion segment. These injuries are usually associated with life-threatening visceral injuries to the abdomen or thorax. Open reduction and fixation of the injuries facilitates the general care of the patient with multiple injuries. Lateral distraction injuries are also purely ligamentous and soft-tissue injuries and they are unlikely to heal without surgical intervention.

Burst Fractures

Burst fractures are caused by axial loading of all three columns of the spine.[14] The anterior and posterior cortices of the vertebral body are fractured. Secondary forces following the primary axial loading of the spine produce the

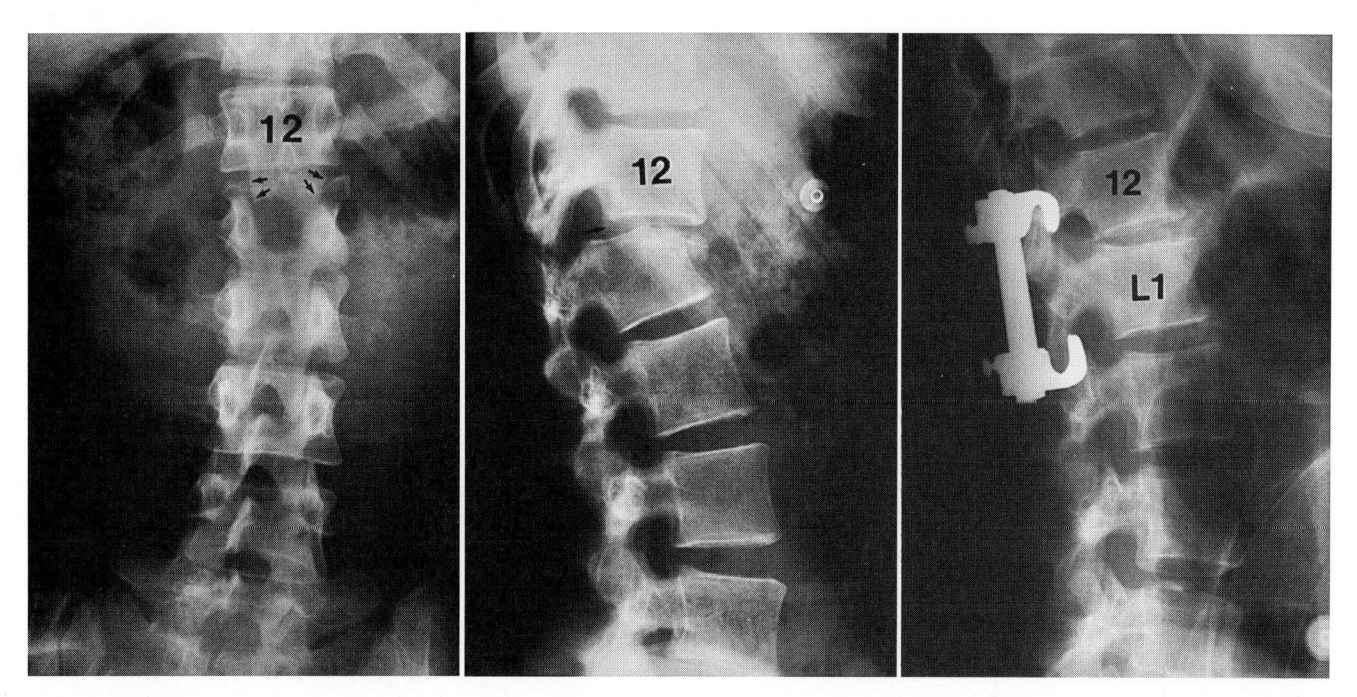

Fig. 3 **Left,** Anteroposterior radiograph at the thoracolumbar junction shows a lapbelt flexion-distraction injury. The posterior elements are not fractured; the interspinous process distance is significantly enlarged between the spinous processes of T12 and L1. Arrows show that the facets remain intact and are not dislocated. **Center,** Lateral radiograph of the thoracolumbar junction shows the facet joints perched in flexion. There is a mild compression injury to the anterior column but there is no significant sagittal plane translation (arrow). **Right,** Lateral radiograph shows a single-level compression montage holding the reduction and acting as a tension band.

various patterns of burst fractures: sagittal plane angulation (most commonly seen in Denis type B), frontal plane angulation (Denis type E), or rotation (Denis type D). In burst fractures, there is no sagittal plane translation of the vertebral bodies; the facet joints are widened but not dislocated.

Most burst fractures at the thoracolumbar junction can be treated nonsurgically.[3] Patients with a significant or progressive neurologic deficit require surgical stabilization and spinal canal decompression. In the neurologically intact patient, the fracture patterns that commonly require surgical intervention have loss of the anterior vertebral height of more than 50%, spinal canal compromise from retropulsed bony fracture fragments of more than 50%, and local kyphosis of 30° or more.

Posterior instrumentation can be used in burst fractures to clear the spinal canal, restore vertebral body height, correct angular deformity, and maintain normal sagittal alignment. Both distraction and angular deformity correction must be used to clear the spinal canal adequately and to restore normal spinal alignment.[29-31] Both rod-hook and pedicle screw constructs have been effectively used to treat burst fractures.[19,22,32-36] The intact anterior longitudinal ligament acts as a tension band and prevents overdistraction from posterior instrumentation. Posterior distraction can effectively restore vertebral body height and can partially clear the spinal canal. Distraction is the main force used to indirectly clear the retropulsed bone fragments from the spinal canal. Distraction indirectly and partially clears the spinal canal by tightening all of the ligamentous structures, including the posterior longitudinal ligament, the anterior longitudinal ligament, and the anulus fibrosis. However, distraction alone will not correct the sagittal angular deformity and will not completely clear the spinal canal. Constructs that produce distraction and lordosis are best at restoring the normal sagittal contours and providing maximal indirect clearance of the spinal canal.[29,31] Indirect techniques for fracture reduction most effectively clear the spinal canal of retropulsed bone fragments when the surgical reduction is performed within 48 hours after injury.

Rod-hook constructs apply distraction above and below the injured motion segment through the infralaminar and supralaminar hook placement on adjacent uninjured motion segments. The angular deformity is corrected by the rod exerting an anterior force on intact posterior spinal elements. This anteriorly directed force can be increased by using rod sleeve connectors[22] or by bending the rod in situ. Square-ended hooks or sublaminar wiring must be used in these constructs to prevent lateral displacement of the contoured rods. Intraspinal hooks and sublaminar wires should not be placed on the lamina adjacent to the area of spinal canal compromise from retropulsed bony fragments.

Long posterior instrumentation constructs that incorporate three levels above and below the injured motion segment have also been used.[37-39] The fusion is not extended the entire length of the instrumentation but rather incorporates only the injured motion segment and one level above and below. The distraction rod can be removed 12 to 24 months after the initial surgery. This "rod-long fuse-short" technique uses the longer lever arms of the distraction rods to apply an anteriorly directed force over multiple motion segments. This allows for an improved reduction of the sagittal plane angular deformity and decreases the force exerted by the distraction rod on the laminar hook sites. Clinical studies have shown no deleterious effects on the facet joints of the unfused motion segments at long-term follow-up. However, this technique does require an extended posterior dissection of the thoracolumbar spinal elements and requires that the patient undergo two separate surgical procedures.

Pedicle screw constructs have also been used in burst fractures.[9,23,32] In some patients, pedicle screw devices can enable the surgeon to instrument and limit the immobilization to only the motion segment above and below the fractured vertebra. The short-segment pedicle screw constructs allow the surgeon to exclude the uninvolved, normal spinal motion segments from incorporation into the fusion. This is especially important in the lumbar spine where hook placement in the lower lumbar spine is associated with late complications.[40] The sagittal angular deformity can be corrected by manipulation of the pedicle screws. Distraction across the injured motion segment can also be achieved through the pedicle screws. Some short-segment pedicle constructs have shown an early failure rate,[41] while others have produced good results.[9,32] Pedicle screws placed one level above and one level below the fractured vertebra do not restore the injured spinal segment to its normal stiffness in axial loading or in torsion. Using two screws above and two below increases the axial and torsional stiffness of the construct.[18]

Both pedicle screw and rod-hook systems have been shown to be effective in clearing the spinal canal and re-establishing vertebral body height.[33,34] Constructs incorporating pedicle screws at the caudal end and hooks in the cephalad portion have also been used. These constructs have the advantage of immobilizing fewer lumbar motion segments than dual rod-hook constructs. All posterior constructs used in the treatment of burst fractures show loss of sagittal angular correction over time. This loss of correction occurs whether or not the implants are removed and occurs in the presence of a solid posterior arthrodesis. This increase in kyphosis has not been found to lead to deteriora-

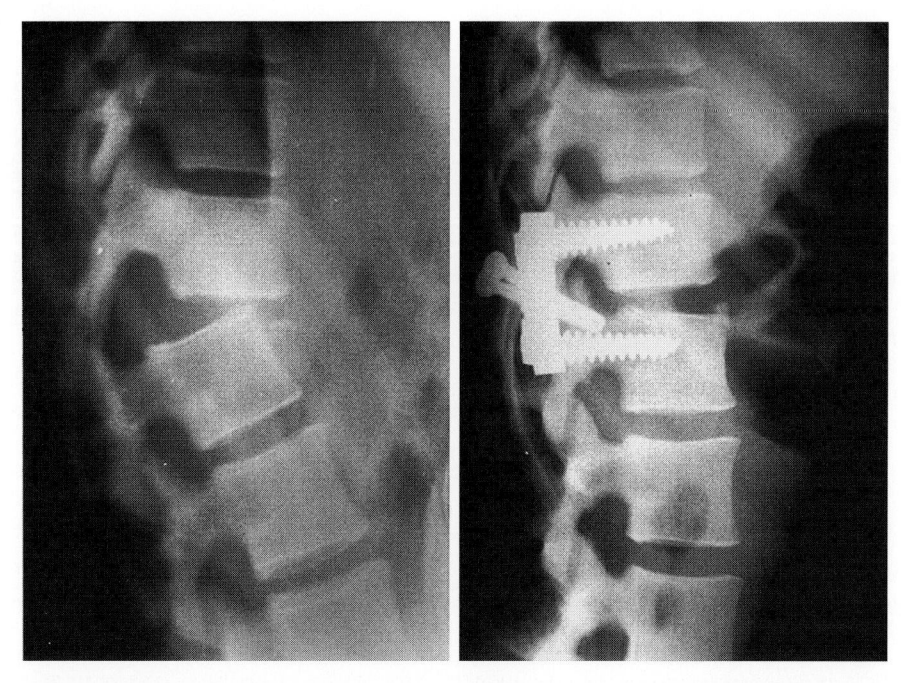

Fig. 4 Left, Lateral radiograph of the thoracolumbar junction shows a flexion-distraction fracture-dislocation. The facet joints are dislocated and there is significant sagittal plane translation of the vertebral bodies. **Right,** Postoperative lateral radiograph shows an anatomic reduction of the fracture-dislocation. A single-level pedicle screw construct supplemented with transarticular facet screws is used.

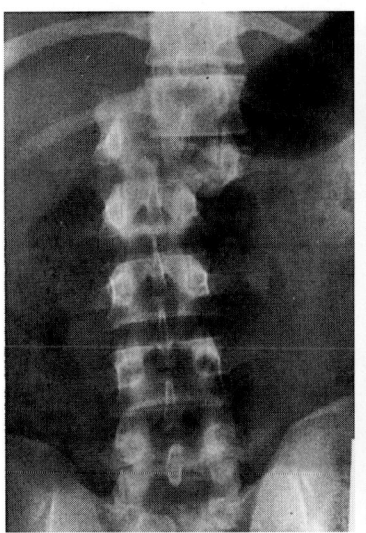

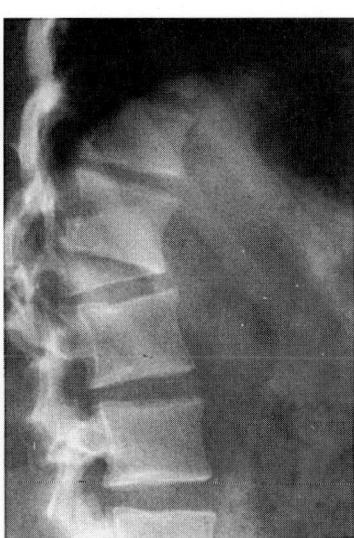

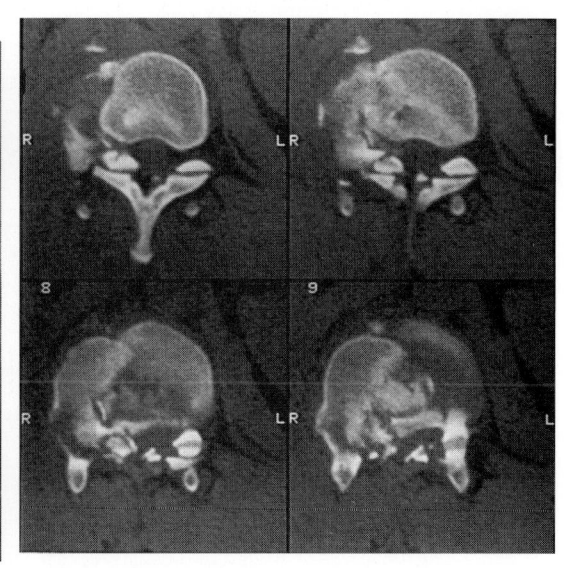

Fig. 5 **Left,** Anteroposterior radiograph at the thoracolumbar junction shows a flexion-rotation (slice fracture) fracture-dislocation. The facet joints are disrupted and there is significant lateral displacement of the spine. **Center,** Lateral radiograph shows loss of vertebral body height and no sagittal translation. **Right,** CT scan at the level of the injury shows comminution of the posterior spinal elements and severe compromise of the spinal canal.

tion of clinical results.[32,42] This loss of reduction is secondary to the failure of the posterior instrumentation to fully reconstruct the anterior and middle columns of the spine.

Posterior instrumentation is effective in re-establishing the spinal canal by indirect reduction of retropulsed bone fragments. For maximal neurologic recovery in patients with partial neurologic deficits, the spinal canal must be reconstituted to at least 75% of its original area. The local kyphosis at the fracture site must also be reduced to within 15° of the normal sagittal contour. If these goals are not achieved through ligamentotaxis, direct decompression of the spinal canal should be undertaken. Posterolateral decompression of the spinal canal can be completed after the insertion of posterior instrumentation.[43-45] An anterior decompression can also be performed after the posterior procedure.

A posterior decompression must be the initial surgical procedure if there is evidence of posterior entrapment of cauda equina rootlets in a laminar fracture.[46,47] The lamina fracture occurs in approximately half of burst fractures. The posterior dural laceration occurs in approximately 18% of burst fractures and cauda equina rootlet entrapment in the lamina fracture occurs in approximately 6% of burst fractures. Cauda equina entrapment occurs most commonly in lower lumbar burst fractures. The cauda equina elements should be extracted from the lamina fracture and the dural laceration must be repaired before any reduction maneuver is begun.

Fracture-Dislocations

Fracture-dislocations result from translational forces that disrupt the bony and ligamentous structures of the three columns of the spine.[14] Failure occurs from a combination of shear, rotational, tension, and axial compression forces. The three major injury patterns are flexion-distraction, flexion-rotation (slice fracture), and shear (anterior-to-posterior and posterior-to-anterior).

The flexion-distraction fracture-dislocation is similar in appearance to the lap-belt injury. In the fracture-dislocation pattern, the facet joints are entirely dislocated and there is usually some sagittal plane translation of the vertebral bodies. The anterior longitudinal ligament is often intact but is stripped off the vertebral body. If the articular processes are not fractured and if the spine can be reduced anatomically, a short, pedicle screw montage can be used for fixation (Fig. 4). However, if the posterior arch is comminuted, then a longer, multilevel compression construct should be used.

In flexion-rotation injuries, the posterior and middle columns fail under a combination of compression and rotation. The rotational component of the injury forces occasionally ruptures the anterior longitudinal ligament. There usually is displacement of the spine in both the sagittal and frontal planes (Fig. 5, *left* and *center*). The spinal canal is compromised not from retropulsed bony fracture fragments but rather from the translational displacement of the spinal column (Fig. 5, *right*).

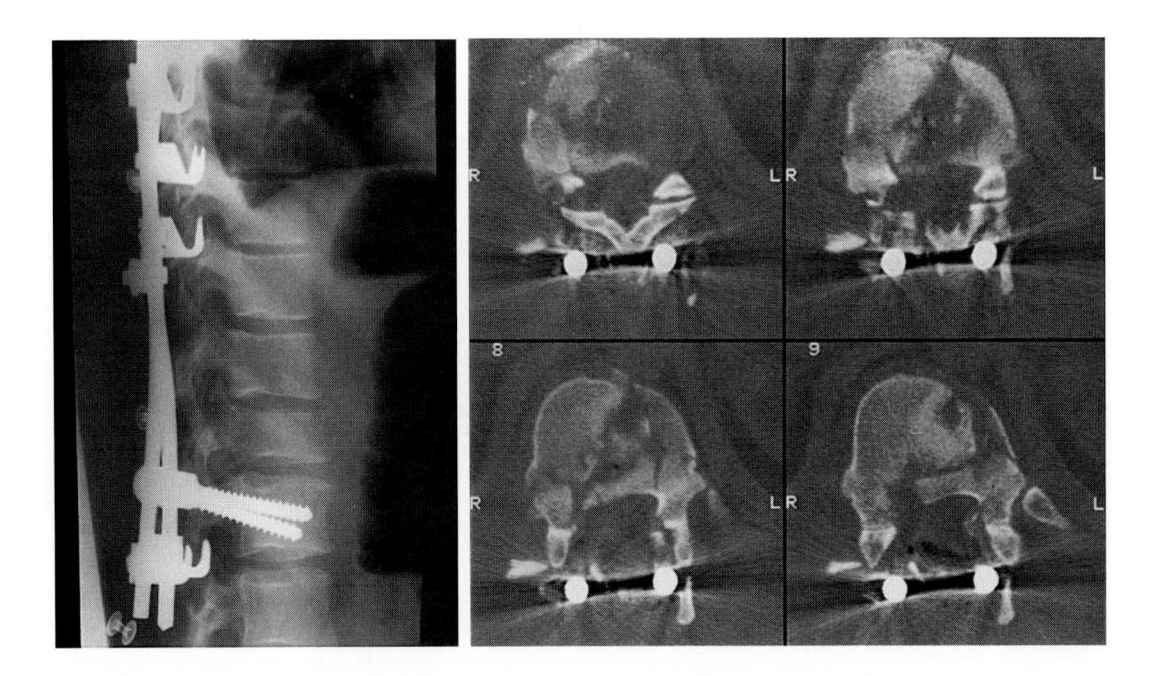

Fig. 6 **Left,** Postoperative lateral radiograph of patient shown in Figure 5 shows the reconstitution of the vertebral body height with no overdistraction. A multilevel rod-hook and pedicle screw montage was used to re-establish the vertebral body height but prevent overdistraction. **Right,** Postoperative CT scan of patient shown in Figure 5 shows reconstitution of the spinal canal by realignment of the spine in the frontal and sagittal plane.

In the shear fracture-dislocation patterns, all three spinal columns are disrupted as well as the anterior longitudinal ligament.[48] In these fracture patterns, the spine is translated in the sagittal plane without wedging or comminution of the vertebral bodies. Often, there are multiple fractures of the posterior elements. Again, the spinal canal is compromised primarily by the displacement of the spinal column.

The flexion-rotation and shear fracture-dislocations require multilevel segmental fixation that neutralizes flexion, extension, and rotational forces.[10,20,49] In these fracture patterns, the anterior longitudinal ligament is often disrupted and cannot be relied on to aid in the reduction of the fracture or to prevent overdistraction of the spine (Fig. 6).

At the time of this writing, bone screws placed posteriorly into vertebral elements have not been cleared for general use in this specific manner by the Food and Drug Administration (FDA). These are Class III devices. This category includes screws placed transfacetally, within pedicles, or in articular, lateral masses. Some screws have been approved for use within the sacrum as Class II devices. Some companies have received Class II clearance for use of screws in lumbar pedicles specifically to supplement fusions in the treatment of grade III and IV spondylolisthesis with the proviso that these devices are removed after the arthrodesis has healed. Anterior vertebral body screws (cervical, thoracic, and lumbar) are Class II devices and can be used as labeled in vertebral bodies. Many of the posterior screw-based devices have been shown in laboratory and clinical testing to be useful and can be used in an off-label manner if the physician feels this is appropriate and important for the treatment of the patient. As with all surgeries, informed consent should explain the procedure and why a particular technique has been chosen, as well as its risks and benefits. The question of whether informed consent regarding pedicle screws must include a discussion of the device's FDA clearance status is currently being litigated in several jurisdictions.

References

1. Davies WE, Morris JH, Hill V: An analysis of conservative (non-surgical) management of thoracolumbar fractures and fracture-dislocations with neural damage. *J Bone Joint Surg* 1980;62A:1324–1328.
2. Frankel HL, Hancock DO, Hyslop G, et al: The value of postural reduction in the initial management of closed injuries of the spine with paraplegia and tetraplegia: Part I. *Paraplegia* 1969;7:179–192.
3. Weinstein JN, Collalto P, Lehmann TR: Thoracolumbar "burst" fractures treated conservatively: A long-term follow-up. *Spine* 1988;13:33–38.
4. Jacobs RR, Asher MA, Snider RK: Thoracolumbar spinal injuries: A comparative study of recumbent and operative treatment in 100 patients. *Spine* 1980;5:463–477.
5. Knight RQ, Stornelli DP, Chan DP, et al: Comparison of operative versus nonoperative treatment of lumbar burst fractures. *Clin Orthop* 1993;293:112–121.
6. Willen J, Lindahl S, Nordwall A: Unstable thoracolumbar fractures: A comparative clinical study of conservative treatment and Harrington instrumentation. *Spine* 1985;10:111–122.
7. Bradford DS, McBride GG: Surgical management of thoracolumbar spine fractures with incomplete neurologic deficits. *Clin Orthop* 1987;218:201–216.
8. Dall BE, Stauffer ES: Neurologic injury and recovery patterns in burst fractures at the T12 or L1 motion segment. *Clin Orthop* 1988;233:171–176.
9. Esses SI, Botsford DJ, Kostuik JP: Evaluation of surgical treatment for burst fractures. *Spine* 1990;15:667–673.
10. Hu SS, Capen DA, Rimoldi RL, et al: The effect of surgical decompression on neurologic outcome after lumbar fractures. *Clin Orthop* 1993;288:166–173.
11. Ferguson RL, Tencer AF, Woodard P, et al: Biomechanical comparisons of spinal fracture models and the stabilizing effects of posterior instrumentations. *Spine* 1988;13:453–460.
12. Ashman RB, Galpin RD, Corin JD, et al: Biomechanical analysis of pedicle screw instrumentation systems in a corpectomy model. *Spine* 1989;14:1398–1405.
13. Mann KA, McGowan DP, Fredrickson BE, et al: A biomechanical investigation of short segment spinal fixation for burst fractures with varying degrees of posterior disruption. *Spine* 1990;15:470–478.
14. Denis F: The three column spine and its significance in the classification of acute thoracolumbar spinal injuries. *Spine* 1983;8:817–831.
15. Heller JG, Garfin SR, Abitbol JJ: Disk herniation associated with compression instrumentation of lumbar flexion-distraction injuries. *Clin Orthop* 1992;284:91–98.
16. Gurr KR, McAfee PC, Shih CM: Biomechanical analysis of posterior instrumentation systems after decompressive laminectomy: An unstable calf-spine model. *J Bone Joint Surg* 1988;70A:680–691.
17. Gurwitz GS, Dawson JM, McNamara MJ, et al: Biomechanical analysis of three surgical approaches for lumbar burst fractures using short-segment instrumentation. *Spine* 1993;18:977–982.
18. Gurr KR, McAfee PC, Shih CM: Biomechanical analysis of anterior and posterior instrumentation systems after corpectomy: A calf-spine model. *J Bone Joint Surg* 1988;70A:1182–1191.
19. Bryant CE, Sullivan JA: Management of thoracic and lumbar spine fractures with Harrington distraction rods supplemented with segmental wiring. *Spine* 1983;8:532–537.
20. Phillips DL, Brick GW, Spengler DM: A comparison of Harrington rod fixation with and without segmental wires for unstable thoracolumbar injuries. *J Spinal Disord* 1988;1:151–161.
21. McAfee PC, Werner FW, Glisson RR: A biomechanical analysis of spinal instrumentation systems in thoracolumbar fractures: Comparison of traditional Harrington distraction instrumentation with segmental spinal instrumentation. *Spine* 1985;10:204–217.
22. Edwards CC, Levine AM: Early rod-sleeve stabilization of the injured thoracic and lumbar spine. *Orthop Clin North Am* 1986;17:121–145.
23. Lindsey RW, Dick W, Nunchuck S, et al: Residual intersegmental spinal mobility following limited pedicle fixation of thoracolumbar spine fractures with the fixateur interne. *Spine* 1993;18:474–478.
24. Daniaux H, Seykora P, Genelin A, et al: Application of posterior plating and modifications in thoracolumbar spine injuries: Indications, techniques, and results. *Spine* 1991;16:S125–S133.
25. Anderson PA, Henley MB, Rivara FP, et al: Flexion distraction and chance injuries to the thoracolumbar spine. *J Orthop Trauma* 1991;5:153–160.
26. Gertzbein SD, Court-Brown CM: Rationale for the management of flexion-distraction injuries of the thoracolumbar spine based on a new classification. *J Spinal Disord* 1989;2:176–183.
27. Levine AM, Bosse M, Edwards CC: Bilateral facet dislocations in the thoracolumbar spine. *Spine* 1988;13:630–640.
28. Denis F, Burkus JK: Lateral distraction injuries to the thoracic and lumbar spine: A report of three cases. *J Bone Joint Surg* 1991;73A:1049–1053.
29. Fredrickson BE, Edwards WT, Rauschning W, et al: Vertebral burst fractures: An experimental, morphologic, and radiographic study. *Spine* 1992;17:1012–1021.
30. Harrington RM, Budorick T, Hoyt T, et al: Biomechanics of indirect reduction of bone retropulsed into the spinal canal in vertebral fracture. *Spine* 1993;18:692–699.
31. Zou D, Yoo JU, Edwards WT, et al: Mechanics of anatomic reduction of thoracolumbar burst fractures: Comparison of distraction versus distraction plus lordosis, in the anatomic reduction of the thoracolumbar burst fracture. *Spine* 1993;18:195–203.

32. Benson DR, Burkus JK, Montesano PX, et al: Unstable thoracolumbar and lumbar burst fractures treated with the AO fixateur interne. *J Spinal Disord* 1992;5:335–343.

33. Crutcher JP Jr, Anderson PA, King HA, et al: Indirect spinal canal decompression in patients with thoracolumbar burst fractures treated by posterior distraction rods. *J Spinal Disord* 1991;4:39–48.

34. Doerr TE, Montesano PX, Burkus JK, et al: Spinal canal decompression in traumatic thoracolumbar burst fractures: Posterior distraction rods versus transpedicular screw fixation. *J Orthop Trauma* 1991;5:403–411.

35. Gertzbein SD, Jacobs RR, Stoll J, et al: Results of a locking-hook spinal rod for fractures of the thoracic and lumbar spine. *Spine* 1990;15:275–280.

36. Stephens GC, Devito DP, McNamara MJ: Segmental fixation of lumbar burst fractures with Cotrel-Dubousset instrumentation. *J Spinal Disord* 1992;5:344–348.

37. Akbarina BA, Crandall DG, Burkus JK, et al: Use of long rods and a short arthrodesis for burst fractures of the thoracolumbar spine: A long-term follow-up study. *J Bone Joint Surg* 1994;76A:1629–1635.

38. Dekutoski MB, Conlan ES, Salciccioli GG: Spinal mobility and deformity after Harrington rod stabilization and limited arthrodesis of thoracolumbar fractures. *J Bone Joint Surg* 1993;75A:168–176.

39. Gardner VO, Armstrong GW: Long-term lumbar facet joint changes in spinal fracture patients treated with Harrington rods. *Spine* 1990;15:479–484.

40. Hales DD, Dawson EG, Delamarter R: Late neurological complications of Harrington instrumentation. *J Bone Joint Surg* 1989;71A:1053–1057.

41. McLain RF, Sparling E, Benson DR: Early failure of short-segment pedicle instrumentation for thoracolumbar fractures: A preliminary report. *J Bone Joint Surg* 1993;75A:162–167.

42. Myllynen P, Bostman O, Riska E: Recurrence of deformity after removal of Harrington's fixation of spine fracture: Seventy-six cases followed for 2 years. *Acta Orthop Scand* 1988;59:497–502.

43. Garfin SR, Mowery CA, Guerra J, et al: Confirmation of the posterolateral technique to decompress and fuse thoracolumbar spine burst fractures. *Spine* 1985;10:218–223.

44. Hardaker WT Jr, Cook WA Jr, Friedman AH, et al: Bilateral transpedicular decompression and Harrington rod stabilization in the management of severe thoracolumbar burst fractures. *Spine* 1992;17:162–171.

45. Vincent KA, Benson DR, McGahan JP: Intraoperative ultrasonography for reduction of thoracolumbar burst fractures. *Spine* 1989;14:387–390.

46. Camissa FP Jr, Eismont FJ, Green BA: Dural laceration occurring with burst fractures and associated laminar fractures. *J Bone Joint Surg* 1989;71A:1044–1052.

47. Denis F, Burkus JK: Diagnosis and treatment of cauda equina entrapment in the vertical lamina fracture of lumbar burst fractures. *Spine* 1991;16:S433–S439.

48. Denis F, Burkus JK: Shear fracture-dislocations of the thoracic and lumbar spine associated with forceful hyperextension (lumberjack paraplegia). *Spine* 1992;17:156–161.

49. Sasso RC, Cotler HB: Posterior instrumentation and fusion for unstable fractures and fracture-dislocations of the thoracic and lumbar spine: A comparative study of three fixation devices in seventy patients. *Spine* 1993;18:450–460.

41

Anterior Thoracolumbar Instrumentation for Burst Fracture

Introduction

The anterolateral approach to the thoracolumbar spine, first described by Hodgson and Stock, was a retroperitoneal muscle-splitting approach. The procedure was developed primarily to drain tuberculous abscesses. In the 1950s, the anterior approach began to be used for anterior fusion in the treatment of scoliosis. Capener advocated anterior disk space fusion of the scoliotic curve. In 1953, Wenger described an anterior distraction device to help reduce scoliotic deformity. Dwyer, Hall, and Zielke each developed anterior instrumentation devices for correcting scoliosis. These fixation devices generally included a single vertebral body screw placed laterally, connected by a flexible cable or threaded rod, which could then be compressed to help reduce the convexity of the scoliotic curve. This fixation was not rigid, but was primarily a device used for reduction.

In 1985, Bohlman developed the retroperitoneal approach to the thoracolumbar spine for the decompression of malunited burst fractures. These fractures were primarily treated late, after healing with a kyphotic malunion. McAfee and associates[1] noted substantial neurologic recovery with late anterior decompression. Anterior strut grafting alone, however, cannot stabilize an acutely fractured spine that has posterior column disruption. When anterior fusion is performed without instrumentation, the reported nonunion rate ranges from 18% to 40%, but averages 10% to 20%. Because of this, several surgeons have begun to recommend a two-stage surgical procedure. Typically, this procedure entails use of posterior instrumentation with distraction followed by intraoperative studies, such as myelography or ultrasonography, to assess canal clearance. If compression of the canal persists, an anterior or posterolateral decompression is carried out.

To reduce the morbidity of a two-stage operation, anterior instrumentation after anterior decompression has been advocated as a single-stage procedure. Initial anterior instrumentation systems consisted of those previously used for scoliosis surgery. However, single vertebral body screws connected by cables or threaded rods are not rigid enough to provide adequate fixation following trauma. Fixation systems using two points of fixation to each vertebral body were independently developed by Dunn,[2] Kaneda, and Kostuik. An anterior fixation device designed by Dunn initially had excellent results in both the reduction and fixation of thoracolumbar burst fractures. This device was applied in the anterior/anterolateral spine using a screw and staple for fixation. Although this device was eventually withdrawn because of late vascular injuries, other surgeons were more successful with the use of anterior thoracolumbar devices. Rigid low-profile devices that do not interfere with magnetic resonance imaging (MRI) have been developed and have profoundly improved the results of anterior fixation for burst fractures of the thoracolumbar spine.

Basic Research

Few animal studies have focused on the efficacy of anterior fixation followed by corpectomy. In one study of a dog model of burst fractures treated by anterior corpectomy, the authors concluded that, in the unstable spine, anterior bone grafting alone led to a high rate of nonunion and less mechanical rigidity than anterior grafting plus instrumentation.

A number of studies have been conducted using benchtop testing to determine the initial stability of anterior thoracolumbar fixation devices.[2] The biomechanical stiffness of spinal constructs has been tested using simulated spine injuries.[3] Although anterior vertebral body plates were tested, the report did not show their effectiveness. In a study comparing the mechanical stiffness of the Kaneda device construct with traditional posterior spinal constructs in a calf spine model, the authors found that posterior pedicle screw systems spanning five levels gave equivalent stability as the Kaneda device spanning three levels.[5] In a study in which four anterior fixation systems were tested (the Slot-Zielke, the Kostuik-Harrington, the ASIF T-Plate, and the broad compression plate), the authors found that the broad dynamic compression plate was stiffer in axial load and torsion than the other systems tested.[6] In particular, the Kostuik-Harrington system was found to be less stiff in torsion.

In a comparison of an anterior Kaneda-type device with posterior Harrington compression rods and a transpedicular

Table 1. Comparison of the advantages of anterior and posterior burst fracture fixation

Relative Advantages	Anterior Approach	Posterior Approach
Short segment fixation	X	
Ease of approach		X
Immediate stability	X	
Prevents kyphotic settling	X	
Direct neurologic decompression	X	
Rigidity in 3-column injury		X
Hardware prominence	X	

external fixator, the external fixator was found to be superior in returning spinal stability in flexion-extension and rotation (Table 1).[7] The Kaneda device, although performing well in flexion and extension, was not believed to be as stable in rotation. This device did not include crosslink bars. However, in another study, the biomechanical stiffness of the Kaneda device, the Kostuik-Harrington device, the TSRH vertebral body screw construct, and the Armstrong contoured anterior spinal plate (CASP) in a calf spine model were compared under torsion, flexion-extension, and axial compression.[8] In torsion, the Kostuik-Harrington device was unstable, while the Kaneda device was most rigid. In axial loading and flexion, the Kaneda device and the Texas Scottish Rite Hospital (TSRH) construct were the stiffest. The authors concluded that the TSRH anterior vertebral body screw construct or the Kaneda device were most effective in restoring the acute stability to the lumbar spine after corpectomy.

In comparing posterior VSP pedicle screw plates with anterior Kaneda device plus strut graft, the latter system was found to be stiffer than the intact spine in axial load and both systems were equally stiff in torsion.[9]

When properly applied, rigid anterior instrumentation is as rigid as, or more rigid than, posterior pedicle screw instrumentation. Anterior instrumentation spans only one level above and below the injured vertebra and allows single-stage complete canal decompression and stabilization.

Classification of Devices

The devices that have been used for anterior fixation after acute burst fracture include simple bone plates, rigid and semi-rigid rod/screw combinations, and advanced locking plate designs. Simple bone plates applied to the lateral thoracic or lumbar spine are low-profile devices with the ability to perform only in situ fixation. They are not considered to be rigid devices because there is no constraint between the screw and the plate. These devices are best used for in situ fixation in cases of tumor reconstruction.

Fixation devices in which two screws within each vertebral body are connected by rods provide more rigid fixation. Dunn[2] designed one of the initial anterior fixation devices using collars and interconnecting rods. However, his device had a high profile anteriorly and was eventually withdrawn because of late vascular injury. Kostuik[10] used a combination of Harrington screws, compression rods, and distraction rods in designing a fixation system with two screws within each vertebral body connected by two rods. This device had no cross-link member between the rods. Early clinical results were excellent; of 80 sequential patients treated with single-stage anterior decompression, bone grafting, and stabilization using the Kostuik-Harrington device, excellent neurologic recovery was noted in those patients with incomplete neurologic deficit and the nonunion rate was only 4%, although 16% had some type of hardware failure.

Kaneda and associates[11] have developed an anterior fixation device that employs vertebral body staples and screws connected by two threaded longitudinal rods that are cross-linked. In the first 100 cases in the United States, 96% of patients have had some neurologic recovery and the nonunion rate is 6%. More importantly, no vascular or neurologic complications have occurred with this device. In further follow-up, Kaneda has reported on long-term results in more than 500 cases that show a high success rate in terms of neurologic recovery, solid arthrodesis, and lack of hardware failure.

Recent reports of early results using the TSRH screw and rod system as an anterior fixation device following corpectomy have shown low rates of hardware failure, high fusion rates, and excellent neurologic recovery.[12,13] Finally, dynamic and rigid plate devices have been developed that provide a low-profile, MRI compatibility, rigid fixation, and the ability to compress and distract. These devices have had excellent early clinical results.

Other less rigid devices have not fared as well. In a review of the first 62 patients treated with the Slot-Zielke device, of those patients who had only anterior decompression and stabilization with this device, 41% lost reduction of more than 5°.[14] With additional posterior instrumentation, only 3% of patients lost reduction. This is in comparison to a recent survivorship analysis of 21 burst fracture patients treated with posterior VSP implants and fusion.[15] In those patients, if anterior bone graft augmentation was performed, 100% of the implants survived through 22 months. Without anterior augmentation only 50% of the posteriorly instrumented patients had instrument survival. This correlates with more recent data by Gaines and associates,[16] showing that in those cases with severe vertebral body comminution or spreading of the fragments, posterior instrumentation alone will lead to a high incidence of implant failure.

Neurologic Recovery

The primary indication for combined anterior decompression and instrumentation remains neurologic deficit. Although authors have been able to perform canal decompression via a transpedicular or posterolateral approach, direct anterior decompression certainly ensures the most complete canal clearance. In one study that compared 20 patients treated by anterior decompression and stabilization with 39 patients treated by posterior decompression and stabilization, the neurologic recovery rate was greater for those with anterior surgery (88% versus 64%) and inferior results correlated with residual bony canal stenosis identified without using postoperative computed tomography scans.[17]

In a study that compared the rates of neurologic recovery in those patients who underwent a formal vertebrectomy for decompression with those patients who had indirect reduction via posterior instrumentation using the American Spinal Injury Association motor index score, the authors found an average improvement in the motor index of 9.9 points was found in those patients undergoing vertebrectomy, compared to only 4.2 points of improvement in those patients having fusion without formal decompression.[18] This difference was significant. This information has been further refined in a study in which it was found that in patients who underwent anterior decompression and stabilization for burst fractures with neurologic deficit, those patients having early decompression, ie, within 48 hours of injury, had a significantly better rate of neurologic recovery than those patients having late decompression.[19]

Clinical Indications

Anterior decompression and stabilization does play a significant role in the treatment of thoracolumbar burst fractures. For those fractures without neurologic deficit and with mild deformity, postural reduction followed by bed rest and casting is still indicated. Those patients with less than 20° of local kyphosis and less than 50% canal compromise generally can be adequately treated in this manner. With greater degrees of deformity but without neurologic deficit, posterior reduction and stabilization with fusion is the treatment of choice. In burst fractures in the proximal thoracolumbar spine, stabilization is best performed with either rod and hook devices or pedicle screw and rod devices. In the mid to lower lumbar spine, pedicle screw fixation of one level above and below the fracture is indicated. With severe comminution or spreading of the burst fragments, posterior pedicle screw fixation devices may fail, and anterior load sharing is recommended. This can be obtained with either anterior strut grafting or instrumentation.

There is no absolute indication for anterior instrumentation after burst fracture. However, there are several excellent indications for surgery. In those patients with neurologic deficit from a thoracolumbar burst fracture, anterior decompression and stabilization may be indicated. This recommendation is based on the higher degree of neurologic recovery following anterior decompression, the restoration of the height of the anterior and middle columns possible with the anterior approach, and the lower incidence of late collapse and settling with restoration of the anterior and middle columns.

If nonsurgical treatment is chosen initially, a plateau in neurologic recovery would be a relative indication for then proceeding with anterior decompression and stabilization. A plateau in neurologic recovery or a loss of neurologic status following posterior stabilization would also be an indication for anterior treatment. Other relative indications include marked comminution of burst fracture fragments, involvement of both the superior and inferior endplate of the burst fracture fragments, open wounds of the posterior skin, and extremely thin patients with predicted prominence of posterior hardware.

Complications

It is necessary to prevent any contact of an anterolateral fixation system with the great vessels. Reports following the extensive use of the Dunn device included six cases of late aortic rupture from vascular erosion. All currently available systems are placed laterally and not on the anterior aspect of the spine. Prolonged bleeding from anterior exposure, great vessel injury, and pulmonary insufficiency are all potential complications from anterior instrumentation. The expected hardware failure rate and nonunion rate should be low if proper grafting and instrumentation technique is utilized. Should graft or hardware failure occur, salvage surgery with posterior instrumentation may be necessary. Postoperative bracing should be used following anterior instrumentation. Without postoperative bracing for 10 to 12 weeks, some settling and recurrence of kyphosis may occur.

Single-stage anterior decompression and stabilization requires that the most rigid system be used. However, there are numerous perceived difficulties of the current anterolateral fixation devices. Although the Kaneda device and the anterior TSRH system were rigid under biomechanical testing, both are high-profile systems with difficult insertion of the rods and cross-link. In addition, both devices are stainless steel, which makes postoperative imaging difficult. In those cases of fracture, imaging for postoperative syringomyelia is best achieved with MRI, which is precluded by the use of a stainless steel fixation device. For patients with tumor decompressions, following the tumor with either computed tomography or MRI is difficult with these stainless steel devices. Although plate devices such as the contoured anterior spinal plate or the Yuan plate are low profile and easier to insert, they have shortcomings as well. With either plate device, the device cannot be used to reduce the kyphotic deformity, that is, for distraction. In addition, once the device is placed, placing compression across the bone graft further increases the stability that can be achieved. Neither of these plate devices allows bone graft compression. Newer designs, such as the Z plate and the University plate, solve some of these design shortcomings.

Contraindications for the use of primary anterior instrumentation for spine fractures include significant chest trauma, flexion distraction injuries, fracture dislocations of the spine, and L4 or L5 burst fractures. Because primary anterior fixation to either L5 or the sacrum is difficult, the treatment of low lumbar burst fractures is a relative contraindication.

Summary

There is a role for anterior decompression and stabilization for thoracolumbar burst fractures. The best surgical indications are for patients who have significant burst fractures with neurologic deficit and canal compromise and for those who have marked comminution and displacement of the burst fracture fragments. In these patients an improved neurologic recovery and a lower spine implant failure rate can be expected if anterior decompression and load sharing with strut grafting and instrumentation is carried out.

Annotated References

1. McAfee PC, Bohlman HH, Yuan HA: Anterior decompression of traumatic thoracolumbar fractures with incomplete neurologic deficit using a retro-peritoneal approach. *J Bone Joint Surg* 1985;67A:89–104.

2. Dunn HK: Anterior stabilization of thoracolumbar injuries. *Clin Orthop* 1984;189:116–124.

3. Zdeblick TA, Shirado O, McAfee PC, et al: Anterior spinal fixation after corpectomy: A study in dogs. *J Bone Joint Surg* 1991;73A:527–534.

    The authors created a dog model of burst fracture treated by anterior corpectomy. They performed anterior corpectomy and spacer application in seven dogs, anterior corpectomy followed by anterior arthrodesis with an ulnar strut in seven dogs, and an ulnar strut plus an anterior Kaneda-type instrumentation in seven dogs. They analyzed the rate of fusion, biomechanical rigidity, neuropathologic findings, and histomorphometric data and found that the rate of fusion was significantly higher in the group having anterior instrumentation. In addition, the spines with instrumentation were stiffer in torsion than spines that were not instrumented. Minimal device-related osteopenia occurred in spines treated with the anterior fixation device.

4. Jacobs RR, Nordwall A, Nachemson A: Reduction, stability, and strength provided by internal fixation systems for thoracolumbar spinal injuries. *Clin Orthop* 1982;171:300–308.

5. Gurr KR, McAfee PC, Shih CM: Biomechanical analysis of anterior and posterior instrumentation systems after corpectomy: A calf-spine model. *J Bone Joint Surg* 1988;70A:1182–1191.

6. Ashman RB, Bechtold JE, Edwards WT, et al: In-vitro spinal arthrodesis implant mechanical testing protocols. *J Spinal Disord* 1989;2:274–481.

7. Abumi K, Panjabi MM, Duranceau J: Biomechanical evaluation of spinal fixation devices: Part III. Stability provided by six spinal fixation devices and interbody bone graft. *Spine* 1989;14:1249–1255.

8. Zdeblick TA, Warden KE, Zou D, et al: Anterior spinal fixators: A biomechanical in-vitro study. *Spine* 1993;18:513–517.

9. Gurwitz GS, Dawson JM, McNamara MJ, et al: Biomechanical analysis of three surgical approaches for lumbar burst fractures using short-segment instrumentation. *Spine* 1993;15:18:977–982.

10. Kostuik JP: Anterior spinal cord decompression for lesions of the thoracic and lumbar spine, techniques, new methods of internal fixation results. *Spine* 1983;8:512–531.

11. Kaneda K, Abumi K, Fujiya M: Burst fractures with neurologic deficits of the thoracolumbar spine: Results of anterior decompression and stabilization with anterior instrumentation. *Spine* 1984;9:788–795.

12. Heller JG, Zdeblick TA, King DA, et al: Spinal instrumentation for metastatic disease: In vitro biomechanical analysis. *J Spinal Disorders* 1993;6:17–22.

13. Lowry GL, Zdeblick TA, O'Leary PF, et al: Titanium mesh for vertebral body defects. Presented at the 28th Annual Meeting of the Scoliosis Research Society, Dublin, Ireland. 1993;9:18–23.

14. Been HD: Anterior decompression and stabilization of thoracolumbar burst fractures using the Slot-Zielke-device. *Acta Orthop Belg* 1991;57(suppl 1):144–161.

15. Ebelke DK, Asher MA, Neff JR, et al: Survivorship analysis of VSP spine instrumentation in the treatment of thoracolumbar and lumbar burst fractures. *Spine* 1991;16(suppl 8):S428–S432.

16. Gaines RW, Holt B, McCormack T: A classification to predict screw breakage when using short segment instrumentation. Presented at the 28th Annual Meeting of the Scoliosis Research Society, Dublin, Ireland. 1993;9:18–23.

17. Bradford DS, McBride GG: Surgical management of thoracolumbar spine fractures with incomplete neurologic deficits. *Clin Orthop* 1987;218:201–216.

18. Hu SS, Capen DA, Rimaldi RL, et al: The effect of surgical decompression on neurologic outcome after lumbar fractures. *Clin Orthop* 1993;288:166–173.

19. Clohisy JC, Akbarnia BA, Bucholz RD, et al: Neurologic recovery associated with anterior decompression of spine fractures at the thoracolumbar junction (T12-L1). *Spine* 1992;17(suppl 8):S325–S330.

42
Sacral Fractures

Introduction

The sacrum forms the caudad continuation of the lumbar spine and serves as the anchoring structure of the posterior pelvic ring. The sacrum is firmly connected to the surrounding bony structures by strong ligaments, such as the iliolumbar, sacroiliac, sacrospinal, and sacrotuberal ligaments. Because of the strength of these surrounding structures, significant energy is required to injure the sacrum. Usual injury mechanisms include motor vehicle accidents, falls from heights, and crush injuries. Pathologic bone conditions such as those found in severe osteoporosis, rheumatologic conditions, or neoplasia may lead to spontaneous fractures of the sacrum. Sacral fractures have been found in 17% to 85% of pelvic fractures[1,2] and are reported to be missed in 50% of patients with neurologic damage and in 70% of patients without neurologic deficits.[3] A systematic approach to the assessment, classification, and treatment of sacral injuries is necessary to minimize the occurrence of bladder, bowel, and sexual dysfunction, neurologic impairment of the lower extremities, and chronic pain.

Assessment

As for all patients with a significant injury mechanism, taking a history and performing a thorough physical examination are the first management steps. Clinical assessment aimed at identifying areas of tenderness, swelling, and bruising in the lower torso, the perineum, and the dorsum is followed by examination of the stability of the pelvic ring. Patients with known disruption of the pelvic ring require aggressive resuscitation and close monitoring because of the inherent risk of catastrophic bleeding from this area. Mortality rates of up to 50% persist for some types of pelvic ring disruptions despite best treatment efforts. Application and inflation of military antishock trousers or emergency placement of a pelvic clamp or anterior external fixation device have been recommended for the initial management of patients with severe pelvic disruption and hypotension. For patients with persistent hypotension despite external stabilization of the pelvic ring, embolization of arterial bleeders has been recommended. The urogenital tract should be assessed for injury in the emergency room. Occult open fractures of the pelvic ring should be looked for by performing vaginal and rectal examinations. Neurologic evaluation of the injured patient with pelvic disruption should include examination of the lumbar and sacral plexus. Lower sacral root function is evaluated by the quality of anal sphincter tone and the presence of voluntary contraction, the bulbocavernosus reflex, and perianal sensation. The cause of bladder dysfunction may be difficult to differentiate in cases of concomitant anterior pelvic disruptions and sacral fractures, because anterior pelvic disruptions are frequently associated with bladder and urethral injuries.[4-7]

In polytrauma patients an anteroposterior (AP) radiograph of the pelvis is recommended during the initial assessment. Injuries to the sacrum may be obscured on the AP pelvic radiograph because of the 45° posterior inclination of the upper sacrum relative to the frontal plane and because of overriding soft tissue and bowel gas shadows. Subtle radiographic signs of possibly significant pelvic ring or lumbosacral injuries include lumbar transverse process fractures, displaced anterior pelvic ring fractures without an obvious posterior pelvic ring fracture, disruption of the arcuate lines of the sacral foramina, or asymmetry of the sacral foramina or sciatic notch. A Ferguson AP radiograph obtained at a 30° cranial projection angle shows the upper sacrum but not the lower sacrum. Pelvic inlet and outlet views are helpful in identifying sacral ala fractures, shortening of the sacrum, and any AP displacement of one hemipelvis in relation to the other. A lateral view of the pelvis can help to identify transverse fracture patterns of the sacrum and obstruction or malangulation of the sacral spinal canal but is limited by the overriding posterior iliac wing. Computed tomography (CT) has become the standard of care in the assessment of suspected posterior pelvic injuries.[8] In cases of complex sacral fractures, sacral CT scans with narrow sections and gantry angles corrected to remain perpendicular to the sacral inclination angle are recommended. This technique also allows sagittal or coronal reconstructions, which can further enhance understanding of the fracture. Myelography and postmyelography CT play limited roles in the evaluation of sacral fractures because the dura ends above where the majority of injuries occur. Magnetic resonance imaging (MRI) can be used to visualize the cauda equina and sacral roots; however, its clinical role in the treatment of sacral fractures remains to be established. Bone scintigraphy with technetium is useful for identifying occult

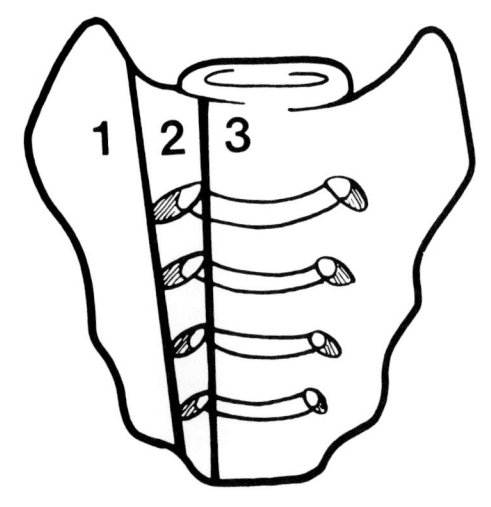

Fig. 1 Classification of sacral fractures according to Denis. Three zones of injury are differentiated. Zone I, sacral ala. Zone II, foraminal region. Zone III, spinal canal. The most medial fracture extension is used to classify an injury. (Reproduced with permission from Denis F, Davis S, Comfort T: Sacral fractures: An important problem. Retrospective analysis of 236 cases. *Clin Orthop* 1988;227:67-81.)

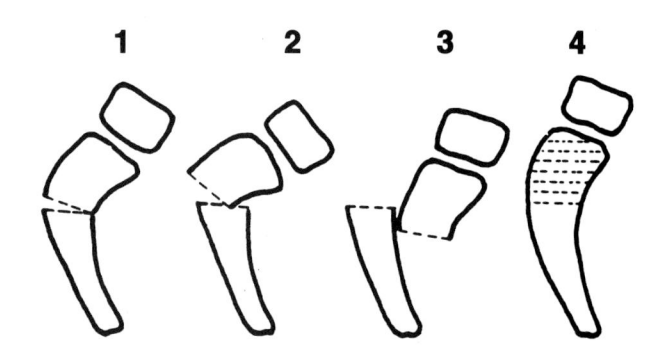

Fig. 2 Classification of transverse sacral fractures by Roy-Camille and associates as modified by Strange-Vognsen and Lebsen. Type 1, flexion fracture without translation. Type 2, flexion fracture with posterior displacement. Type 3, extension fracture with anterior displacement. Type 4, segmental comminution of upper sacrum. (Reproduced with permission from Strange-Vognsen HH, Lebech A: An unusual type of fracture in the upper sacrum. *J Orthop Trauma* 1991;5:200-203.)

fractures, such as pathologic fractures. Cystomyography has been recommended for early diagnosis and follow-up of possible neurogenic bladder injury.[3,7]

Classification

To date there is no single comprehensive classification system that addresses trauma to the surrounding pelvic ring or lumbosacral junction and effectively differentiates sacral injuries. Several morphologic classification systems of sacral injuries have been proposed but do not address the risk of neurologic compromise and the implications for treatment. Determination of the stability of the sacrum and pelvic ring, which is crucial for treatment considerations, can be difficult to do. Radiographic studies are helpful in demonstrating instability, but they are limited in their ability to predict instability accurately. Obvious signs of instability are any significant displacement or shear injury, such as is found in vertically displaced fractures.

The Denis three-part classification system correlates with neurologic injuries and treatment recommendations (Fig. 1). A 30% incidence of sacral fractures was found in 776 patients with pelvic fractures assessed with radiography and later with CT.[3] Zone I (alar) injuries (50% incidence) were subdivided into two major types, either minimally displaced (ie, open book or lateral compression injuries) or severely displaced (ie, vertical shear fractures). Neurologic injuries were found in only 5.9% of patients with zone I injuries and involved either the sciatic nerve or the L5 nerve root. Zone II (transforaminal) fractures were found in 34% of patients and were associated with neurologic deficits in 28% of patients. A variety of abnormalities involving the L5, S1, and S2 roots were identified in this group. Some 97% of undiagnosed injuries were minimally displaced zone I or II injuries. Sixteen percent of injuries involved zone III (spinal canal), and 57% of patients with zone III injuries had neurologic damage. Bowel, bladder, and sexual function were affected most frequently (76.1%) in this group.

Transverse fractures of the sacrum, which usually are Denis type III injuries, were divided into three categories by Roy-Camille and associates,[9] depending on the degree of displacement in terms of sagittal plane translation and angulation (Fig. 2). A fourth category was recently added to describe a severely comminuted upper sacral burst fracture without malalignment.[10] The implication of the level of a transverse sacral fracture is that upper sacral fractures (S1-3) are more frequently associated with bladder dysfunction than lower sacral injuries (S4-5).

The anatomic correlation of nerve injuries in pelvic ring disruptions was studied in postmortem dissections.[11] In 22 of 42 cadavers with pelvic ring fractures, 40 neural injuries were found. Forty percent of these injuries were root avulsions that were associated with vertical shear fractures in the transforaminal region. Of six cadavers with transverse sacral fractures, five had root avulsions.

The importance of obtaining a CT scan with appropriate technique as an aid for diagnosis and treatment has been established. A new classification system based on CT findings has been introduced but has not been further validated in clinical studies.[2]

In conjunction with the classification of sacral fractures, the integrity of the pelvic ring must be evaluated. The pelvic ring classification introduced by Tile[12] does not specifically address the sacrum but has important implications for the stability of the pelvic ring. Determination of pelvic ring stability is crucial for treatment considerations and is based on bony displacement and injury pattern. Although radiographic studies can demonstrate pelvic instability, predicting instability in minimally displaced posterior pelvic ring injuries remains difficult.

Sacral injuries may also be associated with injuries to the lumbosacral articulation. In a study of 193 patients with pelvic ring fractures, 6% were found to have lumbosacral injuries. Based on these findings, three injury categories were described: type 1—extra-articular L5–S1 injuries; type 2—disruption of the L5–S1 joint; and type 3—complex irregular fracture patterns between the lumbosacral junction secondary to a dislocating hemipelvis. The long-term significance of these injuries is unknown.

Treatment

General Considerations

Because of the anatomic location of the sacrum and the involved injury mechanisms, discussion of the treatment of sacral fractures includes consideration of the pelvic ring. The goals of treatment are to reestablish a pain-free, stable pelvic ring without deformity and to create an environment for optimal neurologic recovery. Nonsurgical treatment methods consist of bed rest, protected weightbearing, casting or bracing with a hip spica cast, and skeletal traction. In polytrauma patients, early fixation of skeletally unstable pelvic fractures has been associated with improved outcome.[13,14] Surgical stabilization methods described for the sacrum include indirect anterior pelvic ring stabilization using external fixation or open reduction and internal fixation.[3] The sacral ala can be accessed anteriorly through an iliac approach. Posterior approaches use single midline or bilateral longitudinal or transverse incisions. Extensive posterior surgical exposures and dissection through the frequently severely contused dorsal soft-tissue envelope have been associated with infection rates of up to 25%.[15] Therefore, transverse incisions or extensive parallel longitudinal approaches are not recommended in a trauma setting. Recently, a percutaneous reduction and posterior instrumentation technique has been described.[16] In 68 patients, misplaced screws were found in five patients without bowel or vascular injuries. One patient was found to have a transient L5 radiculopathy. Of 35 sacral fractures (27 transforaminal), five sacral malreductions and one instance of loss of fixation were found postoperatively. All of these problems occurred in the group with transforaminal injuries. Because direct surgical stabilization of the sacrum is very difficult, most fixation techniques engage the sacrum through one or both iliac wings.[12,16] Suggested methods of stabilization include plates placed across the sacroiliac joint anteriorly, sacral bars using compression rods placed through the posterior iliac crests, plates placed as tension bands across the posterior iliac crests, and percutaneous screws placed across the sacroiliac joint with the patient supine or prone.[14] For transverse sacral fractures, sacral lateral mass plates have been described.[9]

Patients with neurologic deficits benefit from decompression, which may be achieved either indirectly, by realignment and stabilization of a displaced neural canal or neuroforamina, or directly, by sacral laminectomy and ventral sacral foraminotomy if needed. In a clinical study of 23 patients with neurologic deficits resulting from sacral fracture, 88% of patients improved following surgical decompression, compared to 20% of the nonsurgically treated group.[1]

Treatment Algorithm

The literature addressing sacral fractures specifically consists largely of case reports and anecdotal reviews. The most extensive series of sacral fractures has been retrospectively compiled and reviewed by Denis and associates.[3] Based on their experience, the following treatment protocol is recommended.

Zone I Stable injuries can be successfully treated with bed rest and early ambulation, with weightbearing as tolerated. Neurologic damage is rare with zone I injuries and usually recovers spontaneously. External fixation can be successful in patients with mainly bony disruption of the anterior pelvic ring. Unstable injuries with symphyseal disruption require open reduction and internal fixation. Early mobilization with protected weightbearing can be permitted unless unstable injuries such as a vertical shear injury are identified.

For vertically displaced (unstable) zone I injuries, closed reduction with skeletal traction and subsequent anterior and posterior fixation is recommended, followed by bed rest if postoperative stability remains doubtful. Difficulty in obtaining and maintaining fracture reduction can be anticipated if definitive care is delayed for 72 hours or if the fracture displacement is greater than 2 cm.

Zone II Zone II injuries can be treated conservatively if the foraminal fractures are minimally or nondisplaced and if the anterior pelvic ring remains intact. In cases of persistent neurologic symptoms or foraminal compression of 75% or more at S1 and S2, early decompression, within 2 weeks, is recommended to minimize epidural fibrosis. Unstable zone II injuries benefit from stabilization of the anterior and posterior pelvic ring, because anterior stabilization alone has little effect on posterior ring stability.[17] Early fracture reduction with traction of surgical means and stable posterior fixation is recommended. Because of the location of the fracture and concomitant comminution, anterior alar plating usually is not feasible. Posterior tension band plates or sacroiliac screws remain options for internal fixation.

Zone III In zone III injuries without neurologic damage, stability of the pelvic ring dictates the treatment decision. In case of neurologic deficits, early decompression of neural tissue, either indirectly, through fracture reduction, or directly, with laminectomy or foraminotomy, has been reported to yield better results than either conservative treatment alone or late decompression. Preservation of even unilateral lower sacral roots has been shown to allow for adequate bowel and bladder sphincter control.[6] Conservative options include placement in a hip spica cast with an attempt at indirect reduction of the sacrum. Displaced transverse fractures of the sacrum that cannot be treated conservatively can be stabilized with lateral mass plates on the sacrum.

Lumbosacral Injuries

Dislocated facet joints may prevent an anatomic reduction of sacral injuries. Unrecognized injuries to the lumbosacral junction may contribute to persistent pelvic pain. Treatment recommendations to date are anecdotal and range from conservative treatment in a hip spica cast to posterior open reduction and internal fixation using segmental instrumentation of displaced unreducible or unstable injuries.

Summary

Sacral fractures are significant injuries that are often overlooked on standard plain radiographs. Initial treatment efforts are directed toward resuscitation of the patient because of the frequently associated life-threatening injuries. Sacral injuries are best evaluated with fine-section sacral CT with reconstructed views. The Denis classification is simple and correlates with the incidence of neurologic trauma and suggested treatments.

Treatment decisions are based on the skeletal injury to the sacrum and pelvic ring and the neurologic status of the patient. The stability of a sacral fracture may be difficult to assess. In general, the literature to date supports conservative care in the form of bed rest and protected weight-bearing for minimally displaced injuries without neurologic deficit. No uniform agreement on the ideal form of surgical treatment for sacral fractures exists. Combined anterior and posterior instrumentation offers biomechanical advantages for the stability of displaced pelvic ring disruptions. For patients with neurologic deficits, reduction of fracture deformity with decompression of compressed neural elements, especially in the absence of signs of early recovery, appears to yield better results than nonsurgical care.

References

1. Gibbons KJ, Soloniuk DS, Razack N: Neurological injury and patterns of sacral fractures. *J Neurosurg* 1990;72:889-893.

2. Kaehr DM, Anderson PA, Mayo KA, et al: Classification of sacral fractures based on CT imaging. *J Orthop Trauma* 1989;3:163-164.

3. Denis F, Davis S, Comfort T: Sacral fractures: An important problem. Retrospective analysis of 236 cases. *Clin Orthop* 1988;227:67-81.

4. Dowling T, Epstein JA, Epstein NE: S1-S2 sacral fracture involving neural elements of the cauda equina: A case report and review of the literature. *Spine* 1985;10:851-853.

5. Fisher RG: Sacral fracture with compression of cauda equina: Surgical treatment. *J Trauma* 1988;28:1678-1680.

6. Gunterberg B: Effects of major resection of the sacrum: Clinical studies on urogenital and anorectal function and a biomechanical study on pelvic strength. *Acta Orthop Scand* 1976;162(suppl):1-38.

7. Schnaid E, Eisenstein SM, Drummond-Webb J: Delayed post-traumatic cauda equina compression syndrome. *J Trauma* 1985;25:1099-1101.

8. Rommens PM, Vanderschot PM, Broos PL: Conventional radiography and CT examination of pelvic ring fractures: A comparative study of 90 patients. *Unfallchirurg* 1992;95:387-392.

9. Roy-Camille R, Saillant G, Gagna G, et al: Transverse fracture of the upper sacrum: Suicidal jumper's fracture. *Spine* 1985;10:838-845.

10. Strange-Vognsen HH, Lebech A: An unusual type of fracture in the upper sacrum. *J Orthop Trauma* 1991;5:200-203.

11. Huittinen VM: Lumbosacral nerve injury in fracture of the pelvis: A postmortem radiographic and pathoanatomical study. *Acta Chir Scand* 1972;429:3-43.

12. Tile M: Pelvic ring fractures: Should they be fixed? *J Bone Joint Surg* 1988;70B:1-12.

13. Browner BD, Cole JD, Graham JM, et al: Delayed posterior internal fixation of unstable pelvic fractures. *J Trauma* 1987;27:998-1006.

14. Latenser BA, Gentilello LM, Tarver AA, et al: Improved outcome with early fixation of skeletally unstable pelvic fractures. *J Trauma* 1991;31:28-31.

15. Kellam JF, McMurtry RY, Paley D, et al: The unstable pelvic fracture: Operative treatment. *Orthop Clin North Am* 1987;18:25-41.

16. Routt MLC Jr, Meier MC, Kregor PJ, et al: Percutaneous iliosacral screws with the patient supine technique. *Oper Techn Orthop* 1993;3:35-45.

17. Stocks GW, Gabel GT, Noble PC, et al: Anterior and posterior internal fixation of vertical shear fractures of the pelvis. *J Orthop Res* 1991;9:237-45.

Index

Page numbers in italics refer to figures or figure legends.

Acetabular fractures
    biomechanics of 235–236
    classification of 215, 229–233, 263–264
    complex 232–233, 263–269
    complications of 274–277
    open reduction and internal fixation for 227, 233
    posterior column 232, 253–254, 256–257
    posterior wall 232, 254–256
    postoperative management 273–274
    radiographic evaluation for 227–229
    simple 231–232
    transfer criteria for 214
    transverse 232, 253–254, 257–258
Achilles tendon rupture 192
Acromioclavicular joint dislocations 10–11
Ada and Miller fracture classification 3–4
Adenosine triphosphate 294
Adolescent femur fractures 131–133
Adult respiratory distress syndrome 218–219, 221
Advanced Trauma Life Support protocol 213, 281
Algorithm
    for femoral neck fractures *117*
    for hemodynamically unstable patients *223*
    for sacral fractures *367–368*
American Spinal Injury Association 303
    motor score *305–306*, 363
Amputation
    foot 207
    and infected pilon fractures 189
    and tibial diaphyseal fractures 177
Anatomy
    atlas 311
    axis 311, 323, 325
    distal femur 137
    distal humerus 36–37
    elbow 36–37, 47
    femoral head 283
    hip 281
    humeral diaphysis 25–*26*
    occipitocervical complex 311
    patella 153
    proximal femur 113–114
    proximal humerus 15–16
    sacrum 365
    shoulder 3
    tibia 171–172
    wrist 83–84
Anderson and D'Alonzo odontoid fracture classification 323–*324*
Anderson technique for posterior cervical plating *337*
Angiography, therapeutic 222, 264
Ankle arthrodesis and pilon fractures 188
Ankle injuries 191–197
Ankle fractures 193–197
    ligament injury 191–192
    tendon injury 192–193
Ankylosing spondylitis 333
Anterior cruciate ligament injury 147–150
Anterior medial collateral ligament 49
AO classification system
    for distal femur fractures 137–*138*
    for distal humerus fractures 37–38, *40–41*
    for distal radius fractures 68, *71*
    for femoral neck fractures *115*
    for femur fractures 127, *129*
    for forearm fractures 57–*58*
    for humeral shaft fractures 25–27
    for proximal humerus fractures *17*–19
    of soft–tissue injury 59
    for tibial plateau fractures 160, *164*
AO plating results 30
AO screws
    for hand fractures *98*
    for metacarpal fractures 102–103
    for scapular fractures 6
Arterial injury (*see also* Blood supply; Neurovascular injury; Vascularity)
    forearm 60
    and knee dislocation 145–147
    and pelvic fracture 221
Arteriography
    and knee dislocation 146–147
    for scapulothoracic dislocation 7
Artery (*see also* Blood supply)
    arcuate 15
    axillary 16
    axillary-brachial *7*
    femoral circumflex 113
    humeral circumflex 15
    popliteal 145
    pudendal 221
    scapular 6
    superior gluteal 265–266
Arthritis, posttraumatic
    and acetabular biomechanics 235
    following acetabular fracture 277
    and hip dislocations 283
    following talus fractures 199
    following tibial plafond fractures 188
    following tibial plateau fractures 167
Arthroscopy
    and fracture reduction 76
    for tibial plateau fractures 165, 167
Atlanto-dens interval 320, 322
Atlanto-occipital injuries, radiologic signs of 313
Atlantoaxial rotatory fixation 321–322
Atlas
    anatomy 311
    fractures 317–320
Axillary nerve 16, 18, 30
Axis
    anatomy 311, 323, 325
    fractures 323–327
    traumatic spondylolisthesis of the 325–*326*
Axons, disruption of 297–298
Babinski test 292–293
Bankart dissection 6
Beevor's sign 291
Bennett's fracture 104
Berndt and Harty staging system 197
Biomechanics
    acetabular 235–236
    pelvic 236–238
Blood loss and pelvic fracture 217–218, 220–221
Blood supply
    extensor mechanism 153
    humeral head 15, 19
    proximal femur 113

scapula 6
talus 199
tendon 77
tibial shaft 172
Bracing, functional
    of distal humeral fractures 42–43
    of distal radius fractures 73
    of forearm fractures 60
    of humeral shaft fractures 27–29
    of thoracic and lumbar fractures 347–349
    of tibial diaphyseal fractures 174–175
Brain injury
    associated with pelvic fracture 219, 221
    occipital cranial injury 311–315
Breuerton views 97, 103
Broden's views 200
Brooker classification 276–277
Brown-Séquard lesions 304, 306
Bulbocavernosus reflex 293, 365
Bunnel sutures 157
Capitellum fractures 38, 52–53
Carpal injury 83–91
    classification 84, 86
    and distal radius fracture 79
Cast immobilization (*see also* Halo vest immobilization)
    for ankle injuries 191–192, 196
    for distal femur fractures 138–139
    for distal radius fractures 73
    for forearm fractures 60
    hanging arm cast 27
    hip spica cast 367–368
    for metacarpal fractures 102
    for tibial diaphyseal fractures 174–175
Cervical spine injuries, lower
    classification 329–333, 335–336
    diagnostic checklist 329–330
    surgical management 335–338
Chance fracture *344*, 348
Chopart amputation 207
Chrisman-Snook technique 192
Classification system
    for acetabular fractures 215, 229–233, 263–*264*
    for acromioclavicular joint separations 10–11
    for atlas fractures 317–320
    for ankle injuries 191, 193
    for axis injuries 323–*326*
    for calcaneal fractures 200–*202*
    for cervical injuries 329–333, 335–336
    for distal clavicle fractures 11
    for distal femur fractures 137–*138*
    for distal humerus fractures 37–*41*
    for distal radius fractures 67–*71*
    for femoral head fractures 284
    for femoral neck fractures 114–115
    for femoral shaft fractures 127–*129*
    for fixation devices 362
    for hip dislocations 282
    for humeral shaft fractures 25–27
    for introchanteric fractures 121–*123*
    for knee dislocation 145–*146*
    for Lisfranc joint dislocations *204*
    for metacarpal fractures *101*
    neurologic classification of spinal cord injury 290–293
    for occipital condyle fractures 312–*313*
    for occipitocervical instability 313–*314*
    for olecranon fractures 50–*51*
    for odontoid fractures 323–*324*
    for patellar fractures 154
    for pelvic fractures 214, 218, *220*–221
    for pilon fractures 183–*184*
    for proximal humerus fractures 15–19
    for ring metacarpal fractures *91*
    for sacral fractures 366–367
    for scaphoid fractures 86–*89*
    for scapular fractures 3–4
    for spinal injury *290*, 303–304, 341–345
    thoracolumbar fractures 341–345
    for tibial diaphysis fractures 172–*174*
    for tibial plateau fractures 160, *162–163*
    for trapezium fractures 86, *90*
Clavicle fractures 9–11
Clay shoveler's fracture 329
Closed reduction
    of metacarpal fractures 102
    of phalangeal fractures 96
    of sternoclavicular dislocations 8
Compartment syndrome
    and calcaneal fractures 203
    and distal radius fractures 77
    of the foot 206–207
    of the forearm 59
    and knee dislocation 145
    of the thigh 133
    and tibial fractures 167, 171–172, 178
Computed tomography
    for acetabular fractures 229
    for atlas fractures 317
    for intracapsular hip fractures 114
    for occipital cranial injuries 312–313, 315
    for occult fractures of the cervical spine *294*
    for pelvic ring trauma 219
    for sacral fractures 365–366, 368
    for thoracolumbar fractures 341
    for tibial plateau fractures 159–*161*
Continuous passive motion 273
Coronoid fractures 49–*50*
Corsets 347
Cotrel-Dubousset multiple-hook rod construct 351–*353*
Cotton test 195
Cuboid fractures 204
Cuneiform fractures 204

D'Aubigne and Postel rating system 268, 277
Danis-Weber scheme 193–*194*
De Quervain tenosynovitis 77
Deep vein thrombosis and pelvic injury 224, 228, 275–276
Deltoid *5–6*, 15–16, *26*
Denis
    burst fracture classification 344
    sacral fracture classification *366*, 368
    three-column spine model 342–*343*, 348
Distal femur fractures 137–142
Distal humerus fractures 35–45
Distal radioulnar joint 58, 78
    and plate fixation 61
Distal radius, fractures of the 67–79
    classification 67–*71*
Dorsal intercalated segmental instability pattern 83, 91
Dunn device 361–363
Dynamic compression plate
    for humeral fractures 30
    removal 62
    for spinal injury 361
    for symphysis pubis disruption 241
    for tibial diaphyseal fractures 175

Elbow
    anatomy 36–37, 47
    dislocation 47–49
    floating 59
    injury 47–54
Ender nail 30

for distal femur fracture fixation 140
for tibial diaphyseal fracture fixation 175
Epidemiology
　ankle injuries 191
　distal femur fractures 137
　distal humerus fractures 35
　distal radius fractures 67
　extensor mechanism injuries 153
　hip fractures 113, 121
　proximal humerus fractures 17
　tibial fractures 159, 171
Essex-Lopresti lesion 52
Evans-Jensen classification for intertrochanteric fractures 121–*123*
Extensor mechanism injury 153–157
External fixation
　of distal femur fractures 140–*141*
　of distal radius fractures 74–75
　of the femur 127
　of forearm fractures 61
　versus intramedullary nailing 177
　and pelvic biomechanics 237–238
　of pelvic ring injuries 222, 249–251
　of phalangeal fractures 97
　of pilon fractures 187–188
　of proximal interphalangeal joint fractures 99–100
　of sacral fractures 367
　of tibial diaphyseal fractures 175–179
　of tibial plateau fractures 166

Femoral
　diaphysis, fractures of 127–134
　head fractures 281, 283–285
　neck fractures 114–115
Ferno-Washington stretcher 289
Foot injuries 197–207
　calcaneal fractures 200–203
　Lisfranc joint injuries 204–206
　navicular fractures 203
　talus injuries 197–199
Foramen magnum 311
Forearm fractures 57–62
Fractures
　acetabular 227–233, 253–259, 263–269, 273–277
　ankle 193–197
　atlas 317–320
　calcaneal 200–203
　carpal 83, 86–91
　clavicle 9–11
　cuboid 204
　cuneiform 204
　distal humerus 35–45
　femoral diaphysis 127–134
　femoral head 281, 283–285
　forearm 57–62
　hand 95–106
　hip 113–125
　humeral shaft 25–31
　iliac wing 242–243
　navicular 203
　occipital condyle 312
　odontoid 323–325
　olecranon 49–50
　patellar 153–156
　pelvic 213–215, 217–224 (*see also* Pelvic fractures)
　pilon 183–189
　proximal humerus 15–21
　pubic ramus 242–*243*
　sacral 245–246, 365–368
　scapular 3–6
　talus 198–199
　teardrop 329, *332*, 338

thoracolumbar 341–345, 347–349
thoracolumbar junction 351–358
tibial diaphysis 171–179
tibial plafond 183–189
tibial plateau 159–167
Frankel score 303

Galeazzi lesions 57–59, 61
Gamma nail 134
Gangliosides 295–296, 300
Garden's classification for femoral neck fractures *114*–115
Gardner-Wells tongs 293, 330
Gartland fracture classification 67–68
Gastrocnemius 137–*138*
Glasgow Coma Score 219
Glenohumeral joint dislocations 17–18
Greenfield filters 228, 275–276
Gross-Kemph nails 175
Gunshot wounds
　to the cervical spine 333
　to the femur 131
　to the forearm 59
　to the hand 105
　and spinal cord injuries 306
Gustilo classification of open fractures 57–59, 172–174
Guyon's canal 76

Haas repair for quadriceps tendon rupture *155,* 157
Hackethal technique 30
Halo vest immobilization
　for atlas vertebral injury 320
　for cervical spine injury 331–332, 335–338
　for C2 vertebral fractures 326–327
　for occipital cranial injury 313, 315
　for odontoid fractures 324
Hand fractures 95–106
　complications of 104–106
　metacarpal 100–103
　phalangeal 95–100
　thumb 103–104
Hardcastle classification of Lisfranc joint dislocations *204*
Harris hip score 268, 277
Hawkins' sign 198–199
Hawkins classification of talar neck fractures *198–199*
Hematoma, retroperitoneal 219, 221–222
Hemodynamically unstable patients 218, 220–*223*
Henry approach, volar 62
Herbert screw 79
　for capitellum fractures 53
　for perilunate injuries 85–86
　for scaphoid nonunions 89
Heterotopic ossification
　and acetabular fracture surgery 273–274, 276–277
　and distal humeral fractures 45
　following intramedullary nailing 133–134
　prevention of 45, 228, 259, 267
　radiographic classification of 276
Hill-Sachs defect 17–18
Hip (*see also* Acetabular fractures; Pelvic fractures)
　dislocations 281–283
　fractures, intracapsular 113–117
Hip spica cast 367–368
Hoffa fractures 141
Hoffman fixators 61, 97
Hook of the hamate fractures 86, 91
Hybrid fixators *166*
Hypovolemic shock 218, 221

Iliac wing fractures 242–243
Indomethacin 45, 228, 259, 274
Infection

and acetabular fractures 274
and distal femur fractures 142
and distal humeral fractures 44–45
and hand fractures 104–105
and intramedullary nailing 133, 178
and pilon fractures 188–189
and plate fixation of forearm fractures 61–62
and tibial diaphyseal fractures 178
and tibial plateau fractures 166
Injury severity score 217
Internal fixation (see also Open reduction and internal fixation)
of complex acetabular fractures 267–269
of humeral shaft fractures 28–31
and pelvic biomechanics 237–238
of pelvic ring disruptions 241–246
of phalangeal fractures 96–97
of sacral fractures 367
of spinal fractures 351–358, 361–364
of tibial plateau fractures 165
International Standards for spinal cord injuries 303–304
Intertrochanteric femur fractures 121–125
Intramedullary nailing
complications 133–134
for distal femur fractures 139–140
for femoral diaphysis fractures 128–*131*, 133–134
for forearm fractures 61
for humeral shaft fractures 29–30
for tibial diaphyseal fractures 175–179
Ipsilateral neck fractures 130–131

Jefferson fractures 317–320
Jewett brace 347–349
Johner and Wruhs classification of tibial fractures *173*
Joint injuries
acromioclavicular 10–11
carpometacarpal 103
elbow 47–54
glenohumeral 15, 17–18
knee 145–151
Lisfranc 204
metatarsophalangeal 206
sacroiliac 243–245
sternoclavicular 7–9
thumb 104
Jones fracture 206
Judet
incision 6
radiographs 213, 219, 227–229
table 267
Judet-Letournel classification 229, *264*

Kaneda device 361–363
Kapandji pinning technique 74
Kelikian technique *157*
Kenny Howard splint 11
Kessler sutures 157
Kienböck's disease 86, 88
Kirschner wires
for distal clavicle fractures 11
for hand fractures 102, 105
for metacarpal shaft fractures 102
for patellar fractures 155
for perilunate injuries 85–86
for phalangeal fractures 96–97
for scaphoid fractures 88–89
for the sternoclavicular joint 8
Knee
dislocation 145–151
ligament injury 147–151, 160–162
Kocher-Langenbeck approach 254, 257–258, 265–266, 273–275
Kostuik-Harrington device 361–362

Krakow sutures 157
Küntscher nails 31, 128

Lachman test 148
Lag screw fixation
for acetabular fracture fixation 236, *257*, 266–267
for distal humeral fractures 43–44
iliosacral 244–*246*
for Lisfranc dislocation *205*
for pilon fractures *187*
for scaphoid nonunions 89
for subtrochanteric fractures *134*
for talar neck fracture *199*
Lateral collateral ligament 36, 147–149
Lateral ulnohumeral ligament 47
Lauge-Hansen scheme for ankle fractures 193–*194*
Letournel classification of acetabular fractures 215
Ligament injury
anterior medial collateral 49
about the axis 320–322
coracoclavicular 10–11
knee 147–151
Ligaments
anterior cruciate 147–150
anterior medial collateral 49
coracoclavicular 10–11
cranial cervical 311
knee 147–151
lateral collateral 36, 147–149
lunotriquetral *83*–84
medial collateral 36, 47, 147–149
pelvic 237
radial collateral 47, 49
radiolunate *83*
radioscaphocapitate *83*–84
radioscapholunate *83*
radiotriquetral, dorsal *84*
radioulnar, dorsal *84*
triquetroscaphoid *84*
ulnocarpal *83*
Lisfranc joint injuries 204–206
Lister's tubercle 77
Load sharing classification for thoracolumbar fractures 342–*343*

Ma technique for patellar fractures *154*
Magerl's
cervical plating technique *337*
classification of thoracolumbar fractures *342*
screw fixation technique 320
Magnetic resonance imaging
of the ankle 191
of cervical spine injury 329–330, 335, 337
of intertrochanteric fracture *121*–*122*
of knee dislocation 148
of osteochondral lesions of the talus 197
of osteonecrosis of the femoral head 114
of quadriceps tendon ruptures 154
of spinal injury 294–*295*, 309, 329–330
of thoracolumbar fractures 341
of tibial plateau fractures 160, *162*, 167
Maisonneuve fracture 196
Mallet fractures 97–99
Malunion
distal femur 142
distal humeral 44
distal radial 71–72, 78–79
femoral diaphysis 133
hand fracture 105–106
talar neck 199
tibial diaphyseal 177
Mangled Extremity Severity Score 177

Mason's classification for radial head fractures 51–52
MAST (Military antishock trousers) 221, 365
McLaughlin wire technique *156–157*
McMurtry and Jupiter fracture classification 68–*69*
Mechanism of injury
    and ankle dislocation 193
    and cervical spine injury 329
    and clavicle fractures 9
    and distal radius fractures 68
    and elbow dislocation 48
    and glenohumeral joint dislocation 18
    and humeral shaft fractures 26
    and intracapsular hip fractures 115
    and knee dislocation 145
    and occipital cranial injury 312
    and odontoid fractures 323
    to the patella 154
    to the pelvis 217
    and pilon fractures 183, 185
    and proximal humerus fractures 16
    and radial head fractures 51
    and sacral fractures 365
    skiing 185
    and sternoclavicular dislocations 7
    and tibial plateau fractures 159
    and tibial shaft fractures 172
Medial collateral ligament 47
    and knee dislocation 147–149
Median neuropathy 69, 76–78
    and the Cotton-Loder position 73
Melone fracture classification 68, *70*
Meniscal injury and tibial plateau fractures 160–161
Mercedes incision 165
Metacarpal fractures 100–103
Metatarsophalangeal joint injuries 206
Methylprednisolone 295, 299–300
Military antishock trousers 221, 365
Monteggia lesions 57–61
Morel-Lavalle lesion 227, 263–264, 267, 274
Motor Index Score 306, 363

Navicular fractures 203
Neer and Rockwood classification of distal clavicle fractures 11
Neer classification of proximal humerus fractures 15–*16*, 18–19
Nerve injury
    and acetabular fractures 274–275
    axillary 16, 18, 30
    and intramedullary nailing 133
    median 69, 76–78
    in pelvic ring disruptions 366
    peroneal 145, 149, 166, 171
    and plate removal 62
    radial 26, 29–30, 62
    sciatic 133, 227, 253, 259, 274–275, 283
    ulnar 47, 76, 85
Neurologic evaluation for spinal injury 290–293
Neurovascular injury
    following forearm fracture 59–60
    and knee dislocation 145–147
Night pain after scapular fracture 4–5
95° dynamic condylar screw 139–140, 142
Nonunion
    of acetabular fractures 276
    of clavicle fractures 9
    of the distal femur 142
    of distal hmeral fractures 44
    of distal radial fractures 79
    femoral 133, 142
    of humeral shaft fractures 31
    of intracapsular hip fractures 115–116
    of odontoid fractures in the elderly 324

    of patellar fractures 156
    scaphoid 88–89
    tibial 167, 177–178

Occipital cranial injuries 311–315
Odontoid fractures 323–325
Olecranon fractures 49–50
Open reduction and internal fixation
    of acetabular fractures 227, 233
    of ankle fractures 195–196
    of capitellum fractures 52–53
    of cervical spine injuries 335–338
    of distal humerus fractures 35, 39, 42–44
    of distal radius fractures 74–76
    of foot injuries 197–*199*
    of forearm fractures 61–62
    of Lisfranc dislocation *205*
    of metacarpal shaft fractures 102–103
    of occipital cranial injuries *314–315*
    of patellar fractures 154–155
    of pelvic ring injuries 241–246, 249–251
    of perilunate injuries 85–86
    of phalangeal fractures 97–*98*
    of pilon fractures 185–187
    of proximal humerus fractures 15, 19–22
    of sacral fractures 367
    of tibial plateau fractures 164
Oppenheim test 293
Orthopaedic Trauma Association 57, 115, 172
Osteonecrosis
    and acetabular fractures 277
    and hip dislocations 283

Paraplegia
    and expected function 307
    motor recovery after 304–305, 308
Parkinson's disease
    and hip fractures 116
    and humeral shaft fractures 28
Patellar injuries 153–157
Pauwel's anterior tension band wiring 153
Pectoralis major 25–*26*
Pedicle screws 351–352, *354, 356–358*, 361–363
Pelvic fractures 213–215, 217–224
    and biomechanics of the pelvis 236–238
    classifications of 214, 218, *220*–221, 249–250
    fixation of pelvic ring disruptions 241–246, 249–251
    injuries associated with 219, 221–222
    open 223–224
    outcomes of pelvic ring injuries 249–251, 365
    physical findings 217–218
    transfer criteria for 214
Pennal classification of pelvic fractures 214, 218, *220*
Percutaneous fixation
    of distal radius fractures 73–74
    of metacarpal shaft fractures 102
    of phalangeal fractures 96
    of proximal humerus fractures *19*, 21
    of sacral fractures 367
    of tibial plateau fractures 165
Perilunate dislocations 84–*86*
Peroneal nerve injury 145, 149, 171
    and tibial plateau fractures 166
Peroneal tendon injury 192–*193*, 203
Pfannenstiehl exposure 241–*243*
Phalangeal fractures 95–100
Pilon fractures 183–189
Pipkin's classification of femoral head fractures 284
Plate fixation
    AO 30
    for cervical spine injuries 336–338

for clavicle fractures 9
for distal humeral fractures 42–44
for forearm fractures 61–62
for humeral shaft fractures 30–31
for metacarpal shaft fractures *102*, 105
for thoracolumbar burst fractures 362–363
Pneumatic antishock garment 222
Polytrauma patients
  hand fractures in 104
  and pelvic fracture 213
  and surgical intervention 28–29
Popliteal artery and knee dislocation 145
Posterior cruciate ligament injury 147–151
Prevention
  of heterotopic ossification 45, 228, 259, 267
  of hip fracture 121
Proximal femur anatomy 113–114
Proximal humerus fractures 15–21
Proximal interphalangeal joint injury 95, 99–100
Pubic ramus fractures 242–*243*

Quadriceps tendon rupture *155*, 157

Radial collateral ligament 47, 49
Radial head fractures 51–52
Radial nerve injury 26, 29–30, 62
Radiocarpal arthrosis 72, 78
Radiographic evaluation
  for acetabular fractures 227–229
  for ankle injury 191, 193–194
  for atlanto-occipital injury 313
  for atlas fractures 317
  for calcaneal fractures 200
  for carpal injury 85, 87–*89*
  for cervical injury 329–330, 335
  for distal femur fractures 138
  for distal humeral fractures 39
  for distal radioulnar joint injury 58–59
  for distal radius fractures 68–71
  for hand fractures 103
  for heterotopic ossification 276
  for hip dislocations 281–282
  for humeral shaft fractures 26
  for intracapsular hip fractures 114
  for knee dislocation 146
  for osteochondral lesions of the talus 197
  for pelvic ring injuries 218–219
  for proximal humerus fractures 16–17
  for sacral fractures 365
  for spinal injury 293–294
  for tibial diaphyseal fractures 173
  for tibial plateau fractures 159, 163
Radioulnar synostosis 57, 62
Rayhack's technique 74
Reaming, intramedullary 130
  for tibial fractures 175–*176*
Reflex sympathetic dystrophy 77
Renal failure and hip fracture 116
Retroperitoneal hematoma 219, 221–222
Rolando's fracture 104
Rotator cuff dysfunction 4–5
Roy-Camille
  classification of transverse sacral fractures *366*
  technique for posterior cervical plating *337*
Ruedi and Allgöwer classification of pilon fractures *184*
Rush pin 140
Rush rod fixation for ankle injuries 195

Sacral fractures 245–246, 365–368
Sacroiliac joint disruptions 243–245
Saltzman method for patellar tendon repair *156*–157

Sanders classification of calcaneal fractures 200–*202*
Scaphoid and distal radius fracture 79
Scapula fractures 3–6
Schanz pins 21, 116
Schatzker's classification
  of olecranon fractures 50–*51*
  of tibial plateau fractures 160–*162*
Sciatic nerve injury
  and acetabular fractures 227, 253, 259
  and hip dislocations 283
  and traction 133
Screws
  AO 6, *98*, 102–103
  for acetabular fractures 255–*258*
  for cervical spine injury 336–*337*
  condylar *125*
  dynamic condylar, 95 139–140
  for hand fractures 95–103
  Herbert 79, 85–86, 89
  hip *124*
  lag 89, *134*, 257 *(see also* Lag screw fixation)
  pedicle 351–352, *354*, *356–358*, 361–363
  polylactide 195
  sacroiliac 367
  for scaphoid fracture 79
  for scapular fracture fixation 6
Shock 218, 221
Shoulder girdle injuries 3–11
Skiing injuries 185
Slot-Zielke device 361–362
Smith-Petersen approach 284–285
Soft-tissue injuries
  AO/ASIF classification 59
  following distal radius fractures 76–78
Somatosensory-evoked potential nerve monitoring
  for posterior wall acetabular fractures 254
  and sciatic nerve injury 253, 259, 275
  and spinal cord injury 308, 331
Spinal injury
  atlantoaxial rotatory fixation 321–322
  atlas fractures 317–320
  axis fractures 323–327
  experimental treatment of 295–296, 299–300
  fixation devices for burst fractures 361–364
  International Standards 303–304
  lower cervical injuries 329–333, 335–338
  pathophysiology 297–299
  patient assessment in 289–296
  prognosis 303–309
  thoracolumbar fractures 341–345, 347–349, 361–364
Splenic injury associated with pelvic fracture 219, 221
Splint
  coaptation 27
  Kenny Howard 11
spur sign 263
Sternoclavicular dislocations 7–9
Stretch test *293*
Stretcher, Ferno-Washington 289
Suave-Kapandji procedure 78
Subtalar dislocation 203
Subtrochanteric fractures *132*, 134
Sunrise radiographs 153
Superior gluteal artery 265–266
Surgical approaches
  for acetabular fractures 254–259
  for acromioclavicular injury 10–11
  for cervical spine injury 336–338
  Chrisman-Snook technique 192
  for complex acetabular fractures 265–268
  for distal humeral fractures 39, 42–44
  for femoral head fractures 284–285

for forearm fractures 61–62
Haas repair for quadriceps tendon rupture *155,* 157
for humeral shaft fractures 29–31
iliofemoral, extended 265–267
ilioinguinal 265–267, 273–276
Judet incision *6*
Kocher-Langenbeck 254, 257–258, 265–266, 273–275
Letournel's extended iliofemoral exposure 266
Ma technique for patellar fractures *154*
Mercedes incision 165
for patellar tendon repair *156*–157
Pfannenstiehl exposure 241–*243*
for proximal humerus fractures *20–21*
for sacral fractures 367
Smith-Petersen 284–285
Stoppa *267–268*
Thompson 62
Watson-Jones 284
Syme's amputation 207
Symphysis pubis disruption 241–*242*
Synostosis, radioulnar 57, 62

Talus
    fractures 198–199
    osteochondral injuries of the 197–198
Tarsometatarsal joint injuries 204–206
Teardrop fracture-dislocation 329, *332,* 338
Technetium bone scan 173
    for osteochondral injuries of the talus 197
Tendon injury
    Achilles 192
    following distal radius fracture 77
    patellar 157
    peroneal 192–193
    quadriceps *155,* 157
Tenosynovitis, after distal radius fracture 77
Tension band wiring technique
    for olecranon fractures 50
    Pauwel's 153
    for proximal humerus fractures *20–22*
Tetraplegia
    and expected function 307
    motor recovery after 305–306, 308
Texas Scottish Rite Hospital (TSRH) construct 362–363
Thompson surgical approach 62
Thoracolumbar fractures
    classification of 341–345
    fixation devices for burst fractures 361–364
    nonsurgical management of 347–349
Thoracolumbar junction fractures 351–358
Thoracolumbosacral orthosis (TLSO) 347–349

Thromboembolism 224, 228, 275–276
Thumb fractures 103–104
Tibia
    anatomy 171–172
    fracture classifications 160–*164,* 172–*174,* 183–*184*
    in knee dislocation 145–*146,* 150
Tibial diaphyseal fractures 171–179
Tibial plafond fractures 183–189
Tibial plateau fractures 159–167
    and computed tomography 159–160
    surgical indications for 163–164
Tile's classification of pelvic ring injuries 249–250, 366
TLSO (Thoracolumbosacral orthosis) 347–349
Total contact orthoses 347–349
Tourniquet use
    for distal humeral fractures 42
    and knee dislocation 147
Traction
    for acetabular fractures 265
    for cervical spine injury 330–331, 335–338
    for femoral fractures 127
    for hip dislocations 282
Trapezial body fractures 86, *90*
Triangular fibrocartilage complex 78
Triliazoid 295
TSRH (Texas Scottish Rite Hospital) construct 362–363
Turf toe 206

Ulnar neuropathy 45, 76, 85
University plate 363

Vascularity (*see also* Blood supply)
    humeral head 22
    and knee dislocation 145–147
    lunate 86, *89–90*
    tibial shaft 172
Velpeau dressing
    and fractures of the humeral shaft 27
    for sternoclavicular dislocation 8
Volar intercalated segmental instability pattern 84

Watson-Jones approach 284
Weaver and Dunn surgical technique 11
Winquist classification of femoral shaft fractures 127–*128,* 172, *174*

Y incision 165
Young & Burgess pelvic fracture classification 214, *220*
Yuan plate 363

Z deformity 5
Z plate 363
Zickel nail 140